NEW FOUNDATIONS IN

Therapeutic Massage and Bodywork

Jan L. Saeger
BA, LMT, NCTMB, CESMT, RYT
Keiser University, West Palm Beach, Florida

Donna Kyle-Brown
Ph.D, RMA, AHI, CSC, RM
Blue Cliff College, Gulfport, Mississippi

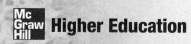 **Higher Education**

Boston   Burr Ridge, IL   Dubuque, IA   New York   San Francisco   St. Louis
Bangkok   Bogotá   Caracas   Kuala Lumpur   Lisbon   London   Madrid   Mexico City
Milan   Montreal   New Delhi   Santiago   Seoul   Singapore   Sydney   Taipei   Toronto

The McGraw·Hill Companies

McGraw Hill **Higher Education**

NEW FOUNDATIONS IN THERAPEUTIC MASSAGE AND BODYWORK

Published by McGraw-Hill, a business unit of The McGraw-Hill Companies, Inc., 1221 Avenue of the Americas, New York, NY 10020. Copyright © 2008 by The McGraw-Hill Companies, Inc. All rights reserved. No part of this publication may be reproduced or distributed in any form or by any means, or stored in a database or retrieval system, without the prior written consent of The McGraw-Hill Companies, Inc., including, but not limited to, in any network or other electronic storage or transmission, or broadcast for distance learning.

Some ancillaries, including electronic and print components, may not be available to customers outside the United States.

This book is printed on acid-free paper.

1 2 3 4 5 6 7 8 9 0 QPD/QPD 0 9 8 7

ISBN 978–0–07–302582–7
MHID 0–07–302582–8

Publisher: *David T. Culverwell*
Director of Development: *Kristine Tibbetts*
Developmental Editor: *Connie Kuhl*
Senior Marketing Manager: *Nancy Bradshaw*
Senior Project Manager: *Sheila M. Frank*
Senior Production Supervisor: *Sherry L. Kane*
Senior Coordinator of Freelance Design: *Michelle D. Whitaker*
Cover/Interior Designer: *Elise Lansdon*
(USE) Cover Image: *©Keith Brofsky/Photodisc Green*
Lead Photo Research Coordinator: *Carrie K. Burger*
Photo Research: *Pam Carley*
Compositor: *Carlisle Publishing Services*
Typeface: *10/12 Minion*
Printer: *Quebecor World Dubuque, IA*

The credits section for this book begins on page CR-1 and is considered an extension of the copyright page.

Library of Congress Cataloging-in-Publication Data

Saeger, Jan L.
   New foundations in therapeutic massage and bodywork / Jan L. Saeger, Donna
Kyle-Brown. – 1st ed.
      p. cm.
   Includes index.
      ISBN 0–07–302582–8 — ISBN 978–0–07–302582–7 (alk. paper)
      1. Massage therapy–Textbooks. I. Kyle-Brown, Donna. II. Title.

RM721.S137 2008
615.8'22–dc

2006046969

www.mhhe.com

Dedication

To my students who provided the impetus for this work,

To my parents who encouraged me in my work but who passed before

seeing this book come to fruition,

To Alfred who led me to become a massage therapist.

Jan L. Saeger

To my students, past, present, and future, and to the instructors who

face the many challenges of changing lives through education.

Donna Kyle-Brown

About the Authors

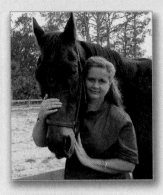

JAN L. SAEGER Jan L. Saeger is an internationally trained and certified massage therapist. She received her license in Florida after fulfilling that state's rigorous requirements at the Florida College of Natural Health, a school approved by the American Massage Therapy Association and accredited by the Commission on Massage Therapy Accreditation; she graduated with a degree in advanced soft tissue therapeutics. Ms. Saeger is also nationally certified in therapeutic massage and bodywork by the National Certification Board of Therapeutic Massage and Bodywork. She also received training and certification in Thai massage from the Traditional Medicine Hospital and the International Training Massage Institute (ITM) in Chiang Mai, Thailand. Ms. Saeger also received certification in *sen* therapy from ITM.

Ms. Saeger is currently a full-time instructor and the massage therapy program coordinator for Keiser University in West Palm Beach, Florida, a 1000-hour massage therapy and associate of science degree program. She has owned and operated a successful massage and yoga therapy practice for more than a decade, working on amateur and professional athletes such as marathon runners, triathletes, and ballet dancers. Ms. Saeger specializes in the equestrian industry, working with professional trainers, riders, and show horses. Along with a partner, she formed an entrepreneurial company importing unique and exotic gifts from Thailand for massage therapists.

As one of the first therapists in the country to work on horses, she was certified by Equissage® in equine sports massage in 1994. A yoga practitioner for 31 years, she is a registered yoga teacher recognized by the Yoga Alliance and has taught yoga for the School District of Palm Beach County Adult Education/Community School. She is certified in Reiki and also works with Qi Gong.

Ms. Saeger was led into the alternative health field by one of her horses, Alfred, a young thoroughbred who was suffering from an idiopathic lameness. Having long recognized the benefits of therapeutic massage for herself, she set out on a quest to find a specific massage modality that would make her dressage horse rideable again. She found therapeutic massage and acupressure point massage were most effective in her horse's recovery. She has since successfully combined therapeutic massage with Thai massage to rehabilitate countless show and pleasure horses, and she teaches other therapists these phenomenal techniques.

Before working in the massage therapy field, Ms. Saeger was an editor and production manager in the magazine publishing industry in New York City. The majority of her time was spent with the American Kennel Club as managing editor and production manager for its monthly publications. She was one of the prime movers in overhauling the magazine's design and purpose by splitting the magazine into three different publications, creating two statistical periodicals and one editorial or content-based magazine.

Ms. Saeger also was production supervisor for Ziff-Davis, at the time New York City's largest magazine publisher. In that capacity, she was responsible for such notable titles as *Car and Driver, Modern Bride, Runner, Flying, Boating, PC, PC jr.,* and *Creative Computing.* Besides directly supervising production managers for these titles, she played a role in accounting for the four-color production costs on all 75 Ziff titles. With the sale of Ziff-Davis, Saeger moved to a Wall Street investment firm, Lord, Abbett & Co., where she was production director for the Marketing Communications Department. At Lord, Abbett, she was responsible for a $2 million marketing budget and, as with her previous positions, she continued to provide the creative impetus behind editorial concepts through to printed pieces.

Work in publishing was a natural step for Ms. Saeger, who graduated from Alfred University with a Bachelor of Arts in English literature and grew up in her family's graphic arts and typesetting business.

Ms. Saeger currently lives in Loxahatchee, Florida, with her two Newfoundland dogs and two horses, an Irish draught and the thoroughbred, now age 27, whose injury led her into the healing arts.

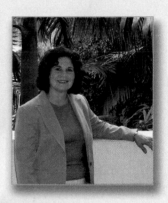

DONNA D. KYLE-BROWN

Donna Brown has enjoyed 32 years of working and studying in the allied health field and has over 20 years' experience as a published writer. Ms. Brown began her health career by receiving a scholarship to Providence Hospital School of Radiological Technology in Mobile, Alabama. That began many years of working in hospitals, medical offices, and centers for chiropractic care. She received her Registered Medical Assistant Certification from the American Medical Technologists, a national certifying agency for the allied health profession, and has worked as an x-ray technician, medical office manager, insurance collection specialist, chiropractic assistant, physical therapy assistant, and lab technician in the medical field.

She was chosen at an early age to study shamanism from the Cherokee perspective and is a Certified Shamanic Counselor. She received certification as a Master Herbalist and in reflexology, and she is a Reiki Master/Teacher of the Usui Shiki Ryoho tradition. Ms. Brown currently owns Pathways, a business centered on natural health care practices. She also practices indigenous massage and crystal therapy of the Cherokee tradition.

Donna Brown received a doctor of philosophy degree in religion in 1997 and a doctorate in motivation therapy from a nondenominational seminary in 2001. She has taught kindergarten, physical education classes for middle-school girls, writing classes, medical assisting classes, and massage lecture classes, and was the director of education for several years at an allied health vocational training center that included massage therapy as a program. In that role, she wrote the material for the massage therapy program and also taught anatomy and physiology, business and marketing, Reiki, reflexology, and CPR in the massage therapy program. She has received her Allied Health Instructor Certification from the American Medical Technologist Association.

During the past 15 years, Ms. Brown has given numerous seminars and workshops promoting natural health care. She currently teaches for the Mobile (Alabama) County Parks and Recreation Department and is the Campus Director at Blue Cliff College of Gulfport, MS.

Ms. Brown currently lives in Vancleave, Mississippi, a small town just north of the Gulf Coast, where she is active in many community endeavors. She is an avid naturalist, and when not writing or teaching, she enjoys spending time with friends, pets, and family.

Brief Contents

PART ONE

Basic Concepts of Therapeutic Massage and Bodywork

CHAPTER 1   History of Therapeutic Massage

CHAPTER 2   Equipment, Environment, and Safety Practices

CHAPTER 3   The Massage Therapy Session

CHAPTER 4   Therapeutic Massage Techniques

CHAPTER 5   Physiological Effects of Therapeutic Massage

PART TWO

Kinesiology, Anatomy, and Pathophysiology

CHAPTER 6   Biomechanics of Movement

CHAPTER 7   General Overview of the Skeletal System

CHAPTER 8   Muscular System

CHAPTER 9   Other Body Systems

PART THREE

Beyond The Basic Curriculum

CHAPTER 10   Maternity, Infant, and Pediatric Massage

CHAPTER 11   Massage for Special Populations (Children with Special Needs, Geriatric, and Hospice and Palliative Care)

CHAPTER 12   Massage for Survivors of Abuse

CHAPTER 13   Sports Massage for Amateur and Professional Athletes

CHAPTER 14   Spa Therapy: Peace, Beauty, and Massage

PART FOUR

Complementary Massage and Bodywork Modalities

CHAPTER 15   Eastern Practices and Energy Work

CHAPTER 16   Introduction to Other Modalities

PART FIVE

Wellness for Body and Mind

CHAPTER 17   Body-Mind Connection

CHAPTER 18   Nutrition and Wellness

CHAPTER 19   Eastern and Western Principles of Movement

PART SIX

Ethics and Professional Business Practices

CHAPTER 20   Law, Ethics, and Professionalism

CHAPTER 21   Business Development, Marketing Success, and Community Education

PART SEVEN

Pharmacology and Specific Pathology Routines

CHAPTER 22   Common Medications and Effects in Clients

CHAPTER 23   Special Massage Routines for Common Pathologies

Quick Reference Guides

QUICK GUIDE A   State-by-State Requirements

QUICK GUIDE B   Resource List

QUICK GUIDE C   Reference List

QUICK GUIDE D   Medical Terminology and Anatomical Abbreviations for Massage and Bodywork

QUICK GUIDE E   Muscular System Tables with Origin, Insertion, Innervation, and Actions

QUICK GUIDE F   Aromatherapy and Herbal Preparations

QUICK GUIDE G   Commonly Prescribed Medications

Contents

PART ONE

Basic Concepts of Therapeutic Massage and Bodywork

CHAPTER **1**
History of Therapeutic Massage 5

Introduction 6

Massage in the Ancient World: An International Phenomenon [5000 BCE–500 AD] 6

The Earliest Civilizations 7

Massage in Ancient Greece and Rome (700 BCE–476 CE) 11

The Middle Ages: (500–1500 CE) 14

The Renaissance 15

The Nineteenth Century 15

The Twentieth Century 19

The Philosophical Foundation of Massage 21

Chapter Summary 23

Applying Your Knowledge 23

CHAPTER **2**
Equipment, Environment, and Saftey Practices 25

Introduction 26

Equipment (Tables, Chairs, Mats, Accessories, Heat & Cryotherapy Sources, Linens and Lubricants) 26

Environment (Room Set-up, Color and Music Selection) 36

Safety First in the Massage Environment 39

PROCEDURE 2.1 Hand Washing Technique 40

Pathogens and Transmission of Diseases 43

Health Crises (AIDS/HIV, Hepatitis Types B and C, SARS, and TB) 50

Chapter Summary 52

Applying Your Knowledge 52

Case Studies/Critical Thinking 52

CHAPTER **3**
The Massage Therapy Session 55

Introduction 56

The Massage Therapy Session (Draping, Special Bolstering) 56

PROCEDURE 3.1 Special Bolstering for Postural Deviations 59

Assessment (Postural Analysis, SOAP Notes) 61

PROCEDURE 3.2 Postural Analysis 64

PROCEDURE 3.3 Narrative Report 66

Medical Terminology 66

PROCEDURE 3.4 Common Medical Abbreviations for Massage Therapists 67

Managing Physician Referrals and Insurance 68

Chapter Summary 72

Applying Your Knowledge 72

Case Studies/Critical Thinking 72

CHAPTER **4**
Therapeutic Massage Techniques 73

Introduction 74

Indications and Contraindications 74

Areas of Endangerment 76

Directional Terms 76

The Art of Skeletal Muscle Palpation 76

THINK ABOUT IT Areas of Endangerment 78

Introduction to Massage and Bodywork 80

Sequence and Flow 88

Body Mechanics 89

Table Massage Sequence 92

Chair Massage Sequence (By Peter Joachim, LMT, NCTMB) 107

Chapter Summary 110

Applying Your Knowledge 110

Case Studies/Critical Thinking 111

CHAPTER **5**
Physiological Effects of Therapeutic Massage 113

Introduction 114

Principal Physiological Mechanisms 114

Effects of Massage on Body Systems (Cardiovascular System, Lymphatic System, Nervous System, and Muscular System) 115

THINK ABOUT IT General Principles 119

THINK ABOUT IT Adenosine Triphosphate 122

Reflex Mechanisms of Massage 123

Physiological Effects of Massage Techniques 125

Effects of Hydrotherapy (Cold and Heat Applications) 126

Chapter Summary 128

Applying Your Knowledge 128

Case Studies/Critical Thinking 129

PART TWO

Kinesiology, Anatomy, and Pathophysiology

CHAPTER 6

Biomechanics of Movement 133

Introduction 134

Terminology and Basic Concepts 134

Body Movements and Ranges of Motion 137

Biomechanics of the Musculoskeletal System (Connective Tissue, Muscle, and Joints) 143

Anthropometry 145

Biomechanics and Ergonomics 145

Kinesiology and Movements 145

Posture and Equilibrium 146

Prevention of Musculoskeletal Injuries 148

Biomechanics and Massage 149

Chapter Summary 150

Applying Your Knowledge 150

Case Studies/Critical Thinking 151

CHAPTER 7

General Overview of the Body and the Skeletal System 153

Introduction 154

Terminology and Basic Concepts 154

Basic Structure and Systems of the Human Body (Cells, Tissues, and Organs) 157

Skeletal System (Overview, Bone Formation and Growth, Classification of Bones, Palpation and Bony Landmarks, and Joints,) 163

PROCEDURE 7.1 Palpation Exercises 172

A Detailed Look at Skeletal Components (Skull, Pectoral Girdle, Carpals, Ribcage, Spine, Vetebrae, Pelvis, Legs, Knee, and Tarsal) 176

Chapter Summary 189

Applying Your Knowledge 190

Case Studies/Critical Thinking 192

CHAPTER 8

Muscular System 193

Introduction 194

Anatomy and Physiology of Muscle Tissue 194

Naming Muscles 198

Muscle Contractions (Face and Head, Torso, Respiration, Abdomen, Back, Arm, Hip and Femur, Legs, and Feet) 198

Common Pathology of the Muscular System 214

PROCEDURE 8.1 Palpation Exercises 217

Chapter Summary 218

Applying Your Knowledge 218

Case Studies/Critical Thinking 222

CHAPTER 9

Other Body Systems 223

Introduction 224

Cardiovascular System 224

Nervous System 232

Endocrine System 237

Lymphatic System 241

Digestive System 245

Respiratory System 248

Urinary System 250

Reproductive System 251

Integumentary System 252

The Senses 254

Chapter Summary 258

Applying Your Knowledge 258

Case Studies/Critical Thinking 260

PART THREE

Beyond The Basic Curriculum

CHAPTER 10

Maternity, Infant, and Pediatric Massage 265

Introduction 266

Prenatal, Labor, and Postpartum Massage (By Carla DiMauro, LMT) 266

Applications of Theory and Practice for Massage During Pregnancy: Organized by Body System 274

Infant and Pediatric Massage (By Carla DiMauro, LMT) 279

Applications of Theory and Practice for Infant and Pediatric Massage 281

Massage for Children (By Carla DiMauro, LMT) 286

Chapter Summary 287

Applying Your Knowledge 287

Case Studies/Critical Thinking 288

CHAPTER 11

Massage for Special Populations (Children with Special Needs, Geriatric, Hospice and Palliative Care) 289

Introduction 290

Special Needs Children (By Carla DiMauro, LMT) 290

Applications of Theory and Practice for Specific Needs Massage 290

Working with Elderly Clients 296

Applications of Theory and Practice for Geriatric Massage 297

PROCEDURE 11.1 Toolbox of Modalities for Senior Clients 298

Massage for Hospice and Palliative Care (By Carla DiMauro, LMT) 299

Applications of Theory and Practice for Hospice and Palliative Care Massage 302

Chapter Summary 304

Applying Your Knowledge 304

Case Studies/Critical Thinking 305

CHAPTER 12

Massage for Survivors of Abuse 307

Introduction 308

Working with Survivors of Sexual Abuse (By Donna Cerio) 308

Applications of Theory and Practice for Massage of Survivors of Abuse: Organized by Category of Clients 313

Chapter Summary 318

Applying Your Knowledge 318

Case Studies/Critical Thinking 319

CHAPTER 13

Sports Massage: For Amateur and Professional Athletes 321

Introduction 322

Sports Massage (Definition, Indications and Contraindications, Strokes, Timing Parameters, Stretching and Joint Movement, PNF Techniques, Muscle Testing) 322

PROCEDURE 13.1 Sports Massage Techniques and Timing 331

Injury Pathology (Four Step Healing Process, Strains and Sprains, Spasms and Cramps, Hydrotherapy for Injuries) 339

Sports Massage at Events 346

Rehabilitative/Maintenance Massage (Shoulder Routine, Elbow Routine, Quadriceps Routine, Anterior Lower Leg/Shin Splints Routine, Lower Leg Routine, Hamstring Routine, Low Back Routine, and Knee Routine) 347

Chapter Summary 358

Applying Your Knowledge 359

Case Studies/Critical Thinking 359

CHAPTER 14

Spa Therapy: Peace, Beauty, and Massage 361

Introduction 362

Types of Spas 362

Types of Service 363

PROCEDURE 14.1 Performing a Basic Facial Treatment 367

PROCUDURE 14.2 Performing a Friction Bath 376

PROCEDURE 14.3 Performing a Basic Paraffin Treatment 378

PROCEDURE 14.4 Performing a Parafango Treatment 379

PROCEDURE 14.5 Performing a Basic Herbal Wrap 384

Chapter Summary 384

Applying Your Knowledge 385

Case Studies/Critical Thinking 385

PART FOUR

Complementary Massage and Bodywork Modalities

CHAPTER 15

Eastern Practices and Energy Work 389

Introduction 390

Chinese Medicine, Meridians, and Acupressure (By Marc H. Kalmanson, BSN, MSN, ARNP, LMT, RYT) 390

The Meridian System 394

Acupressure 405

Shiatsu 410

Jin Shin Do 410

Amma 411

Moxibustion 411

Cupping 411

Ayurveda (By Donald J. Glassey, MSW, DC, LMT, NCTMB) 411

Thai Massage 414

Lomi Lomi 418

Energy Work 418

Chapter Summary 424

Applying Your Knowledge 424

Case Studies/Critical Thinking 425

CHAPTER 16

Introduction to Other Modalities 427

Introduction 428

Trigger Point Therapy 428

PROCEDURE 16.1 Performing Trigger Point Therapy 429

Intuitive Neuromuscular Massage (By Lewis Rudolph, BS, AAS, LMT) 430

PROCEDURE 16.2 Performing an Intuitive Neuromuscular Massage 433

Rolfing (By Don Curry, LMT, Certified Advanced Rolfer) 434

Hellerwork 438

Myofascial Release (By John F. Barnes, PT) 438

Bindegewebmassage 444

Trager (By Deane Juhan, MA) 444

Alexander Technique 449

Feldenkrais 449

Lymphatic Drainage Therapy (By Bruno Chikly MD, DO (Hon.)) 449

Cerebrospinal Fluid Technique Massage (By Donald J. Glassey, MSW, DC, LMT, NCTMB) 452

Craniosacral Therapy (By Don Ash, PT, CST-D) 457

Chapter Summary 460

Applying Your Knowledge 460

Case Studies/Critical Thinking 460

PART FIVE

Wellness For Body And Mind

CHAPTER 17

Body–Mind Connection 465

Introduction 466

Fight-or-Flight Response 466

Placebo Effect 467

Methods that Connect Body and Mind (Meditation, Balancing the Spirit, Chakra Balancing, Energy Work and Guided Imagery) 468

Indigenous Massage and Native American Practices 472

Visualization/Guided Imagery Technique for Relaxation 473

Chapter Summary 474

Applying Your Knowledge 474

Case Studies/Critical Thinking 475

CHAPTER 18

Nutrition and Wellness 477

Introduction 478

Food and Health 479

Vitamins and Minerals 481

Digestion, Absorption, and Metabolism 486

Nutritional Pathology 489

Food and the Mind 490

Chapter Summary 492

Body Mass Index 493

Applying Your Knowledge 493

Case Studies/Critical Thinking 494

CHAPTER 19

Eastern and Western Principles of Movement 495

Introduction 496

Yoga (Prana and Chakras, Meditation) 497

Tai Chi 513

Traditional Western Stretching Exercises (Strength, Mobility, and Flexibility, Stretching, and Maintenance) 514

Chapter Summary 525

Applying Your Knowledge 525

Case Studies/Critical Thinking 526

PART SIX

Ethics and Professional Business Practice

CHAPTER 20

Law, Ethics, and Professionalism 531

Introduction 532

Codes of Ethics and Laws 532

Therapeutic Massage and Bodywork Codes of Ethics 533

AMTA Code of Ethics 533

Associated Bodywork and Massage Professionals 533

International Massage Association 534

National Certification Board for Therapeutic Massage and Bodywork 534

Scope of Practice (Right to Privacy, HIPAA, Right of Refusal and Informed Consent, Working Smart, Working Safely, and Professional Appearance and Demeanor) 535

Boundaries and Professional Relationships (Personal and Professional Boundaries, Multidimensional Relationships, and Emotional Release) 543

Chapter Summary 545

Applying Your Knowledge 545

Case Studies/Critical Thinking 546

CHAPTER 21

Business Development, Marketing Success, and Community Education 547

Introduction 548

Keys to Success 548

Entrepreneur or Employee 548

Marketing Yourself (Marketing material, marketing yourself through chair massage, networking and community volunteer work) 553

Personal Care 556

Types of Business (Sole proprietorship, Partnership, Corporations, and Selecting a business name) 558

Chapter Summary 560

Applying Your Knowledge 561

Case Studies/Critical Thinking 561

PART SEVEN

Pharmacology and Specific Pathology Routines

CHAPTER 22

Common Medications and Effects in Clients 565

Introduction 566

Pharmacology Basics 567

Understanding Pharmacology Terminology 569

Sources of Drugs 570

How Drugs Are Processed by the Body (Route of Administration, Pharmacokinetics, and Drug Excretion) 570

Drug Classifications (Non-Controlled and Controlled Drugs, Topical Medications, Psychotropic Medications, Recreational Drugs, and General Contraindications) 573

Vitamins And Minerals 579

Using a Drug/Medication Guide 583

Chapter Summary 584

Applying Your Knowledge 585

Case Studies/Critical Thinking 585

CHAPTER 23

Special Massage Routines for Common Pathologies 587

Introduction 588

Carpal Tunnel Syndrome 588

PROCEDURE 23.1 Performing a Massage Routine for Carpal Tunnel Syndrome 590

Thoracic Outlet Syndrome 590

PROCEDURE 23.2 Performing a Massage Routine for Thoracic Outlet Syndrome 591

Torticollis/Wryneck 592

PROCEDURE 23.3 Performing a Massage Routine for Torticollis (Wryneck) 593

Temporomandibular Joint Dysfunction 593

PROCEDURE 23.4 Performing a Massage Routine for Temporomandibular Joint Dysfunction 594

Fibromyalgia Syndrome 595

PROCEDURE 23.5 Performing a Massage Routine for Fibromyalgia Syndrome 596

Chapter Summary 597

Applying Your Knowledge 597

Case Studies/Critical Thinking 597

Quick Reference Guides

QUICK GUIDE A   State-By-State Requirements A-1

QUICK GUIDE B   Resource List B-1

QUICK GUIDE C   Reference List C-1

QUICK GUIDE D   Medical Terminology D-1

QUICK GUIDE E   Complete Muscle System Tables E-1

QUICK GUIDE F   Aromatherapy, Herbal Preparations, and Supplements F-1

QUICK GUIDE G   Common Medications G-1

Glossary GL-1

Contributors' Biographies CO-1

Credits CR-1

Index I-1

Foreword

It is indeed an honor to address a foreword to this new and important textbook for massage training programs. During the past 20 years massage therapy has been burgeoning, with hundreds of new schools and thousands of new practitioners. It is in fact the fastest-growing profession among the alternative, or complementary, approaches to health care. With this rapid expansion there has been a growing need for an authoritative text that presents to students a full picture of the history, the science, and the art of massage therapy, and that informs them of the wide variety of modalities and professional opportunities toward which their initial training may lead them. Jan L. Saeger and Donna D. Kyle-Brown have collaborated, along with a number of contributing authors, to produce just such a book. It is an enormous project, and it is informed by their decades of experience in massage and health care as practitioners and instructors. It is also much enhanced by their extensive professional involvement in publishing, which has given them the skills to write and assemble a mass of information into a very well organized and accessible book.

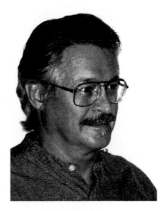

The authors' intentions go well beyond writing an informative and easily readable text. Their broader goal is to influence the direction of future developments in the therapeutic massage profession. Growth in the field has been so rapid, and has been spurred by many different training programs and modalities, with many different approaches and philosophies, a mutually agreed upon definition of the profession, one that encompasses all of its sources and possibilities, has been elusive. The authors feel—and I wholeheartedly agree—that it is time to develop a clear and comprehensive description of the work in all its diversity, one that honors both the uniqueness of the profession as a whole and the wide variety of techniques and application. As it emerges, this coherent sense of the field of massage will serve students who are entering it by lending clarity and inspiration to their endeavor, serve training programs by giving them a sense of mutual purpose rather than competitiveness, and serve the public at large by educating them about the effectiveness of massage therapy and about the numerous kinds of treatment that are available.

The authors have placed light emphasis on "teaching massage" through their text, wisely leaving most of the hands-on details to the discretion, talents, and experience of individual programs and instructors. Instead, the bulk of their work is devoted to the fundamentals of anatomy, physiology, and psychology that underlie all modalities, to the historical, sociological, and therapeutic aspects of massage, and to the complex issues of professionalism in an intimate, touching practice. These are to me the broad and necessary basics around which any specific program can be designed.

Especially welcomed are the chapters describing a wide variety of modalities and a wide variety of applications, inclusive of Eastern disciplines of therapeutic touch and movement. Exclusive specialization in this or that modality is becoming less and less the norm in the profession, and students increasingly need to absorb knowledge and experience of many different approaches to deepen both their effectiveness and their appreciation for the diversity and ingenuity of the world history of massage.

Massage needs to be informed by science, but it will always be essentially an art, a deep communication between individuals. The beauty of this book is its balance between these two aspects of the work, and its emphasis on the soul that must inhabit the art. More than a comprehensive text (which it emphatically is), this book is a testimony to the efficacy and versatility of touch and the deep contact with our fundamental humanity, which it arouses and nourishes. It is both a summing up of past developments in therapeutic massage and a beacon toward future ones. My greatest hope for it is that it will nudge that future in the directions the authors have in mind. Massage is a unique and important part of health care and well-being, and as a profession it very much deserves—and needs—to be viewed by its members and by the public in the light that Saeger, Kyle-Brown et. al. have cast upon it.

Deane Juhan

Contributors

This book offers the knowledge and expertise from many contributors that are known in their field. You will enjoy reading their excerpts throughout the book. To learn more about each contributor look for their biographies at the end of the book on page CO-1.

Dr. Medhat Alattar, MB.BCh, DC., MS
Don Ash, PT, CST-D
John F. Barnes, PT
Donna Cerio
Burno Chikly, MD, DO (Hon.)
Don Curry, LMT, Certified Advancer Rolfer
Carla DiMauro, LMT
Dr. Donald J. Glassey, MSW, DC, LMT, NCTMB
Daniel A. Heidel, BS, LMT

Peter Joachim, LMT, NCTMB
Deane Juhan, MA
Marc Kalmanson, BSN, MSN, ARNP, LMT, RYT
Dan Rowlands, LMT, NCTMB
Linda Rowlands, LMT, NCTMB
Lewis Rudolph, BS, AASm LMT
Valerie Wohl
Christian M. Wright, DC, BsHB

Preface

This important new work that you are holding, *New Foundations in Therapeutic Massage and Bodywork,* is unique in approach and format. In writing this text, our objective is to provide a concise, focused, and practical approach to massage technique for students of massage therapy. No matter what connection you have with therapeutic massage—beginning student, practicing massage therapist, sports therapist, massage instructor, alternative healing practitioner, or medical health practitioner—this text will serve for both training and reference purposes.

The system of study within this book will enable the reader to employ a vast amount of up-to-date knowledge toward practical applications for successful healing techniques. We have incorporated well-illustrated and well-organized material relevant to an optimized application of massage therapy principles and techniques. We also developed numerous pedagogical aids for use by students and instructors wishing a complete program for the study of therapeutic massage.

Objectives

We reviewed and analyzed information and perspective from practicing therapists, instructors of massage therapy, and massage therapy students to present the following objectives:

- Provide a focused examination of anatomy with an emphasis on physiology as it applies to therapeutic massage. We combined anatomy and the physiology of body systems to give the student or practitioner a complete guide to the function and structure of the human body, and then the ability to use precise medical/professional terminology in describing them.

- Continue the learning process by giving in-depth information on how massage can benefit the body by maintaining health and eliminating certain disease processes. Specific chapters explain the role of massage in increasing circulation of blood and lymph and the direct mechanical effects of rhythmic applied pressure toward blood flow. With this objective in mind, we have included chapters that are massage-specific in regard to injury and rehabilitation. Also discussed are the effects of increasing the body's ability to remove waste material, toxins, and impurities through the lymphatic and integumentary systems, and better manage disease and debility.

- Present information, perspective, and practical guidance for working with all segments of the population—from the very young to the very old, from those who have to live with disabilities to those who have endured hardships.

- Provide a thorough and comprehensive explanation of therapeutic massage and complementary bodywork modalities (both Eastern and Western), written by the developer or recognized expert in the field, as enhancements to or a launching point for specialization in the therapist's massage practice.

- Give the student a foundation for proper handling of client relationships and documentation, such as HIPAA guidelines, and professional and ethical standards, along with an understanding of successful business practices.

Pedagogical Features and Special Ancillaries

We have incorporated the following features to make the text more practical and valuable:

- Full-color photographs and illustrations throughout the text give the student a realistic view of the application or point being studied.
- A number of "how to" photographs and illustrations to show step-by-step procedures and techniques.
- Numerous reference mentions to assist the student or practitioner in accessing material located elsewhere in the text.
- Repetition is used throughout the text to enforce learning and build clinical terminology and confidence in the beginning student.
- Learning Outcomes at the beginning provide a glimpse ahead to important sections for quick understanding of flow and organization.
- Key Terms at the beginning of each chapter and bolded when first introduced in the chapter familiarize the students of important concepts.
- An Introduction for each chapter gives the students an idea of what is going to be taught.
- Technical Emphasis boxes in each chapter incorporate counseling, ethics, and teaching skills for positive application of massage techniques.
- Exam Point boxes highlight critical areas of understanding for certification and review.
- Special Application (Procedures) boxes demonstrate real-life experiences and provide informative sidebars.
- A Summary at the end of each chapter gathers key points that are presented in the chapter.
- Applying Your Knowledge questions at the end of each chapter help to reinforce the information the student just read in that chapter.
- Case Studies at the end of each chapter give the students an opportunity to apply the concepts and learn by discussion.

There is a website for both students and instructors. The students can benefit from additional quiz questions, animation exercises, and labeling exercises. The instructor can view the Instructor's Manual, PowerPoint presentations for each chapter, and an image bank of all the illustrations in the text, which can be printed and used as handouts.

An Instructor's CD-ROM is available. The CD contains the Instructor's Manual, PowerPoint presentations for each chapter, and EZ Test questions for each chapter. McGraw-Hill's EZ Test is a flexible and easy-to-use electronic testing program. The program allows instructors to create tests from book specific items. It accommodates a wide range of question types, and instructors may add their own questions. Multiple versions of the test can be created and any test can be exported for use with course management systems such as WebCT, BlackBoard, or PageOut. EZ Test Online is a new service and gives instructors a place to easily administer their EZ Test-created exams and quizzes online. The program is available for Windows and Macintosh platforms.

The Instructor's Manual includes an overview/introduction to massage therapy, instructor teaching tips, two sample syllabii, an answer key for all chapter review questions with feedback, and a lesson plan for each chapter.

Summary

While writing this text, our guiding principle was that therapeutic massage has become a core discipline in the modern health care continuum and that it will continue to grow in importance through more rigorous training and certification of its practitioners and through more research into its obvious benefits. These benefits, which include the prevention or treatment of certain diseases and the contribution to overall health, vitality, and well-being, are being better understood each day. We have attempted to create a work that teaches fundamental concepts as well as effective reasoning and decision-making skills, so that our readers may go on to fruitful and rewarding positions in professional practice. Therapeutic massage deserves its rightful place in a health care continuum that respects modalities that can save health care dollars while dramatically improving the quality of individual lives.

We hope we have created a valuable new resource for educators and students in the classroom setting, for massage and bodywork practitioners in the field, and for all requiring a continuing education resource.

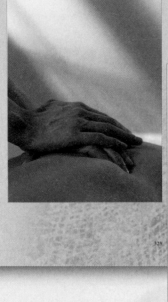

Every chapter opens with the Learning Outcomes, Key Terms, and an Introduction that helps prepare the students for the learning experience.

A thorough explanation of massage modalities written by the developer or expert provides the students with a working knowledge of these specialties.

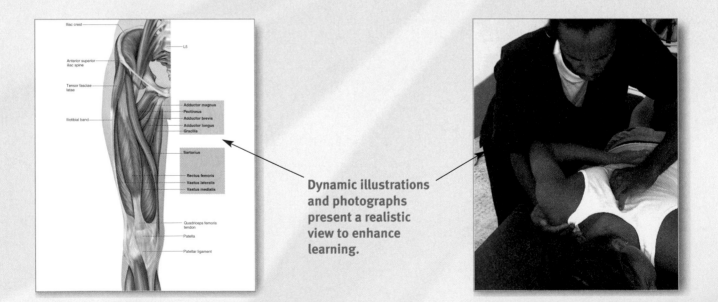

Dynamic illustrations and photographs present a realistic view to enhance learning.

"The depth of information and tone of the authors' voice is obvious to me that they care deeply for the profession and all the future clients as well as for the student and professional therapist." *Sheryl Daniel–Academy of Natural Therapy, Eaton, CO.*

EXAM POINT Given all of these applications, effleurage is considered the most versatile stroke of all.

Exam Point boxes highlight critical areas of understanding for certification and review.

Technical Emphasis boxes incorporate counseling, ethics, and teaching skills for positive application of massage techniques.

TECHNIQUE EMPHASIS When you palpate, remember the acronym PALPATE, or "*Press Always Lightly, Perceive At The Exterior.*"

Chapter Summary

Being an accomplished massage therapist involves far more than setting up an office and hanging out a sign. You should possess good communication skills so that you are aware of your clients' needs and comfort level and can explain to your client what to expect during the massage session. You also need to be motivated to compile and keep accurate records so that you are able to run a smooth and organized office. It is likewise important for you to understand basic medical terminology and insurance procedures.

The key points in Chapter Summaries help students retain what was just learned.

Review questions at the end of every chapter reinforce massage therapy competencies.

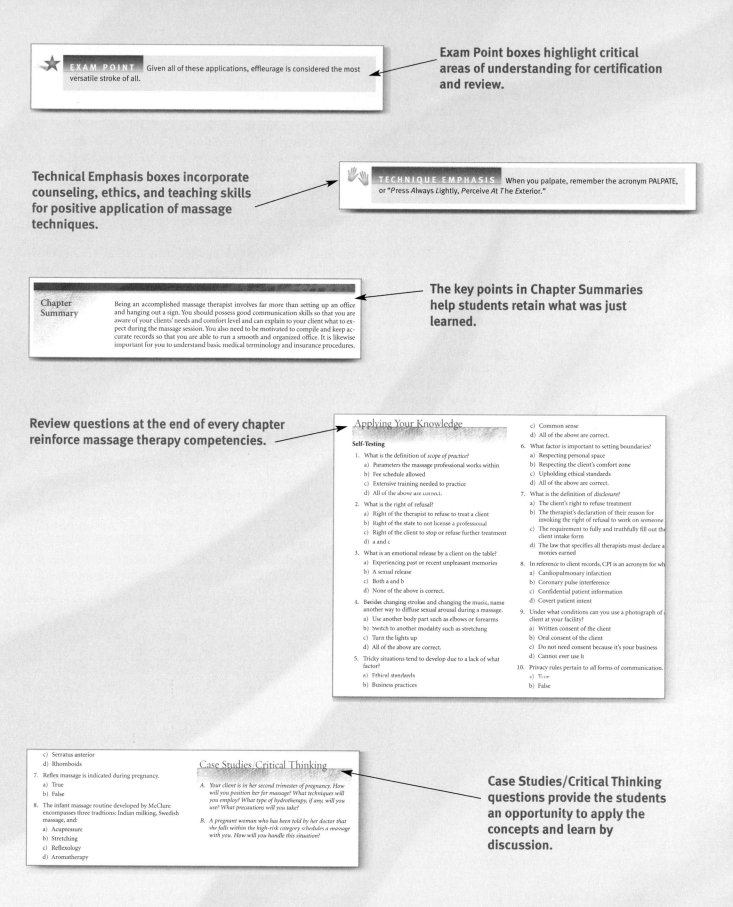

Applying Your Knowledge

Self-Testing

1. What is the definition of *scope of practice*?
   a) Parameters the massage professional works within
   b) Fee schedule allowed
   c) Extensive training needed to practice
   d) All of the above are correct.

2. What is the right of refusal?
   a) Right of the therapist to refuse to treat a client
   b) Right of the state to not license a professional
   c) Right of the client to stop or refuse further treatment
   d) a and c

3. What is an emotional release by a client on the table?
   a) Experiencing past or recent unpleasant memories
   b) A sexual release
   c) Both a and b
   d) None of the above is correct.

4. Besides changing strokes and changing the music, name another way to diffuse sexual arousal during a massage.
   a) Use another body part such as elbows or forearms
   b) Switch to another modality such as stretching
   c) Turn the lights up
   d) All of the above are correct.

5. Tricky situations tend to develop due to a lack of what factor?
   a) Ethical standards
   b) Business practices

   c) Common sense
   d) All of the above are correct.

6. What factor is important to setting boundaries?
   a) Respecting personal space
   b) Respecting the client's comfort zone
   c) Upholding ethical standards
   d) All of the above are correct.

7. What is the definition of *disclosure*?
   a) The client's right to refuse treatment
   b) The therapist's declaration of their reason for invoking the right of refusal to work on someone
   c) The requirement to fully and truthfully fill out the client intake form
   d) The law that specifies all therapists must declare all monies earned

8. In reference to client records, CPI is an acronym for wh...
   a) Cardiopulmonary infarction
   b) Coronary pulse interference
   c) Confidential patient information
   d) Covert patient intent

9. Under what conditions can you use a photograph of a client at your facility?
   a) Written consent of the client
   b) Oral consent of the client
   c) Do not need consent because it's your business
   d) Cannot ever use it

10. Privacy rules pertain to *all* forms of communication.
    a) True
    b) False

c) Serratus anterior
d) Rhomboids

7. Reflex massage is indicated during pregnancy.
   a) True
   b) False

8. The infant massage routine developed by McClure encompasses three tradtions: Indian milking, Swedish massage, and:
   a) Acupressure
   b) Stretching
   c) Reflexology
   d) Aromatherapy

Case Studies/Critical Thinking

A. *Your client is in her second trimester of pregnancy. How will you position her for massage? What techniques will you employ? What type of hydrotherapy, if any, will you use? What precautions will you take?*

B. *A pregnant woman who has been told by her doctor that she falls within the high-risk category schedules a massage with you. How will you handle this situation?*

Case Studies/Critical Thinking questions provide the students an opportunity to apply the concepts and learn by discussion.

"This text is very thorough and well written. I really like the quizzes at the end of the chapters and the pathology for the systems. It also connects to everyday life." *Susan Hughes-Miller–Motte Technical College, Wilmington, NC.*

Author Acknowledgments

Jan L. Saeger—I would like to thank George Stamathis for his foresight and vision that brought us all together to create this work and Christine Ambrose for her unending patience, guidance, and belief in what we were doing.

I would like to thank Don Glassey for encouraging me to keep writing and for spending countless hours reviewing my content, which furthered this work.

I would like to thank all of the contributors who took the time to write for us and share their specialties or modalities, making this book truly a collaborative effort by some terrific people.

I would like to thank Miriam Morgan, who gave me hours of her time always working magic with the art grids.

I would like to thank Shaana, our photographer, and all of my students who were the models for many of the photographs.

I would like to thank Scott Stein CPA for checking the business details in the business chapter and Vinny Aquilino of the Miami Heat for being my sports massage mentor and reviewing that chapter.

Donna Kyle-Brown—I would like to thank George Stamathis for giving me the opportunity to work on such an important text and invaluable marketing research and advice, and Christine Ambrose who cheerfully tackled the job of bringing our words into book form and brought encouragement to the project when I faced difficulties. My very special thanks go to Ben Johnston, who spent hours trying to find just the right text for my classes and telling me, "Why don't you just write one?"

I would especially like to thank the contributors and reviewers for their outstanding work and the time they spent helping to make this book an asset to massage programs across the nation.

I would like to thank Joan Cerny for training me to teach when my career first began and for being a sounding board for my ideas for this text, and Denise Comptom, Shanita Peoples, Misty Spahr, Luana Kowalski, and Donna Bell, whose support as fellow instructors and friends helped make this project possible.

I would like to thank massage therapists Charlene Russell, Todd Koch, Linda Martin, Elizabeth Evans, Donald Klugg, Lee Williams, and Kay Deason for advice and information regarding massage curriculum development.

And a very special thanks to my husband, family, friends, and pets for their patience and support during the writing of this text. I could not have done this without them.

Reviewer Acknowledgement

Laura Abbott, MS, NCTMB
Georgia State University
Atlanta, GA

Don Ash
Upledger Institute
Palm Beach Gardens, FL

William Ashmall, MA, LMT
Onondaga School of Therapeutic Massage
Syracuse, NY

Jennifer Barrett, BS, LMT
Queensborough Community College
Bayside, NY

Mary Berger, CMT
Kirtland Community College
Roscommon, MI

Paul Bolton, DC
National Holistic Institute
Emeryville, CA

Susan L. Bova, NCMT, CMMMT
Penn Commercial, Inc.
Washington, PA

Michelle Burns
Advanced Holistic Healing Arts
Austin, TX

Steve Capellini
Miami, FL

Sheryl D. Daniel, BA, CMT, NMT, BMT, HNC,
  Reiki Master
Academy of Natural Healing
Eaton, CO

Tim L. Davidson
Heritage Institute
Jacksonville, FL

Julie A. DeJoe, NCTMB
Westfield, NY

Jennifer M. DiBlasio, AST, ACMT
Career Training Academy, Inc.
New Kensington, PA

Dana J. Douglas, NCTMB
Mount Nittany Institute of Natural Health
State College, PA

Charlotte Elipoulos, RN, MPH, ND, PhD
Glen Arm, MD

Elizabeth Fegley
International Academy of Daytona Beach
Daytona Beach, FL

Alexandria M. Fialka
Southeastern School
North Charleston, SC

Lora Freeman
Chicago College of Healing Arts
Chicago, IL

Judith Gawron, MSPT, LMT
Berkshire Community College
Pittsfield, MA

Donald J. Glassey, MSW, DC, LMT, NCTMB
International Academy
South Daytona, FL

Cher Goldman, LMT, MBA
New York, NY

Melissa J. Grey
Miller-Motte Technical College
Wilmington, NC

Patricia M. Grimm, PhD, RW, CMT
Baltimore School of Massage
Baltimore, MD

Ramona Gruber-Hester
Miller-Motte Community College
Wilmington, NC

Amy R. Holibaugh
Community College of Vermont
Morrisville, VT

Colleen Holloway
Success Beyond Work
Grasonville, MD

Susan L. Hughes
Miller-Motte Technical College
Wilmington, NC

Holly Huzar, LMT
Center of Natural Wellness School of Massage
Albany, NY

Robert J. Ianacone
Sonoma College
San Francisco, CA

Lisa Jakober, Director of Education
National Massage Therapy Institute, LLC
Philadelphia, PA

Marc H. Kalmanson, MSN, ARNP, LMT, RYT
Dragon Rises College of Oriental Medicine
Gainesville, FL

Dawn E.R. Kirby, CMT
Denver Career College
Thornton, CO

Kimberly Konrad
Valparaiso, IN

Julianne Lepp
Rising Spirit Institute of Health
Atlanta, GA

Theresa Lowe, LMT
Central Maine School of Massage
Lewiston, ME

Catherine A. Mastroianni, DC, CCSP
Ashmead College
Seattle, WA

Donald McCann, MA, LMT, LMHC, CSET
Structural Energetic Therapy
Lutz, FL

Lisa Mertz, PhD, LMT
Queensborough Community College/City University
  of New York
Bayside, NY

Karen A. Mitchell, NCTMB, LMT, ACMT
St. Louis College of Health Careers
Fenton, MO

Jay M. Nelson, LMT, LMP (Member ABMP, NCTMB)
Concorde Career Institute
Portland, OR

Deborah Ochsner, MS, CMT
Institute of Business and Medical Careers
Fort Collins, CO

Jody L. Olson, LMT
Minnesota State Community & Technical College
Wadena, MN

Cassandra E. Orem
Oasis Health Systems, Inc.
Baltimore, MD

Lesley M. Pearl
McKinnon Institute
Oakland, CA

Anita Phillips, CMT
Sonoma College
San Francisco, CA

Susan Pomfret, MA, LMT, Program Coordinator
Central Arizona College
Apache Junction, AZ

Dr. Grace Reischman, BA, DC, LMBT#1149NC
South Piedmont Community College
Monroe, NC

Keven Robinson
Virginia College
Homewood, AL

Selena Royal Mayes, LMBT
Miller-Motte Technical College
Cary, NC

Dorothy Sala, LMT, CIMI
Teamwork, LLC
Salem, CT

Jill Sanders Stanard, ND
Oregon School of Massage
Portland, OR

Gregory Scelsi
Baltimore School of Massage
Baltimore, MD

Theodore M. Schiff, LMT, CR Instructor
Branford Hall Career Institute
Springfield, MA

Suann M. Schuster, MA/LCMT
Great Lakes Institute of Technology/Massage
Erie, PA

Shana Scott
Georgia Medical Institute
Norcross, GA

Shanwnte Simmons, CMT
Rising Spirit Institute of Massage Therapy
Atlanta, GA

Cheryl L. Siniakin, PhD, LMTI, NCTMB
Community College of Allegheny County
Pittsburgh, PA

Cherie Sohnen-Moe
Sohnen-Moe Associates, Inc.
Tucson, AZ

Tina A. Sorrell, RMT, LMT, MTI, NCTMB
Plano, TX

Michael A. Sullivan, BS, CMT
Anne Arundel Community College
Arnold, MD

Susan B. Thomasson, Med., MT(ASCP)SH, LMBT
Therapeutic Massage Training Institute
Charlotte, NC

Dr. Marilyn S. Veselack
Institute of Therapeutic Massage of Western Colorado
Grand Junction, CO

Efthimios Vlahos
Northwestern Business College
Chicago, IL

Sara J. Wallace
Miller-Motte Technical College
Wilmington, NC

John Neil Wheatley
Rising Spirit Institute
Atlanta, GA

Laura Woitte, Therapeutic Massage Program
    Coordinator
National American University
Sioux Falls, SD

Kim Woodcock, NCTMB
McCann School of Business & Technology
Sunbury, PA

Kevin C. Zorda, LMT
Branford Hall Career Institute
Windsor, CT

Therapeutic Massage: An Overview and Introduction

Massage is fundamentally based on the desire to heal, give comfort, and promote relaxation. From its early beginnings, the profession traversed back and forth over a wide chasm of acceptability to disfavor. The earliest writings were of Chinese and Japanese massage, followed by Hippocrates' mention of massage as treatment for various ailments. Massage was held in high esteem for decades until a series of unfortunate circumstances removed this therapeutic art from the limelight. These unfortunate events include scandals that erupted in Roman culture—and later in England—that led to the proliferation of sexual favors and "massage parlors." The Middle Ages, a historical period marked by superstition of anyone who sought to heal others, brought persecution to those who practiced massage. These circumstances contributed to driving massage underground and out of the mainstream of accepted health care (see chapter 1, History of Therapeutic Massage).

With the help of professional organizations such as the American Massage Therapy Association and many dedicated therapists, massage therapy has once again been elevated to a prestigious vocation. In fact, increasing acknowledgement by physicians and the insurance industry is proof we have come full circle in our perception of massage therapy as a legitimate profession. Of course, the individual client has always been the therapist's most ardent supporter. Many people who are drawn to the field suggest they have experienced a "calling" to do such work: massage therapists innately hold the desire to heal. "Laying on of hands" or possessing the "healing touch" is a powerful guiding force.

Of our five senses, touch is our primary and greatest sense. Every living organism responds to touch, even if hearing or sight is not present. Without touch, we cannot, as human beings, procreate naturally. Our skin touches the air and determines the correct response to heat and cold, pain or pleasure. And when touch is withheld, we become depressed, confused, and may experience feelings of abandonment. With touch, not only do we heal, we also thrive, becoming more physically and emotionally balanced individuals.

In children, touch is so important that babies who are deprived of touch tend to have stunted growth and may even die. Untouched and seldomly held children who survive may continue to be emotionally damaged throughout their lifetime. Touch affects our entire being; it reaches out from us to touch others, whether it is in the form of a pat on the back, a high five, or a handshake (see chapters 10, Maternity, Infant, and Pediatric Massage; 11, Massage for Special Populations; and 12, Massage for Survivors of Abuse).

When we are touched, many physical changes take place within our body. With appropriate touch, our heart rate stabilizes, body temperature normalizes, brain wave patterns are more connected and controlled, and our immune system jumps into action.

Touch plays such a large role in our lives that we include it in our verbal vocabulary. We say "someone has lost his touch" or is "out of touch," or "I will get in touch." We have "touchy subjects," and we can want something so badly that we can "almost touch it." Amazingly, the effect of touch can now be scientifically measured. Many studies by health care professionals have proven that touch is vital to a healthy life. Touch has mutual benefits for both the giver and receiver. You feel better when you receive touch, but you can feel equally as good when you touch someone else.

Massage is a form of **professional touch.** Professional touch is defined as touch from a skilled practitioner that is performed to bring about a specific therapeutic outcome. Massage professionals have the joy of serving others through their desire for the most innate and basic need—touch (see chapter 20, Law, Ethics, and Professionalism).

The Benefits of Massage

It is widely recognized that the first benefit of massage is an increase in circulation, thereby promoting overall good health. For the whole body to be healthy, the individual parts and the sum of those parts must also be healthy. The individual cells of the body depend on an abundant supply of blood and lymph. These fluids supply nutrients and oxygen to the body as well as carry away wastes and toxins. It is easy to understand why good circulation is so important to health and why massage can be so beneficial.

Knowing about the physiological effects of massage makes it possible to better understand the overall health and fitness benefits (see chapter 5, Physiological Effects of Therapeutic Massage). What takes place under a massage therapist's hands has profound importance not only for those interested in general health and fitness, but also for those wishing to "tune up" their bodies for sport and exercise. By helping to reduce physiological fatigue and aid recovery from the exertion of working out or playing sports, massage enables better training with longer, more effective workouts, thus facilitating better performance and preventing injury.

Massage also aids recovery from soft tissue injuries such as sprains and strains, whether such an injury is to a professional athlete or "weekend warrior." This recovery is possible because the growth and repair of tissues are accelerated by efficient circulation in the injured areas and appropriate stimulation of the healing tissues. Therefore, massage therapy can often help accelerate and improve recovery as well as reduce discomfort from such mishaps (see chapter 13, Sports Massage for Amateur and Professional Athletes).

Massage and Body Systems

Massage fosters homeostasis, or balance, in the body by directly and indirectly influencing all body systems. Specifically, touch facilitates the smooth flow of energy and communication among the cardiovascular, digestive, urinary, respiratory, lymphatic, and nervous systems, to name a few.

One of the most profound affects of massage is on the lymphatic system. Lymph fluid carries impurities and waste away from the tissues and passes through glandlike structures spaced throughout the lymphatic system that act as filtering valves. The lymph does not circulate as the blood does, so its movement depends largely on the squeezing effect of muscle contractions. Consequently, inactive people fail to stimulate lymph flow. Massage can dramatically aid the movement of lymph in active or inactive persons. Besides increasing venous flow and lymph drainage, massage can increase the body's secretions and excretions.

Massage can aid nutrition by improving circulation. Greater overall health awareness has also increased nutrition awareness, yet many do not understand that the most carefully planned diet is partly wasted if blood vessels are not developed and open so that nutrition can reach the cells. Massage promotes an increase in the production of gastric juices, saliva, and urine. There is also increased excretion of nitrogen, inorganic phosphorus, and sodium chloride (salt). This suggests that the metabolic rate (the utilization of absorbed material by the body's cells) increases after massage.

Massage can often enhance skin condition. Massage directly improves the function of the oil and sweat glands that keep the skin lubricated, clean, and cooled. Tough, inflexible skin can become softer and more supple following massage.

Massage is also known to affect internal organs. By indirectly or directly stimulating nerves that supply internal organs, massage causes the blood vessels of these organs to dilate, bringing a greater supply of blood to them.

Adherents of massage therapy realize that they have found a form of drugless therapy. Headaches, insomnia, digestive disorders including constipation and spastic colon, arthritis, asthma, carpal tunnel syndrome, sinusitis, and minor aches and pains are some of the problems that can respond to massage therapy. Massage can have a calming effect on nervous people who have been dependent on pharmaceuticals for rest and relaxation—or worse, for basic functioning. Massage balances the nervous system by soothing or stimulating nerves and neural pathways, depending on which effect is needed by the individual at the time of the massage.

Simply stated, the foundation stone of therapeutic massage is what Hippocrates, the "father of medicine," defined as ***vis medicatrix naturae,*** or the body's natural recuperative powers (see chapter 1, History of Therapeutic Massage). Massage therapy essentially promotes health by boosting the body's own processes and its Chi (Qi, Ki) or vital life force.

Relationship of Massage to Other Manual Therapies

Many "manual therapies" are used in the practice of modern medicine and allied health care, such as chiropractic, osteopathy, physical therapy, sports medicine, and massage. All incorporate some form of manipulation or movement of the body in the process of healing or creating health optimization. There are also many "manual therapies" in use in alternative or complementary forms of healing and health maintenance, such as those used in yoga, qi gong, tai chi, Aryuvedic medicine, Chinese medicine, Rolfing, and acupuncture/acupressure. Massage therapists, like many healing practitioners, manipulate the soft tissues of the body to "normalize" those tissues, or restore healing energy that optimizes the function and the relationship of the mind and body. In doing so, massage therapists seek to promote overall health and treat specific illness through the alleviation of physical tension and energy blockage in the body (see chapters 15, Eastern Practices and Energy Work; 16, Introduction to Other Modalities; and 19, Eastern and Western Principles of Movement).

Massage has powerful and positive psychological effects. Since massage animates the tactile sense—the body's primary sense—it brings people into the "here and now" and away from tension generated by constant preoccupation with problems. It also loosens muscle tension or "armoring," the physical counterpart to how we defend and protect ourselves from psychological pain. Massage can rid the body of these holding patterns, thus contributing to a release of repressed emotions (see chapter 17, Body-Mind Connection).

Modern and alternative therapies may differ dramatically in their orientation, focus, and approach, but all share the goal of restoring the body's inherent healthy energies via "laying on of the hands."

The above-mentioned therapies were intended to be used without additional medical support or intervention. The reason massage therapy has evolved into such an attractive healing option is that it can be applied as a stand-alone therapy *or* as part of a continuum of modern, multimodality health care practice.

With such a valued position in modern health care comes the need for standards, certification, and training. What may become confusing are the many forms of massage therapy and which of those forms are accepted (and certified) within modern health care. We should first consider the varied curriculum and certification process.

Massage and Bodywork

There are so many different disciplines, schools, variations, and techniques of massage and so many relationships between massage and other healing arts that a complete list of "massage forms" becomes difficult to produce. As a first step, the term *massage therapy* is often replaced with *massage and bodywork* in an attempt to be more inclusive of these various related, overlapping, or continuous approaches.

Many modern massage and bodywork techniques were developed out of a need to better heal injuries or establish well-being, while others developed as a cultural tradition. Many practitioners developed their own techniques after studying one therapy and deciding there was a better way. Often, therapies were combined to come up with a new way of doing something and to make it "new" or proprietary. Still others, particularly those wrapped around strict obedience to an individual's philosophical bent, were developed to do nothing more than make money. From a potential quagmire of confusing forms of professional massage therapy and bodywork has come a narrowed field that will no doubt be further refined to serve modern health care, with many other forms remaining outside of that arena. Thus, more consistent standards will be the rule in massage and bodywork performed in the world of reimbursable health care, while less formal or accepted forms of practice will remain in the realm of out-of-pocket alternative health care.

American Massage Therapy Association

Founded in 1943, the American Massage Therapy Association (AMTA) is the oldest and largest international, member-driven organization representing the massage therapy profession. It has more than 54,000 members in 27 countries.

On an ongoing basis, the AMTA develops and reexamines guidelines for the ethical practice of massage to keep such guidelines current and to reflect needs of the profession and the consumer. The AMTA has a *Practice Standards* document and a Code of Ethics, and is developing behavioral guidelines for its members. Such standards help to ensure a safe and nurturing environment for all who seek the benefits of massage.

The AMTA further upheld massage therapy standards with establishment of the Commission on Massage Therapy Accreditation (COMTA) in 1989. Operating independently, COMTA is determining benchmarks of massage therapy education. COMTA-accredited educational programs must demonstrate compliance with COMTA standards through a comprehensive self-study, onsite observation by external professionals and educators, and evaluation by an independent commission.

The AMTA is a key contributor to the advancement of the art, science, and practice of massage therapy through promoting and providing for continuing education in the profession.

Commission on Massage Therapy Accreditation (COMTA) and Other Accrediting Bodies

The stated mission of the Commission on Massage Therapy Accreditation, a nonprofit independent body recognized by the US Department of Education, is to maintain and improve quality assurance in massage therapy and bodywork education by recognizing postsecondary schools and programs through an accreditation process. Schools and programs achieve this recognition by continually demonstrating their compliance with and commitment to standards developed and monitored by the commission. This process ensures that students receive quality education, the industry receives competently trained practitioners, and the public receives quality services.

Additional national and regional accrediting bodies exist to ensure quality in education. For example, the ACCSCT, Accrediting Commission of Career Schools and Colleges of Technology awards national accreditation while SACS, Southern Association of Colleges and Schools accredits schools in the South (northern and western regions are handled by separate bodies). The ACCSCT visits schools yearly to review the curriculum. Along with an independent, unbiased observer, a team from ACCSCT observes classes and clinics in session, inspects labs and clinics, and interviews students currently enrolled in the program. Additionally, there are bodies such as the Commission on Occupational Education that govern smaller occupational schools.

National Certification Board for Therapeutic Massage and Bodywork

The National Certification Board for Therapeutic Massage and Bodywork (NCBTMB) was created in 1992 as an independent, not-for-profit organization whose National Certification Exam has become the standard for licensure used by the majority of the 36 states (and the District of Columbia) that regulate the practice of massage therapy or bodywork. The goal of NCBTMB is to ensure a high level of proficiency in the practice of massage and bodywork. Certain standards of ethical practice are adhered to by those who have received NCBTMB certification. NCBTMB recognizes the importance of maintaining the public trust. Each candidate for certification must read and agree to uphold NCBTMB's **Standards of Practice** and **Code of Ethics.** The code stresses professional conduct, consumer protection, and integrity of services. Currently, more than 80,000 massage therapists have national certification.

The NCBTMB Certification Program is accredited by the National Commission for Certified Agencies, the accrediting branch of the National Organization for Competency Assurance. A nine-member board of directors is elected by the certificant population and includes a wide range of practitioners. Of the nine-member board, two are public members that represent the public interest of consumers.

Federation of State Massage Therapy Boards

Another milestone in the profession of massage therapy and bodywork was reached in late 2005, when the Federation of State Massage Therapy Boards (FSMTB) was established as an organization through which the various massage therapy state boards could communicate with each other. Besides supporting its member boards, the FSMTB's goal is to ensure that the practice of massage therapy is provided to the public in a safe and effective manner.

An important focus of this new organization is to work with the National Certification Board for Therapeutic Massage and Bodywork to address all issues concerning certification, including allowing for state boards to have input into the makeup of the exam and creating a standardized curriculum that would be upheld from state to state. The most exciting outcome of the FSMTB's work may very well be the portability of licenses from state to state.

FSMTB researched 10 different board federations in other professions, such as nursing, physical therapy, and medicine, as models of successful organizations providing the highest levels of quality assurance and protection of the public. The FSMTB recognizes that the majority of well-run professions have a national licensing exam that is owned and operated by its member boards. With this in mind, FSMTB is actively exploring the option of creating a new massage therapy credentialing examination that would meet the specific needs of entry-level licensure at the state level as well as attempting to work with the current exam's board, the NCBTMB.

Educational Requirements and Coursework

At present, close to 800 massage schools and many more community and private colleges offer diploma and associate degree programs in massage therapy in the United States. Generally, individual states create statewide standards and determine total hours of training required for licensure or registration, although a few states, such as California, have different standards in different counties and cities. Some types of massage and bodywork, such as Reiki, polarity therapy, Trager, and structural integration work such as Zentherapy and Rolfing, are exempt from massage licensing. Adoption of the possible FSMTB outcomes for the profession of massage and bodywork would create standardized curriculum and criteria across the nation.

Every massage therapy school will have different entrance requirements and a school-specific curriculum to follow. Some programs are quite robust, requiring 1000 hours of study, while others are more relaxed with a less rigorous program. The majority of schools that graduate certifiable students require at least 500 hours of study. Almost all schools will require an incoming student to have a high school diploma, and a postsecondary education is very useful for the more advanced programs.

Many well-rounded programs require an interview to assess personal qualities and characteristics such as communication skills, empathy/compassion, trust and understanding, and listening skills. Some schools may also require prior knowledge or training in certain subject areas, such as the basic sciences (anatomy, physiology), psychology, the humanities, and business. Many schools offer supervised clinics, which are available to the general public, allowing students the opportunity to work on a variety of clients and conditions.

Current National Certification Exam

The National Certification Examination in Therapeutic Massage and Bodywork (NCE) is the exam component. As of June 1, 2005, the NCBTMB began administering two exams and certifications. The National Certification in Therapeutic Massage (NCTM) is directed toward the more minimal 500-hour massage program, while the National Certification in Therapeutic Massage and Bodywork (NCTMB) continues to denote passage of a comprehensive, 1000 hour-type program that often includes training in Eastern modalities. Students have the option of taking either the NCTM exam or the NCTMB exam, depending on their intent and their state's requirements (e.g., Florida continues to use the NCTMB exam only for licensure). Both exams reflect the increased criteria for massage therapy at the national certification level. However, it must be remembered that even after certification, practitioners still have to comply with state and local laws that regulate the profession.

Endnotes

Note 1: Explorations in the theory and practice of massage and bodywork
http://www.thebodyworker.com/typesofmassage.html

Note 2: American Massage Therapy Association
http://www.amtamassage.org

Note 3: The National Certification Board for Therapeutic Massage and Bodywork
http://www.ncbtmb.com

Note 4: Federation of State Massage Therapy Boards
www.fsmtb.org

NEW FOUNDATIONS IN

Therapeutic Massage and Bodywork

PART I

Basic Concepts of Therapeutic Massage and Bodywork

CHAPTER 1 History of Therapeutic Massage

CHAPTER 2 Equipment, Environment, and Safety
Practices

CHAPTER 3 The Massage Therapy Session:
Preparations for Before, During,
and After

CHAPTER 4 Therapeutic Massage Techniques

CHAPTER 5 Physiological Effects of Therapeutic
Massage

History of Therapeutic Massage

LEARNING OUTCOMES

After completing this chapter, you will be able to:

- List the names and locations of early civilizations that used massage.

- Describe the historical records and artifacts that tell us about massage in ancient times.

- Identify the "father of Western medicine," and explain why his approach to health care was so revolutionary.

- Trace the development of Swedish massage, identifying who is most closely associated with it today, and when and where it originated.

- Identify who is closely associated with the Battle Creek Sanitarium, and explain how it differed from other institutions.

- Explain how bathhouses and massage parlors become associated with the sex industry, and describe how that history resulted in early regulation of professional therapeutic massage.

- Recognize the importance the nursing industry had in the development of massage as a profession.

- List elements of vitalistic philosophy.

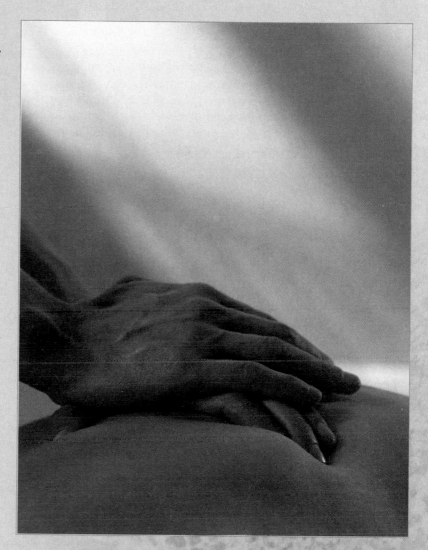

KEY TERMS

American Massage Therapy
   Association (AMTA) *(p. 19)*
Amma (p. 10)
Avicenna *(p. 14)*
Ayur Veda (arts of life) *(p. 11)*
Ayurvedic medicine *(p. 10)*
bathhouses *(p. 12)*
Battle Creek Sanitarium *(p. 18)*
Federation of State Massage
   Therapy Boards
   (FSMTB) *(p. 20)*
Graham, Douglas *(p. 17)*
gymnasiums *(p. 12)*
herbal massage *(p. 7)*

Hippocrates *(p. 11)*
Hippocratic oath *(p. 11)*
Hippocratic tradition *(p. 11)*
Jensen, Kathryn *(p. 19)*
Kellogg, John Harvey *(p. 18)*
Ling, Per Henrik *(p. 15)*
Lomi lomi (p. 6)
manual medicine *(p. 6)*
Maori massage *(p. 6)*
McMillan, Mary *(p. 19)*
Metu(p. 7)
Nei Jing *(p. 10)*
oral tradition *(p. 6)*
papyrus *(p. 7)*

Pare, Ambrose *(p. 15)*
Qi *(p. 10)*
Rawlins, Maude *(p. 19)*
Renaissance *(p. 15)*
Roth, Mathias *(p. 20)*
sanitariums *(p. 17)*
shamans *(p. 7)*
shiatsu *(p. 15)*
Swedish movement cure, Swedish
   treatment cure, or Swedish
   massage *(p. 15)*
Taylor, Dr. Charles Fayette *(p. 20)*
vitalism *(p. 21)*

INTRODUCTION

This chapter examines the history of massage, tracing its progression from ancient roots in religious ceremonies and mystical traditions to contemporary applications in traditional and alternative health care, and an increasingly important role in medical research. Any subject with a history as old as massage is not easily summarized in a few pages. This chapter will only touch upon some of the more significant episodes and individuals who influenced the way massage is practiced and regulated today (figure 1.1). Many excellent resources for studying more about this subject matter exist. Be sure to consult the many books and references listed in appendix C on page C-1.

Massage in the Ancient World: An International Phenomenon (5000 BCE – 500 CE)

Many varieties of massage have been practiced by different groups of people around the world throughout much of human history. Evidence of the practice exists on nearly every continent on earth—Africa, Asia, Australia/Oceania, Europe, North America, and South America—and while massage is not common to all cultures, its prevalence among so many diverse populations suggests to many a universality, as though the impulse to rub a sore muscle or bruise might be rooted in human instinct.

People in ancient times recognized the therapeutic benefits of massage and incorporated it into their cultures. Over many generations, each distinct tradition of massage was shaped by countless powerful and subtle forces, leading to the development of many unique massage traditions throughout the world.

It is not known how many ancient cultures practiced some form of healing through **manual medicine**, the use of the hands to treat illness or physical damage. Before the invention of writing, massage was taught and preserved in **oral tradition**, memorized and passed down by word of mouth from one designated individual in a generation to the next over many centuries. Ancient traditions are visible in the contemporary practice of *Lomi lomi* (Hawaiian massage), for example, and traditional **Maori massage** of New Zealand. Both techniques originated in ancient Polynesia about 5000 years ago and migrated to neighboring islands along with members of the population. Over many generations, the Polynesian method evolved into three distinct but related massage traditions.

The first great civilizations grew from small encampments along riverbeds, where settlers were drawn to a sure source of water in times of drought as well as the means to irrigate their crops. These earliest civilizations are the Sumerians of Mesopotamia, from the Tigris-Euphrates River Valley, in what is now Iraq; the people of the Indus River Valley, in present-day Pakistan and India; the Shang people of the Yellow River Valley, in what is now China; and the people of the Nile River Valley, in Egypt. Figure 1.2 indicates the geographic location of these early civilizations.

The Earliest Civilizations

Mesopotamia

The Sumerians of Mesopotamia (meaning "land between two rivers"), in the Tigris-Euphrates River Valley, developed the first known writing system as early as 3100 BCE (BCE stands for "before the common era," an acceptable format used today). Clay tablets carved with wedge-shaped symbols, called cuneiform, and cultural artifacts, remnants of things they made and used, tell us that the Mesopotamians, like the people before them, combined beliefs in the supernatural and religious ideology with medical know-how, developing complicated healing traditions and rituals.

Early medicine men and women, known as **shamans**, were religious leaders, mystics, and physicians, all in one. They were believed to possess special healing abilities and the power to influence gods or evil spirits responsible for illness and disease. A Sumerian shaman, for example, might use sorcery to discover the identity of an inhabiting spirit and then attempt to drive it out of a body or destroy it using a variety of tools, including herbal remedies and plasters, charms and incantations, and touch or manipulation of the body.

Healers of the time often applied ointments and salves in conjunction with other medical treatment. Describing this practice, the earliest medical records use a term that means literally "to smear or rub on" and can be interpreted as either "anoint" or "massage" (from the Latin *inungere*). This common practice—performed for cosmetic and ritual, as well as medical, purposes—involved the combination of olive and other oils with fragrant substances such as cinnamon and myrrh. The mixture was applied to the skin with a rubbing action, much the way we use moisturizer today. It is difficult to assess whether the Sumerians considered rubbing a significant medical action in and of itself or practiced it only in conjunction with the application of salves or ointments.

Succeeding populations (such as the Babylonians) who inhabited Mesopotamia after the Sumerians and borrowed much of their ideology also used touch and manipulation of the body along with the use of herbal salves and ointments to alleviate discomfort. The Assyrians, another population living around the same time, are credited with the invention of **herbal massage**, a unique practice of massage and anointing, and an ancestor of the contemporary custom.

Ancient Egypt

The Egyptians of the Nile Valley, like the Mesopotamians, initially considered illness or disease the result of evil spirits or hostile adversaries, living and dead. As Egyptians learned more about the human body through scientific study, their medical ideology evolved, and they began to use clinical methods. The Egyptians considered the heart the center of all bodily function and compared the cardiovascular system to channels of the Nile River, called *metu*. They believed good health depended on free flow through these channels in the body, and sickness was the result of blocked *metu*.

While ancient Egyptian medicine had questionable curative value, it was a highly regarded and influential practice in its time. Visitors traveled great distances to be treated by Egyptian physicians, who were trained at exclusive medical schools (and typically specialized in one specific organ or part of the body). Egyptian medical traditions and ideology were detailed in a vast system of historical and medical records written on **papyrus**, a durable plant fiber that was preserved by the dry Egyptian climate. The

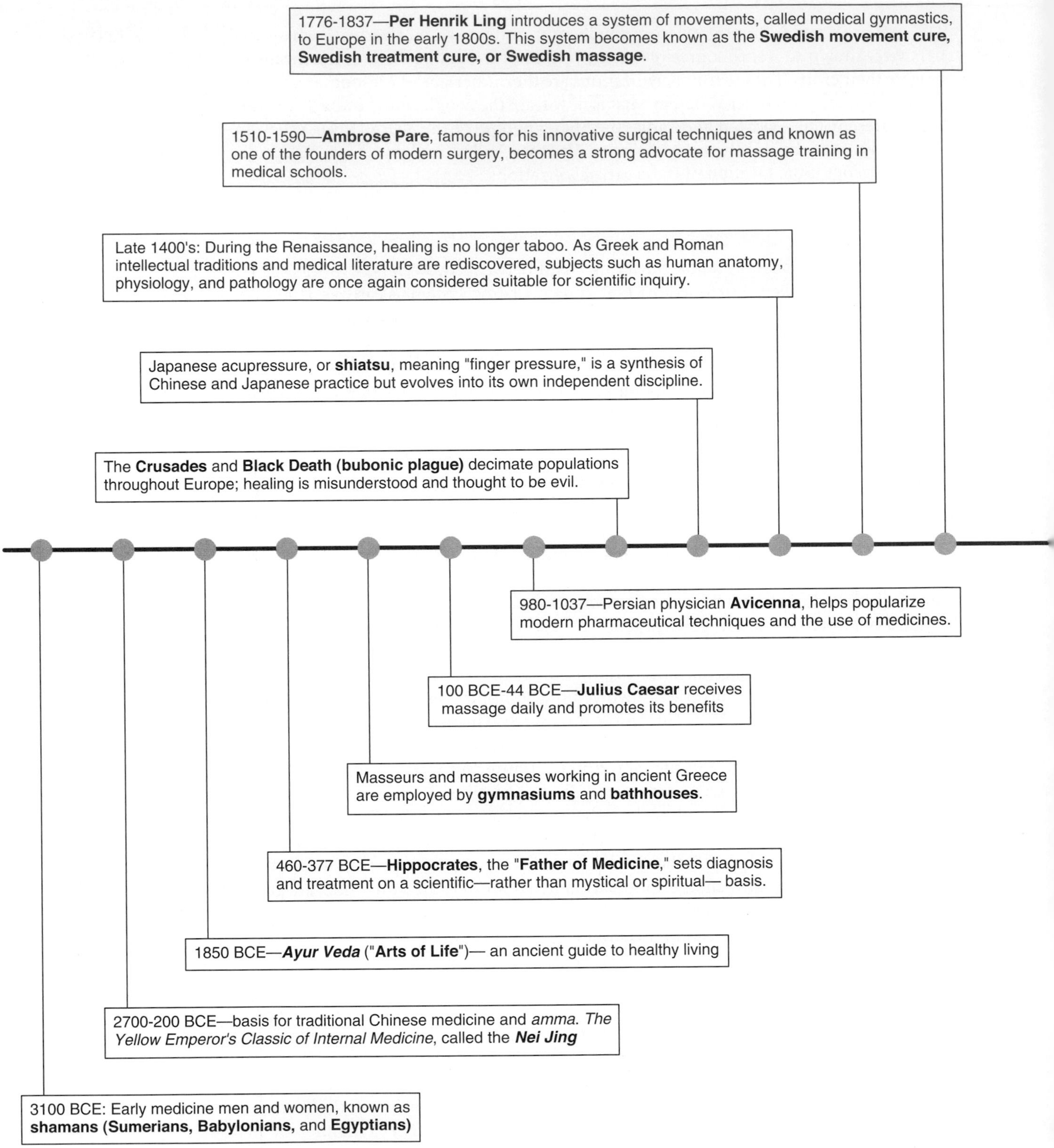
1776-1837—Per Henrik Ling introduces a system of movements, called medical gymnastics, to Europe in the early 1800s. This system becomes known as the Swedish movement cure, Swedish treatment cure, or Swedish massage.
1510-1590—Ambrose Pare, famous for his innovative surgical techniques and known as one of the founders of modern surgery, becomes a strong advocate for massage training in medical schools.
Late 1400's: During the Renaissance, healing is no longer taboo. As Greek and Roman intellectual traditions and medical literature are rediscovered, subjects such as human anatomy, physiology, and pathology are once again considered suitable for scientific inquiry.
Japanese acupressure, or shiatsu, meaning "finger pressure," is a synthesis of Chinese and Japanese practice but evolves into its own independent discipline.
The Crusades and Black Death (bubonic plague) decimate populations throughout Europe; healing is misunderstood and thought to be evil.
980-1037—Persian physician Avicenna, helps popularize modern pharmaceutical techniques and the use of medicines.
100 BCE-44 BCE—Julius Caesar receives massage daily and promotes its benefits
Masseurs and masseuses working in ancient Greece are employed by gymnasiums and bathhouses.
460-377 BCE—Hippocrates, the "Father of Medicine," sets diagnosis and treatment on a scientific—rather than mystical or spiritual— basis.
1850 BCE—Ayur Veda ("Arts of Life")— an ancient guide to healthy living
2700-200 BCE—basis for traditional Chinese medicine and amma. The Yellow Emperor's Classic of Internal Medicine, called the Nei Jing
3100 BCE: Early medicine men and women, known as shamans (Sumerians, Babylonians, and Egyptians)

Figure 1.1 Historical highlights in massage and bodywork

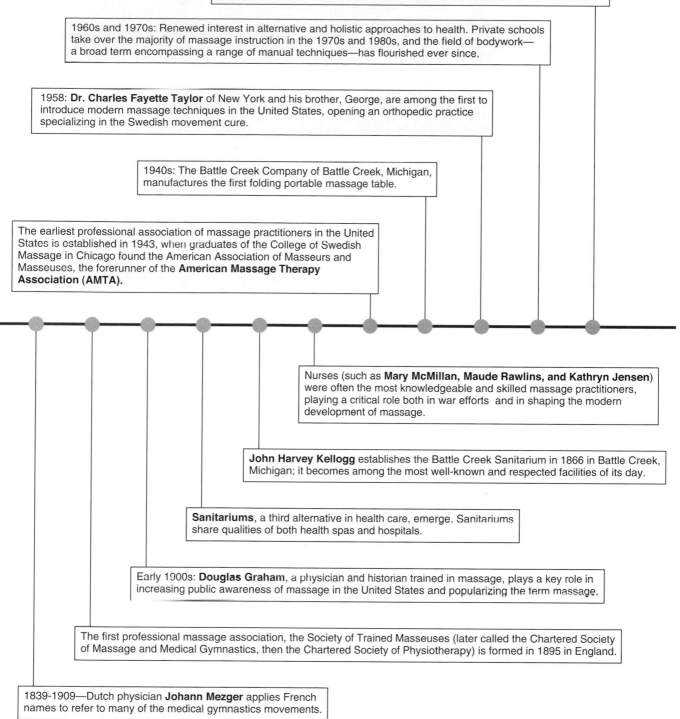

The creation of the American Massage Therapy Association (AMTA) and National Certification Examination (1992) further solidify professional ethics and standards.

1960s and 1970s: Renewed interest in alternative and holistic approaches to health. Private schools take over the majority of massage instruction in the 1970s and 1980s, and the field of bodywork—a broad term encompassing a range of manual techniques—has flourished ever since.

1958: **Dr. Charles Fayette Taylor** of New York and his brother, George, are among the first to introduce modern massage techniques in the United States, opening an orthopedic practice specializing in the Swedish movement cure.

1940s: The Battle Creek Company of Battle Creek, Michigan, manufactures the first folding portable massage table.

The earliest professional association of massage practitioners in the United States is established in 1943, when graduates of the College of Swedish Massage in Chicago found the American Association of Masseurs and Masseuses, the forerunner of the **American Massage Therapy Association (AMTA).**

Nurses (such as **Mary McMillan, Maude Rawlins, and Kathryn Jensen**) were often the most knowledgeable and skilled massage practitioners, playing a critical role both in war efforts and in shaping the modern development of massage.

John Harvey Kellogg establishes the Battle Creek Sanitarium in 1866 in Battle Creek, Michigan; it becomes among the most well-known and respected facilities of its day.

Sanitariums, a third alternative in health care, emerge. Sanitariums share qualities of both health spas and hospitals.

Early 1900s: **Douglas Graham**, a physician and historian trained in massage, plays a key role in increasing public awareness of massage in the United States and popularizing the term massage.

The first professional massage association, the Society of Trained Masseuses (later called the Chartered Society of Massage and Medical Gymnastics, then the Chartered Society of Physiotherapy) is formed in 1895 in England.

1839-1909—Dutch physician **Johann Mezger** applies French names to refer to many of the medical gymnastics movements.

Figure 1.2 Map of the ancient world

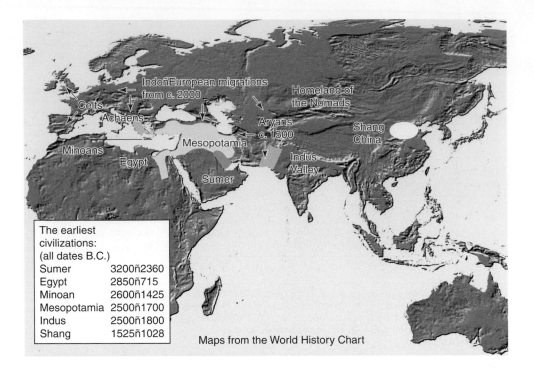

The earliest civilizations: (all dates B.C.)

Sumer	3200ñ2360
Egypt	2850ñ715
Minoan	2600ñ1425
Mesopotamia	2500ñ1700
Indus	2500ñ1800
Shang	1525ñ1028

Maps from the World History Chart

longest document, at 110 pages, is the Ebers Papyri, a collection of many different medical texts written from 3000 to 1534 BCE. Organized by medical ailment, the compilation includes magic spells, diagnostic information and treatments, and sections on anatomy and physiology.

Although an abundance of medical papyri and artifacts have been found over the years, specific details regarding Egyptian massage are still largely a mystery. An Egyptian wall painting from the Tomb of the Physician (Ankhmahor, 2323–2291 BCE) is thought to depict the practice of massage or reflexology. It illustrates how the thumb or finger can be used to exert pressure on specific points of the feet, with each point corresponding to a different part of the body. Pictographs from 1279 to 1213 BCE show images something that look like massage—Egyptians tending to the feet of soldiers on a long military march—and the Kahun Medical Papyrus (dated 1825 BCE) recommends a mud massage to treat a woman with aching legs and calves; but no artifacts or records provide any details regarding the theory or techniques used in Egyptian massage.

Ancient Asia: China, India, and Japan

The earliest known mention of massage in China is a prescription in *The Yellow Emperor's Classic of Internal Medicine*, called the **Nei Jing**. The work is attributed to the Yellow Emperor (Huang Di), who lived as early as 2700 BCE. Passed down by oral tradition for thousands of years, it was first put into writing around 200 BCE. This text is the philosophical basis of Traditional Chinese Medicine (TCM) and forms the foundation for many schools of acupuncture and acupressure, as well as massage.

Early Chinese massage, known as **Amma,** is thought to have originated in the Chinese practice of rubbing and pressing cold hands and feet to warm them. *Amma* is built on a knowledge of pressure points and organized around the concept of **Qi**, (also spelled *Chi*) an energy or life force traveling through pathways, or meridians, in the body. Practitioners release blocked Qi from energy centers (pressure points) along the meridians, allowing Qi to flow uninterrupted throughout the body and restoring good health and peace of mind.

Chinese techniques shaped the growth of massage throughout Asia and the rest of the world, and are thought to have been an influence in the development of **Ayurvedic medicine**, a system based on the idea of chakras (energy centers in the body) and *doshas* (general tendencies). The *Ayur Veda* ("Arts of Life") is an ancient guide to healthy living that includes prescriptions for herbal treatments and massage techniques that may have originated in China, but, today, is most associated with India. Written around 1850 BCE, the *Ayur Veda* is one of a set of sacred Sanskrit texts called the *Vedas*. The word *massage* is probably related to the Sanskrit term *makeh*, meaning, "to press softly."

In contrast to earlier medical traditions that relied heavily on magical words and actions, Greek medicine did not consider supernatural phenomena the source of most illness and disease. The prevailing medical philosophy in ancient Greece attributed sickness to imbalances in four essential properties of the human body, known as The Four Humours. Also known as essentialism, this theory asserted that every living thing was composed of a mixture of air, earth, fire, and water, which produced humours (blood, phlegm, yellow bile, and black bile) associated with specific physical, emotional, or intellectual characteristics in an individual.

Hippocratic Tradition

This ideological shift is most closely identified with the Greek physician **Hippocrates** (460–377 BCE). Known as the "Father of Western Medicine," Hippocrates of Cos (figure 1.3) is considered the first physician in the modern tradition. He set diagnosis and treatment on a scientific, rather than mystical or spiritual, basis. Hippocrates' philosophy of medicine characterized the healthy human body as a natural system in perfect equilibrium. Effective medical treatment, according to Hippocrates, allowed the body's natural restorative powers to work. Encouraging the humours to return to their natural balance, he felt, would restore the patient to good health.

A great deal is known about medicine of this time (known as the Hellenistic era) because Hippocrates documented its status in the *Hippocratic Corpus*, a vast medical encyclopedia of case histories, surgical practices, pharmacological treatments, anatomy, and physiology of the day. The **Hippocratic tradition** refers to philosophical tenets and ideals originating with or popularized by Hippocrates and his followers. Many have become an integral part of Western medical practice. Even today, medical students pledge to follow a professional code of ethics called the **Hippocratic oath**, which is based on his doctrine.

Massage in Ancient Greece and Rome (700 BCE – 476 CE)

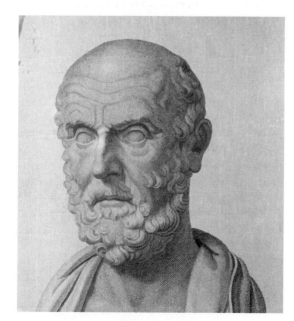

Figure 1.3 Greek physician Hippocrates of Cos

Most of the masseurs and masseuses working in ancient Greece were employed by **gymnasiums** and **bathhouses**. Massage played an important role in both of these Greek cultural institutions. At the public baths, massage was provided to patrons before or after a bath, and later, when the baths grew more elaborate, in conjunction with steam or hot water baths. Even exfoliation and oil massages were a common part of daily exercise and bathing routines in ancient Greece. At the gymnasium, athletes employed personal assistants to provide their massage before and after training sessions and during competitions.

Originally, gymnasiums were used for athletic and military training, but they eventually grew to accommodate intellectual and artistic, as well as physical, activities. Similar to parks today, gymnasiums were situated among open fields that could be used for sporting events. Many were located near a body of water, providing a place to wash up after competitions and games. While baths were initially a small part of gymnasiums—a room or rooms with small tubs of water or a cold-water pool—they grew increasingly elaborate as Greece grew more affluent. Gymnasiums became grand institutions, housed in palatial buildings, with extraordinarily luxurious bathing facilities and services.

While massage was a common practice in the gymnasiums and bathhouses, Hippocrates stressed its therapeutic benefits, encouraging its use for medicinal purposes. He considered massage a highly effective and underutilized medical tool, and one requiring a substantial degree of skill and knowledge.

Unlike many who lived before and after him, Hippocrates directed practitioners of massage to rub in an upward motion (anatripsis), rather than the downward movement favored by most shamanic healing practices known around the world. Many traditions hypothesize that a downward motion moves the source of illness from the core of the stricken body, toward and out the extremities, through the tips of the fingers and toes. Hippocrates concluded, after some length of study, that massage in an upward motion, from the limbs toward the core of the body, would be more effective, as it utilized the body's natural system of waste disposal, encouraging the body to rid itself of toxins through the alimentary tract. This philosophical turning point was significant. Years later, Hippocrates' innovative ideas would resurface, and the Hippocratic model of medicine, with its "modern" understanding of the human body, would meet a receptive audience.

Rome

When Rome conquered Greece in 146 BCE, Roman citizens had little regard for medical practitioners. Rome had no system of medical licensing as did Greece, and purported healers were often found to be frauds. It was only after Greek citizens were made slaves by the conquering Roman army (as was the custom) that this perception began to change. Greek slaves were far superior to their Roman counterparts at providing basic medical care and tending to the ill, and it was not long before Roman citizens recognized the superiority of Greek medical practices.

According to Robert Noah Calvert's *The History of Massage*, Julius Caesar (100–44 BCE) is said to have learned about the benefits of Greek massage in a letter that claimed it "cured many...by the process of rubbing and anointing." The letter's author beseeched the Roman leader to grant all Greek slaves their freedom, reasoning that they would work far more effectively for Roman health as free citizens than as slaves. In 46 BCE, Caesar granted this request, giving Greeks their freedom and the privileges of Roman citizenship on the condition they remain in Rome serving the needs of their Roman patients. Caesar himself is said to have received a daily massage for relief of neuralgia.

In Rome, the Hippocratic tradition carried on in the work of two Roman physicians: *De Medicina,* by Aulus Cornelius Celsus (25 BCE–50 CE), enlarged upon massage theory and practice, recommending effective techniques for relief of common ailments

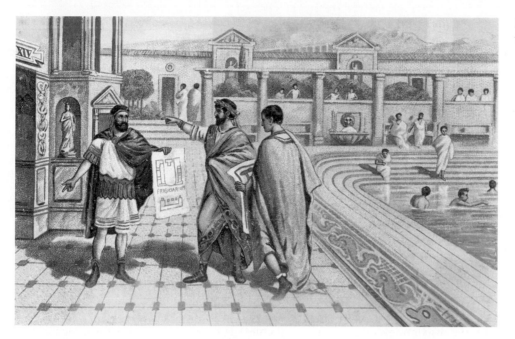

Figure 1.4 Athletic conditioning in the Roman bath

such as headaches and upset stomachs; and *De Sanitate Tuenda* (*Hygiene*), by Claudius Galenus (Galen, 129–199 CE), discussed the function and structure of ligaments, tendons, muscle, and bone, and explained the anatomical basis of massage—a subject he knew well from treating gladiators wounded in the arena.

The Romans adopted many Greek cultural institutions, including the gymnasium and public bath. In Rome, gymnasiums grew to house whole libraries and were the location for civic functions, worship services, public sacrifice, feasting and parties, athletic events, and competitions. As gymnasiums became the center of Roman cultural, social, and educational life, the baths within them grew even more ornate and magnificent than those in Greece. Made of beautiful and expensive materials, public bathhouses (figure 1.4) grew to house multiple pools of varying temperatures and were even equipped with wet and dry steam rooms.

Demand for massage (and qualified practitioners to meet that demand) grew enormously over these years, with the increase in gymnasiums, public baths, and doctors' offices often outstripping the supply of skilled workers. Practitioners varied significantly in training, experience, and skill. Roman physicians prescribing massage for their patients needed the services of specially trained medical masseurs; professional athletes (such as wrestlers and gladiators) and gymnasiums needed attendants with some knowledge of sports massage; bathhouse attendants were typically poorly trained but might offer a variety of massage options, depending on the needs of their clientele.

As the empire grew, Roman bathhouses were more often associated with debauchery, and massage practitioners, with prostitution. Roman culture became increasingly indulgent and devoted to pursuits of sensual pleasure. Bathhouses offered private rooms and personal services of many kinds. Initially, bath attendants were typically female slaves with minimal training who were expected to serve patrons food and wine, and massage them with fragrant oils. Over time, these attendants were increasingly expected to cater to their patrons' sexual appetites as well.

Roman influence and power over the region gradually disintegrated from the beginning of the common era (CE) to the fifth century (500 CE), when Germanic forces deposed the last emperor seated in Rome. This point, the so-called "Fall of Rome," refers to the end of the Greco-Roman era, a time when Rome fell into a weakened, fragmented state and the Greco-Roman medical tradition fell into disuse.

The Middle Ages (500–1500 CE)

For many years, massage had been associated with three practices: exercise, the baths, and medicine. All fell out of favor during medieval times. Early Christianity condemned exercise as glorification of the body and excessive attention to the physical self; Roman Emperor Constantine declared the baths dens of indecency and decadence, and abolished them (along with the gymnasiums) after his conversion to Christianity; and the study of medicine became taboo, highly suspicious, and even sinful.

Europe

While the four humours remained a prevalent ideology for centuries, medical practice regressed during the Middle Ages (also known as medieval or "Dark Ages"), replaced by superstition, fear, and ignorance in matters regarding the human body. The Crusades and Black Death (bubonic plague) decimated populations throughout Europe—killing tens of thousands of people and taking a terrible toll on those who survived. Disease was poorly understood; many thought illness was the result of sinful thoughts and actions. Aside from prayer, the most common medical prescriptions involved the loss of body fluids—thought the best way to restore balance to the body. Common treatments included frequent bloodletting and the use of laxatives, diuretics, and purgatives.

Midwives had commonly used massage for hundreds, if not thousands, of years to ease the discomforts of pregnancy and childbirth. Now, its use was forbidden and, if discovered, penalized harshly. Estimates suggest that close to 1500 midwives were executed as witches during this period. At a time when physicians were scarce and rarely attended childbirth, the policy against midwives further victimized mothers and infants, as midwives played a critical role in complicated pregnancies and deliveries. All across Europe, the practice of massage was forcibly suppressed, surviving only where it was hidden. Although the healing traditions and folk cultures of the Slavs, Finns, and Swedes, and the Arabic tradition endured, the Greco-Roman medical tradition disappeared from Europe.

The Arabic Tradition

The Arabic tradition was the Greco-Roman medical tradition preserved in the writings of the Persian physician **Avicenna** (980–1037). Avicenna (figure 1.5) is largely responsible for popularizing modern pharmaceutical techniques (such as chemical

Figure 1.5 Persian physician Avicenna

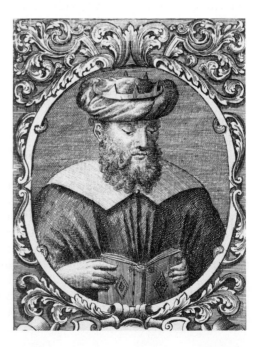

preparation and distillation) and the use of medicines, such as camphor and iodine, bringing these practices to a wider audience. His 16-volume medical encyclopedia was a synthesis of Hippocratic and Arabic medical traditions, and its influence was considerable. Five hundred years after he wrote it, the text was still in mainstream use, renewing interest in the Hippocratic tradition of medicine. Originating near Constantinople, Avicenna's synthesis of the Arabic and Greek traditions, known as "unani medicine," transformed Damascus, Cairo, and Baghdad into important medical centers and traveled with the spread of Islamic traditions to regions and people far away.

Asia

Ayurvedic and Chinese traditions continued to gain influence across Asia during this period. Traditional Chinese Medicine was held in such high regard that Japanese medical students commonly traveled to China for lengthy periods of training. Japanese acupressure, or **Shiatsu**, meaning "finger pressure," is a synthesis of Chinese and Japanese practice that evolved into its own independent discipline. Shiatsu stimulates the same pressure points used in acupuncture, but finger pressure is used in place of needles.

The Renaissance

The **Renaissance**, meaning "rebirth," was a cultural transformation that began in Europe around the late 1400s. Also known as the Enlightenment, the Renaissance was characterized by a revival in intellectual curiosity. No longer taboo, Greek and Roman intellectual traditions and medical literature were rediscovered. As a result, human anatomy, physiology, and pathology were once again suitable subjects for scientific inquiry.

Celsus' *De Medicina* was rediscovered under Pope Nicolas V (1397–1455) and published in 1478 on the newly invented Gutenberg printing press. It was one of the first medical textbooks ever published and one of the most popular of the Renaissance. A French physician named **Ambrose Pare** (1510–1590), famous for his innovative surgical techniques and known as one of the founders of modern surgery, was a strong advocate for massage training in medical schools. Pare popularized and lent credibility to massage, famously treating Mary Queen of Scots. By the 1600s, medical schools commonly offered massage instruction, due in some part to Pare's influence.

The Nineteenth Century

The nineteenth century is dominated by the work of Per Henrik Ling and Johann Mezger. Their techniques and treatments helped to repopularize massage as a viable treatment option.

Europe and the Swedish Movement Cure

Per Henrik Ling (1776–1837) introduced a system of movements called medical gymnastics to Europe in the early 1800s (figure 1.6). Known by many names—most commonly, the **Swedish Movement Cure, Swedish Treatment Cure**, or **Swedish massage**, Ling's system had three main parts and used French terminology (learned from Dutch physician Johann Mezger [1839–1909]) to refer to many of the movements. The first part of the system explained the underlying mechanics of physical movement in the body, and the second introduced specific actions for use in rehabilitation and treatment. It is mainly the third part of the Swedish Treatment Cure that evolved into what is now known as massage.

Ling found massage an effective treatment for his own symptoms of rheumatism. He pursued its further study enthusiastically, traveling extensively, observing and training in different types of massage, and compiling information about the use of

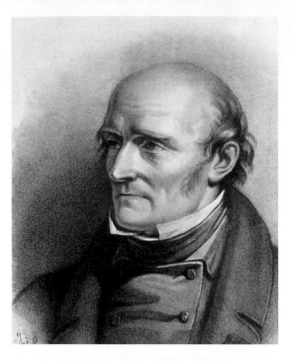

Figure 1.6 Per Henrik Ling, Founder of the Swedish movement cure

massage in countries around the world. While Ling introduced Swedish massage as his own invention, much of the system was a clever repackaging of existing traditions. Ironically, Swedish massage is most likely Chinese in origin, based on principles Ling learned in Asia.

Swedish massage became tremendously popular and was eventually taught in schools throughout Europe. Its success owes much to Ling's skillful combination of modern medical knowledge and time-honored massage techniques. His real innovation, however, was the meticulous, systematic testing of single movements or sets of movements against specific physical conditions or disabilities, from which he developed a theory of the anatomical and physiological mechanics of movement, turning the treatment into a modern discipline based on scientific principles.

Early Regulation

Police crackdowns on prostitution in the late 1800s drove prostitution out of many bars, hotels, and restaurants, which were subject to strict legal enforcement of antiprostitution measures, and into massage parlors and bathhouses, which were not. Prostitutes began to identify themselves as masseuses, describe their services as "massage," and operate out of brothels advertised as "massage parlors" and "bathhouses," causing some degree of public confusion and tarnishing the reputation of legitimate massage and massage practitioners.

The confusion between legitimate massage services and prostitution was exacerbated by public ignorance: "A good deal of misconception exists in this country on the subject of massage," wrote English physician William Murrell in 1886. Murrell also wrote that "many people think that it is only a kind of 'rubbing'...while others associate it ... with the idea of a Turkish bath...Another common mistake is to suppose that anyone can 'do massage,' and that the whole art can be acquired in one or two easy lessons...."

As massage was increasingly associated with prostitution, the need to distinguish massage—the respected therapeutic practice requiring specific training, skills, and knowledge—from a euphemism for sexual services, became increasingly evident, turning attention to the larger issue of professional credentials and guidelines for the field of massage. Health care professionals called for standards to ensure the safety of individuals receiving massage. At minimum, they argued, patients or clients needed to be able to distinguish between medical and nonmedical credentials. Then, as now, the question of regulation was complicated by the existence of many different types of massage, each with its own ideology and standards of practice.

The first professional massage association, the Society of Trained Masseuses (later called the Chartered Society of Massage and Medical Gymnastics, then the Chartered Society of Physiotherapy) was formed in 1895 in England. The organization was founded by four women, British nurses concerned about the reputation of legitimate massage in light of numerous "massage parlor scandals" featured heavily in the news of the day. The society established the first rules of professional conduct, guiding doctrine, prerequisites for educational training, curriculum, and qualifying criteria for massage education, and clearly delineated the difference between therapeutic massage in the hands of trained professionals and everything else.

Many questions and issues hotly debated at those early meetings, over 100 years ago, remain contentious even today: Who determines the legitimacy of one massage method or another? What is medical versus nonmedical massage? How, if at all, should practitioners be trained? What, if any, formal medical study should be required? How much, if any, practical experience is necessary? How long an apprenticeship, if any, is appropriate? Should physicians, nurses, and other medical personnel be required to learn massage? Should massage be taught in medical or trade schools, or should it develop as an independent discipline with its own governing body?

The United States of America

In the early 1900s, **Douglas Graham**, a physician and historian trained in massage, played a key role in both increasing public awareness of massage in the United States and popularizing the term *massage*. He wrote for academic audiences, publishing articles in scholarly peer-reviewed journals, as well as for the general public in popular magazines. His most comprehensive work, *Manual Therapeutics, A Treatise on Massage: Its History, Mode of Application, and Effects* (1902), discussed contemporary massage theory and practice but also explored massage from a number of historical and ethnographic perspectives, describing its use throughout history by many cultures around the world.

Graham considered the study of anatomy an essential part of massage training, warning that unskilled practitioners could do more harm than good. This was an important point, as mainstream medicine in the United States had not progressed much beyond the use of bleeding, purgatives, and laxatives. Wounds easily became infected because medical personnel knew nothing of sterilization, and the best anesthetic, ether, was unpredictable to the point of being deadly. Most health care and convalescing took place in the home. Hospitalization was an option for the very ill but was of questionable benefit.

Sanitariums, a third alternative in health care, shared qualities of both health spas and hospitals. Like health resorts today, they varied widely in philosophical approach, the quality of their health-related services, diet and exercise programs, accommodations, and other amenities, including massage. Many sanitariums made outrageous claims in print and advertising, lauding "exclusive miracle treatments" unavailable from their competitors.

American practitioners confronted the same obstacles met by their European counterparts. With no regulation or standardized criteria for massage training and practice, and no legal penalties for fraudulent claims, inadequate training and false advertising tended to penalize the massage industry as a whole. While massage was increasingly respected as a medical modality in the late 1800s, it also evoked greater skepticism, undermining that newfound legitimacy.

Figure 1.7 Battle Creek
Sanitarium

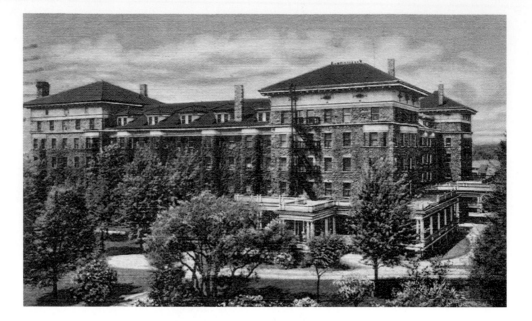

The Battle Creek Sanitarium

Many sanitariums offered massage, but few took the time to train practitioners in any formal method. Institutions often used attendants for double duty; the masseur might also be the maid, the cook, or the dishwasher. The **Battle Creek Sanitarium** (figure 1.7), by contrast, was among the first to implement professional standards for massage and develop a rigorous training program for practitioners at the facility.

Established in 1866 in Battle Creek, Michigan, the Battle Creek Sanitarium was among the most well-known and respected facilities of its day. Like many sanitariums, it stressed natural healing, encouraging the body's self-restoring abilities with fresh air, rest and relaxation, exercise, and a healthy diet. Its emphasis on massage was the work and influence of **John Harvey Kellogg** (1852–1943), a young doctor at the sanitarium in the 1870s and an energetic advocate of massage.

After completing his medical education in the United States, Kellogg (figure 1.8) traveled in Europe, observing and learning massage techniques largely unknown in the United States from experts in Sweden, Germany, and France. On his return to Battle Creek, Kellogg took charge of the sanitarium and implemented sweeping changes patterned after a European model.

Kellogg's first inclination was to hire experienced practitioners, but he found new employees, even licensed nurses, minimally skilled and poorly trained in massage. Few textbooks or training manuals for massage existed at the time, and those that did fell short of Kellogg's high standards, so he set about developing his own formal curriculum and text. *The Art of Massage* (1895), later subtitled *A Practical Manual for the Nurse, the Student, and the Practitioner,* was the fruition of 20 years' study and clinical research in the field of massage, and remained the standard for massage instruction for many years.

As the head of a food and fitness empire, Kellogg was an influential and powerful figure in American health care, and his endorsements wielded considerable promotional power. Greatly enamored of the Swedish Movement Cure, Kellogg established Ling's reputation as an authority in the United States by commending Ling's system of medical gymnastics as an excellent model.

Kellogg was charismatic, vigorous, opinionated, and eccentric, and his close association with massage was both beneficial and detrimental to the discipline's reputation. While he published scholarly articles based on substantive research, he was also an avid merchandiser with an interest in gadgetry; he endorsed products and treatments of highly questionable therapeutic value, including dunks in electrified water, celibacy, daily enemas, and the use of a vibrating chair.

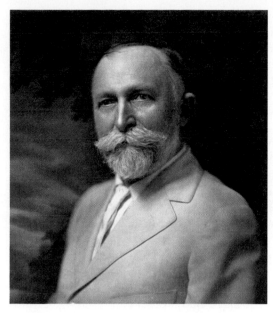

Figure 1.8 John Harvey Kellogg (1852–1943)

While countries such as Japan, China, Germany, and the Soviet Union continued to use massage throughout the 1900s, even integrating it into their medical systems, use of massage in England and the United States tended to decline. The American Medical Association took a stand against massage in the early 1900s. This decision was influenced by a British Medical Association report that found that massage schools in the United States and England were issuing phony credentials and individuals and businesses involved in the sale of sexual services were falsely identifying themselves as massage practitioners and parlors.

Massage experienced a modest revival during World War I (1914–1918) and World War II (1939–1945), when medical personnel had fewer options available to them and relied more heavily on inexpensive, low-technology treatments. Nurses were often the most knowledgeable and skilled massage practitioners, playing a critical role in both war efforts and shaping the modern development of massage. **Mary McMillan**, a nurse during World War I, wrote *Massage and Therapeutic Exercise* (1921), a primer in basic anatomical and physiological information, to inform nonmedical personnel assisting in army hospitals throughout the United States. Later, she developed a program for the U.S. Army Reconstruction Department and became a leading physiotherapist, establishing the American Physical Therapy Association in 1921.

At the turn of the century, many nursing schools and hospitals recommended some knowledge of massage, but requirements varied tremendously from school to school. By the early 1930s, massage was more often a compulsory—rather than an elective—part of the nursing curriculum, but no standard text or course guide existed. A nurse named **Maude Rawlins** wrote *A Textbook of Massage for Nurses and Beginners* in the early 1930s to be used in teaching the required 16 credit hours of practical massage needed for matriculation in New York. **Kathryn Jensen**, a nurse educated in Europe, wrote *Fundamentals in Massage for Students of Nursing*, based on the European model of massage instruction, which emphasized anatomical and physiological understanding, as well as theoretical and practical applications of massage.

One of the earliest professional associations of massage practitioners in the United States was established in 1943, when graduates of the College of Swedish Massage in Chicago founded the American Association of Masseurs and Masseuses, the forerunner of the **American Massage Therapy Association (AMTA)**. The status of massage in medical education and practice was still ambiguous; should massage be taught only in

The Twentieth Century

medical schools and used exclusively by doctors and nurses, or should it be an independent discipline with its own regulation and credentialing?

Massage became more closely associated with sports and exercise throughout the 1940s and 1950s. Endorsed by professional athletes and trainers, it was commonly available at YMCAs. As mainstream medicine tended to emphasize pharmaceutical and surgical innovations over manual techniques, doctors and nurses more frequently turned the responsibility of massage over to their assistants—considering it too time-consuming or old-fashioned for the modern era.

In 1958, **Dr. Charles Fayette Taylor** of New York and his brother, George, were among the first to introduce modern massage techniques in the United States, opening an orthopedic practice specializing in the Swedish movement cure, based on the teachings of an English physician named **Mathias Roth**, who had been a student of Ling's. The 1960s and 1970s saw a renewed interest in alternative and holistic approaches to health. Private schools took over the majority of massage instruction in the 1970s and 1980s, and the field of "bodywork," a broad term encompassing a range of manual techniques, has flourished ever since. The creation of the American Massage Therapy Association (AMTA) and National Certification Board further solidified professional ethics and standards (see Overview and Introduction). Today, several organizations, such as the International Massage Association, Associated Bodyworkers and Massage Professionals, and the International Spa Association, exist to meet the needs of this everchanging and evolving profession. You will find a complete listing of these organizations and their contact information in Quick Guide B at the end of this book.

Another milestone in the profession of massage therapy and bodywork was reached in late 2005, when the **Federation of State Massage Therapy Boards (FSMTB)** was established as an organization through which the various massage therapy state boards could communicate with each other. An important focus of this new organization is to give state boards input into the makeup of the national exam, create a standardized curriculum, and ensure the portability of licenses from state to state.

In this chapter, we have covered the history of massage from its earliest beginnings through the start of the twenty-first century. The last several decades have seen many notable touch researchers, such as Ashley Montague and Tiffany Fields, who will, no doubt, assume their rightful place in history. Montague, a noted anthropologist, recognized the connection between a mother's nurturing and her offspring's ability to survive, while Fields, a professor of pediatrics and psychology, has conducted extensive research on the ability of premature infants to gain weight and thrive with the presence of touch (see chapter 10). Present-day students acknowledge the great strides their profession has taken due to the foresight of these two individuals. Students of massage in years to come will read Montague's and Fields' research material as history, and perhaps they will expand upon such important bodies of work.

Massage Tools and Equipment

Massage implements of many kinds have been used throughout history. More than 3000 years ago, in a practice that mirrors contemporary treatments, the Longshan culture of ancient China placed heated and cooled stones on aching muscles to soothe them. Later, Asian cultures would form precious materials, such as jade and marble, into massage implements and carve pieces of wood or bone into sharpened tips that could be worked into specific areas or pressure points more accurately and easily than fingers or dull instruments.

Both the Mesopotamians and Egyptians used sticklike staves in massage—instruments that evolved as they were refined over many generations. The Greeks and Romans employed a similar tool, called a strigil, that was used with a piece of cloth to scrape sweat, dirt, and oils off the body after exercising, as well as to apply pressure, in a tradition much like tapotement today.

Massage tools and equipment can be categorized as manual, mechanical, or electrical implements. Some manual implements are virtually the same today as they were generations ago, as effective now as then. In Hawaii, for example, *lomi-lomi* sticks are still carved of guava tree wood and used with lava rocks, called *lomi*-balls, in a form of traditional massage developed generations before by the Laau of the Pacific Islands. Today, many different companies imitate the look and feel of ancient instruments in their attempts to replicate successful manual tools used in less technologically advanced times. The introduction of mechanical and electric implements in massage treatment meant massage therapy with vibrating or rolling implements was increasingly delegated to physician's assistants. Although electrical devices can imitate many manual gestures and actions, they have never been able to replace manual tools.

Massage tables made of marble and wood were used in the lavish gymnasiums of Greece and Rome as early as 800 BCE. Until the 1920s, massage tables were referred to as "couches." During the Victorian era, they were typically upholstered in velvet and stuffed with horsehair—more commonly used than cotton or straw because of its resistance to pests—and covered with leather. These couches were used for physical exams as well as massage. Eventually, this type of upholstered couch was used less and less, giving way to wooden examination tables with adjustable settings. The Battle Creek Company of Battle Creek, Michigan, manufactured the first folding portable table in the 1940s, around the same time that the face cradle that attaches to the end of the massage table was developed. Today, massage tables with face cradles commonly adjust in a variety of ways, with a number of settings for sitting and reclining positions.

The Philosophical Foundation of Massage

What makes the profession of massage a healing art is its historical philosophical foundation. A philosophy can be defined as a group of beliefs or values that are the basis for a person's or group's practice or conduct. The person, persons, or cultures who are the founders of a healing art establish its central area of interest and mission, and thereby define its philosophy.

The historical roots of massage have shamanistic or priest-physician origins that are the most ancient of healing practices. These ancient healers used "massage" or the laying on of hands as part of their magic rituals to cleanse the body of demons by rubbing downward toward the extremities and out.

Interwoven with the physical practices of massage as a healing art is a cosmological, metaphysical philosophy. This metaphysical philosophy is separate and distinct from the materialistic philosophical reflections concerning medicine that reach back to the beginnings of Greek philosophy. Shamanistic and priestly healing practices were closely connected to their spiritual or religious rituals. In ancient China, a cosmological view of the spirit world brought forth the concept of the Tao composed of two souls, Yin and Yang. The ancient Chinese called massage *moshou*, or "hand rubbing." The *Amma*, or "press and rub" technique, was later developed as an integral part of their early healing arts recorded in the book *The Cong-Fou of the Tao-Tse* (around 5000 BCE). This is the historical starting point of modern Swedish massage.

Similarly, the founders of East Indian healing arts based their practices on the classical Indian mystical document called the *Ayur Veda*. Ayurvedic philosophy emphasizes the trinity of mind, body, and spiritual awareness as the basis of healing. Massage was, and is, an essential component in ayurvedic healing practices.

As you learned earlier in this chapter, two great Roman physicians of antiquity—Celsus and Galen—were followers of the Hippocratic philosophical tradition. Galen also applied the central themes of Aristotle's (384–322 BCE) natural philosophy to healing and was the first to pronounce the principle of **vitalism**. Galen's precept of vitalism maintained that the body was imbued with "vital spirits."

Historically, the modern vitalistic principle was introduced in the eigtheenth century when Johann Fredrich Blumenbach (1752–1840) maintained that there is an "innate" impulse in living creatures toward self-development. This principle of vitalism holds that life cannot be explained fully in terms of chemical and physical forces alone. According to vitalism, there is a third separate and distinct "vital force" (*élan vitale*) necessary to any explanation of life. The life of the organism and its functions depend on this vital force that is always a part of physical processes. The early eighteenth-century vitalists agreed that this vital force was the very source not only of life but also of health and healing. The late nineteenth and early twentieth century saw science continue to quantify in an age where objective measurement meant everything. This period also witnessed the expansion of electrical and mechanical therapies that led not only to a decline in massage as a healing art but also to the dismissal of the idea of "vital" energy. "Scientific" medical doctors in the early 1900s relied on bioscience to explain life and treat disease, and consequently discredited vitalism. However, the later twentieth century witnessed a resurgence of both massage therapy and the vitalistic philosophy of its foundation. Central to modern vitalistic philosophy is the principle that a benign source of well-being supports life and that the organism tends to self-regulate—neither building up nor breaking down too much. This homeostatic balance depends on the flow of "life force"—chi or Qi (Chinese), *ki* (Japanese), or *prana* (Indian)—to continually reestablish equilibrium.

The modern theory of homeostasis or physiological adaptation emerged with the French scientist Claude Bernard (1813–1878). Bernard proposed that the fluids and cells in the body of higher animals and man continue in an essentially constant state despite the many and varied changes in their external environment.

American physiologist Walter B. Cannon (1871–1945) coined the word *homeostasis* in his book *The Wisdom of the Body*. He introduced the term to indicate that under "normal" conditions, the human body is capable of maintaining its internal processes in a state of equilibrium by constantly compensating for the upsetting effects of external forces. The concept of homeostasis is a basic premise of vitalism, as it implies both an awareness of and the ability to respond appropriately to external or internal environmental changes. This includes a human being's ability to express both self-awareness and self-regulation.

Massage as a healing art and its historical vitalistic philosophy gained increasing credibility among Western scientists in the later twentieth century, as is evidenced in a number of groundbreaking books. Both the imminent anthropologist Ashley Montague's *Touching* (1971) and Pulitzer prize-winning pathologist and microbiologist Rene Dubos' *A God Within* (1972) speak to the closing of the philosophical distance between mainstream mechanistic science and vitalistic healing arts.

Today, the principle of vitalism is grounded in the holistic concept that the human body is greater than the sum of its parts. The basic assumption of contemporary vitalism is that there is an intelligent force, distinct from all internal physical and chemical forces, that creates and sustains all living organisms.

Present-day vitalism assumes that life is self-determining and self-evolving. The fundamental principle of modern vitalism is that there is inherent or innate intelligence within the body that animates, motivates, heals, coordinates, and inspires living beings, and that this wisdom within guides and directs the life of each individual on his or her path of healing.

According to current vitalistic philosophy, healing is a process of personal evolution, growth, self-development, and self-discovery. As a person heals holistically, a closer communication among mind, body, and spirit comes about. Genuine healing gives individuals the opportunity to see themselves more clearly and thereby get more in touch with themselves physically, mentally, emotionally, and spiritually.

This inherent healing force and power of the body is referred to variously in both Eastern and Western healing arts. In chiropractic, it is called the "innate intelligence;" in traditional Chinese Medicine, it is qi or *chi;* in ayurvedic medicine, it is *prana.* Consequently, the vitalistic philosophy of massage is shared by many disciplines and healing arts from acupuncture to yoga.

Accordingly, both parallel ancient doctrines and modern international cross-cultural and cross-disciplinary theories affirm the existence of a universal life force that intelligently animates and guides the functioning of the human mind, body, and spirit. These references validate and support the philosophical foundations of massage and its place today and historically as a healing art.

The information in this chapter shows how throughout history, various massage precepts have had an impact on health and wellness. As you have read, massage has come full circle, reclaiming its rightful place within the health care continuum. What contribution will you make to massage theory, technique, philosophy, and practice?

Chapter Summary

Applying Your Knowledge

Self-Testing

1. The earliest medicine people or healers were known as
   _____.

2. Where was the first depiction of the use of thumb or finger for massage and reflexology?_____

3. What text first mentions Chinese medicine and acupuncture/acupressure?_____

4. Ancient Greece attributed sickness to imbalances in
   _____.

5. _____ philosophy of medicine characterized the healthy human body as a natural system in perfect equilibrium.

6. What was the definition of gymnasiums in ancient Greece?_____

7. Who wrote *De Medicina?*_____

8. Why did the Greco-Roman medical tradition disappear from Europe?_____

9. When did medical schools begin to offer massage instruction, due in some part to Pare's influence?_____

10. Who introduced medical gymnastics?_____

11. Who applied French terms to Swedish movements?_____

12. _____ was among the first to implement professional standards for massage and develop a rigorous training program for practitioners.

13. What was the original name for the AMTA, and when was it formed?_____

14. The tool called a strigil was used by Greeks and Romans for what purpose?_____

15. What were the first massage tables made of? _____

16. Doctors were often the most knowledgeable and skilled massage practitioners during World Wars I and II.
    a) True
    b) False

17. Traditional Chinese medicine is the foundation for many schools of acupuncture, acupressure, and massage.
    a) True
    b) False

18. *Lomi-lomi* (Hawaiian massage) and traditional Maori massage of New Zealand are the basis of the Swedish movement cure.
    a) True
    b) False

19. During the medieval or "Dark Ages," illness was thought to be the result of sinful thoughts and actions.
    a) True
    b) False

20. In ancient Greece, massage was associated with the gymnasium and public baths.
    a) True
    b) False

21. During the Middle Ages, midwives discovered using massage could be executed as witches.
    a) True
    b) False

References for information in this chapter can be found in Quick Guide C at the end of the book.

CHAPTER 2

Equipment, Environment, and Safety Practices

LEARNING OUTCOMES

After completing this chapter, you will be able to:

- Choose a massage table based on the outlined criteria, including intended use, weight, portability, durability, and cost.

- Adequately give consideration to various accessories for the massage room such as heat sources, lighting, and music.

- Familiarize yourself with and make economical purchases of linens and other accessories.

- Select a pleasing color palate to work with for the massage environment.

- Describe how to maintain a safe and healthy environment.

- Understand viruses such as AIDS/HIV, hepatitis, SARS, and tuberculosis and their transmission.

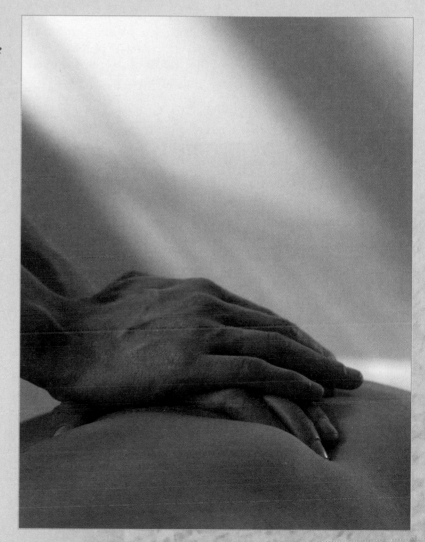

KEY TERMS

ABCs of CPR *(p. 41)*
bacteria *(p. 44)*
blood-borne pathogens *(p. 46)*
carrier *(p. 45)*
contagious disease *(p. 45)*
contaminated *(p. 47)*
CPR (cardiopulmonary
    resuscitation) *(p. 41)*
cycle of infection *(p. 45)*
direct transmission *(p. 46)*
disinfection *(p. 48)*
environmentally transmitted
    pathogen *(p. 45)*

Escherichia coli (E. coli)
    bacteria *(p. 47)*
"glideability" *(p. 36)*
Hydrocollator® *(p. 33)*
incubation period *(p. 48)*
indirect transmission *(p. 46)*
microorganisms *(p. 46)*
Noncomedogenic *(p. 35)*
opportunistic infection *(p. 50)*
opportunistically transmitted
    pathogen *(p. 45)*

person-to-person contact *(p. 45)*
sanitation *(p. 48)*
sexually transmitted diseases
    (STDs) *(p. 47)*
Standard precautions *(p. 48)*
sterilization *(p. 48)*
streptococci bacteria *(p. 47)*
susceptibility *(p. 47)*
Universal Precautions *(p. 48)*
virus *(p. 44)*

INTRODUCTION

Setting up a comfortable massage environment goes well beyond purchasing a table and linens. There are many factors to consider when purchasing equipment, selecting linens, and choosing colors with which to work. The following guidelines will help you set up your first massage room or improve on existing office space. From thread count in the sheets to choices in music, you will get a glimpse of the seemingly small details that combine to create a successful business environment. How you approach your client is also of great importance. Effective communication is an art. Cultivate the ability to listen rather than just hear. Develop the verbal skills necessary to convey clear, concise information or instructions. Furthermore, as a massage professional, you must always consider the health and well-being of your clients and yourself. It is *your* responsibility to make sure you have provided a safe and sanitary environment within your facility. Even if you are renting space or working on a trade basis, your area and how you work can have a great impact on your clients and coworkers.

Equipment

To function as the talented choreographer that you are and create artful massage, you need the proper "stage" for the performance. Recalling (and paraphrasing) Shakespeare's image of the world as a stage, carefully chosen equipment will provide the perfect backdrop to deliver a memorable therapeutic massage performance.

Massage Tables

The workhorse of the massage professional is the massage table. Lending credence to the old adage "Necessity is the mother of invention," most table manufacturers were once therapists themselves; they recognized and filled the need for affordable and quality equipment. The primary criterion of selection is intended use; other considerations are table weight and portability, weight-bearing capacity, durability, and cost.

Massage tables are, for the most part, uniform in basic appearance and structure but differ widely in their manufacturing process and available options. Most table frames are either wood or a lightweight metal (figures 2.1 and 2.2) such as aluminum. Deciding between wood or metal depends on specific criteria, which are detailed in the section on table selection criteria in this chapter. Therapists who work primarily with energy modalities, such as Reiki, often prefer a table with a wooden frame as any metal will disturb the energy flow.

Tables are covered with a variety of fabrics ranging from vinyl to soft faux leather, and are available in dozens of colors to fit any office decor. Most manufacturers offer at

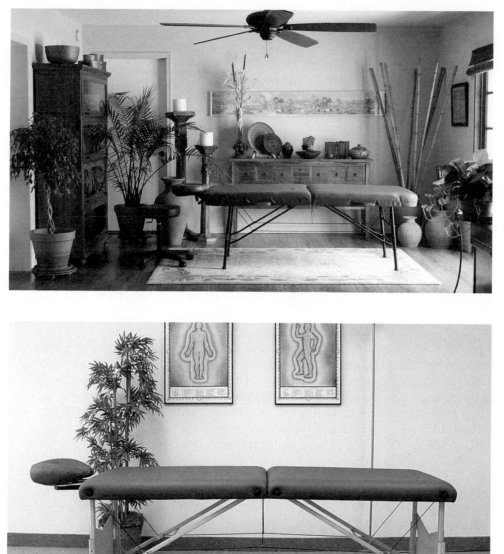

Figure 2.1 Lightweight-frame portable table

Figure 2.2 Wooden frame table

least two or three different widths, with varied styles of corners and indented sides, and other specific attributes such as removable arms for larger clients. The purpose or modality for which the table will be used will dictate the specifics of the table. The amount of padding or cushioning is also often determined by intended use.

Although massage tables can be purchased with a hole in one end of the table for the client's face when lying prone, the majority of tables manufactured today are equipped with a removable face cradle. On some tables, these face cradles may be inserted on either end, while others have placement holes only on one end. Removable face cradles have an advantage over holes in the table in that they are adjustable, moving and/or tilting both up and down. This range of adjustment is necessary for particular work (on the neck, for example) and for larger clients who need the cradle raised up to align the cervical spine.

The top of the line in massage tables is the hydraulic table (figure 2.3). Therapists who work on a wide variety of clients or perform several modalities appreciate the convenience of using a table that raises and lowers at the touch of a button or foot pedal, allowing them to add pressure during any *one* massage session without exerting undue

Figure 2.3 Hydraulic table with wooden frame

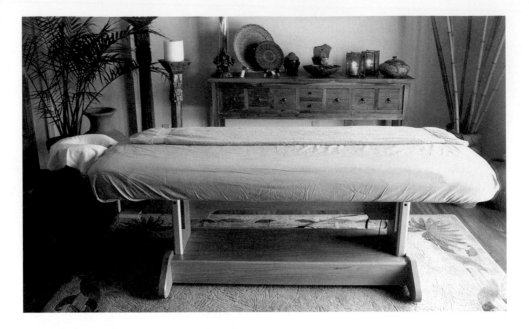

force on their body. These tables also offer tilt options that are good for clients with specific concerns such as someone who has sinus problems when lying down. Hydraulic tables have extreme weight-bearing capacity, owing to their stationary structure and the positioning of the motor. Both wood and metal frame construction can be found on these tables, with the design being one that moves straight up and down or opens and closes like a scissor. Of consideration here is the motor. Some brands are extremely quiet, while others can be somewhat disruptive to the serene massage environment. A hydraulic table can cost between $1500 and $4500.

Unless you have a large start-up budget to open an office, you will probably begin your practice by purchasing one portable table. A portable table will give you flexibility to set up an at-home office, zoning permitting, as well as travel to clients' homes to perform outcalls.

Table Selection Criteria

The primary criterion for selecting a table is its intended purpose or use. For example, if you are going to work with deep tissue modalities such as sports or neuromuscular therapies, you should select a less padded table that can be set lower to the floor. If you will be performing Swedish relaxation massage or any modality requiring little to no pressure, such as Trager® or Reiki, you can choose a table that is made of a more plush material for added comfort with a greater height range. Many therapists do more than one type of massage, so try to choose a table that will fit a broad spectrum of needs—especially for your first table purchase.

A second criterion for table selection is table weight and portability. Most portable tables weigh from 21 to more than 39 pounds. Added to that weight will be bolsters and face cradles as well as linens, lubricants, and other accessories. Before selecting your table, decide how often you will need to move it around: are you primarily doing outcalls, going to several houses a day, or are you working out of one location with the occasional outcall? The more frequently you need to transport the table, the lighter it should be.

A real back-saver for the therapist is the rolling table cart (figure 2.4), which is designed to carry the massage table, linens, and other supplies. This may be a particularly important consideration for therapists who are small in stature because lugging around a table that weighs almost as much as they do can spell injury down the line. These special carts work better than standard luggage carts because the table is carried in a posi-

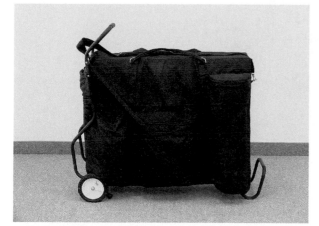

Figure 2.4 Rolling table cart

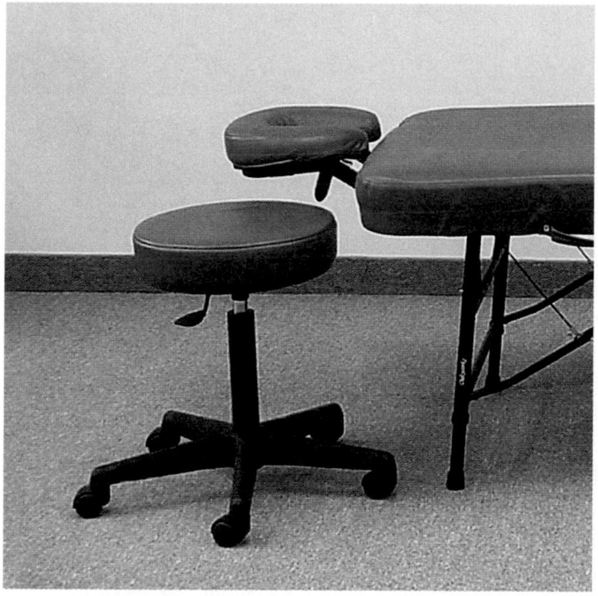

Figure 2.5 Pneumatic stool with castors

tion that allows it to fit through doorways without having to take it off the cart. Further, these carts are fitted with large wheels that prevent the cart from tipping over. Most carts fold up for easy storage.

Weight-bearing capacity and durability are the third and fourth criteria. The frame and general construction of the table will vary from manufacturer to manufacturer. Again, consider your clientele; if you are working on bodybuilders in your local gym, you will need a substantial table with a greater weight-bearing capacity. A practice of predominantly outcalls will require a solid, well-built table, perhaps with a more durable fabric, while a table set up in an office setting will take less abuse because it is not carted around. In either case, a well-made table will provide several years of service.

Finally, price is the final criterion. Portable tables range from $300 to $900. The cost depends on the whole package: frame, padding, covering, and accessories. Lower-end tables often do not include a face cradle, bolster, or carrying case. Be sure to add up all costs. Many manufacturers offer package deals that may be more cost-effective in the long run, as well as offer student discounts to schools. Check manufacturers' websites for deals and special offers. Also, check local schools offering seminars; they may have tables for sale at a reduced price that were used only once or twice for a seminar.

Along with your table, consider obtaining a stool for use when you are doing foot and head massage or any specific work where sitting for a period of time will be required. A pneumatic stool is a great investment (figure 2.5). These stools easily adjust

Figure 2.6 Thai mat used for Thai massage and shiatsu

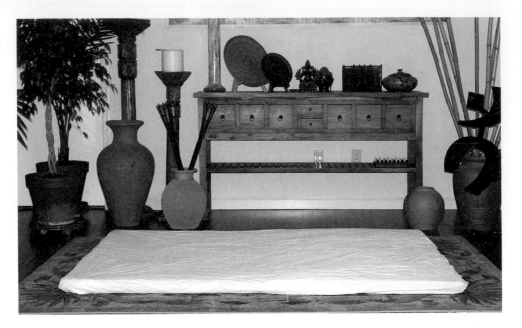

in height and are set on rolling casters, both of which allow for a therapist position or angle change. Several manufacturers produce lightweight portable or foldable stools that can be easily transported with your table for outcalls.

A substitute for the massage table is the massage mat (figure 2.6). Mats are used for modalities performed on the floor such as Thai massage and Shiatsu and are available in a variety of thicknesses and colors. The material inside the mat is most important. It should be dense, allowing for comfort during an extended period of time on the floor. The outer covering should be easily washable and durable.

Table manufacturers are beginning to manufacture "table" versions of mats, which may prove to be very popular in Western markets. These mats are usually much wider than a standard table, are sturdy like a table, and have adjustable legs that allow them to be set just off the floor. Setting the mat just off the floor makes it more accessible to clients and keeps them out of any drafts. It is also easier for therapists to move around on or change positions. Although the typical Thai massage in Thailand is two to two and a half hours long, most clients in the United States tend to be comfortable on the floor for no more than one and a half hours, even with a good floor mat. The unique construction of these "table" mats will be appreciated by both therapists and clients.

Massage Chairs

Massage chairs are specifically made for seated or corporate massage (figure 2.7). Office workers can slip into these chairs without getting undressed for a tension-relieving session. Many therapists choose to perform an entire one-hour massage on a chair because it gives them great flexibility with respect to positioning, time, and location. Many of the same criteria for table selection hold true for massage chairs.

Frames for massage chairs are usually metal, with some designs being easier to collapse and transport than others. Besides portability, consider stability and the frequency with which the chair will be used. Prices range from $300 to $900. As with the massage table, the more it is used, the more you will probably need to invest.

Some chair designs (figure 2.8) have been engineered to posture the client at an angle from 45 to 180 degrees (horizontal). This allows the therapist to work the posterior neck, back, and legs with greater ease and is ergonomically sound for the manipulation of deep tissue normally not seen in more traditional chair massage routines.

Some chairs have a wider range of adjustments for seats and chest plates and may be easier to change settings between each client. Try out colleagues' chairs or visit trade

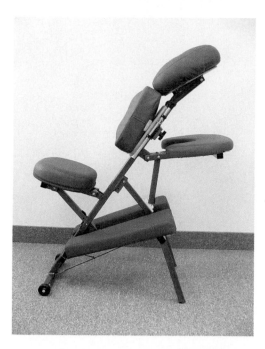

Figure 2.7 Chair made specifically for seated or corporate massage

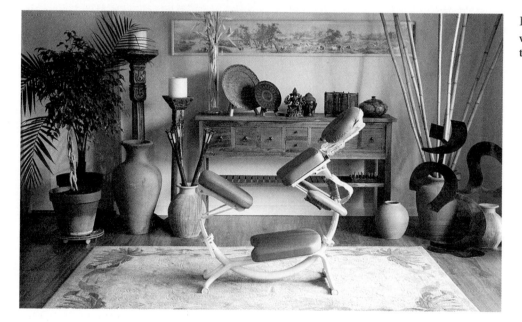

Figure 2.8 Dolphin chair with capability of adjusting to a horizontal position

shows before purchasing a chair. Therapists who are tall may have difficulty working long hours with a chair that is set lower to the ground and vice versa. Also, consider your clientele; some seniors or less mobile clients will have a harder time using some chairs than others.

Cushions and Bolsters

A variety of body cushions, pregnancy cushions, and bolsters are available to suit all client needs. Pregnancy cushions allow for women to safely receive massage in the second and third trimesters. Cushions such as the one pictured in figure 2.9 provide effective treatment for all types of massage. Cushion segments can be used for clients requiring additional support or compensatory bolstering. Wedge bolsters give comfort for low-back sufferers.

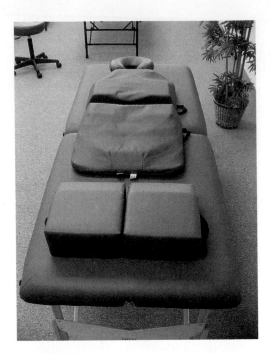

Figure 2.9 The bodyCushion™ for supportive and pregnancy massage

Figure 2.10 (Left to right) Wedge bolster, 6-inch round bolster, 8-inch round bolster, and breast cushion

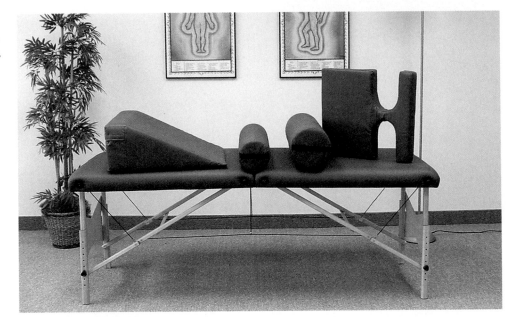

 EXAM POINT Half-round bolsters can be placed under the hips in prone position to reduce a lordotic curve, while clients with kyphotic curves are made comfortable in supine position by placing bolsters under the neck and shoulders.

Large-breasted women, especially those with implants, are made more comfortable by using breast cushions (figure 2.10).

Moist Heat Hydrotherapy Sources

Thermophores® and Fomenteks® (figure 2.11) are portable heat sources that are easily used during outcalls. The Thermophore is an electrical heating pack that looks like the standard dry heating pad but differs in that it draws moisture from the air. Special flan-

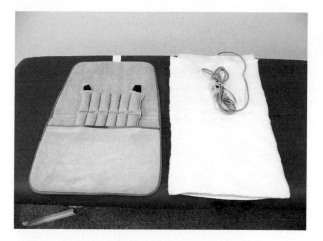

Figure 2.11 Moist heat sources: Hydrocollator® pack and Thermphore®

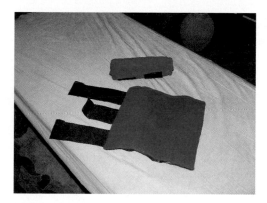

Figure 2.12 Convenient-to-use ice wrap with Velcro straps

nel coverings with a rubber lining for insertion of a wet towel are available to provide added moisture. The Fomentek is a large plastic bag that is filled with warm water much like a hot water bottle. Some clients enjoy the feeling of the extra weight of the Fomentek. The Fomentek can also be used cold.

For office use, the best device is the **Hydrocollator®**, a stainless steel tank that holds hot water. "HotPaks" are soaked in the hot water, which is regulated by a thermostat. These packs are put in heavy terry cloth covers before being placed on the client's body. Hydrocollators are most often found in chiropractor's and physical therapist's offices.

Cryotherapy Sources

Many varieties of ice packs are available, ranging from vinyl gel packs to cloth-covered packs. Many of these ice packs also double as heat packs, making them economical to use. Several brands of compression ice wrap systems (figure 2.12) are convenient to use and easily adapted to individual clients because they have Velcro straps that hold each wrap in place (see chapter 13 for further discussion on cryotherapy choices).

Massage Tools

Many massage therapists and bodyworkers use a variety of tools such as T-Bars, Knobbles, Bongers, and wooden rollers. These tools allow therapists to work deeply and hold pressure points without putting undue pressure on their joints (usually the thumb). Hand-held mechanical massagers are also popular and can further enhance any session. Implements shaped like an S are designed for the therapists to use on themselves, for example, to release tension around the scapula after working.

Supplemental Equipment Sources

Depending on individual state regulations, some massage therapists are now able to use ultrasound equipment, electrical stimulation devices, and cold lasers. All of these pieces of equipment serve to increase circulation and speed healing in a localized area. Use of any form of ultrasound, electrical stimulation, or laser should be performed with specific training in the respective device and under the attending physician's direction. Most therapists will encounter such equipment in a medical doctor's, chiropractor's, or physical therapist's office.

Equipment Care

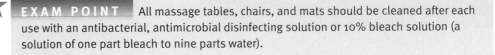 **EXAM POINT** All massage tables, chairs, and mats should be cleaned after each use with an antibacterial, antimicrobial disinfecting solution or 10% bleach solution (a solution of one part bleach to nine parts water).

Various antibacterial "wipes" are now available that are convenient to use and easily transportable for cleaning tables and chairs.

EXAM POINT The most effective deterrent to spreading germs is thorough and constant washing of equipment and hands.

If a hand-washing facility is not available, such as at a sporting event, therapists can clean their hands on site using wipes or antibacterial gels. For further cleanliness and safety procedures, see the section titled "Safety First in the Massage Environment" (p. 39).

All equipment in the massage room should be maintained with regularly scheduled checks. Make repairs as often as necessary. Follow manufacturer's recommendations for any and all repairs. Do not use any equipment that is structurally unsound.

Draping Materials

Whether you use a massage table or mat, it will need to be covered with a draping material (figure 2.13) for hygiene purposes. Most often used on tables are twin-size flat or fitted sheets. The twin size is large enough to cover the table and be pulled up over the client for warmth, yet not so big it falls on the floor, creating a tripping hazard. Fitted

Figure 2.13 Table setup with appropriate draping materials

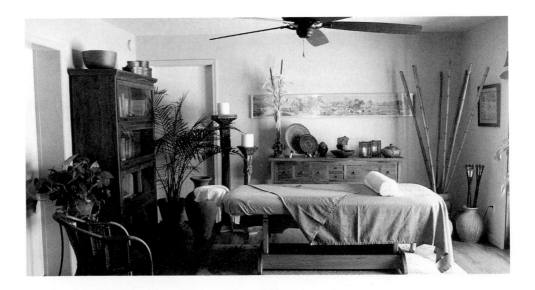

sheets work well to provide a covering for the table; they also do not shift as the client moves. A fleece cover or a fitted sheet can also be used under a flat sheet to keep it in place. In some cases, a full-size fitted sheet may be needed to cover a mat.

Sheets should be durable and able to withstand repeated washing in hot water. Therefore, take into consideration color and thread count. Darker colors will run or fade, while white sheets will show stains from oils and crèmes. Subtle patterns work well for hiding stains; take care to not use any pattern that is too busy if you are trying to set a calming tone. A higher thread count, above 300, will indicate more durable linens; these are often called "hotel linens" by stores. Hotel linens can have a thread count as high as 600. Lower thread counts, 260 and below, are the least expensive linens but will not be as soft or comfortable to the touch. Since linens are washed in hot water repeatedly, a higher thread count is best. Flannel sheets, fleece table covers, and table warmers are good choices for northern climates. Small flannel blankets, similar to those used by the airlines, are ideal for keeping clients warm while on the table.

Washing linens in hot water, harsh soaps, and bleach will definitely cause damage, and it won't be long before you are replacing them, so make sure you consider this in your budget. An alternative to bleach (to which some clients may be allergic) is to use a few drops of lemon, lemongrass, or any citrus-blend essential oil as a disinfectant in the hot wash water along with soap. (Never add essential oil to sheets directly placed in the dryer; it is a fire hazard.)

Either sheets or towels can be used for top drapes. The determining factor will be room temperature. A heavy bath sheet (beach-towel size) will provide the client with privacy and warmth. Flat sheets can be used if warmth is not necessary; however, using a flat sheet can be cumbersome because of the amount of material you will have to position.

Face cradle drapes can be purchased precut in paper or flannel. Flat pieces work best as some fitted face cradle covers have seams that will press into a client's face. Another method of covering the face cradle is to use a folded hand towel or pillowcase.

Initially, you will probably wash your own linens. As your practice grows, it may be necessary to hire a laundry service. Keep in mind these services can be expensive as they often charge by the pound. At this point, you may want to reevaluate the draping materials used; large bath sheets are heavy and can be expensive to launder. Consider using as an alternative a twin flat sheet cut in half; bind the edges on a sewing machine to prevent raveling. This will give you a smaller, lighter-weight drape that can then be covered with a light blanket for warmth and will help you to save considerably on the laundry bill.

A small pillow made of buckwheat or flaxseed, similar to ones sold in airports, is a nice way to pamper your client in the supine position. The pillow can be covered with a small hand towel or the face cradle cover when placed under the client's head.

Massage chairs do not require draping materials other than on the face cradle. Disposable face covers, 100 count per package, are easy to transport to an office environment or sporting event.

Lubricants

Four basic types of lubricants are made especially for massage: oils, crèmes, lotions, and gels. These lubricants are **noncomedogenic**, meaning they do not clog the pores of the skin. A fifth "lubricant" is powder. Certain modalities, such as trigger point work and myofascial release, require a minimal amount of drag or glideability.

Although it is a matter of preference as to which type you choose to work with, some clients will express a preference for a certain lubricant. Products can be found at a discount in beauty supply stores, ordered directly from a company or manufacturer, or ordered from various massage catalogs. Use caution when purchasing massage products at various "body and bath" stores.

★ **EXAM POINT** These products often are made using a mineral oil or other unsuitable base for professional massage; such products will clog pores.

Any commercially prepared massage lubricant should be noncomedogenic and hypoallergenic. Do not simply accept the manufacturer's claim that the product is for massage; read the label.

All lubricants should be stored in a cool, dry place; do not keep lubricants in a linen bag in your car. Oils have a shorter shelf life than crèmes or lotions and can go rancid. Gels and powder are the most stable and will not deteriorate as quickly. Discard any oil, lotion, or crème that shows signs of separation. Mix up only a very small amount of lubricant with an essential oil for specific clients.

Oils, Crèmes, Lotions, and Gels

When using oils for a lubricant, choose vegetable-based oils such as almond or a manufactured massage oil. A few drops of an essential oil can be added to any oil to create a pleasing scent. A cautionary note here: it is important to not use any aromatherapy in the lubricant—or the room—to which clients may be allergic. Always keep a bottle of fragrance-free massage oil on hand for clients with allergies.

Oils can be slippery but give the best **"glideability"** (ease of movement over skin without drag). They are especially useful with clients who have copious amounts of body hair. The drawback will be your client may need to schedule time for a shower immediately after the massage session, especially if the massage is early in the day. Keep a spray bottle handy with a mixture of distilled water and witch hazel for the client to sponge off with. This mixture is also handy for spritzing on a client's feet before working on them.

Crèmes offer an excellent choice for glideability without being too greasy or slippery. Their consistency can range from silky to thick. Choose thicker crèmes when working with sports massage.

Lotions tend to get sticky when used. Gels are a good compromise between oils and crèmes or lotions. These also work well on individuals who have a large amount of body hair.

Environment

Create a warm and friendly environment by taking into account every seemingly little detail. Careful consideration of all elements, from color to lighting to linens, will indicate a level of professionalism and thoroughness (figure 2.14).

Figure 2.14
Attention to detail creates a warm and friendly environment and indicates professionalism.

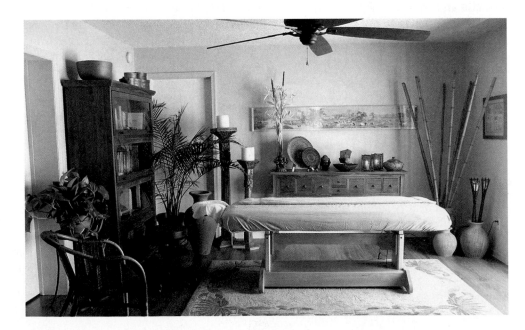

Working in a *Vastu* Environment

With my dedication to yoga, its principles, and practices, I follow *Vastu* in my home and office. My massage room is in the very center of the house, with the remainder of the rooms all falling around the massage room. In *Vastu*, the center of the house is considered the God-center and an area of healing. My table is positioned southwest to northeast, with the head of the table in the southwest. This is the position in which Brahma is believed to be lying. The massage room also happens to be the "safe room" where I rode out several hurricanes in Florida in 2004 and 2005! My writing desk is in the southwest corner of the house, the creative area; and the room where I teach yoga classes is in the northeast corner, the area for meditation. All of my clients comment on their experiences in the massage room, and I truly believe they are experiencing the power of *Vastu*, not the massage alone. Following a prescribed arrangement for each room encourages peacefulness, harmony, well-being, and, most important for your office, prosperity.

Realize that clients sense the energy, the vibration, in your room. We live in a high-stress time when our senses are assaulted by many things: constantly ringing cell phones, a barrage of e-mails, ever-increasing commuting times. There are natural forces that govern the space around us and the space in which we place ourselves. Aligning with and honoring this space creates an environment that not only is free of physical and mental clutter but also is one of respect. Whether your massage room is more clinical or spiritual in nature, clients will appreciate the positive forces they feel in it.

Massage Room Environment

In setting up your massage room, you may want to take into consideration the principles of *Vastu Vidya* or Feng Shui. *Vastu* is known as the Indian version of Feng Shui and is, in fact, the precursor to Feng Shui. *Vastu* is also aligned with the Five Elements (see chapter 15). Feng Shui is a popular topic today, and an entire industry has sprung up from the public's interest in it. Local consultants as well as numerous books can be found on the subject.

The Basics

An important, albeit often overlooked, criterion for the massage room is size. Remember that the massage table is 6 feet long without the face cradle inserted. Additionally, you will need approximately 4 feet of working space all around the table. Choose a room size that accommodates the table and all other equipment comfortably.

Be diligent about keeping the room clean and safe. Make sure there are no electrical cords to trip over, hanging lights to bump into, or slippery floors. If the room has tile or hardwood floors, cover the area under the massage table with a nonslip area rug. The lighting should be adjustable. You may need to turn lights up for the initial greeting and interview, and lower the lights to create the appropriate atmosphere during the massage. Being able to turn lights up also allows you to examine any cuts or bruises on your client so you can avoid working over those areas, as well as clearly observe your client's range of motion or demonstration of problem areas.

As with the lighting, any music played should be subtle or soothing. This does not mean, however, that strictly "massage music" or "elevator music" has to be played. It simply means the music should be appropriate for the environment. Taste in music is a personal thing. You may be inspired by some types of music and not by others. Further, your client may enjoy some music but be irritated by others. Choose your music wisely, selecting music that appeals to both of you. The most common problem encountered with playing popular music is coming across a track with an undesirable or inappropriate subject or tempo. After purchasing a CD or downloading music from a legal site, you can burn a CD that excludes any inappropriate tracks. New Age stores and the New Age/Alternative section of your local book or record store will have a selection of appropriate music for massage sessions.

Color and Ambience

Color vibrates or interacts or resonates, with our own energy. Many people hold certain associations for specific colors. Some colors attract and soothe us, while others repel and irritate us. Certain colors are associated with chakras (*chakra* is a Sanskrit word meaning "energy center" or "wheel"; see chapter 19). The color palate you choose for the massage room, from linens to walls, can directly affect a client's receptivity and response to treatment.

Soft colors are best for the walls, but if you are working on a variety of clients, refrain from a gender-specific decor; you want men and women—young and old—to equally feel comfortable in your massage room. Greens, blues, violets, and amethyst-whites are associated with the upper chakras. People who work with energy-based modalities recognize these colors as possessing a high vibration and being spiritually oriented. Reds, oranges, and yellows are associated with the lower or base chakras, where our survival to self-empowerment instincts are.

Amethyst, ranging from indigo to violet to white, affects the pituitary gland, with the violet end of the spectrum asserting direct influence on the brain. Indigo strengthens imagination and intuition, which is why it helps us in meditation. Indigo is stabilizing. Violets intensify the properties of indigo and are considered powerful healing colors. Violets lead us along the path to enlightenment. White represents purity and the unification of mind, body, and soul.

Blues are colors of harmony and calm, and are especially calming to our emotions. Lighter hues of blue denote simplicity, while darker hues suggest magnetism.

Greens are traditionally thought of as nourishing colors and aid in balancing as well as general healing. Green is associated with the heart chakra and represents unconditional love. In Asia, jade green is thought to be a healing color, hence the popularity of jade. Greens create harmony and balance. As part of nature, greens represent renewal. Subtle greens are thought to affect blood pressure and cranial nerves.

Yellows are associated with the solar plexus chakra, resonate warmth, and are thought to have a stimulating affect on the glands. Yellow increases creativity and curiosity. It represents the spiritual light that illuminates the truth.

Oranges and reds are strong, energetic colors that are often too intense for a massage room but are warming. Oranges and reds can increase energy and vitality as well as immunity in the human body. In Hinduism, orange burns impurities and represents the quest for enlightenment.

According to Hinduism mythology, Vedic scholars believed all seven colors in the visible spectrum to be created by the sun's energy. Knowing the properties that are associated with each color can help restore balance to a person's *dosha* or mind-body constitution (see chapter 15).

Additional Considerations

A ceiling fan or small oscillating fan is an excellent way to keep air circulating during the massage. The air in the room can quickly become warm and stagnant when you are working. Be sure, however, that your client is sufficiently covered with extra draping material if necessary to prevent him from getting chilled. Be cautious in using aromatherapy; what one client likes is not necessarily what the next one likes. It is very difficult to get scents out of a room.

One of the most valuable tools for the small business owner is an office computer with industry-specific software (see chapter 21). Do not, however, have the computer or a phone in your massage room. If this is unavoidable, use an inaudible answering machine or voice mail and turn off the computer screen. Further, make sure you have a file cabinet with a lock; federal regulations require that client intake/history forms and SOAP Notes be kept in a locked cabinet. Try to handle the business end of the massage—setting appointments and collecting payment—in another room.

If the massage is an outcall—in the client's house—you do not have as much control over the environment. You will have to set your table up in the location specified by the client. Be candid with your client as to whether or not the area is appropriate. You know the amount of space needed and the temperature required to effectively perform your best work. The client will usually provide whatever background music she likes or allow you to play a CD you have brought along on the stereo. Children, phones, spouses, and pets can all be disruptive. If any of these presents a problem, you will have to diplomatically discuss this with your client.

It cannot be stressed enough that it is crucial for you, the massage professional, to follow cleanliness practices both in your clinic or office and on outcalls. Along with good hygiene, you and any employees should be familiar with basic CPR (cardiopulmonary resuscitation), precautions concerning the transmission of AIDS/HIV (acquired immunodeficiency syndrome/human immunodeficiency virus), hepatitis, SARS (severe acute respiratory syndrome), and tuberculosis, and procedures to follow in case of accidents.

Personal Hygiene

Personal hygiene is a very important part of professionalism and the safety of your clinic. An unkempt or unclean practitioner is a breeding ground for microorganisms that can lead to infection or illness. Jewelry that can harbor germs, long fingernails, and unwashed hair can contribute to the spread of disease. Your clients expect professionalism and the highest level of care for their time and money. Failing to make personal hygiene and clinic cleanliness a main priority can turn away clients.

Proper Hand Washing

You must wash your hands at the beginning of your day, after breaks or eating, and before and after using the restroom. Always wash your hands before you leave the clinic (or therapy room) for the day. Hands should also be washed before and after each client, after cleaning the therapy room or doing laundry, and before and after using the appointment book. Washing your hands properly is an easy and very effective way to prevent harmful microorganisms from spreading. Be sure to wash your hands after you sneeze or cough; a hand is effective in stopping droplets of breath going into the air during a sneeze, but the hand must be washed to retard transmission.

TECHNIQUE EMPHASIS A good practice is to stock alcohol-based hand sanitizer and antibacterial wipes in the therapy room so you do not need to interrupt the flow of the massage.

The Healthy Physical Environment: Clinic, Spa, or Home Office

Regardless of the physical environment in which you practice massage—clinic, spa, home office, or other—this environment has to be healthy and safe. While you want the environment to be hospitable for your clients, you also want to avoid making it too comfortable for germs and pathogens. Pathogens will survive and be passed on only if their environment is hospitable. For example, if your clinic or home office has very warm waiting areas, the chance for airborne transmission from a cough or sneeze is very probable. If, however, the room's temperature is below 70°F, the pathogens in the air and on surfaces may die from the cold. In most spas and massage clinics, the temperature is often above 75 degrees in order to make the experience comfortable for the client and help the muscles to relax; however, this warm temperature can contribute to the survival of pathogens. If spills are cleaned up quickly and laundry washed promptly, then

PROCEDURE 2.1 Hand Washing Technique

> **Objective** To learn how to properly wash your hands to remove dirt and microorganisms

Items to be used:
- Liquid soap
- Nail brush
- Paper towels
- Sink

Procedure Steps:

1. Turn on sink faucets using a paper towel. Use moderately warm water.

2. Wet your hands and apply liquid soap.

3. Lather both hands completely with the soap for two minutes. Keep your hands lower than your forearms (figure 2.15).

4. Use the nailbrush to clean under and around your fingernails and cuticles (figure 2.16).

5. Rinse your hands well.

6. With the water still running, dry your hands thoroughly with clean, dry paper towels and then turn off the faucets using another clean, dry paper towel.

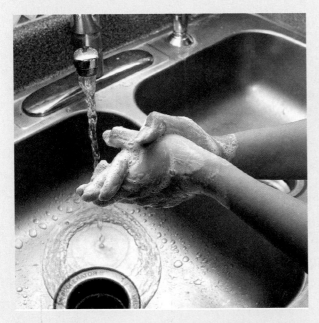

Figure 2.15
When you wash your hands, be sure to clean all surfaces, including the palms, between the fingers, and under the nails.

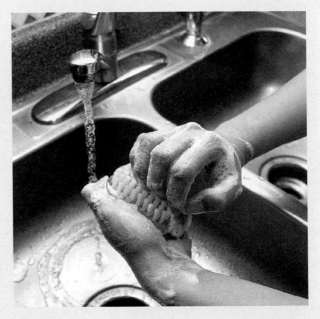

Figure 2.16
The nails and cuticles require additional attention to ensure that all dirt and microorganisms are removed.

pathogens will have less time to multiply and may be eradicated more easily. Holding clinic laundry until you have a full load can result in cross contamination of linens and is an unacceptable practice.

In addition to the hygiene and cleanliness procedures already mentioned, the following cleanliness practices should be followed in your home office, clinic, or spa:

- The reception area must be clean and orderly.

⭐ **EXAM POINT** The temperature should remain at 72°F and be well-ventilated and -lit.

- Facial tissues should be placed in the reception room and in other areas for easy access.
- Hand sanitizer should be in all bathrooms, massage, and laundry rooms.
- All door knobs and phone mouthpieces should be cleaned daily.
- Floors should be cleaned daily; check local health regulations regarding the use of carpet or tile in the various areas of the clinic.
- Toilets and all tub areas should be disinfected daily.
- A "no eating policy" should be strictly enforced and "no drinking" areas delineated. Shared food such as snacks in spas should be individually presented and kept refrigerated, if necessary, between clients. Uneaten fruit and other snacks must be discarded at the end of the day.
- Regular pest control must be utilized as insects can transmit disease.
- Trash should be removed daily.
- Emergency information and phone numbers must be posted for employees and clients.

CPR and General First Aid

Every practicing massage therapist should be certified in basic first aid and **CPR (cardiopulmonary resuscitation)**, even if such certification is not required by licensing. Several organizations train allied health and laypersons in basic first aid and CPR. The most common are the American Red Cross, the American Heart Association, and the National Safety Council. Most massage therapy schools include CPR and first aid in their curriculum. Both CPR and first aid programs require a number of hours of hands-on training and a short test to be sure you are proficient in handling emergencies. Certification renewal can be done through the organization that provided the original training. Figure 2.17 shows you the equipment and techniques of a typical CPR class.

Basic First Aid Steps

Always call 911 before performing any emergency care. The 911 rescue team can immediately send help and talk you through virtually any procedure that is needed. Be aware that in some instances, a delay in transport or in advanced life support procedures can result in death.

If a client appears to be having a heart attack (myocardial infarction) or stroke (cerebrovascular accident), call 911 and begin the **ABCs (airway, breathing, circulation) of CPR**. If a client feels faint, have him lie down, loosen his clothing, and elevate his legs. You can also have him sit in a chair and lower his head between his legs.

If the client experiences leg or other muscle cramps along with heavy sweating, move him to a cooler area, give him tepid water, and do not massage. If the client's skin is cold to the touch and he is sweating heavily, follow the same procedure and call 911.

These are only a few of the emergency situations that may occur. A basic first aid course will also cover choking, burns, strains and sprains, cuts or abrasions, and swelling. Remember, it is your responsibility to have the knowledge to take the right action required in an emergency situation. Failure to act appropriately can result in a liability to your practice, although Good Samaritan laws protect you, should your good intentions to give aid result in harm to your client.

Health Department Criteria

Your local health department can familiarize you with the pathogens that may be prevalent in your area, as well as the laws governing your clinic, office, or spa. A health inspector often will visit a new clinic before licensing it for business and will periodically make random visits to ensure the clinic is maintaining a safe environment for its clients

Figure 2.17

(*a*) Basic life support/health care provider CPR course provided by certified American Heart Association instructor. (*b*) CPR rescue breathing. (*c*) Infant CPR and first aid techniques. (*d*) Bag mask and CPR technique. (*e*) Automatic electronic defibrillator (AED) device used in CPR.

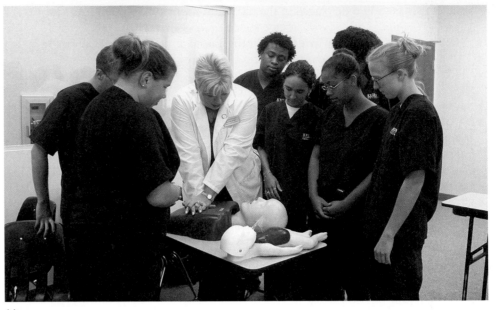

(a)

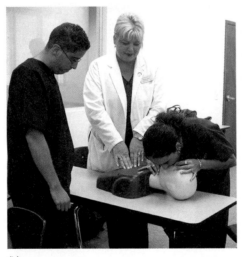

(b)

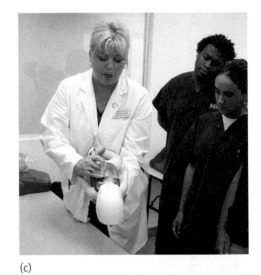

(c)

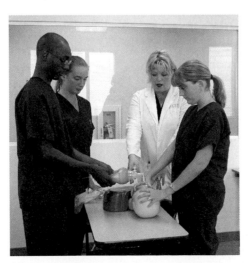

(d)

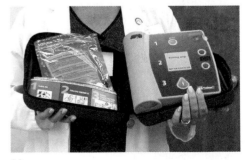

(e)

Figure 2.18 Sample
accident report form

```
                    ACCIDENT REPORT FORM
                    FOR NEWFOUNDLAND SPA
                         123 Koda Road
                        Ajna, Florida 33470




  Client's name:                              Date:
  Massage therapist's name:                   Time:
  Description of accident/incident:


  Actions taken:




  _____          _____
  Signature of massage therapist / Date    Signature of client / Date

  Reviewed and resolved:                     Date / Time:


  Those in attendance during review and resolution of accident:

```

and employees. It is up to you, however, to implement a regular program of sanitization in your facility.

Accidental Injury Reports for Police or Insurance

When opening your clinic, spa, or office each morning (or before your first client), briefly inspect the parking lot, waiting area, treatment rooms, and any other areas to be used. You must make sure that the areas you and your client are using are free of hazards. Accidents can and do happen even in the most carefully maintained and inspected facilities. It only takes a small spill or something such as a trash can or mop left in the path of a client or therapist to cause an injury. When an accidental injury occurs, it is very important to fill out an accident report. Figure 2.18 is a sample accident report that you can adapt for use in your spa or clinic. These reports must be kept on the premises for insurance, health department, and federal Occupational Safety and Health Administration (OSHA) purposes. All repairs or steps needed to correct a situation after an accident must be implemented immediately and included in the report. Exits must be clearly marked, and signs giving emergency instructions must be posted where clients can see them, usually in the waiting or reception area. Many states require fire extinguishers on the premises and posting of an evacuation plan, especially if it is a large facility.

Pathogens and Transmission of Diseases

As stated earlier in this chapter, you must always consider the health and well-being of your clients and yourself. Your clients expect to be treated in a safe and sanitary manner as possible, and state health laws establish mandatory guidelines for the protection of your clients, yourself, and your coworkers.

Pathogens

There are four main classes of pathogens: bacteria, viruses, fungi, and protozoa. Each of these pathogens has its own set of characteristics.

Bacteria

Among the significant pathogens that can invade your clinic are bacteria. **Bacteria** are microorganisms that have both plant and animal characteristics. Often called germs or microbes, they are found in dirt (plants in the clinic), discarded waste items (face cradle paper, paper cups), unclean water, and diseased tissues (skin breaks or eruptions, saliva from the client on the table). Bacteria are everywhere all the time. These pathogens exist on the skin, in the air, in our bodies, underneath fingernails and toenails, in the body hair, and on every inanimate surface.

Bacteria are classed as either nonpathogenic (harmless) or pathogenic (harmful). Nonpathogenic bacteria are very beneficial to us in the performance of many processes such as digestion, metabolizing vitamins and enzymes, and keeping harmful bacteria at bay.

Pathogenic bacteria produce disease. Parasites also belong to this group because they must have living tissue to grow and reproduce. Three main forms of pathogenic bacteria are cocci, bacilli, and spirilla. These bacteria are of no threat to us until they invade the body and begin to reproduce. When a person is healthy, they have a strong immune system that is supported or enhanced by massage. Keep in mind, however, that circulatory massage can overwhelm the body's ability to fight infection.

Viruses

A **virus** is a class of submicroscopic organisms that are pathogenic agents capable of causing disease. Viruses cannot survive without the presence of a host. They make us ill by invading living cells and taking over their duties. Secretions from the virus cause the cell to accept the virus as part of itself. This disables the usual immune response and allows the virus to replicate. The invaded cell will die and release the virus to other cells, allowing the virus to quickly and methodically grasp hold of the entire body. Viruses are very hard to treat because they mutate easily to survive. Viruses are responsible for the common cold, small pox, viral pneumonia, and many childhood diseases. They also cause AIDS and hepatitis (see the sections on AIDS/HIV and hepatitis in this chapter).

Fungi

Many types of fungi can cause disease in a massage clinic and especially within a spa facility. The most common fungi, molds, are parasitic plants that depend on other life forms for food. Molds reproduce by budding into spores that are released into the air. These spores attach to damp areas on any surface and spread. Mold spores that are inhaled can cause mild to serious respiratory distress in clients. Clients with asthma, emphysema, or an immune system disorder are at a greater risk for an adverse reaction when exposed to the spores.

Spa facilities have a greater chance of mold infestation due to the warmer temperatures and a higher density of moist air from hot tubs, hydrotherapy equipment, and showers. The spores of mold attach to damp areas on any types of surface, from floors to towels, to tubs, and spread very quickly. If left untreated, mold, which is unsightly in appearance, destroys the surface it is attached to, and the materials must be removed and destroyed. Simply cleaning a surface after the spore has attached will not rid the area of mold. The mold also releases unpleasant odors as the surfaces decay, which change the esthetics of any clinic.

Other fungi that must be eliminated from massages/spa clinics are *tinea pedis* (athlete's foot), *tinea corporis* (ringworm), *tinea capitis*, (scalp fungus), and *tinea cruris* (jock itch). Fungal skin infections are caused by dermatophytes that live on the skin surface proteins. They especially love to live under fingernails and toenails. These fungal infections are highly contagious and can be passed by direct skin-to-skin contact. They can also be passed by contact with the outside of massage crème bottles, unwashed or improperly stored sheets, damp floors and any pets that are allowed in the clinic area. Itching can cause skin breaks when fungal areas are scratched and gives an opportunity for a secondary infection to occur. Massage therapists must avoid contact with any areas of fungal growth when massaging a client.

Protozoa

Protozoa are the lowest forms of life in the animal world. They differ from most microorganisms in that they can move purposely on their own. Most protozoa are harmless and reside in soil and water, but several forms are parasitic and able to live within a host, causing discomfort and illness. Of these types, the ones that could infect clients and therapist are: *Entamoeba histolytica*, which causes amoebic dysentery; *Trichomonas vaginalis*, which can live on wet towels and causes infections of the male and female genital tracts; and *Giardia lamblia*, which can be transmitted by unwashed hands and causes a severe gastrointestinal infection.

Means of Infection Transmission

Transmission of diseases and infection occurs through various methods. Knowledge of the basic methods of transmission is important for all massage therapists. Special precautions must be taken with a client who has a **contagious disease** or infection in order to protect the massage practitioner and other clients from contracting the disease. A more detailed understanding of disease transmission and the cycle of infection is necessary for anyone working in a hospital, hospice, or large clinic setting.

Primary Transmission

EXAM POINT The primary means for transmission of diseases are through the environment, opportunistic infections, and person-to-person contact.

Although primary transmission methods seem to be similar, there are minor differences.

An **environmentally transmitted pathogen** is one that lives in the environment—in food, water, and soil—and is picked up from direct contact with these surfaces.

An **opportunistically transmitted pathogen** is one that naturally occurs on the skin and in mucous membranes, but changes in the body's "environment" render these pathogens disease-producing.

Person-to-person contact, including through any item handled by an infected person, is a common method of transmitting viruses such as colds and flu. Direct contact with an infected person's blood or other bodily fluid is in this category as well.

The Cycle of Infection

Medical guidelines further break down the means of transmission into five elements as a **cycle of infection**. These elements are a reservoir host, a means of exit from the host, a means of transmission, a means of entrance to another, and a susceptible host. At any time, this cycle of infection (figure 2.19) can be broken before the pathogen infects the new host and the cycle begins again. The reservoir (holding) host can be an animal or insect, as well as a human body. If the reservoir host does not provide a climate with the proper conditions, such as heat, moisture, or food, the cycle can stop at the host. If the host is a suitable breeding ground, however, then the pathogen can be spread to others. Sometimes hosts have no symptoms of infection and are not aware that they are a **carrier** of a disease- or infection-producing pathogen.

To continue the cycle, the pathogen must have a method of exit from the host. The most common such methods are:

- Exit through the nose, mouth, eyes, or ears, such as through a sneeze, cough, tears, or drainage.
- Exit through feces or urine.

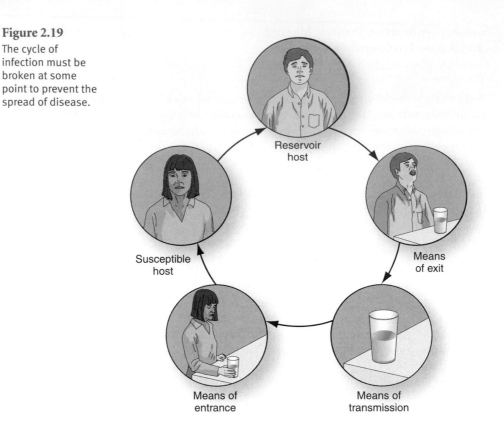

Reservoir host

Means of exit

Means of transmission

Means of entrance

Susceptible host

- Exit through sexual contact as in semen, vaginal fluid, or other discharge from the reproductive tract.
- Exit through blood or blood components in open wounds. Pathogens that are found in the blood and use blood loss or injury for transmission are called **blood-borne pathogens**.

After a pathogen has exited the host, it must spread to another host by transmission. When the infected host or discharges from the infected host come into contact with the new host, the process is called **direct transmission.** When the pathogen exits the host and lives or lies dormant outside a host, such as bacteria in a rain puddle or parasite eggs in carpet or sand, the resulting infection is called **indirect transmission**. Indirect transmission can occur when a susceptible host comes in contact with insects or objects such as towels, unclean massage table surfaces, and floors that are contaminated with the pathogen.

Airborne Transmission

Indirect transmission can also occur when a sneeze, cough, or speaking expels droplets into the air. We expel large volumes of air as we breathe. If you have seen the vapor from your breath when the air is cold, then you can understand how much and how far pathogens might travel.

Not only can we pick up influenza or other respiratory diseases from the air, but we can also inhale **microorganisms** from the soil, a cat litter box, or bird cage droppings. In some southern states, it is against the law to spit on a public street due to the high infection rates for tuberculosis in humid climates.

Blood-Borne Transmission

When a pathogen enters a new host through contact with blood or blood products, the transmission can be direct (through broken skin of one individual coming in contact with broken skin of another or blood splashing into the eyes or mucous linings of the nose or mouth). Another direct contact for blood-borne pathogens occurs when a mother transmits pathogens in her blood through the placenta to her fetus. Indirect blood-borne pathogen transmission occurs through blood transfusions, needle sticks, or improperly sterilized dental or surgical equipment.

Transmission by Ingestion

A new host may become infected by pathogens by eating food or drinking a liquid that has been **contaminated**. Food that has been handled by infected persons who do not practice safe hygiene may become contaminated. Such contamination can lead to serious disease processes. If you ingest food that contains *Escherichia coli* (**E. coli**) **bacteria**, food poisoning could occur. Parasites that cause diarrhea, bloating, weight loss, and fatigue can be ingested from poorly washed foods. Bacteria-contaminated seafood that is ingested can lead to paralysis or even death. Water sources must also be thoroughly clean as *E. coli* can reside inside faucets, on sloppily washed dishes, or in water pools around a hand-washing basin. Spa equipment such as pedicure tanks, facial treatment towels, and face cradles on massage tables and chairs can harbor bacteria and viruses that grow in moist areas.

Transmission by Touch

Transmission by touch is of grave concern for massage therapists because of the amount of touch associated with a massage. Every time skin-to-skin contact is made, bacteria and other organisms are passed. If the bacteria are harmless or if the recipient has skin that is intact, then no harm is done. If, however, the skin is open or broken out and draining, a transmission can occur. Some species of **streptococci bacteria** can actually live on the surface of intact skin and cause skin eruptions that spread. You may also become infected if you touch items (such as table surfaces) that have been touched by an infected person or if you drink from the same glass or cup.

Persons with **sexually transmitted diseases (STDs)** transfer the pathogens when they come in contact with mucous membranes (such as those that line the mouth, nose, penis, vagina, urethra, or anus). STDs may also be transmitted to a fetus through the placenta or the birth canal.

Means of Entrance to a New Host

Without a way to enter a new host, the pathogen that is transmitted can go no farther. Pathogens can enter the new host through mucous membranes—such as the mouth, nose, eyes, throat, penis, vagina, or rectum—or they can enter the intestinal tract, urinary tract, or reproductive tract. The most common method of entry is through breaks in the skin. Our hands travel over many surfaces throughout the day. Hands then find their way into our mouths, on objects or food that enters the mouth, or onto other areas of our bodies or the bodies of others that may have skin breaks.

★ **EXAM POINT** For these reasons, the most common method of transmission and infection is through the hands.

The End of the Cycle: Susceptible Host

The last element in the cycle of infection is that of the susceptible host. If the person that the pathogen is transmitted to has a limited immunity to infection, then the pathogen has a new home. If the person has a healthy immune system, the infection cycle will cease. Some of the factors that determine **susceptibility** include the person's overall health, age, genetic predisposition, nutritional status, other disease processes already present (such as AIDS or diabetes), stress levels, and hygiene habits.

Incubation

The pathogen has some factors of its own that regulate its ability to infect, such as number, virulence (strength), and point of entry. When the new host becomes infected, the cycle begins again. The type of pathogen sets the rate of speed of transmission and infection. The amount of time between exposure and infection of a pathogen and the first occurrence of symptoms of disease varies and is called the **incubation period**. Chickenpox usually takes from 7 to 21 days between infection and symptoms; tuberculosis has an incubation period of 4 to 12 weeks. Some tropical diseases have an incubation period of less than 12 hours. The longer the incubation time, the less likely it is to pinpoint where or how the pathogen was transmitted to the infected person.

Methods of Decontamination

Although it is neither possible nor necessary to remove all pathogens from the massage facility, you must at least maintain a sanitary level. There are three levels of decontamination: sterilization, disinfection, and sanitation.

Sterilization is the most thorough process for removing pathogens. This process destroys all living organisms on surfaces and equipment, including the spores of bacteria. Sterilization is seldom necessary within a massage practice; however, if you are involved in therapeutic treatment in a hospital or hospice setting—especially with sports injuries that require surgery—you will need to know about sterile technique.

Disinfection is the next level of decontamination and is nearly as effective as sterilization. Disinfection will destroy most viruses, fungi, and bacteria but will not usually kill bacterial spores. Professional-strength disinfectant solutions must be used safely and always according to the manufacturer's guidelines. Disinfectants are not to be used on the body or as hand cleaners because they may damage the skin or cause irritation if inhaled or splashed into the eyes. Common disinfectants used in a clinical setting are phenols such as Lysol®, chlorine bleach in a 10% solution, and 70% alcohol.

★ **EXAM POINT** For massage therapists, following universal precautions requires using gloves and masks. Most important, though, be sure to use a 10% bleach solution, which is made by adding one part bleach to nine parts water.

The 10% bleach solution must be mixed daily to be effective because the strength of the solution diminishes with time. As with all potentially dangerous products, disinfectants must be stored away from food or water and kept out of the reach of clients and children.

Sanitation is the third level of decontamination and is the method used in all massage clinics and public facilities. Sanitation involves removing pathogens on a surface by cleaning with soap and general detergents. Hand washing is considered a form of sanitation, as is using antibacterial soaps. Make sure you read the directions carefully as some soaps and detergents may discolor or damage surfaces.

Universal and Standard Precautions

Universal precautions are rules and guidelines set forth by the U.S. Department of Health and Human Services Centers for Disease Control. They are mandated by the Occupational Safety and Health Act (OSHA). These rules to protect health workers are designed to save lives and prevent injury. Universal precautions apply to blood and blood products, human tissue, semen, vaginal secretions, saliva (if it contains blood), other bodily fluids, and breast milk from mothers who are HIV-positive. Because they apply mostly to blood-borne pathogens, there is no real need to follow universal precautions in most massage practice settings.

Standard precautions are generally used by hospitals and medical clinical settings. These precautions apply to blood, all bodily fluids, secretions, and excretions (except sweat), nonintact skin, and mucous membranes.

Within the massage setting, you only need to disinfect equipment, add bleach to laundry, store laundry in air-tight containers to prevent bacterial spores and fungi from growing, and wash your hands vigilantly. Wear disposable nonlatex gloves when cleaning up any potentially contaminated area. Figure 2.20 details how to don disposable gloves. These gloves are worn only once and then discarded. It is also important to properly remove the disposable gloves (figure 2.21) and thoroughly wash your hands.

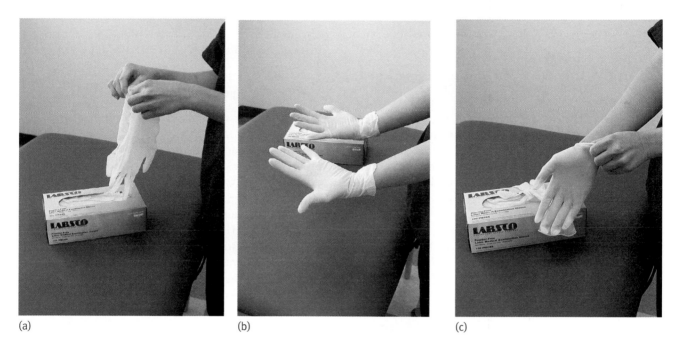

(a)   (b)   (c)

Figure 2.20

(a) Don gloves. *(b)* Make sure that your gloves have no holes and are free of tears. *(c)* Make sure that the gloves are the correct size. They shouldn't pull tight against the skin; the glove must cover your wrist.

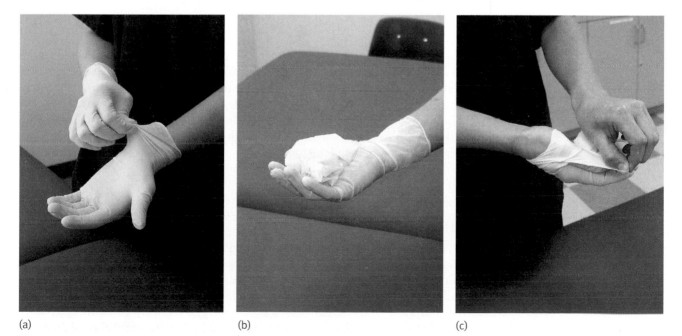

(a)   (b)   (c)

Figure 2.21

(a) Grasping above the cuff, pull off one glove. *(b)* Place the glove you removed in the center of the gloved hand. *(c)* Remove the other glove while still holding the removed glove in the center of the gloved hand by slipping the fingers under the cuff next to the skin. Throw away the used gloves.

Health Crises

Some of the potentially fatal diseases that massage therapists must be fully informed of are AIDS/HIV, hepatitis, SARS, and tuberculosis. Knowledge of such diseases will help you to be prepared when working with clients who are either infected or at risk of being infected with these diseases.

AIDS/HIV

Acquired immunodeficiency syndrome (AIDS) is a fatal disease that can be transmitted from one person to another through body fluids.

> ⭐ **EXAM POINT** AIDS is caused by human immunodeficiency virus (HIV).

Since viruses are only capable of replicating (multiplying) while inside a living cell, the HIV pathogen invades the cells and transforms them into reproducing agents to produce more of the virus and invade the entire body. HIV prefers to invade the white blood cells (lymphocytes) that defend the body from infection. The cells are tricked into recognizing the virus as a normal component, so the body's natural defense mechanism, the lymphocytes, do not attack or contain the virus. The immune deficiency caused by the virus depletes the lymphocytes and causes the immune system to collapse, making the body susceptible to any **opportunistic infection** it encounters. Therefore, it is most important that you do not perform a massage on a client with AIDS if you are sick with a cold, flu, pneumonia, or shingles. These common illnesses can be fatal to a client with a weakened or nonexistent immune system.

Everyone is susceptible to HIV infection. A rapid HIV test is being developed, but at this time, there is no vaccination that will prevent AIDS.

> ⭐ **EXAM POINT** Since HIV is transmitted by bodily fluids such as whole blood or blood components, semen, seminal fluid, saliva, and vaginal secretions that have blood within them, the best plan of action is to treat all bodily fluids you come in contact with as a possible source.

Many of your clients—even coworkers and close friends—may have been infected with HIV. Infected persons are sometimes not aware that they have been infected, or if they are aware, they may not be willing to share the information. The Centers for Disease Control and Prevention recommends that you take universal precautions when coming into contact with any bodily fluids. Body fluids such as sweat, tears, and urine without the presence of blood or semen usually do not transmit HIV. The World Health Organization has documented the transmission of HIV to infants who are breast feeding, so it may be wise to use universal precautions if breast milk is present on linens or equipment.

Hepatitis: Type B and Type C

Hepatitis is an infection of the liver that is caused by a virus. This virus causes cell destruction and the failure of the liver to function properly. At present, hepatitis types A, B, C, D, E, and G have been identified and named. There is no virus named Type F. Type A is usually transmitted by organisms found in human or animal wastes that contaminate food sources—most often unclean water. Seafood taken from contaminated water is responsible for most of the Type A hepatitis cases in North America. Type A can be treated, and the liver will repair itself, leaving the body immune from contracting the infection again. Types B and C are of greatest concern to massage therapists as they can be more easily transmitted by human contact. Scientists continue to research hepatitis and are likely to uncover other viruses in the hepatitis family, as well as more information on types D, E, and G.

Hepatitis B (HBV) is transmitted through contact with an infected person's body fluids. HBV is slow to respond to treatment and leads to liver damage and sometimes cancer. A vaccination is available for HBV; all individuals who are likely to come into direct contact with clients should be vaccinated. Hepatitis C (HCV) also causes cancer and at this time cannot be prevented by vaccination or cured. It is transmitted in the same manner as HBV. An HBV vaccination is required in most states for all allied health care workers. It is mandated by OSHA that all persons working within a medical clinic, spa, or athletic facility be certified by the local health department as being free of blood-borne pathogens. Before beginning to practice, make sure you visit your local health department to see what regulations regarding blood-borne pathogens might apply to you. If you are infected, you must let your state health officer know and follow the state regulations regarding where and how you are allowed to work.

SARS

Severe acute respiratory syndrome (SARS) causes respiratory failure; it is sometimes fatal and extremely contagious. SARS is caused by viruses associated with the common cold as well as by viruses as yet unidentified. It can be prevented by thoroughly washing your hands, wearing a mask, and avoiding exposure to an individual who is infected. At this time, no vaccination exists for SARS; treatment primarily consists of rest and antiviral drugs. The World Heath Organization believes that SARS will regularly make an appearance around the world, but no one knows what may be the future of this illness. Over the past decade, many diseases such as SARS that were prevalent in Asia or in tropical rain forests have made their way into the rest of the world courtesy of travelers. Massage therapists who work on cruise lines or in resort areas may be at an increased risk of possible infection and must be very diligent in using precautionary measures to prevent disease transmission.

TB

Mycobacterium tuberculosis (TB) is the bacteria responsible for the respiratory disease known as tuberculosis. This disease is still quite common, especially in southern climates, where hot, damp temperatures increase TB's ability to spread. Tuberculosis is most commonly transmitted through inhalation of airborne droplets from a sneeze or cough. However, close contact with the breath or sputum of an infected person can also cause contamination. Most allied health professionals, including massage therapists, are required to be tested routinely. The testing (sometimes called a TB tine test) involves an injection under the skin and then a reading of the results at the injection site after three to four days.

Therapeutic Value and Confidentiality Issues

The diseases discussed in this chapter can be devastating physically and emotionally to the infected individuals. Massage is of high therapeutic value in treating some of the physical pain and loss of physical strength associated with the disease processes. Many infected persons no longer receive touch and possibly may not be supported emotionally by their friends or family members. The benefits of massage offered by a compassionate massage therapist will help them deal with depression, stress, and fear. Before attempting massage on these persons, evaluate your own feelings and value systems concerning the diseases. Honestly examine your comfort level. Remember that individuals with AIDS are protected under the Americans with Disabilities Act, and any information regarding their condition, even a phone message or SOAP Note, must be handled with the utmost confidentiality.

Chapter Summary

There is more to setting up your massage practice than buying and setting up a table. Every detail must be considered. Color, lighting, linens, and music all play an integral part in creating the total massage experience. Be mindful that it is often the little things that count. Always strive to provide your client with that little extra that makes your massage worth remembering and coming back for time and again.

Be diligent in protecting the client and yourself at all times: obtain the knowledge required to enable you to practice safely. You can also use this knowledge to educate your clients on safe health and hygiene practices. Knowing where and how harm can occur and acting to prevent or limit the possibility of disease transmission and accidental injury are your responsibilities.

Applying Your Knowledge

Self-Testing

1. What is the *single* most effective deterrent to spreading disease?
   a) Heat
   b) Blue light
   c) Use of fans
   d) Hand washing

2. The 10% bleach solution for cleaning is made by using:
   a) 10% bleach and 90% white vinegar.
   b) 10% bleach and 50% water.
   c) 10% bleach and 90% water.
   d) 10% bleach and 10% bleach.

3. Lubricants are used to:
   a) reduce friction on the skin.
   b) help the massage go faster.
   c) keep the client's skin soft.
   d) All of the above are correct.

4. What are the four common categories of lubricants?
   a) Oil, lotion, water, wax
   b) Oils, creams, gels, lotions
   c) Vegetable oils, fruit oils, mineral oils, baby oils
   d) None of the above is correct.

5. Which grouping represents positions on the table?
   a) Prone, supine, side-lying
   b) Prone, supine, upside-down
   c) Side-lying, kneeling, standing
   d) Sitting, prone, supine, kneeling

6. A portable heat source to be used on your clients is a
   _____.
   a) Hydrocollator pack.
   b) Thermophore.
   c) Fomentek.
   d) b and c

7. Which disinfectant can be used to clean the massage room?
   a) Antibacterial wipes
   b) Lysol or Pinesol
   c) 10% bleach solution
   d) All of the above are correct.

8. What element is part of a *safe* massage room?
   a) Ceramic tile floors
   b) Extension cords
   c) Good lighting
   d) Used linens stored under the table

9. What is acceptable as a face cradle cover?
   a) Pillow case
   b) Hand towel
   c) Precut disposable cloths
   d) All of the above are correct.

10. What colors are considered healing colors?
    a) Greens
    b) Reds
    c) Violets
    d) a and c

Case Studies / Critical Thinking

A. *You plan to start a massage practice near a retirement community. What factors do you need to consider when purchasing equipment (table, etc.) for your practice?*

B. *Jim, a massage therapist in a spa facility, noticed a slimy, greenish substance floating on the surface of the water in the hydrotherapy tub. He was in a hurry to place his client into the tub since his next client was waiting. He skimmed the substance from the water with a paper cup and called his client into the room. He assisted his client into the tub, and after checking the temperature of the water, he left the room to complete his SOAP Notes. What was Jim's first mistake? Does Jim have a time/scheduling problem?*

Should he check the water temperature before his client gets in? What should Jim do to prevent a dirty hydrotherapy tub? Is it wise to leave clients unattended while they are using equipment? List the health and safety hazards apparent in this situation.

C. While rubbing on hand sanitizer, Ella felt a burning sensation and noticed scratches on her hands that probably came from playing with her new kitten. She washed off the sanitizer and applied lotion to stop the burning, then readied her room for her next client. Ms. Jacobs, her client, has an abraded rash covering her abdomen and shoulders. What should Ella do to protect herself and her client from contact with broken skin? Should Ella be more careful with her hands since she uses them in her profession? Should Ella touch a client with her scratched, bare hands, even if they do not have evidence of skin infections? How should she prepare before going from performing a massage on this client to the next massage?

References for information in this chapter can be found in Quick Guide C at the end of the book.

CHAPTER 3

The Massage Therapy Session

LEARNING OUTCOMES

After completing this chapter, you will be able to:

- Effectively communicate with the client before, during, and after the massage.
- Understand proper draping and positioning procedures.
- Properly use client intake and history forms.
- Perform a postural analysis.
- Write clear and clinically effective SOAP Notes.
- Create an effective treatment plan.
- Properly conduct a posttreatment assessment.
- Recognize the common medical abbreviations that massage therapists are most likely to encounter.
- Manage physician referrals.
- Understand procedures for filing insurance claims.

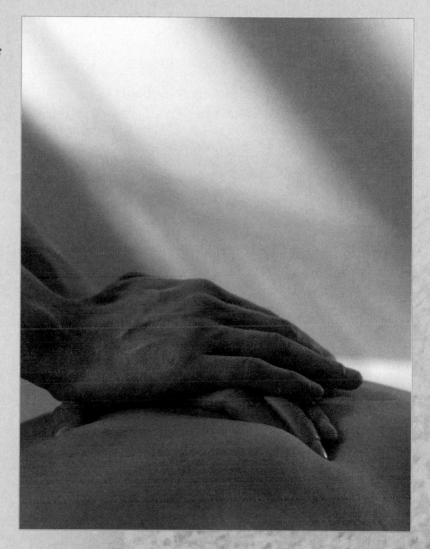

KEY TERMS

abbreviations and acronyms *(p. 66)*

assignment of benefits
  claim form *(p. 71)*

benefits *(p. 70)*

carrier *(p. 71)*

coinsurance *(p. 72)*

co-pay *(p. 72)*

Current Procedural Terminology
  (CPT) *(p. 72)*

deductible *(p. 72)*

entrainment *(p. 60)*

health insurance claim *(p. 70)*

hold harmless clause *(p. 70)*

International Classification of
  Diseases, Ninth Revision,
  Clinical Modification
  (ICD9-CM) *(p. 72)*

kyphosis *(p. 59)*

lordosis *(p. 59)*

physician or doctor referral *(p. 68)*

preauthorization *(p. 70)*

prefix *(p. 68)*

scoliosis *(p. 59)*

suffix *(p. 68)*

INTRODUCTION

The massage table is prepared with linens, the music has been selected, and the lights are set: you are ready for the client. Whether or not this is the first time you have seen this client, there are standard questions to be asked each time. You will need to inquire about any change in health—including any new cuts or bruises, changes in medications, and worsening or improvement in medical conditions.

The Massage Therapy Session

Greeting the Client

Introduce yourself in a kind yet professional tone of voice (figure 3.1). The first question to ask is: "Have you ever had a massage before?" The three possible answers will dictate the next step. If the client responds, "No, never," you will need to explain what massage is, what it can do, what it cannot do, and describe in detail the procedure you will follow. New clients should fill out a detailed client intake form that will give you knowledge of their medical history and current concerns. An example of a simplified intake form is found in figure 3.2; a client history form with SOAP Notes is detailed in figure 3.10 (p. 65).

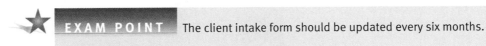

★ **EXAM POINT** The client intake form should be updated every six months.

The second possible answer to your initial question is, "Yes, once or twice." This response usually is indicative of someone who has received a gift certificate for a massage;

Figure 3.1

Introduce yourself in a warm manner to set the tone for the client interview.

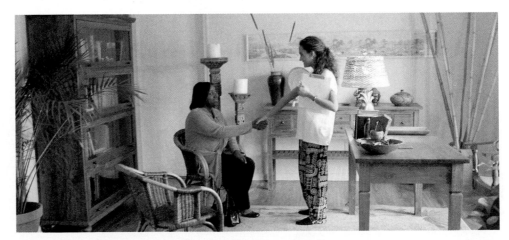

CLIENT INTAKE FORM

NAME _____ DATE _____

Address _____

Phone _____ Cell Phone/pager _____

Email _____

Occupation _____

Referred by _____

Physician _____

Are you currently being treated?_____

Are you taking any medications, if so, what?_____

HAVE YOU HAD ANY OF THE FOLLOWING DURING THE PAST YEAR?

__SEVERE HEADACHE__FAINTING__DIZZINESS__CHEST PAINS__HEART PROBLEMS
__NUMBNESS/TINGLING OR SWELLING IN HANDS/FEET__HIGH/LOW BLOOD PRESSURE
__PREGNANT__HERNIATED DISCS__OTHER

Is this a result of an auto accident or work related? _____

I AM SEEKING TREATMENT FOR: _____

Have you ever had a massage before?_____

How often? _____

I hereby request and consent to massage therapy and any other therapies that are included within the scope of the professional treating me. I understand I will be receiving massage for therapeutic reasons and understand there are some risks to treatment including—but not limited to—soreness, bruises, and inflammatory pain. I do not expect the therapist to be able to anticipate or explain all risks and complications, and wish to rely on the therapist to exercise reasonable skill during the course of treatment.

I understand that massage therapy may involve some undressing. I understand that at all times the therapist will abide by my wishes with regards to my comfort level of undress. I also understand that I can request an area not to be treated or exposed.

I have read, or have had read to me, the above consent. I have also had the opportunity to ask questions regarding its content, and by signing below I agree to the above named procedures. I intend this consent form to cover treatment for my present, as well as all future conditions (and will notify therapist of such).

PATIENT'S SIGNATURE _____

Figure 3.2 A basic client intake form

they have experienced a massage but are probably not familiar with massage. You will still need to get a detailed client history, inquire what the chief complaint is (the reason for coming), and give some basic instructions for the procedure.

The third possible answer comes from someone who gets a massage regularly, say once a week or a couple times a month. A client intake form is filled out and the reason for the visit is determined. Since the client is knowledgeable about massage (having received it regularly), less time may be needed giving specific information (such as the benefits of massage and detailed instructions). Keep in mind, however, that the client will be new to you and your massage methodology, so be sure to cover specifics on the modality (or modalities) you work with and the procedure you follow for delivering the massage. With returning clients, it is not necessary to repeatedly fill out client intake forms; instead, you need only, and document, any changes since their last visit.

Draping and Positioning During the Massage

After the interview, you will be leave the room to allow your client to disrobe and get onto the table. Wait an appropriate amount of time, knock on the door, and ask if the person is ready for you to enter the room. Over time, you will be able to gauge what an appropriate amount of time will be for each individual—but always knock first and get permission to enter the room. Also, make sure you tell your client that the amount of undressing is up to them (undergarments on or off) and offer specific instructions for getting on the table (such as sit first, then lie down, rather than crawling onto the table on their knees).

Clients likely will not be familiar with the terms *prone* (face down) and *supine* (face up). Before you leave the room, if you are starting prone, tell them to lay face down on their stomach with their face in the face cradle (patting the face cradle as you do so) under the top drape (sheet or towel). If the bolster is already positioned at the end of the table, tell them it is for the ankles as new clients may mistake the ankle bolster for a pillow. Especially if you are starting in the prone position, be careful when you reenter the room that you do not startle the person with an abrupt touch. Keep in mind that when prone, the client cannot see you and therefore will not be aware of when you are beginning the massage. As you reenter the room, it is best to ask if the client is comfortable and mention you will adjust the drape or place heat on their back. In that way, the client will be aware of your presence and ready for your touch. You certainly do not want to start off your massage session with a startled client. With the client in the prone position, adjust the face cradle for comfort to the cervical spine and place a bolster under the ankles.

> **TECHNIQUE EMPHASIS**   For clients who easily get sinus congestion from lying prone, try the following techniques: adjust the face cradle a little higher, tilt the head end of the table up if using a hydraulic table, omit the use of the face cradle and allow the client's head to be turned sideways on the table, or even use a drop of peppermint oil on a tissue placed on the floor under the face cradle.

If starting in the supine position, place a pillow under the neck and a bolster under the knees to take pressure off the low back. For clients with postural deviations, see Procedure 3.1 for recommended bolstering; for pregnant women, refer to chapter 10.

Take great measures to keep your client adequately covered at all times to ensure privacy and warmth. First-time clients may be a bit tentative and require extra care and concern with draping. It is a good idea to explain to them that they will be covered at all times with only the single body part being worked on (such as a leg or an arm) being uncovered and then recovered at any given time. With respect to choice of draping materials, here is where you will recognize the importance of the large bath sheet or flat sheet. Both of these options will provide sufficient material to wrap around any body part, such as a leg or arm, that is being stretched.

With the client in the prone position, fold the towel or sheet back off the leg to the upper thigh, leaving the buttocks covered, and tuck the excess drape under the other leg (figure 3.3). In the United States, we always keep both women's and men's breasts covered as well as the abdomen and buttocks. To perform abdominal massage or work on the intercostals, a small towel is placed over the breasts while the larger towel or sheet is folded down to the navel or slightly below; the gluteals can be worked on over the drape or with the drape folded back slightly. To work on the back, fold the drape back to the low back area. If an undergarment is being worn, tuck the drape just under the edge of the garment; this keeps the drape in place and the garment protected from damage by lubricants.

With the client in the supine position (as with the legs in prone), fold the drape over to mid- or upper thigh and tuck the excess under the other leg. Place the arms on top of the drape, tucking the drape under the armpit to secure it over the chest; this allows for work on arms, upper chest (under the clavicle), neck, and head.

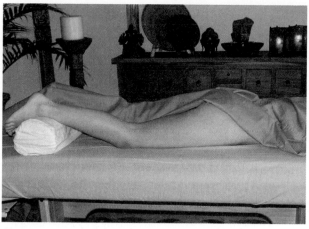
(a)

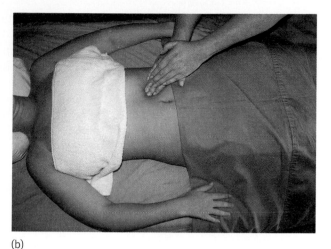
(b)

Figure 3.3

(*a*) Undrape only the body part being worked on. (*b*) Cover breast area with a small towel to access intercostals and abdominals.

P R O C E D U R E   3.1   Special Bolstering for Postural Deviations

Kyphosis—an exaggerated curvature of the thoracic spine commonly seen in elderly people (figure 3.4): In prone position, place a bolster under the chest. In supine position, place bolsters under the arms and neck.

    Lordosis—an exaggerated curvature of the lumbar spine, known as "swayback" (figure 3.5): In prone position, place a half-round bolster under the hips.

Scoliosis—an exaggerated S or C curve in the cervical, thoracic, or lumbar spine (figure 3.6), named for the convexity or the side the curve bends away from. For example, a right thoracic curve has the curve bending away from the right side. Bolstering is according to each client's needs. If there is a "rib hump" on one side, a rolled-up towel or small bolster may need to be placed under the shoulder for support in prone and supine positions.

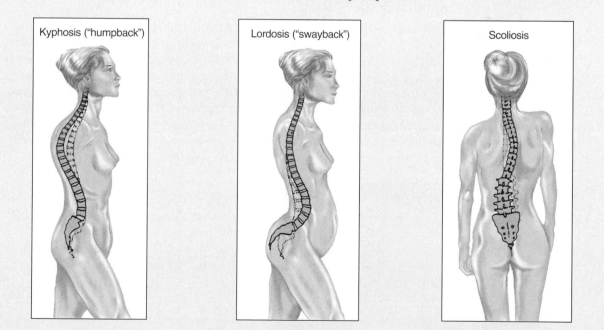

Figure 3.4 Kyphosis spinal deviation
This is also known as "humpback."

Figure 3.5 Lordosis spinal deviation
This is also known as "swayback."

Figure 3.6 Scoliosis spinal deviation

In the side-lying position, used for specific work on IT Bands, pregnant women, and people with postural deviations, the client is positioned on one side, bottom leg straight and top leg bent and placed on a bolster; a small neck pillow is helpful. It may be advantageous to use a sheet or two towels for top drapes to maintain privacy.

Large-breasted women or women with implants may be made more comfortable by using a special breast cushion (see chapter 2) or a rolled-up towel. Pregnant women should be placed in a side-lying position with a bolster under the top leg or between the legs (see chapters 2 and 10). Persons with postural deviations such as kyphosis or lordosis should be made comfortable with the bolster (see Procedure 3.1 for suggestions on bolster placement).

Remember that whatever bolstering or support is needed can be accomplished with prefab bolsters, pillows, or rolled towels. It is important that the client be comfortable as well as supported and in a safe position.

Communicating Throughout the Massage

Check with the client during the massage to make sure you are meeting his or her needs. You will want to know if the pressure is correct and if you are addressing the chief complaint. Often clients are reluctant to say anything during the massage. Watch for signs of discomfort, such as clenched fists or holding the breath. Some people think that since you are the professional, you know what is best.

Allow the client to guide you in regards to conversation. If the client wants to talk, respond in kind. If the client is silent, respect that and do not talk unless you need clarification on something you are doing (see chapter 20 concerning acceptable conversation). Remember to maintain your focus and intent throughout the massage.

As you move through the massage, pay attention to your breathing as well as that of your client. Truly artful massage therapists fall in sync with their client: breathing becomes relaxed and rhythmic; movements become fluid and effortless; and a delightful symbiotic relationship issues forth. Some texts refer to this occurrence as **entrainment**, or synchronization to a rhythm.

Completing the Massage

On completion of the massage, pause for a moment and sit quietly. This gives a nice finish to the massage. Depending on your philosophical or spiritual inclinations, you may silently offer a prayer. Tell the client you are finished and recommend that he or she take time in getting up and dressing. A considerate touch is to have water available; be sure to explain it is beneficial to drink water after a massage to flush out toxins released by work on the muscles and to help alleviate soreness. Before leaving the room, instruct your client on the proper (safe for the back) way to get up and off the table. Explain that he should roll over onto his side; use the upper arm to push the torso up off the table, coming into a sitting position; then drop the legs off the side of the table.

 TECHNIQUE EMPHASIS Mention they should sit quietly for a moment on the table before coming onto their feet. Realize that your client may be a little light-headed, although you do not want to alarm them with that suggestion. If you are working on someone who needs assistance getting up from the table, help them while making sure the drape is fully covering their torso and leave the room only after they are safely in a seated position.

In an outside room, ask your clients for feedback: what they liked; what in particular they enjoyed; what, if anything, did not suit them. Remind them that your intent for the massage was to address their needs, and you would like to design subsequent sessions especially for them. Even if you are a recent graduate, no doubt you have been exposed to, and had practice with, many types of massage. Your experience with a variety

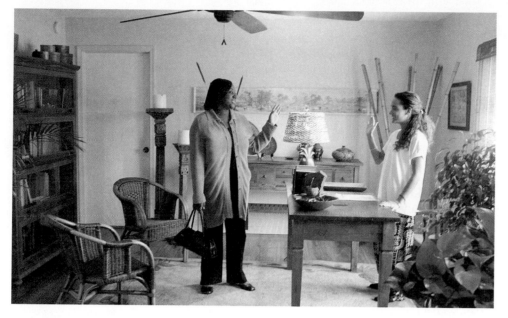

of techniques will serve you well in choreographing a routine. As mentioned in the two modality chapters (chapters 15 and 16), therapists and clients alike have an affinity for one type of massage or another. The more you are acquainted with different types of massage, the better you will be able to meet any client's needs.

Always try to schedule the next appointment before the clients leave (figure 3.7). Thank them for their patronage.

TECHNIQUE EMPHASIS Many therapists will follow up the session with a call the next day to see how the client is doing.

Always tell clients to feel free to call you if they have any questions about the massage or the effects they are experiencing afterward (also see the section on SOAP Notes in this chapter). Again, handle the business end of the massage in a room other than the massage room. Acceptable forms of payment or compensation are currency, personal checks, or credit cards. Be aware, however, that accepting a credit card for payment requires you have a contract with a bank's merchant services department. This usually is profitable only if you do a larger volume of business or also sell products, such as in a spa.

Assessment

It is advantageous for any massage therapist to learn basic orthopedic assessment. This knowledge will aid you in determining whether or not you should work on a particular client or refer that person to another therapist.

Thorough knowledge of skeletal and muscular systems, biomechanics, and kinesiology will help you address muscular problems that you may be able to work on. A good massage therapist must understand how the body works: what muscles produce specific movements. For example, if you determine through basic questioning that the client experiences pain when lifting the arm up and you know that the supraspinatus muscle is responsible for initiating this movement (from 0 to 15 degrees), then you can better assess and design a plan of action (treatment plan). Keep this in mind as you proceed through your particular course of instruction; begin to get an idea of what you are observing in someone's posture and build on this as you gain more detailed knowledge of the skeletal and muscular systems, biomechanics, and kinesiology.

A Client's File

The following information should be included in any client file: Client Intake/History form, Postural Analysis, SOAP Notes, written narrative, and physician prescription or referral. Each of these items alone is important; all of these documents together allow for proper treatment for the client. Some or all of these documents make it possible for you to work with a team of health care providers (including keeping other therapists up-to-date on a particular client if more than one therapist is on the team) and to adequately file for insurance reimbursement. Further, these documents will support your testimony, should you be asked to give a deposition or testify in court.

Client Intake/History Forms

New clients will fill out a detailed form providing contact information, insurance information if applicable, referring physician, medical history, reasons for getting a massage, and any other information or documentation that may play a role in the decision to receive massage. This form usually clearly defines the massage process, expectations, and possible ramifications (such as bruising), and includes an area for a signature (signature of parent or guardian if the client is a minor) and date. Figure. 3.2 shows an example of such a form.

Postural Analysis

One of the first things a massage therapist learns to recognize is how a client walks into the office or treatment room. Does the client enter the room with an air of strength and confidence, suggesting tone and flexibility, or bent over, walking with one shoulder "leading" the other, or feet turned out or in? All of these observations suggest specific postural imbalance due to shortened or contracted muscles—muscles that may be that way because of injury, compensation, or even the stresses of everyday life. One shoulder leading the other may suggest contracted pectoralis or a more severe spinal deviation, while feet pointing out may indicate tight lateral rotators.

You will want to do a postural analysis (figure 3.8) on the first visit to help identify such problem areas. A follow-up postural analysis should also be done after a number of treatments.

Figure 3.8
A postural analysis is a useful element of the client intake.

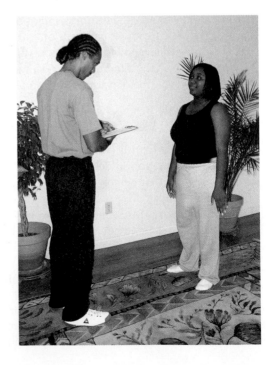

Client's name: Date of postural analysis: Massage therapist's name:	
	Notes
1. ac joint to ac joint:	
2. inferior angle of scapula to inferior angle of scapula:	
3. iliac crest to iliac crest:	
4. spine (curvature or other deviation):	
5. ASIS to opposite ASIS:	
6. ASIS to PSIS:	
7. body alignment (posture):	
8. cervical spine (curvature):	
9. leg length (lying supine on table) • knee comparison: • ankle comparison:	

Figure 3.9 A sample format for performing postural analysis

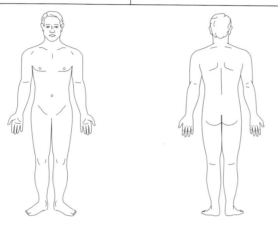

Look at the client as a whole, and then break your observations down into measurable sections. Refer to figure 3.9 for a sample form to use in assessing your clients. See Procedure 3.2 for details of a simple format to follow. In some states, massage therapists may not perform a formal postural analysis, so they learn to eyeball clients. Whether or not you conduct a formal analysis, you should continually hone your observation skills. After practicing postural analysis on other students in school, you will find it second nature to look at every body this way—on the beach, at the mall, or anywhere you can observe people.

Always compare both sides of the body. If you notice a difference, ask the client if there are any preexisting conditions or injuries that may account for the difference. If the client has a problem, such as limited range of motion in the right shoulder, palpate for differences in the muscles of the affected side and the unaffected side, and perform basic muscle testing on all of the muscles or groups of muscles that affect the shoulder for strength and range of motion. All of these findings should be included in the observation section of your SOAP Notes.

SOAP Notes

No matter where you work—in a spa, a clinic, or your own office or—you will want to become proficient in writing SOAP Notes. SOAP is an acronym for *s*ubjective *o*bjective, *a*ssessment (or *a*ction taken) *p*lan. SOAP Notes should be used to chart all massage and bodywork sessions with every client with whom you work, even outcalls. Make sure you bring Client Intake/History forms with you to a client's house. Either have a SOAP Note

PROCEDURE 3.2 Postural Analysis

(Ask client to remove shoes and stand in bare feet.)

1. Check acromioclavicular (ac) joint to opposite ac joint by standing behind the client, placing index fingers on each ac joint.

2. Check inferior angle of scapula to inferior angle of opposite scapula by placing index fingers on point.

3. Check iliac crest to opposite iliac crest by placing thumbs on left and right.

4. Check if spine is curved or rotated by asking the client to bend forward; run fingers down spinous process from superior to inferior.

5. Check anterior superior iliac spine (ASIS) to opposite ASIS to detect elevation or rotation by placing thumbs on left and right.

6. Check anterior superior iliac spine (ASIS) to posterior superior iliac spine (PSIS) by placing fingertips on anterior and posterior iliac spine. (Note: Males have a 0 to 5 degree tilt; females have a 5 to 10 degree tilt.)

7. View the client from the side and check that the following are lined up (one on top of another):
   - Ear is over the shoulder.
   - Shoulder is over the hip.
   - Hip is over the knee.
   - Knee is over the ankle.

8. Check cervical spine for unevenness between C1 and occiput by placing the thumbs against the occipital ridge.

9. Ask client to lie supine on the massage table. Check for leg-length discrepancies by comparing both legs:
   - Check patella to opposite patella by placing thumbs on top of the kneecap.
   - Check ankle to opposite ankle by holding heels in your hands with thumbs on lateral ankle.

with you or a composition book with stitched binding to record date, time, and notes (spiral or loose-leaf binders are not accepted in court).

SOAP Notes serve several purposes: they allow another therapist to assume treatment of the client if you are not available, they keep physicians informed of a client's progress, and they are legal documents that may be used in a court of law.

Subjective is what the client tells you; for example, "my right shoulder hurts."

Objective is what you observe. Take into account everything you notice about the client from gestures to a formal postural analysis. Remember to note all findings in this section: anything found during palpation (e.g., right supraspinatus palpates as hypertonic), any observations of gait (how the client walks), any change in range of motion (e.g., right shoulder has decreased or limited range of motion), and anything found during muscle testing (e.g., right supraspinatus and middle deltoid test weak on abduction). (See chapter 6 for a discussion on gait and movements and chapter 13 for a discussion of active and passive range of motion and muscle testing.)

Assessment/action is the combination of **S** and **O**, or your deductive reasoning of the facts in front of you. If this is the second (or more) time you have seen this client, **A** can also represent the action you took last session.

Plan is the treatment plan you have formulated for a specified amount of time.

As with Client Intake/History forms, there are a variety of SOAP Note formats. You will find them within this text (see figures 3.2 and 3.10), as well as in various medical software programs. Refer to figure 3.10 for a sample client history form with SOAP Notes included. This version is a good practice format for writing SOAP Notes. You may adapt your own format based on this and any other forms that work well for you.

Figure 3.10 This client intake form includes SOAP Notes.

```
CLIENT HISTORY FORM WITH SOAP NOTES

Client Name:_____ Date:_____

Address:_____

_____

Date of Birth:_____

Referred by:_____

Physician Name:_____


S:  CHIEF COMPLAINT:

      ONSET

      DURATION

      PAIN LEVEL (Scale 1-10)


      WHAT INCR/DECR PAIN

      PAST MEDICAL HX (that may have an impact on chief complaint)

      FAMILY MEDICAL HX (that may have an impact on chief complaint)

      ACTIVITIES OF DAILY LIVING (ADLs)

O:  ROM

      STRENGTH

      GAIT

A:  ASSESSMENT/ACTION


P:  PLAN/TREATMENT

      MODALITIES

      EDUCATION

      FREQUENCY
```

Making Corrections

Many states have specific policies for handling medical errors as well as required notation for legal documents. As a massage professional, it is essential that you keep clear and accurate records. You rarely will have any extended length of time to write SOAP Notes; most often, you are writing in between clients. Therefore, it is critical that you familiarize yourself with medical abbreviations as well as how to properly correct any mistakes that you may make in client SOAP Notes.

A list of common medical abbreviations for massage therapists is found in the medical terminology section of this chapter.

EXAM POINT Should you make a mistake—such as a misspelling—strike through the mistake with a single line, put your intials next to it, and circle *your initials*. Use of "white-out" or correction tape is absolutely forbidden.

PROCEDURE 3.3 Narrative Report

Clinical Report for: *Jane Smith*
Seeking Treatment for: *Right shoulder pain*

Ms. Smith is a 42-year-old female in good health with no family medical history of diabetes, heart conditions, or arthritis (see Client Intake/History form on file). She has a very active personal and professional lifestyle. Ms. Smith is a high school physical education teacher with a course load of three to four periods of gym instruction at least four days a week.

Ms. Smith complains of right shoulder pain when leading class exercises, particularly "jumping jacks" and any action that requires abduction of the right arm. She has not had any previous injuries involving the right shoulder and is unaware of any in-stance that would cause the current problem other than overuse.

Onset of symptoms occurred approximately one month ago. She has difficulty initiating the abduction movement; pain and difficulty cease when the arm is at shoulder level. The supraspinatus muscle tests positive on active range of motion (when she performs the movement) but not on passive range of motion (when therapist performs movement). The supraspinatus also tests weak and palpates with spasms and tender points. Ice and anti-inflammatories reduce the symptoms.

Treatment plan will include neuromuscular massage and continued cryotherapy program to alleviate pain twice a week for four weeks. Massage will be followed by stretching and strengthening exercises when appropriate.

Written Narrative

Procedure 3.3 is an example of a written narrative to accompany any other documentation in the client's file, such as Client Intake/History forms, Postural Analysis, SOAP Notes, and physician prescription. Depending on the clinic or office, you may or may not be required to include a written narrative in the file. Physicians will find this helpful in getting "the big picture" of the client, while some insurance companies may require a written narrative be included in the file.

Posttreatment Assessment

A good treatment plan also involves a thorough assessment. Take the time to review all SOAP Notes from previous sessions. Decide what worked and what did not, and make appropriate changes. These changes may involve referring the client to someone else if the desired result is not being reached, changing modalities for a different approach, or suggesting a change in frequency of treatment.

Medical Terminology

Knowing and understanding medical terminology is an invaluable asset in the health care industry. The professional health care team includes physicians, nurses, therapists, technicians, dietitians, medical office managers, and other support staff. This medical terminology section will help you to learn the fundamentals of word building needed to understand the basic medical terminology required for communicating clearly with physicians and other health care professionals.

Medical Abbreviations

Abbreviations and acronyms are commonly used by medical professionals. These can often be confusing if you do not have a medical background. When you learn medical terminology, you are learning a new language as well as a new way of communicating. Most of the medical words are taken from Latin or Greek. Many of the diseases and conditions are taken from the name of a person who discovered them or first had the dis-

PROCEDURE 3.4 Common Medical Abbreviations for Massage Therapists

L: mild
M: moderate
S: severe
(L:) left
(R:) right
BL: bilateral
cons.: constant
freq.: frequent
inter.: intermittent
seld.: seldom
C1-C7: cervical spine
T1-T12: thoracic spine
L1-L5: lumbar spine
θ: none, no
c̄ or w/: with
s̄ or w/o: without
arrow up: increase
arrow down: decrease
X: times
XFF: cross-fiber friction
DP: direct pressure
(M:) massage
PNF: proprioceptive neuromuscular facilitation
NMT: neuromuscular therapy
TP: trigger point
SCS: strain-counterstrain
LD: lymphatic drainage
C/S: cranial sacral
MFR: myofascial release
HA: headache
(P:) pain
(Sp:) spasm
PA: postural analysis

ROM: range of motion
    A: active, **P:** passive, **R:** resisted
Adh.: adhesion
Fx: fracture
st: strain
sp: sprain
HT: hypertonicity
I: inflammation
tp: tender point
ten.: tension
Tx: treatment
Hx: history
Rx: prescription
Dx: diagnosis
Px: prognosis
N/A: not applicable
DOI: date of injury
C/O: complains of
CC: chief complaint
pt: patient
ADLs: activities of daily living
MVA: motor vehicle accident
meds: medication
LMP or LMT: licensed massage practitioner/therapist
PT: physical therapist
DC: doctor of chiropractic
DO: doctor of osteopathy
MD: medical doctor
RN: registered nurse
ND: naturopathic doctor
OT: occupational therapist

ease, such as Bell's palsy. Massage therapists, clinicians, and office assistants must be familiar with the abbreviations and acronyms used in their profession. Although most medical institutions have their own list of approved abbreviations for reports and medical records, progress (or SOAP) notes taken in a massage therapist's or physician's office tend to be less formal. Often, use of abbreviations is a matter of personal preference. Procedure 3.4 details the medical abbreviations commonly used by massage therapists or in health care offices where massage therapists work.

Prefixes, Suffixes, and Root Words

Knowing and understanding the suffixes and prefixes used in the health care industry is important as these word parts are the foundation of medical terms. The majority of medical terms in current use are composed of Greek and Latin word parts. Many of these terms are the same words used by Hippocrates and Aristotle over 2000 years ago. Understanding medical prefixes and suffixes helps you build a strong medical vocabulary. This knowledge will help you in understanding medical reports, office chart notes, and progress notes. Understanding reports from laboratory tests and diagnostic studies will also be easier. Medical terminology consists of the following components:

- **Prefix**—word beginning
- **Suffix**—word ending
- Root word— the word that the term is about
- Combining vowel—usually "o" connecting a root word to a suffix or to another root
- Combining form—the combination of a root word and a combining vowel

Managing Physician Referrals and Insurance

Massage therapists who have completed their state's requirements for licensure or registration may accept referrals from medical professionals and file insurance (see chapter 20). Before taking on insurance clients, however, you must be familiar with the policies for managing a physician's referral and the procedures for filing an insurance claim.

Referrals from Medical Professionals

When a chiropractor, physical therapist, or medical doctor sends a patient to you for therapeutic massage, it is called a **physician or doctor referral**. These referrals can be very important to you because they lend a high degree of credibility to your work. Referrals can also open up a door to a relationship with referring physicians that can continually contribute to your client base. But you need to remember that physicians and other health care practitioners require a truly medically acceptable range of care and treatment of paperwork, or they will not use your services.

Three reasons underlie this requirement: physicians are under strict codes of ethical and moral practice and can be charged with malpractice if they refer inappropriately; patients referred out will not return to the physician if they were unhappy with their care; and insurance companies will not pay for their patients' care if you (the massage professional) do not keep adequate and clinically effective documentation.

In this chapter, we have discussed client intake and general SOAP Notes. Such methods of documentation are fine for a therapeutic massage level of care; however, medical insurance companies, rehabilitation agents, and workers' compensation agencies will require SOAP Notes to be more detailed and extensive. They may require as well a written narrative, such as the one detailed in Procedure 3.3. The following information will give you an idea of the type and purpose of clinically effective documentation.

Purpose of Documentation

The general purpose of the treatment records is to:

- Document care and the treatment provided
- Give members of the entire health care team access to information
- Give complete information to insurers and reimbursement agencies
- Allow quick and complete review by concerned agencies
- Substantiate injuries for workers' compensation and disability claims

The patient/client file must include:

- Patient data, such as the name as it appears on the driver's license, insurance card, date of birth, Social Security number, and so on.
- Insurance and billing information (who is paying)
- All consent forms, including assignment of benefits and release of information forms (signed by client or legal guardian)
- A general case history (usually supplied by the referring doctor by letter or prescription pad)
- Preliminary physician examination report
- Intake postural analysis performed by you (massage therapist)

- Any diagnostic test reports supplied by the physician (x-ray, labs)
- Diagnosis supplied by physician (update it if it changes)
- A daily or weekly charting of progress notes
- An account of exact services performed (e.g., heat and deep tissue application through massage to a specified body area)
- A treatment plan (be sure to do another plan if treatment changes)
- Any letters, phone messages, or other correspondence from the physician or client
- Case identification number, if given one by the workers' compensation or other agency

The patient history *must be signed by client* and include:

- Date the history was taken
- Present or chief complaint
- Description of accident, event, or other condition that led to the complaint
- Personal, social, family, work, and recreational activities and a review of systems
- Past and present treatment and any attempts at self-care (e.g., ice pack at night)
- Drawings and diagrams illustrating pain or discomfort locations and levels

The patient/client diagnosis (supplied by the physician) and all modalities used must have:

- Correct ICD-10 and CPT coding
- Any and all applicable diagnoses supplied by physician, such as one for a torn ligament, one for muscle strain, and one for pain

In addition, each chart must:

- Include progress notes of each session in SOAP Note format
- Any changes in care requests
- Any evaluations or reassessment
- A statement in report format at the end of care with a final SOAP Note or reassessment

As well as being careful to include these items in the client/patient chart, you must also ensure the correct order of the material. Insurance companies and government agencies will periodically review physician referral charts and will not pay for services or possibly fine you for not following the regulations. If you always treat referrals in a clinically effective manner, such a review will cause you no trouble and contribute to referrals from many health care professionals. The correct order for material, contained in charts, is as follows:

1. The outside of the chart should have the patient name.

2. Inside on the left side, the chart should contain personal information, the doctor referral form, and financial and payment data. Phone messages and letters from the client are also filed here.

3. Inside on the right side, the chart should contain the history, assessment, and all clinical and therapeutic documentation (such as SOAP Notes and diagrams).

4. All charts must be free of "sticky notes," correction fluid, and informally scrawled notes. They must be filed in a secure place away from access by other staff members or clients. If a mistake is made, the mistake is struck through with a single line, initialed, and the initials circled. If the document is a medical referral, it must be dated in the following manner: 04/06/2008; a single-digit day or month and a two-digit year (e.g., 4/6/08) are not acceptable.

Understanding Insurance

Health care facilities across our nation accept responsibility for filing insurance claims. With some insurance companies, clients with specific needs for massage care can use their insurance benefits to pay for massage sessions from an individual therapist not affiliated with a medical facility and not doing treatment from a physician referral. However, companies that reimburse individual therapists are still very few. As the acceptance and credibility of massage grow, so will the number of massage therapist jobs within medical offices and hospitals; thus, understanding how claims are filed is very important.

One of the benefits of filing an insurance claim is that clients will have more dollars to spend on massage care than they might have had if all the money came from thier own pocket. Some people also believe that if insurance will pay, then massage must be a viable and professional service.

The downsides of seeking insurance payments are the paperwork —filing a claim usually requiries at least 30 minutes per client visit; the control by the insurance company of how much you can charge; and the fact that even if you follow all the rules, you may not receive payment and have to go to litigation to collect. If you are paid, you may have to wait 45 to 180 days in some cases for a check. Such delays can be quite exasperating when you have to pay utilities, rent, and other bills.

Hopefully, someone within the facility where you are employed will have the task of collecting your money. But if not, the following information will give you the knowledge to file an insurance claim on your own or at least understand what the person who has this task in the facility where you are employed is doing for you.

Insurance Terms

There are several important terms that are specific to the industry. The first term to know is **health insurance claim**. This refers to the documentation and forms submitted to an insurer requesting money for the service you, the massage therapist, have provided. Specific claim forms used are the CMS-1500 for private practice and the UB-92 for hospital charges, such as massage in a cardiac rehabilitation setting. These are the universally accepted forms, and most health care insurance companies will not accept a claim or pay if another form is used. The exception to this rule is that accident insurers will use their own forms or method of filing. Verify which forms are to be used by calling the insurer's information number for **benefits** located on the client's insurance card. Ask the benefits representative directly. Always check for yourself if the client's insurance company will reimburse. The client may not know the extent of benefits covered, and you need to be sure so you will be paid.

Specific questions to ask when you call are: Will the insurance company pay for what I will be doing? What forms and documentation should I include? Where should I mail or send the claim? Should I let the physician file and then pay me? Do I need to get preauthorization?

Preauthorization refers to getting permission from the insurer upfront to perform the services for which it will pay. A number of insurers require that you get permission (or a precertification) before treatment starts. You may want to get the insurance information from clients when the appointment is made and call before they come in, so they will not have to wait while you contact the insurer. Make sure you call in a private room; it is a breach of confidentiality for any other persons to hear the information you relay to the insurer's representative about the client.

When you request preauthorization, the insurance company representative will tell you what information you must submit, what type of treatment they will pay for, how many times a client can come for treatment, and how to submit the claim for payment. If you begin treatment or a session before permission is given, you will not be paid for the services. Under the **hold harmless clause** of the insurance contract, a client does not have to pay you if you file the insurance claim inappropriately and fail to get paid.

When you receive a referral or make an appointment for new clients, you need to make a copy of the back and front of the insurance card, ask if they are covered by more than one insurance company, and make a copy of their driver's license. Include these in the client chart on the left-hand side after the client intake information and personal data. You will need information from these cards when speaking with the insurance company.

The insurance company is referred to as the **carrier**. That simply means that it carries the plan for the insurance program. The client will have a carrier identification number, usually displayed on the card as the "Insurance ID#." It may be the client's Social Security number or a different number assigned by the insurance company. If the client's ID number is a Medicare number, it may be the client's Social Security number with a letter such as A, B, or D after it. Always include the letter when listing this type of number.

After the insurance information is clear and both you and the client understand the payment arrangements, you must have the client sign and date an **assignment of benefits claim form**. An example is given in figure 3.11. This type of form includes a release for records as well as a request for the payment to be mailed to the therapist. If this assignment of benefits is not signed, then the check from the insurer may go to the client, and the client may fail to pay you.

Remember that records cannot be released, even to the client's attorney or insurance company, without the client's written consent. If a physician gives you a copy of a test or diagnosis, you do not have the right to pass it on. If the record comes from another person or facility, permission to release it must come from the originator.

Coding

After the client intake forms are filled out and signed, the chart started and treatment given, the claim is ready to be filled out and submitted. All insurance claims use a standardized method of coding that is set by the World Health Organization of the United Nations and translated into alphanumeric groupings that can be read quickly by a

Assignment of Benefits Claim Form

(Dated) _____

To: (Insurance Company Name)

    I hereby authorize _____ (massage therapist's name) _____ to

release to your company or its representatives, any information including the diagnosis

and the records of any treatment or examination rendered to me during the period of such

therapeutic care.

    I also authorize and request your company to pay directly to the above named

massage therapist the amount due me in my pending claim for massage care by reason of

such treatment or services rendered to:

(Patient's name) _____

Patient/insured's signature _____

Witness _____

Figure 3.11 Sample statement for assignment of benefits

computer. The codes for a diagnosis are found in the *International Classification of Diseases, Ninth Revision, Clinical Modification* (**ICD9-CM**). The codes used for the type of service performed are found in the book entitled *Current Procedural Terminology* (**CPT**). If a claim is filed that does not use the accepted coding, the claim will not be processed. A claim not processed will not be paid.

Deductibles, Co-pays, and Coinsurance

There are many forms of insurance policies. Many of the policies require the client to pay a **deductible**, which is a fixed dollar amount that must be paid before the insurance company will cover the charges. The client may also have to pay a **co-pay**, which is a small fee that should be collected at the beginning of each visit. Clients who do not have the co-payment type of insurance, may be required to pay **coinsurance**. With a coinsurance plan, the clients will pay a percentage, usually 20% of the charges, and the insurance company will pay the remaining 80%, but only of the insurer-approved charges.

You also may have clients with disability, accident, liability, vocational rehabilitation, and many other types of insurance coverage. It can be very confusing, but by obtaining the correct insurance or payment information and making a call to the insurer, you can easily get the guidelines you need to file a claim and receive payment for your services.

Chapter Summary

Being an accomplished massage therapist involves far more than setting up an office and hanging out a sign. You should possess good communication skills so that you are aware of your clients' needs and comfort level and can explain to your client what to expect during the massage session. You also need to be motivated to compile and keep accurate records so that you are able to run a smooth and organized office. It is likewise important for you to understand basic medical terminology and insurance procedures.

Applying Your Knowledge

Self-Testing

Define these common medical abbreviations:

1. Tx: _____

2. C/O or CC: _____

3. Pt: _____

4. ADLs: _____

5. HA: _____

6. (P:)_____

7. c̄ or w/: _____

8. s̄ or w/o: _____

9. Who is the "carrier" in insurance?

   a) The physician's office filing the claim

   b) The insurance company

   c) The patient

   d) The HMO

References for information in this chapter can be found in Quick Guide C at the end of the book.

10. Who is the health care provider?

   a) The licensed practitioner who provides health care to patients

   b) The physician

   c) The patient's hospital

   d) a and b

Case Studies/Critical Thinking

A. *Your client has kyphosis. Keeping in mind the discussion of positioning in this chapter, how will you position him for massage? What precautions will you take?*

B. *You have been backed up in your appointments all day. A new client comes for her scheduled massage, fills out the paperwork, and gets on the table. Since you are rushed, you do not fully review the intake form before beginning her massage. After she leaves and while finishing up paperwork for the day, you notice on her form that she indicated that she may be pregnant. What do you do?*

C. *A young and otherwise healthy woman who is diabetic comes in for a massage. She has written on the intake form that she gets regular massages at home. Do you work on her?*

CHAPTER 2

Therapeutic Massage Techniques

LEARNING OUTCOMES

After completing this chapter, you will be able to:

- Identify conditions under which massage is and is not performed, known as indications and contraindications.

- Identify areas of endangerment that are beyond the scope of the entry-level massage therapist.

- Describe the basic anatomical and directional terms in order to begin work on the body.

- Describe the basic Swedish massage strokes that form the foundation of therapeutic massage.

- Outline and begin to incorporate all six considerations of application into the massage strokes.

- Understand and perform skeletal muscle palpation to identify spasms.

- Recognize the difference between massage sequence and flow, and begin to choreograph a massage routine.

- Discuss and demonstrate proper body mechanics for massage and bodywork.

- Practice a full massage routine for both table and chair.

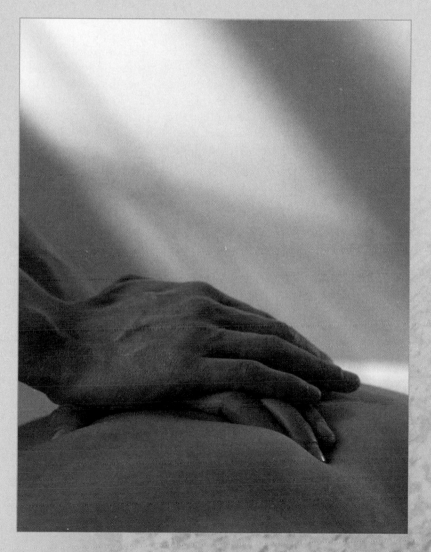

KEY TERMS

areas of endangerment (p. 76)	hypertrophy (p. 79)	rhythm (p. 81)
compression (p. 86)	indications and contraindications	rocking (p. 86)
considerations (p. 74)	(p. 74)	shaking (p. 86)
contusion (p. 79)	massage flow (p. 88)	skin rolling (p. 86)
cramps (p. 79)	massage sequence (p. 88)	spasm (p. 78)
cross-stretch (p. 86)	massage therapist's intent (p. 89)	speed of the stroke (p. 81)
depth or depth of pressure (p. 80)	Meissner's corpuscles (p. 80)	strains (p. 79)
direction (p. 81)	muscle atrophy (p. 79)	supine (p. 88)
duration (p. 81)	nerve stroke (p. 86)	tapotement (p. 85)
effleurage (p. 81)	palpation (p. 76)	thumb presses (p. 88)
fine tremulous (p. 86)	petrissage (p. 83)	vibration (p. 85)
frequency (p. 81)	prone (p. 88)	wringing (p. 86)
friction (p. 84)		

INTRODUCTION

All Western-oriented massage, whether it focuses on relaxation or more highly skilled work, is based on Swedish massage and the strokes first formulated by a Swedish fencing master. The term *Swedish* is often used to refer to a "light" or "relaxation" massage, whereas the term *therapeutic massage* denotes a more contemporary massage that is corrective or rehabilitative.

Certain **considerations** or elements dictate the specifics of each stroke, such as amount of pressure, the speed with which it is applied, and the length of time the stroke lasts. Your ability as a massage therapist to blend these considerations (or mechanics) with fluid movements creates a complete and fully satisfying massage that will appeal to a variety of clients.

For the entry-level massage therapist, general guidelines specify conditions where massage is and is not warranted, commonly known as **indications and contraindications**. Further, there are areas of the body known as **areas of endangerment** that require advanced training and are, therefore, not within the scope of this text. For safety reasons, these precautions must be understood early on in the therapist's training. However, all massage therapists should follow the old adage, "When in doubt, don't" and the medical credo "Do no harm."

Indications and Contraindications

Massage therapists often find themselves in situations where they must ask the seemingly simple question: "Can this person receive a massage at this time?" There are a few guidelines to follow that clearly state instances in which, or conditions where, massage is recommended (indicated) and instances in which, or conditions where, massage is not recommended (contraindicated).

 TECHNIQUE EMPHASIS To complicate matters further, some conditions are local contraindications (so the rest of the body may receive massage), while some conditions may require a different massage modality.

Below are basic guidelines that will aid you in your decision. For an in-depth look at possible ramifications of working with clients taking medications, see chapter 22.

Indications

As mentioned in the Introduction and Overview, there are numerous benefits to receiving a massage and just as many conditions for which massage is indicated. First and foremost, circulatory massage, such as Swedish massage, increases circulation. The individual cells of the body depend on an abundant supply of blood and lymph. These fluids supply nutrients and oxygen to the body as well as carry away wastes and toxins. So, massage simply helps promote overall good health.

Massage facilitates the smooth flow of energy and communication among the cardiovascular, digestive, urinary, respiratory, lymphatic, and nervous systems—creating homeostasis (constancy and balance in the body). With reference to the integumentary system, massage can often enhance skin condition. Massage directly improves the function of the oil and sweat glands that keep the skin lubricated, clean, and cooled. Tough, inflexible skin can become softer and more supple following massage. A healthier, more youthful appearance may be the result.

Massage also aids recovery from soft tissue injuries, such as sprains and strains. The growth and repair of tissues are accelerated by efficient circulation in the injured areas and appropriate stimulation of the healing tissues. Therefore, massage therapy can often help accelerate and improve recovery as well as reduce discomfort from such injuries (see chapter 13).

Finally, massage can have a calming effect on people who are high-strung ("Type A" personalities) and people who have become dependent on pharmaceuticals or alcohol for rest and relaxation (although it should never replace physician-prescribed medications for diagnosed mental or emotional disorders). Massage balances the nervous system by soothing or stimulating nerves and neural pathways, depending on which effect is needed by the individual at the time of the massage.

Common afflictions such as muscle tightness and tension, insomnia, and tension headache caused by stress; spasms and cramps (charley horses) resulting from sports activities; digestive disorders (including constipation and spastic colon) encouraged by a hectic lifestyle; arthritis, asthma, fibromyalgia, sinusitis, and temporomandibular joint dysfunction caused by certain pathologies; carpal tunnel syndrome and thoracic outlet syndrome caused by repetitive motions; and postural imbalances caused by temporary conditions such as pregnancy or genetic conditions such as scoliosis all warrant massage (see Introduction and Overview, and chapter 5). Generally, anytime a massage will be beneficial to the person and no underlying causes of concern such as disease or circulatory problems exist, it is considered an indication.

Contraindications

Contraindications may be general or local, specific to certain modalities, or determined by medication use. Circulatory massage is considered a total contraindication in situations in which any modification, modality, or location would result in unsafe conditions. A circulatory massage is defined as any massage modality, such as Swedish, that directly moves blood and lymph through the body, as opposed to an acupressure massage that works on meridians, and indirectly affects the blood and lymph system.

Anytime a client has a severe condition (e.g., severe insulin-dependent diabetes or high blood pressure), total or full-body circulatory massage is contraindicated. Edema due to any heart, lung, liver, or kidney dysfunction is a contraindication for massage. The response to touch (reflex effect on nervous system) could make the disease worse. In cardiovascular diseases, massage could dislodge a thrombus (blood clot), resulting in an embolus (floating blood clot) and causing heart attack or stroke. Abnormally high body temperature, often an indication of acute infection, is a contraindication for massage.

Modifications to massage such as refraining from working on a certain area (local) can be made to allow massage to the rest of the body. For example, you should not massage distal to (or below) varicose veins so you do not further damage already compromised veins, but you may proceed with massage on the rest of the body (or massage proximal to, above, the veins). Never perform massage over open wounds, lesions, or other potentially infectious sores.

Many grey areas exist in which the therapist must draw on training and practical experience to make an *educated* decision as to whether or not the client may receive a massage. In some cases, it might be a quality of life issue. A terminally ill client, as in the case of a cancer or AIDS patient, would benefit from the touch of a skilled and compassionate therapist. In other cases, under a doctor's guidance, a client may receive a spot—or area-specific—massage to alleviate pain. If you question whether or not you should massage a client or specific area, do not do so until you have further clarification from another health care professional. It is far better to lose one massage than cause harm to a client. If your gut says no, listen!

Depending on the situation, you may be able to switch to another modality, such as Thai massage or Reiki. For example women who are breast cancer survivors may benefit from Thai massage or shiatsu. A small amount of localized acupressure massage and gentle stretching can be both relaxing and balancing for women emerging from a very difficult time. Further, energy work can be an excellent alternative to circulatory massage. Again, conditions that are contraindicated for circulatory full-body massage (such as lupus) may not be compromised by other modalities.

A client on anti-inflammatories (ibuprofen) or analgesics (aspirin and acetaminophen) may not be able to accurately assess pain levels during a massage. A client taking muscle relaxants will have an altered sense of stretch response, prohibiting very deep work. Circulatory massage is contraindicated for any client on an anticoagulant. Medications that slow the clotting process would be compromised by massage that increases blood flow.

Areas of Endangerment

Areas of endangerment are areas of the body where no pressure or no deep application of pressure is recommended because of underlying structures such as nerves, arteries, veins, and vital organs. Most areas of endangerment are located at joints, such as the back of the knee (popliteal region) or inside of the elbow (cubital region). There are a few instances where application of pressure to these areas is acceptable; however, this application requires highly specific training that does not fall within the entry-level massage therapist's scope of practice. The Think About It in this chapter lists areas of endangerment on the body. Figure 4.1 illustrates the location of these sites.

Directional Terms

Before working on the body, a complete understanding of body regions and directional terms is necessary. The body is discussed as it is held in anatomical position: standing erect with head and feet forward, arms at sides with palms facing forward. The extremities refer to the hands, arms, feet, and legs. The torso (or trunk) is the body from the chest cavity to the abdominal cavity, minus the head and neck. Medial refers to toward the midline of the body, while lateral refers to away from the midline. In any circulatory massage, work is done centripetally, which means toward the heart. See chapter 6 for a detailed discussion of directional terms. Also, begin to familiarize yourself with the muscles and their location and bony landmarks by reading chapters 8 and 9.

The Art of Skeletal Muscle Palpation

Simply stated, **palpation** is the art of observing with your eyes, touching with your hands, and identifying with your eyes and hands. When you palpate, you are using the art of touch to evaluate the body. Although there are many types of body palpation, we will focus on accessing the skeletal muscle structure and function. The purpose of the massage therapist's initial palpation evaluation is to determine whether skeletal muscles and their connective tissue coverings are functioning normally or abnormally. This will greatly assist you in determining the type of massage strokes—as well as the amount of pressure applied with the strokes—that are best suited to your client.

Detailed discussions of anatomy, physiology, and kinesiology can be found in part 2 of this text, but for our purposes here, a brief overview of anatomy and physiology re-

Figure 4.1
(*a*) Areas of endangerment
in the supine position.
(*b*) Areas of endangerment
in the prone position.

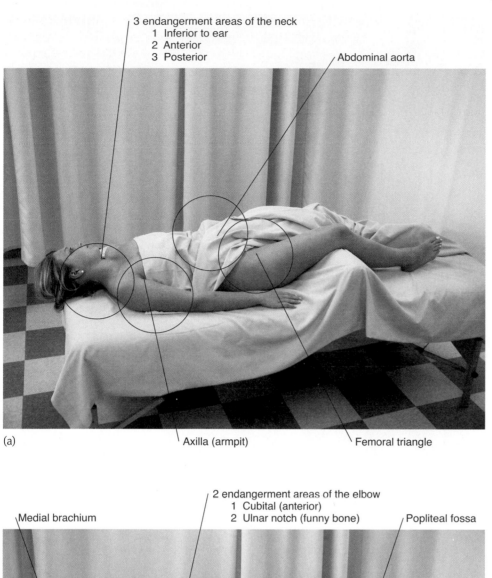

3 endangerment areas of the neck
1 Inferior to ear
2 Anterior
3 Posterior

Abdominal aorta

(a)

Axilla (armpit)

Femoral triangle

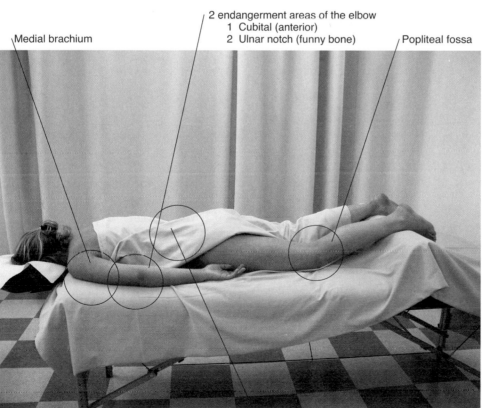

Medial brachium

2 endangerment areas of the elbow
1 Cubital (anterior)
2 Ulnar notch (funny bone)

Popliteal fossa

(b)

(Back) kidneys

1. Inferior to the ear
   Location: notch posterior to the ramus of the mandible
   Structure of concern: facial nerve, external carotid artery, styloid process

2. Anterior triangle of the neck
   Location: borders formed by SCM, trachea, and mandible
   Structures of concern: carotid artery, jugular vein, vagus nerve

3. Posterior triangle of the neck
   Location: borders formed by SCM, trapezius, and clavicle
   Structures of concern: brachial plexus, subclavian artery, jugular, brachiocephalic vein

4. Axilla
   Location: armpit
   Structures of concern: axillary, median, musculocutaneous, and ulnar nerves; axillary artery

5. Medial brachium
   Location: upper inner arm between biceps and triceps
   Structures of concern: ulnar, musculocutaneous, and median nerves; superior ulnar artery, brachial artery, basilic vein

6. Cubital area of the elbow
   Location: anterior bend of the elbow
   Structures of concern: median nerve, radial and ulnar arteries, median cubital vein

7. Ulnar notch of the elbow
   Location: "funny bone" between the medial epicondyle of the humerus and the olecranon process of the ulna
   Structures of concern: ulnar nerve

8. Femoral triangle
   Location: bordered by the sartorius muscle, adductor longus, and inguinal ligament
   Structures of concern: femoral nerve, femoral artery, femoral vein, great saphenous vein

9. Popliteal fossa
   Location: posterior aspect of the knee bordered by gastrocnemius and hamstring
   Structures of concern: tibial nerve, common peroneal nerve, popliteal vein

10. Abdomen
    Location: midabdomen
    Structures of concern: aorta

11. Back (Kidneys)
    Location: against the posterior abdominal wall at the level of T-12 to L-3 (under the twelfth rib); the right kidney is slightly lower than the left
    Structure of concern: kidney

veals that skeletal striated muscles are voluntary and controlled by conscious action of the central nervous system. They are named for the action they do, the region of the body they are found in, and their attachment sites to the skeleton. Skeletal muscles produce movement of body levers. Most massage procedures primarily affect skeletal muscles and their connective tissue coverings.

⭐ **EXAM POINT** Normal muscle contraction is palpated as a slight increase in tension as the muscle shortens.

The most commonly palpated muscle dysfunction is a **spasm**. Spasms are palpated as an increase in muscle tension due to increased shortening (hypertonicity), which the client cannot release voluntarily. This muscle tension prevents lengthening of the muscles involved. Injury, disease, or emotional stress are the usual causes of muscle spasms.

Cramps are involuntary muscle twitches; they are palpable as muscle swelling and usually observable as quivering or palpitating of the muscle tissue. Convulsions are also involuntary spasms of a muscle that usually present a series of jerking movements in the muscle. Minor trauma to the body may cause a **contusion** or muscle bruise.

> ⭐ **EXAM POINT** Internal bleeding caused by the contusion will be palpable as swelling due to inflammation.

Tetonic contracture of muscle tissue results in continuous muscular contractions due to tonic or sustained spasm or fibrosis. It will palpate as a "hardening" of the muscle tissue and is usually observable as persistent twitching or a quick jerking of the muscle.

The most common injuries to muscle tissue are **strains** (torn, overstretched, or hypotonicity) of muscles. Strains are palpated by the degree or grade of strain. Grade I is an overstretching of only a few muscle fibers with minimal or no tearing of the fibers. Grade I may or may not be palpable or visually observable. Grade II consists of a partial tear in less than half of the muscle. Grade II strains show a thickening of the muscle tissue (which is palpable), and there may be some bleeding where the overlying skin may be discolored. Grade III presents tearing of up to 100% of the muscle. It is palpable by a depression or "bunching" of the muscle with very observable skin discoloration.

> ⭐ **EXAM POINT** Strains occur mostly in the belly of the muscle or at musculotendinous junctions.

Muscle atrophy is a wasting away of the tissue and is palpable by a decrease in the overall width of the muscle. **Hypertrophy** is an increase or broadening of the muscle due to vigorous activity or exercise. It is palpable by an enlargement of the muscle fibers. Flaccid muscles diminish in breadth due to a lack of muscle activity or exercise. They palpate as being very relaxed or without normal muscle tone.

The art of muscle palpation is a very important skill to develop as a massage therapist. It requires an understanding of the anatomy and physiology of the "instruments" used in palpation. Recall that these instruments are your eyes and hands (primarily the fingertips). In the clinical artistry of palpation, you must also be aware of how the act of observation and touch may change the anatomy and physiology of the muscle tissue.

Methodology

Many methods of muscle palpation are available to the massage practitioner. They range from intrusive to nonintrusive, active to passive, and very firm contact to little or almost no pressure at all. Firm or heavy pressure may cause muscles to tighten as the body responds to the force of the massage therapist's hand. The information gathered from forceful palpation may indicate more about the body's defense mechanisms than the actual condition of the muscle tissue and its connective tissue coverings.

Noninvasive, light palpation elicits no resistance from the body and more accurately detects the condition of the muscle tissue.

> ✋ **TECHNIQUE EMPHASIS** When you palpate, remember the acronym PALPATE, or "*P*ress *A*lways *L*ightly, *P*erceive *A*t *T*he *E*xterior."

To accurately detect the condition of a muscle, you use the encapsulated nerve endings in your fingertips and pads to relay the information gathered to the brain. When you palpate nonintrusively, you use **Meissner's corpuscles** for fine touch (see chapter 9). These corpuscles are located at the papillae of the dermis right underneath the epidermis (or outer covering of the skin).

Your goal in muscle palpation is to be like a dry sponge placed in a pool of water where information is "absorbed" through your hands. You can then accurately and precisely access the condition of your client's skeletal muscular system and proceed to massage using the most beneficial and effective routine for that individual.

Introduction to Massage and Bodywork

 EXAM POINT Swedish massage was first formulated by Per Henrik Ling, a Swedish gymnastic instructor and fencing master, in the early 1800s. Ling's program provided the foundation for modern-day therapeutic massage and physical therapy.

Extensive travel through Asia gave Ling a background in martial arts and Eastern bodywork practices that he incorporated into Swedish gymnastics. These movements became the basis for body mechanics every Western-oriented therapist uses when working at the massage table.

 EXAM POINT Although a Swede formulated the massage techniques or strokes, it was a Dutch physician, Johann Mezger, who was responsible for applying French and Latin terms to these techniques or strokes.

These terms are still in use today.

EXAM POINT There are five basic Swedish massage strokes, all of which can be used in the varied forms of therapeutic massage: effleurage, petrissage, friction, tapotement, and vibration.

Additional strokes such as compression, skin rolling, rocking, and shaking are derivatives of the basic five strokes. All of the massage strokes can be applied using one or both hands.

Considerations in Applying Massage Strokes

Generally, the application of any massage stroke involves six elements or considerations: depth, speed, rhythm, duration, direction, and frequency. Beginning massage therapists will have to consciously work at incorporating these considerations into their massage. With practice and experience, however, these considerations will become second nature, and the mechanical feeling will evolve into one of fluidity.

Depth or depth of pressure is the amount of force a stroke applies to the tissue. Regardless of what implement is used (thumb, heel of hand, or forearm), the amount of force you apply to the tissue depends on the desired result. If the stroke is performed with the intent of spreading lubricant, the depth of pressure will be less penetrating than if the intent is to reach deep into the tissue and break up adhesions.

Depth of pressure should be increased gradually and with great care. Imagine a friend giving you a "high five" as opposed to a punch in the arm. The "high five" is a warm gesture that is amicably received, whereas the punch is startling. With the punch, the body flinches, recoils, or withdraws in an attempt to protect itself. Muscles react in the same manner; they contract to guard themselves. Muscle contraction produces a protective mode that is counterproductive to effective work on the muscle.

Depth of pressure also depends on the client's tolerance. What is deep pressure to one client may not be deep to another. You should periodically ask your client about the pressure. Always watch for signs of discomfort, such as the client making a fist, holding the breath, or tightening facial muscles. Clients do not often verbalize pain; they believe that you, as the trained professional, know what is best. Finally, depth of pressure may change from one area of the body to another with the same client. Many people can take a good deal of pressure on their back but very little pressure on their legs, for example.

Speed of the stroke is how fast or slow a stroke is performed. Depending on the desired response—relaxation or invigoration—any stroke may be applied slowly or quickly. For example, compression applied with slow, rhythmic presses flushes lactic acid out of a muscle, while compression done quickly pumps fresh blood into the muscle and prepares it for action. In general, slow strokes soothe while fast strokes "wake up."

Rhythm is the regularity or constancy with which a stroke is applied. As with speed, rhythm can be slow or fast, depending on the desired result. Rhythm can speak to the overall tone of the massage; therapists must refrain from working in a herky-jerky fashion.

TECHNIQUE EMPHASIS Recall the analogy of the massage session as a dance; the massage therapist "leads" the dance through fluid steps in keeping with a "beat."

Duration is twofold; it can be the length of time each stroke lasts during its application or the length of time the stroke remains on any given body part. Again, if the desired result is relaxation, a slower and longer stroke is used. *Longer*, here, refers to the amount of tissue traversed, for example, the entire leg from foot to top of thigh. Second, the amount of time spent on any given area, such as the entire time spent on the leg, denotes duration.

Direction is the path or track of the stroke. On the extremities, the direction is centripetally or toward the heart. (Blood flows to the heart through veins, which have one-way valves. Pressure on these valves must be exerted in one direction only; hence, application of any massage stroke pushing blood through these valves must be toward the heart.) For example, effleuraging up the leg is applying effleurage from the foot, over the lower leg, and over the upper leg to the upper thigh (toward the heart).

Frequency is the number of times each stroke is performed. In general, the rule of three's applies: each stroke is performed three times before transitioning to another stroke or area of the body. To spread lubricant, for example, effleurage is applied three times, followed by transitioning to another stroke such as petrissage.

The Strokes

Definition

Effleurage is from the French word *effleurer*, meaning "to glide." Effleurage is considered a warming and gliding stroke and is used in many different ways. This stroke is demonstrated in figure 4.2. Effleurage is used to spread lubricant, to warm up the tissues to prepare them for deeper work, to transition to other strokes or other areas of the body, and to serve as a finishing stroke. Additionally, effleurage can be used during palpation to subtly identify muscles and tendons. In this manner, you palpate with finesse rather than poking or prodding.

EXAM POINT Given all of these applications, effleurage is considered the most versatile stroke of all.

Figure 4.2

(*a*) One-handed effleurage. (*b*) Two-handed effleurage. (*c*) Effleurage using ulnar side of hand. (*d*) Effleurage using thumb. (*e*) Forearm effleurage. (*f*) Proper placement of hands for effleurage on pectoralis. (*g*) Effleurage using a loose fist.

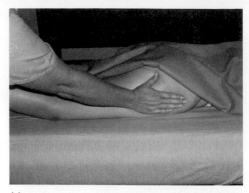

(a)

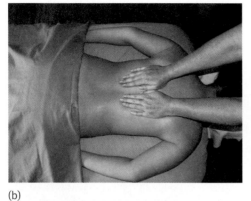

(b)

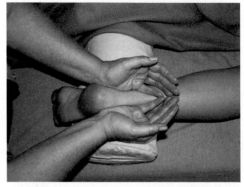

(c)

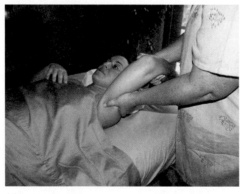

(d)

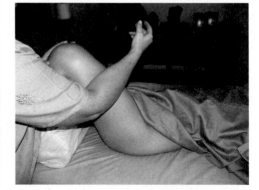

(e)

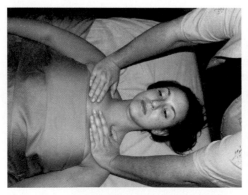

(f)

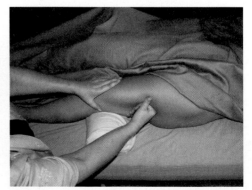

(g)

Application

Effleurage is applied with a flat hand, using the full palmar and finger surface, in a gliding manner. As the hands glide over the body, they fully follow the contours of the body, remaining in constant contact throughout the stroke. Any stroke that glides over the body—whether it is done with the hands, fingers, thumbs, forearms, or any other body part—is considered an effleurage stroke.

Considerations

The depth of an effleurage stroke can be light, moderate, or deep. As the stroke is first applied and lubricant is spread, the depth is fairly light, graduating to more moderate or deeper pressure as the tissue warms and the massage progresses. The speed with which this stroke is applied depends on the intent (i.e., slow to soothe and relax or fast to wake up the muscles). Effleurage is most often performed with constancy lasting an even amount of time. As a general rule, effleurage at least three times at the beginning, in between, and at the end of other strokes or parts of the body (to make sure the lubricant is adequately spread, the tissues are warmed, and to provide a finishing stroke). On the extremities, the direction is always toward the heart—centripetally—or with venous (blood) flow. On the torso or the back, the direction is not restricted to moving toward the heart.

Physiological Effect

Effleurage has the effect of calming down any nerves that may have become irritated. Firmly applied effleurage accelerates blood and lymph flow, and improves tissue drainage, which in turn reduces recent swelling. Rapid strokes, however, have the opposite effect; muscle tone is increased and tissue is stimulated.

Definition

Petrissage is from the French word *patrir*, meaning "to knead"; petrissage is also referred to as "milking" or "wringing" (figure 4.3). This stroke is perhaps the hardest stroke for new students to master since it involves the use of the *C* part of the hand (between the thumb and first finger, or the "webbing") as the primary pressure point. Petrissage almost always follows effleurage to further warm the muscle tissue. It can be applied with two hands or one, and is done toward the heart on the extremities.

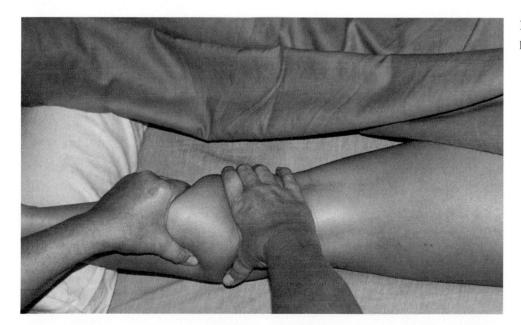

Figure 4.3 Two-handed petrissage

Application

The *C* of the hand is used to push down into the muscle, grasp the muscle, pull it directly up off the bone, and release the tissue in a somewhat backward half-circle motion. In two-handed petrissage, both hands alternate in performing the same motion. The movement is helped with proper body mechanics; bending your left knee helps your left hand to drive down into the muscle, and bending your right knee helps your right hand.

Considerations

By its very nature, the depth of pressure of the petrissage stroke is somewhat deeper than that of other strokes. The speed and duration with which the stroke is performed depend on intent (the desired result being waking up the tissue). In two-handed petrissage, the rhythm is usually consistent between the two hands. Again, the direction on the extremities is always toward the heart. The frequency depends on the surface area covered (generally, it is performed more times on larger muscle groups such as the quadriceps or thigh muscles).

Physiological Effects

Kneading promotes the flow of tissue fluids and encourages increased blood flow by vasodilation. These effects help reduce swelling and resolve inflammation. Rigorous or deep kneading decreases muscle spasms by resetting the muscle spindles and allowing for lengthening of tissues shortened by injury.

Definition

Friction comes from the Latin word *frictio*, meaning "to rub"; friction often follows petrissage.

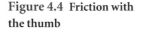 **EXAM POINT** Friction is the best stroke to break up adhesions (or muscle spasms) since it sinks deep into the muscle tissue and works to break apart and realign muscle fibers (figure 4.4).

Figure 4.4 Friction with the thumb

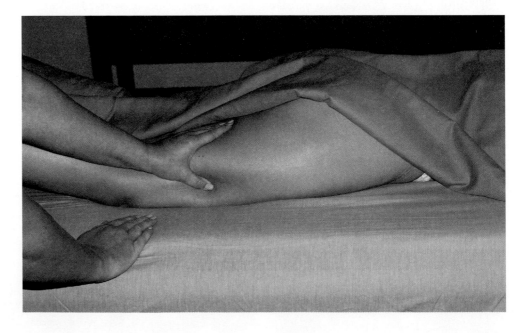

Application

Friction can be done with the thumbs (most common), the heel of hands, and the elbows. This stroke is applied in a parallel (in the direction of the fibers) or cross-fiber (across the direction of—or perpendicular to—the fibers) direction, or circular motion. It is performed with little or no lubricant.

Considerations

Unlike effleurage, the success of friction depends on not gliding over tissue; therefore, depth is important and movement is isolated to the underlying muscle and tendon fibers. As mentioned earlier, friction can be applied in *three ways:* (1) parallel, (2) cross-fiber, or (3) in a circular motion. The rhythm is constant, the speed is slow, and the duration is kept to a minimum as the stroke is intense. The frequency with which this stroke is used depends on your client's needs; suffice it to say, however, that you would not want to do a deep frictioning massage on the entire body!

Physiological Effects

Friction is aimed directly at the site of injury to mobilize muscle; separate adhesions in muscle, tendon, or scar tissue; and restore fibers to a more normal alignment for freer movement.

Definition

Tapotement is derived from the Old French term *tapir,* meaning "light blow." Tapotement is a percussion stroke with the blow being immediately pulled off the muscle as soon as the hand strikes the tissue. There are six types of tapotements: hacking/quacking, beating, cupping, slapping, tapping, and pincement (pinching).

Application

Hacking/quacking are performed using the ulnar side (little finger side) of the hand in alternating blows with the wrists kept loose. Beating is performed with the ulnar side of the hand and loose fists. Cupping is performed with the palmar side of the hand in concave position. Slapping is performed with the palmar side of the with usually more finger surface than palm. Tapping and pincement are both performed using the fingertips.

Considerations

Depending on which of the six tapotements is used and where, the six considerations of application will vary. Tapotements are not performed over the kidneys or bony surfaces.

Physiological Effects

The many variations of tapotement are stimulating initially but can become sedating with prolonged use. In this case, tapotements promote relaxation, desensitize irritated nerve endings, and break up congestion in the lung.

Definition

Vibration comes from the Latin term for "shaker"; vibration is a stroke that ranges from quick shaking to rhythmic rocking. It is an excellent stroke to both wake up tissue and encourage a client to "let go" of a limb that is unconsciously held in partial contraction.

Application

Performed with two hands enveloping the muscle and quickly oscillating back and forth, vibration is a preparatory stroke that increases circulation to get the muscle ready for sports competition. Both fingertips and hands can be used to apply continuous movement.

Considerations

Vibration can be done lightly or vigorously for varying lengths of time. As with the other strokes, use and application depend on the client's needs.

Physiological Effects

Vibration decreases hypertonicity in muscles by interrupting or distracting the receptors in the surrounding tissue or joint. It also stimulates nerve fibers and facilitates neuromuscular reeducation or rehabilitation techniques.

Additional Strokes

There are other strokes that some massage professionals consider to be derivatives or extensions of the five basic Swedish strokes. Other professionals consider these to be strokes in their own right. These strokes often are labeled for the modality with which they are associated, such as sports massage.

Compression is performed with the fist most often but can be applied with thumb, flat hand, elbows, or feet. Compression is performed by pushing directly down into the tissue and may be accompanied by a slight twist (figure 4.5).

Skin rolling is a stroke that addresses the skin and connective tissue. Skin rolling is performed by picking up the skin and connective tissue between the fingers and thumbs and rolling the tissue over the thumbs (figure 4.6).

Rocking is a stroke often used at the beginning and end of the massage to gently soothe the client by affecting the nervous system. Both hands are placed on the body, one on the lower cervical/upper thoracic area and one on the low back; then they generate a gentle, rocking motion.

Although **shaking** is similar to rocking, it is considered a gentler stroke than vibration. Shaking can encourage "letting go" when a client is unconsciously holding onto tension, which can make it difficult to work on a body part.

Fine tremulous is classified by some texts as a shaking stroke, while others list it with vibration. Fingertips are gently placed on the skin with a light, quick, and steady vibration movement stroking downward or outward.

Nerve stroke is a finishing stroke done with the fingertips of both hands lightly stroking down in an alternating fashion. It is sometimes considered an energy technique.

Wringing, a form of petrissage, is actually considered a sports massage stroke. As figure 4.7 shows, this stroke involves a twist (see chapter 13).

Cross-stretch (figure 4.8) is a myofascial release stretch that begins tissue release.

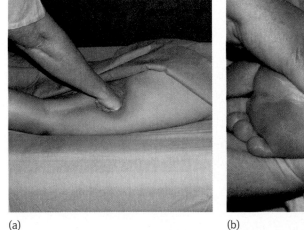

(a)

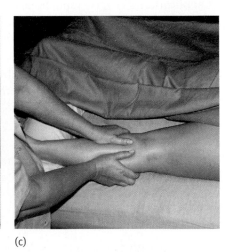

(b)　　　　　　　　　　　(c)

Figure 4.5

(*a*) Compression with back of fist.　(*b*) Direct-sustained pressure with thumb (a compression).　(*c*) Compression broadening (also known as broadening/lifting).

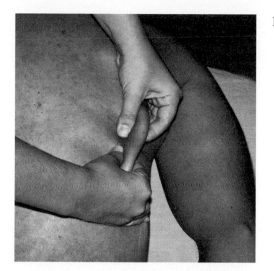

Figure 4.6 Skin rolling

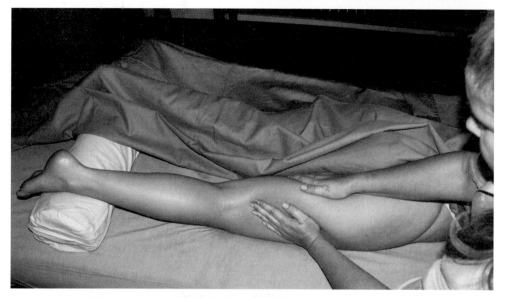

Figure 4.7 Wringing

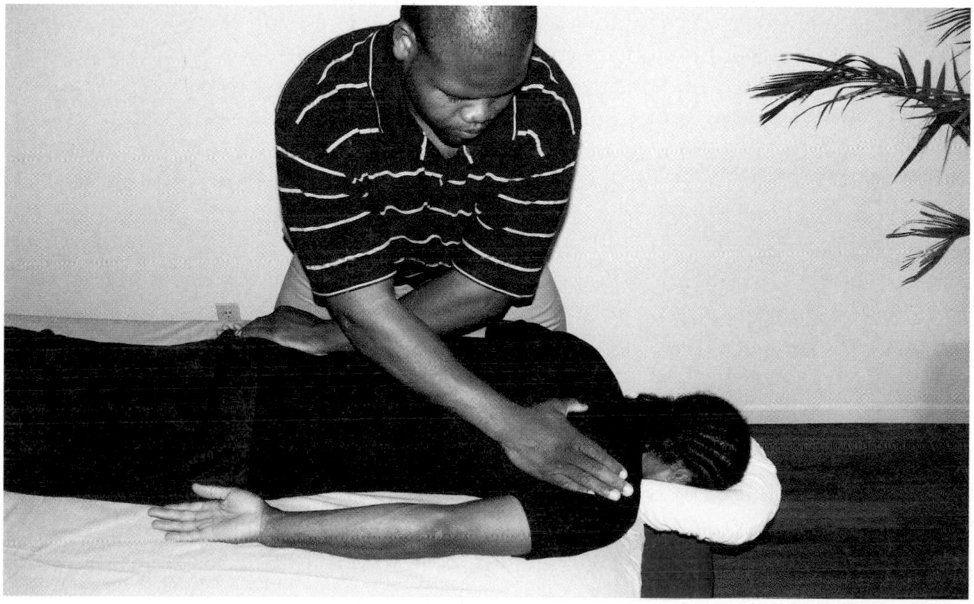

Figure 4.8 Cross-stretch (a myofascial release technique)

Chapter 4 Therapeutic Massage Techniques

Thumb presses originate from Eastern modalities such as Thai massage and shiatsu and are used to hold pressure points. Thumb presses are performed with the pad of the thumb close to the nail (but not the nail).

Today, massage therapists who have furthered their education and extended their practice beyond the basic Swedish strokes perform what is often called therapeutic massage. Such a practice uses the full compliment of strokes or techniques. As you further your studies in both Western therapeutic massage and Eastern modalities, you can blend these techniques for an all-encompassing massage and bodywork session. As you will learn in the sections that follow, massage is an artful dance balancing simplicity with complexity in the integral flow of life.

Sequence and Flow

As a beginning massage student, you must concentrate on the technical aspects of the strokes and the body mechanics that help to deliver those strokes. However, as soon as you are comfortable with the application of strokes, turn your attention to the flow and intent of the massage.

Although a massage can be organized in many ways in terms of sequence or order, it is the flow that unifies the massage. Transitioning from one massage stroke to another or from one body part to another requires fluid movements. A great massage is the result of planning and "feeling." The therapist's intent is to offer to the client a full hour (or whatever the time frame is) of focused work that is nothing short of an artful performance. Using dance as an analogy for the massage, the dance steps falling in a certain order is the sequence, with one number flowing into the next to create the overall performance and work of art. Massage students should view themselves as choreographers of a wonderful dance that without their compassion and spirit would be nothing more than a conglomeration of strokes. Without this choreography, a therapist can be technically correct but not deliver a massage that is memorable and complete.

Descriptive terms for the **massage sequence** are mechanical, technical, thorough, efficient, organized, and logical. Descriptive terms for the **massage flow** are centered, fluid, connected, focused, transitional, and passionate.

Sequence

The client can be positioned on the massage table either **prone** (face down) or **supine** (face up). The decision to start either prone or supine may be dictated by many factors, such as the needs or desires of the client, the purpose of the massage, time parameters, and so on. In general, starting prone works well for most situations since many clients complain of back, shoulder, and neck pain. It is a good idea to address your client's chief complaint first, then work on other areas of the body (time permitting). A typical massage in prone position would begin with work on the back, followed by right leg and foot, then left leg and foot. You can also work on the right foot and leg, then left foot and leg, followed by the back. Starting with the feet and legs allows for application of a heat pack to the back, thereby warming the tissues before working deeply. With Eastern modalities, the work is from the feet up to the crown chakra; the client is turned supine, and work begins on the left foot and leg, followed by right foot and leg, right hand and arm, left hand and arm, chest, neck, and head and face.

A common sequence for beginning massage in the supine position would be to start with the face, head, and neck, followed by the chest, right hand and arm, left hand and arm, left foot and leg, and right foot and leg.

TECHNIQUE EMPHASIS Some therapists choose to work in either a clockwise or counterclockwise direction when working in the supine position (i.e., right hand and arm, right foot and leg, left foot and leg, left hand and foot). The client is then turned prone to work on the back, feet, and legs.

Flow

It is simplistic to say the massage must follow a logical sequence to flow. It is more accurate to say the individual parts must relate to the whole via the therapist's ability to make smooth transitions. Keep in mind that the sequence emanates from what the client's body tells you. Work may move around the body within one session, depending on what the body requires; sometimes, the work will be light, sometimes deep. At times, you may need to ease up on a certain area, move to another body part, and then come back to the area of concern when it is better tolerated or accepted by the client's body. Such an intuitive approach creates a wonderful flow.

All massage therapists approach their work from a nurturing perspective; the very nature of massage requires the therapist possess compassion, concern for others, well-being, and a desire to heal. Whereas the sequence can be considered the more *impersonal* side of massage, the flow can be regarded as the *personal* side. Many clients choose a particular therapist because they feel a certain connectedness or a bond with that person. Indeed, the massage becomes infused with the therapist's personality, philosophy, and spirituality: this is also known as the **massage therapist's intent**.

Strive to maintain continuity throughout the massage by remaining in contact with the client's body as much as possible. Contact here is both physical and mental. It is impractical to always have physical contact; however, it is imperative you maintain mental contact by staying focused on the massage. Resist all interruptions or distractions, such as thinking about what you are doing later that day or what errands you have to accomplish on your way home. A client can tell if your attention is elsewhere.

Body Mechanics

Whether you are performing massage at the table, chair, or on the mat, it is most important to use proper body mechanics at all times. Proper body mechanics ensure that the least amount of stress possible is placed on your body at any given moment. This is especially important if you are working in a setting in which you perform four or five massages back to back. Following proper body mechanics guidelines will also set the stage for a long career in massage therapy. In addition to these guidelines listed below, please read the section in chapter 6 entitled "Prevention and Healthy Living" for further discussion of maintaining good posture at home and work, proper lifting techniques, and improving sleeping habits. See also the section entitled "Biomechanics and Massage" in chapter 6 for further recommendations of proper positioning during massage. Remember, whatever the methodology, good body mechanics have their foundation in working from your center of gravity and establishing balance.

Guidelines

First, and foremost, find your center of gravity. If you are unaware of its presence in your body, develop a feel for it through yoga, T'ai chi, martial arts, dance, gymnastics, or a similar practice.

★ **EXAM POINT** In the martial arts and Eastern modalities, the center of gravity is called the *hara* or *tuntein*.

If you are familiar with yoga and chakras, your center of gravity is found between the solar plexus and sacral chakras.

 TECHNIQUE EMPHASIS Remain centered and grounded in this center of gravity at all times by breathing into and out of this area.

Any and all movements should emanate from this center as well. Keep weight equally balanced over the pelvis and legs, with knees "soft," when standing symmetrically.

When you are standing asymmetrically, such as when performing effleurage up the leg from the side of the table, always keep your weight balanced between your front and back legs with emphasis on the back foot and leg; this corresponds to the yoga asana of the Warrior (*Virabhdrasana*). (See chapter 19 for further information). Do not allow the knee to bend more than 90 degrees, moving past the ankle, as this could cause injury to the knee. Although this is the basic posture for Swedish massage at the side of the table, please note that other modalities (such as *Lomi lomi*) involve specific footwork that has you "dancing" or "flying" around the table, yet operating from a very stable, balanced position.

 TECHNIQUE EMPHASIS Weight on each foot is spread across what is referred to in yoga as the tripod of the foot.

Draw an imaginary line from the big toe edge, horizontally across to the little toe edge, down to the center of the heel, and back up to locate the tripod. Refer to figure 4.9 for some examples of body mechanics. Figure 4.10 illustrates the tripod points.

 TECHNIQUE EMPHASIS Keep the back relatively straight and lengthened by imagining space between each vertebra, rather than straight and stiff in a military fashion.

Shoulders should remain over or slightly in front of hips. The length in the back should continue up through the cervical spine. Remember, the head can weigh up to 6 pounds; occasionally look up and straight ahead rather than down at the body you are working on to lessen neck strain.

Shoulders should be relaxed and down.

 TECHNIQUE EMPHASIS Avoid drawing the shoulders up toward the ears using the upper trapezius.

This action will create tired shoulders after a long day. If using the forearm in a technique, keep the shoulder over or slightly behind the elbow to avoid putting pressure on or damaging the shoulder joint.

 TECHNIQUE EMPHASIS Further, recognize that the strength of each stroke flows from the floor up through your legs, torso, shoulder, and down your arms. Elbows are kept "soft," not locked or hyperextended.

The pad toward the tip of the thumb is used for all work, not the nail tip or first joint.

 TECHNIQUE EMPHASIS If using the thumb for gliding, especially if deep gliding work is done, keeping the thumb joints and wrist in alignment is of the utmost importance.

With developed palpation and usage skills, the elbow is a great substitute for the thumb. Some therapists also find it more comfortable to use a knobble of a T-Bar for holding pressure points. When using the heel of the hand, do not put undue pressure on a hyperextended wrist.

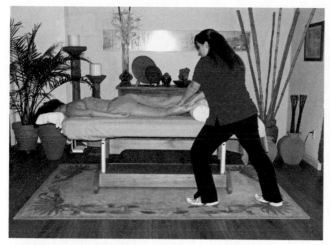

(a) An example of good body mechanics at the table
This therapist is perfectly balanced, keeping shoulders relaxed and down and slightly in front of hips. Her weight is on the back leg and foot, and her head is up.

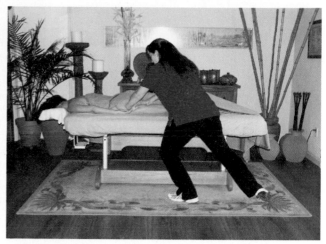

(b) An example of poor body mechanics at the table
The therapist is off balance, having thrown her weight onto the front leg. Shoulders are drawn up, showing tension; elbows are locked with wrists in hyperflexion; and head is down, creating strain on the neck and shoulders.

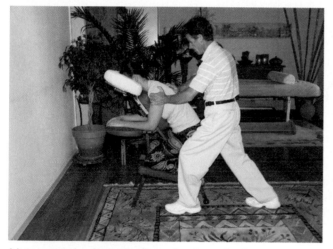

(c) An example of good body mechanics at the chair
This therapist is perfectly balanced, keeping shoulders over hips, weight on the back leg and foot, and head up.

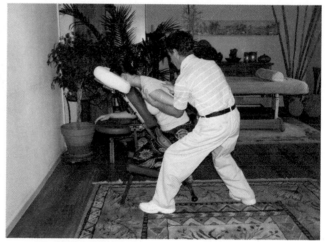

(d) An example of poor body mechanics at the chair
The therapist is off balance; torso is concave, shifting his center of gravity (hara) backward.

Figure 4.9

If you perform any of the bodywork modalities such as Thai massage or shiatsu, you will likely be working on the floor on a dense mat. In this case, it is still important to acknowledge and work from your center of gravity, which is relatively close to the floor. Keep your back as straight as possible without being rigid, with shoulders slightly in front of the hips. Weight can be shifted forward to move a part of the client's body via a lunge (one knee on the floor, one knee off with a 90-degree bend). For any pressure-point holding, position your body above the point with thumbs, wrists, elbows, and shoulders soft and in alignment. Do not allow your head to drop; this will help to prevent the neck muscles from becoming tired.

Remember that the objective of the Eastern modalities is to work effortlessly but effectively by using your body positioning and moving the client's body, rather than using sheer strength from your upper body. For example, with the client in prone position on the mat, cup the front of the shoulder and draw it back against your thumb, which is positioned along the vertebral border of the scapula. With this technique, less

Figure 4.10

To find the tripod of the foot, draw an imaginary line on the bottom of the foot from the ball of the foot under the big toe, over to the little toe edge, down to the center of the heel, and back up to the ball of the foot.

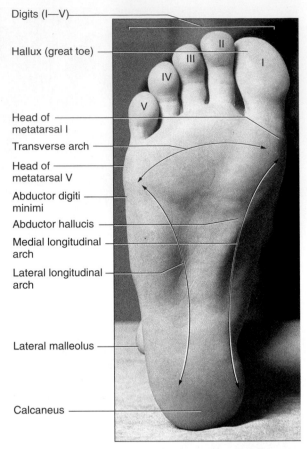

Digits (I—V)

Hallux (great toe)

Head of metatarsal I

Transverse arch

Head of metatarsal V

Abductor digiti minimi

Abductor hallucis

Medial longitudinal arch

Lateral longitudinal arch

Lateral malleolus

Calcaneus

pressure tends to be put on individual joints (such as the thumb) as you are not pushing into the rhomboid attachments at the scapula. Working in this fashion in the Eastern modalities, use the client's body to his or her advantage. It is common in Thailand to massage from sunrise to sunset as a normal workday!

Table Massage Sequence

Set the massage table to the proper height after meeting with the client and determining the appropriate type of massage or modalities you may include. A general rule of thumb is fingertips or knuckles should brush the top of the table as you stand next to it; set it on the higher side for lighter work or smaller bodies and on the lower side for deeper work or larger bodies. Having discussed any recent concerns with the client or reviewed previous session notes, you are ready to choreograph that dance with your client and fully envelop your client in the massage experience. Be sure to familiarize yourself with the basic strokes, elementary anatomy, indications and contraindications, and basic safety precautions before beginning to practice a full sequence.

The sequence described here does not illustrate any spinal deviations and is performed with lubricant, except for the deep tissue sculpting move down the back. It starts with basic thumb glides; this stroke can later evolve into thumb stripping once you have learned about muscle physiology and understand frictioning along or across muscle fibers. Time frames are mentioned only as a guide to help the new student gauge time; the time will be shorter for new students using only a couple of the basic strokes and longer if the client has specific issues, such as a low back or shoulder problem.

Finally, this sequence includes a few pressure points with the work on the feet and hands, abdominals, shoulders, and neck and face taken from Thai massage. It is a great way to begin blending more Eastern-style modalities with Western therapeutic massage. Those who are not comfortable with (or do not choose to work in Eastern modal-

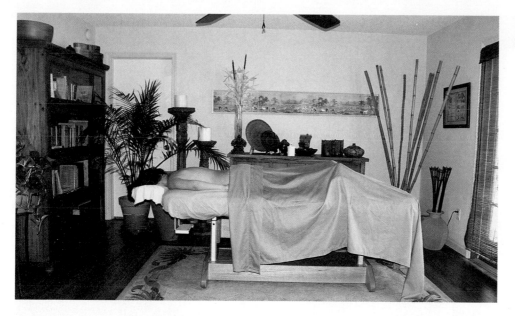

Figure 4.11 Client positioned prone

ities) may simply omit these points. Stretches, based on Eastern and Western principles of movement (see chapters 13 and 19), are not included here but can be added after you become proficient with the strokes, techniques, and draping.

In the sequence, you are the choreographer who—through knowledge, skill, and intent—choreographs the dance and creates the art of massage.

Prone

Ask your client to sit in the middle of the table, then lay on her side, using the arms to support her weight while lying down (figure 4.11). Have her turn onto her stomach with her face in the face cradle. Place a bolster under the ankles and adjust the drape (see chapters 2 and 3 for information concerning positioning, draping, and bolstering).

TECHNIQUE EMPHASIS Begin each massage by taking a few moments to center yourself through deep breathing and focus on the client in front of you.

Deep, rhythmic breathing by you, the therapist, throughout the massage will help you maintain your focus, connect with your client, and facilitate the flow of the massage (see chapter 19).

Feet and Legs (Approximately 10 Minutes)

Figure 4.12 illustrates the prone sequence for feet and legs. Gently place your hands on the client's heels to initiate touch. Undrape the client's right leg. Effleurage the entire foot and leg several times to spread the lubricant and warm the tissues. Work on the bottoms of the feet using alternating one-handed petrissage, horizontal and vertical thumb glides, and static pressure on acupressure points (six points: starting under the middle toe, move one thumb's width down toward the heel for point 2, move one thumb's width down for point 3, move one thumb's width over toward the arch for point 4, move one thumb's width up for point 5, move one thumb's width up to just under the big toe for point 6). Use compression/broadening on the heels, followed by sliding the ulnar side of the hand back and forth over the Achilles heel. Follow with hand over hand up the gastrocnemius and soleus. Petrissage the center, medial, and lateral aspects of the lower leg from ankle to just below the knee; follow with thumb glides, stopping to friction any spasms. Use compression/broadening and effleurage to complete the lower leg.

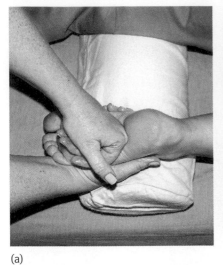
(a)

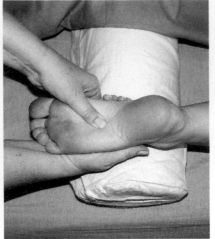
(b)

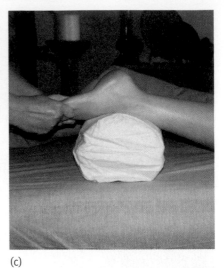
(c)

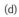
(d)

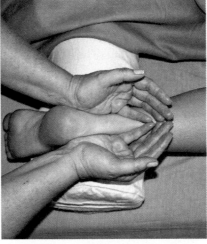
(e)

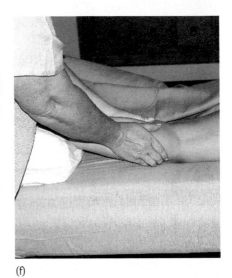
(f)

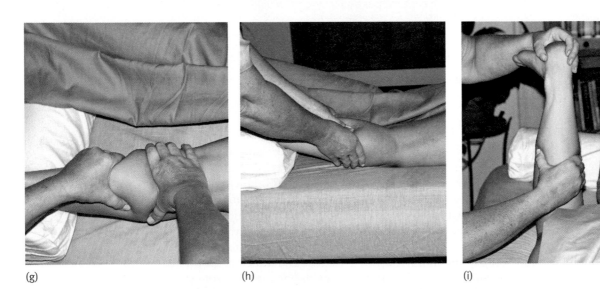
(g)

(h)

(i)

Figure 4.12 Effleurage from foot to leg

(a) Compression on bottom of foot. (b) Acupressure points on bottom of foot. (c) Effleurage entire foot coming off toes.
(d) Compression on heel. (e) Gliding with ulnar side of hand along Achilles tendon. (f) Effleurage on calf. (g) Petrissage on calf.
(h) Thumb glide and friction on calf. (i) Petrissage on calf with knee bent.

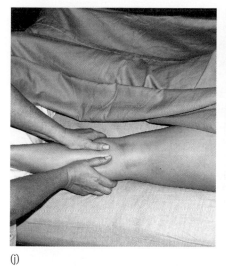
(j)

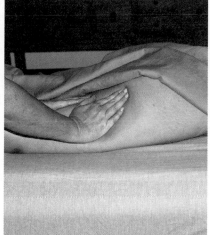
(k)

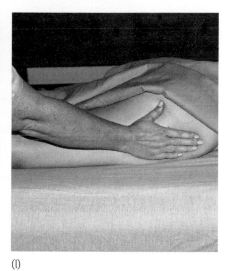
(l)

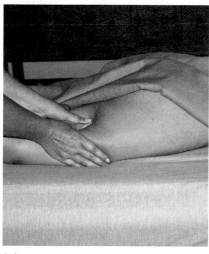
(m)

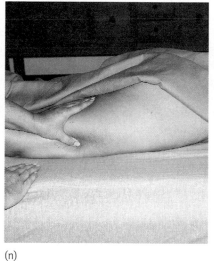
(n)

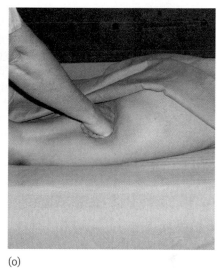
(o)

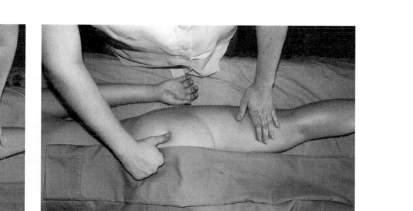
(p)

(q)

Figure 4.12 Effleurage from foot to leg *(continued)*

(*j*) Compression broadening on calf. (*k*) Effleurage on thigh. (*l*) Effleurage on IT band. (*m*) Thumb glide on hamstrings. (*n*) Thumb glide on IT band. (*o*) Loose-fist compression on hamstrings. (*p*) Compression on gluteals. (*q*) Thumb glide on gluteals.

Effleurage up the leg (no pressure on the back of the knee) to transition to the thigh. Use the back of a loose fist (with pressure) to glide from just above the knee to the buttock. Petrissage the center, medial, and lateral aspects of the thigh, follow with thumb glides, and friction all of the hamstring muscles. Follow with compression/broadening and wringing.

Work on the buttocks (gluteal muscles) can be done over the drape with compressions, holding points just off the sacrum on the gluteus maximus, and beating (tapotement). After you have become more proficient with strokes and draping, work on the gluteals undraped (see chapter 13).

To finish, effleurage the entire foot and leg once again, giving it a gentle rocking motion (with no pressure) coming down the leg. Cover with the drape. With the palmar surface of your hand on either side of the knee, stroke away from the knee over the towel toward the foot and toward the buttock; follow with a forearm roll in the same fashion and finish with hacking/quacking. Perform the same movements on the left leg.

Back (Approximately 20 Minutes)

Figure 4.13 illustrates the back sequence. Draw the drape down to the low back/pelvic crest. Place your right hand at the inferior angle of the scapula; cross your left arm over your right arm and place your left hand on the flesh of the buttocks (gluteals) with fingers pointing laterally. Perform a myofascial stretch. Switch. Standing at the head of the table, place your fists on either side of, but not directly on, the spine between the shoulder blades; apply direct pressure for a deep tissue sculpting move (a technique performed without lubricant). Ask your client to inhale and exhale; allow your fists to slide down as the muscle "melts." Change to the ulnar side of the fist before your wrists "break over" and finally to the palmar surface of your hand at the pelvis; hold traction.

With lubricant, effleurage the entire back several times. Effleurage on one side of the spine (over the paraspinals) with one hand placed on top of your other hand; follow with the same movement on the other side. Compress the quadratus lumborum of the low back with fist or forearm; thumb glide crest to twelfth rib. Effleurage the area.

 TECHNIQUE EMPHASIS Follow your hand up on the last effleurage and turn around to thumb glide down the quadratus lumborum from twelfth rib to crest.

Move to the *opposite* side of the table; with palmar surface of the hand, glide laterally and medially over the right quadratus lumborum. This last stroke draws your hand over to the left quadratus lumborum and puts you in position to work on the left quadratus lumborum. Repeat all movements.

From the head of the table, effleurage the entire back as a transition. Step to the right side of the table; with fingertips, glide up the paraspinals and over the lattisimus attachment. If your client has a normal range of motion or is quite flexible, grasp her elbow and hand or wrist; gently draw the elbow directly out and place the hand on the low back. This position allows the scapula to be more visible and accessible for work. If the client is not comfortable with her hand on the low back, allow the arm to remain on the table and slightly draw the elbow out. With right fingers under shoulder at the pectoral attachment and left hand at vertebral border of scapula, traction out. Release and friction attachments at inferior angle of the scapula.

Thumb glide intercostals and up under the scapula. Stepping to the head of the table on the client's left side, use one or both thumbs to glide and friction rhomboid attachments along the vertebral border of the scapula and spine; thumb glide rhomboids. Stepping back to client's right side, carefully remove the client's hand from the low back and lower the arm off the table. Compress the infraspinatus; use thumb glide and friction. Glide your hands down the arm to pick it up and place back on the table. Step to the head and palpate the supraspinatus. Step to the left side of the client and petrissage the right upper trapezius, flowing over to the left. Perform the same movements on the left shoulder.

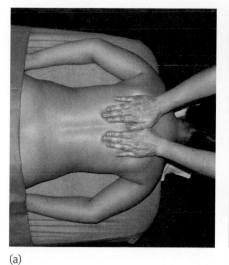
(a)

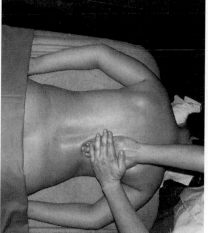
(b)

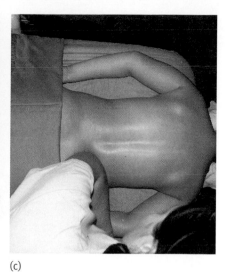
(c)

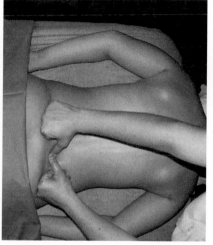
(d)

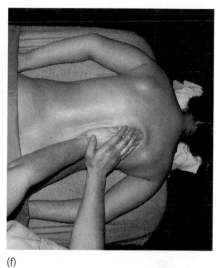
(e)

(f)

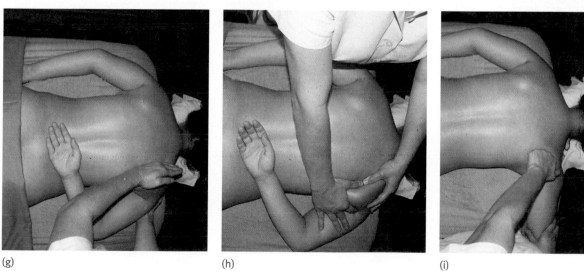
(g)

(h)

(i)

Figure 4.13

(*a*) Effleurage on back. (*b*) Effleurage down paraspinals. (*c*) Forearm compression on quadratus lumborum. (*d*) Thumb glide on quadratus lumborum. (*e*) Acupressure points along pelvis. (*f*) Effleurage up paraspinals. (*g*) Client's hand on low back raises scapula for traction. (*h*) Thumb work on rhomboid attachments. (*i*) Loose-fist compression on scapula.

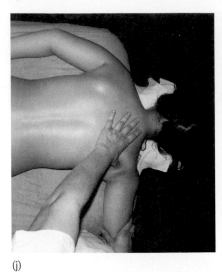
(j)

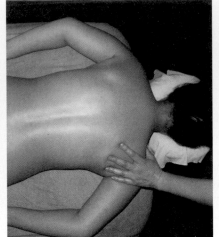
(k)

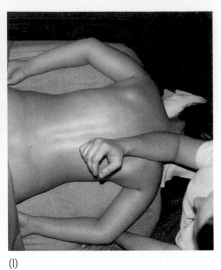
(l)

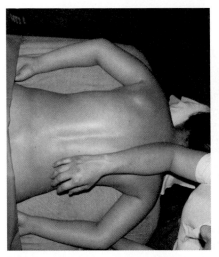
(m)

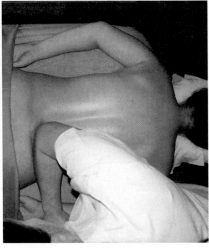
(n)

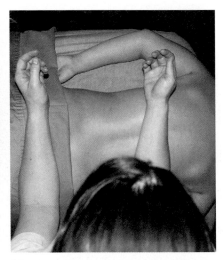
(o)

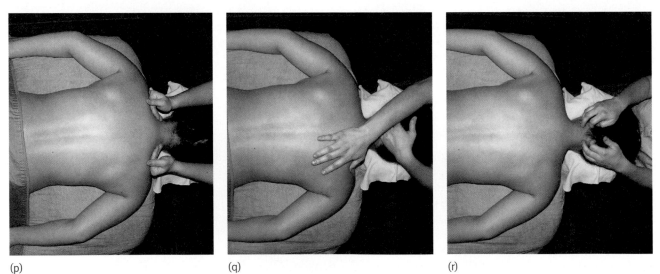
(p)

(q)

(r)

Figure 4.13 *(continued)*

(*j*) Thumb glide on infraspinatus. (*k*) Thumb glide on supraspinatus. (*l*) Forearm work on trapezius. (*m*) Forearm work across rhomboids. (*n*) Forearm work to pelvis. (*o*) Forearm work up back. (*p*) Loose fists on trapezius. (*q*) Thumb glide on upper trapezius. (*r*) Finger glides on levator scapulae.

Effleurage the entire back from the head of the table. Sit on a stool or chair placed at the client's head.

TECHNIQUE EMPHASIS Draw the drape up to keep the client warm while working the upper trapezius and neck.

Effleurage the upper trapezius and neck. Use the back of loose fists to further effleurage. Hold pressure points across the trapezius (using both thumbs, simultaneously hold points nearest the neck, move laterally and hold two more points, move laterally and hold two more points, then move back medially on same points). Effleurage. Glide the palmar surface of your left hand up the neck to the occipital ridge and hold the ridge. With your right thumb, glide from occiput to levator attachment at the scapulae; move laterally and glide from the occiput over the trapezius. The palmar surface of your right hand glides over the shoulder and up the back of the neck to the occipital ridge to position your left thumb to perform the same movements on the left side of the neck. Effleurage the trapezius and neck.

Stand up; move the drape slightly back to effleurage the entire back in completion of the prone position.

Turning the Client

Remove the bolster from under the client's ankles and any other bolstering.

TECHNIQUE EMPHASIS Reach across the client and pick up the towel; hold it up, pinning the edge closest to you between the table and your thigh so that it does not move with the client as she turns over.

Ask the client to roll over by rolling toward you (and the side on which the drape is held up) and move down the table so her head is on the table rather than in the face cradle. Some clients will roll over on the side that is easiest for them, so make sure you stand and hold the drape up on the side that will not exacerbate an injury. For example, in the prone position, if the client has a right arm or shoulder injury, stand on his right side and ask him to roll over toward you using his left arm. In the supine position, if the client has a right arm or shoulder injury, stand on his left side so he will roll onto his left arm (rather than onto the injured right arm). If using a sheet for a top drape, reach across the client and draw the sheet up to a "tent" so that the client can easily and comfortably roll over under the sheet. Reposition the drape and place the bolster under the client's knees.

Supine

Feet and Legs (Approximately 8 Minutes)

Figure 4.14 illustrates the supine sequence for feet and legs. Begin again at the feet. Undrape the left leg. As with the prone position, all strokes are performed with venous flow. Effleurage the foot and leg to spread lubricant and warm the tissues. Use alternating one-handed petrissage and thumb glides between the metatarsals of the foot. Use finger circles around the ankles followed by hand over hand up the shin. There is not much to work on the lower leg; petrissage the medial gastrocnemius again and thumb glide up the tibialis anterior muscle. Effleurage again, gliding up to do a figure eight around the knee: starting above the knee, do three circles toward the knee (similar to a compression/broadening stroke), slide down alongside of the knee and below the knee. Do three circles toward it.

Effleurage up the thigh; petrissage the thigh. Use the back of alternating loose fists to glide from above the knee to the hip, covering each of the quadriceps, adductors, and

Figure 4.14 Client positioned supine
(*a*) Thumb glides between metatarsals. (*b*) Hand-over-hand effleurage up lower leg. (*c*) Petrissage medial aspect of lower leg. (*d*) Thumb glide up lateral aspect of lower leg. (*e*) Figure eight around knee. (*f*) Loose fist on quadriceps. (*g*) Figure eight with loose fists.

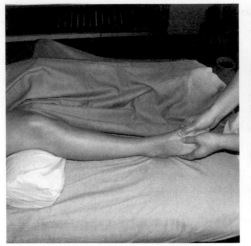

(a)

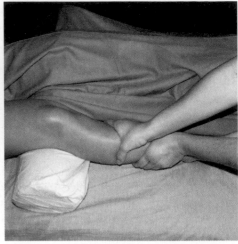

(b)

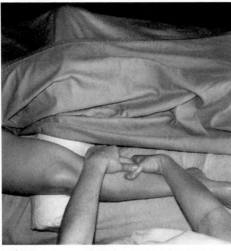

(c)

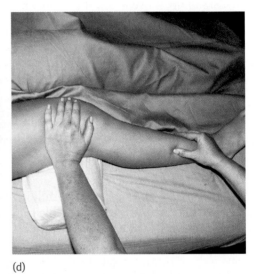

(d)

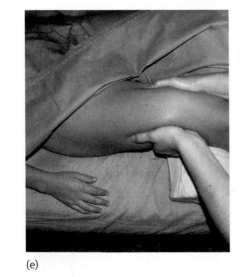

(e)

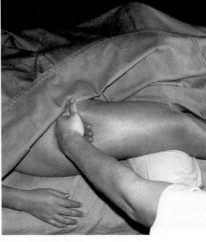

(f)

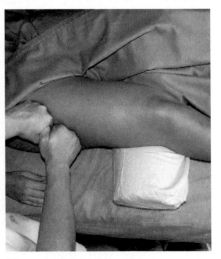

(g)

IT band. Follow with thumb glides and stripping, compression/broadening, or wringing. Effleurage up the entire leg with a gentle rocking motion (no pressure) coming down. Move to the right leg and repeat the movements.

Abdominals and Intercostals (Approximately 1 to 2 Minutes)

Although many massage schools do not teach abdominal massage today, it is well worth your while to familiarize yourself with these techniques. Figure 4.15 illustrates the abdominal sequence. Drape the client as shown; this provides privacy for female clients while allowing easy access to the abdomen and rib cage area. Always massage in the direction of peristalsis (normal rhythmic waves of muscular contraction in the digestive tract) or in a clockwise direction, beginning with palmar circles and followed with more specific work done with the fingertips. Lightly hold six points on the abdomen (1 and 2 are either side of the navel, 2 and 3 are just to the side of the navel, and 5 and 6 are just below the navel). Use thumbs to glide and friction between ribs; be careful not to damage the xiphoid process.

Hands and Arms (Approximately 8 Minutes)

Figure 4.16 illustrates the sequence for hands and arms. Effleurage the client's right hand and arm several times to spread lubricant and warm the tissues. Use alternating one-handed petrissage on the palm and thumb glide between the metacarpals. Turn

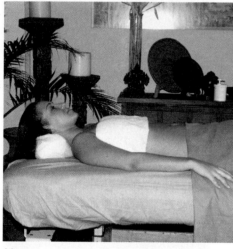
(a)

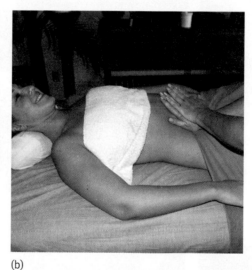
(b)

Figure 4.15
(*a*) Abdominal area undraped for work. (*b*) Palmar circles on abdomen. (*c*) Finger drag in direction of peristalsis. (*d*) Hand glides across abdomen. (*e*) Work on intercostals.

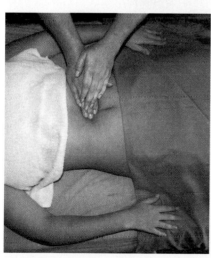
(c)

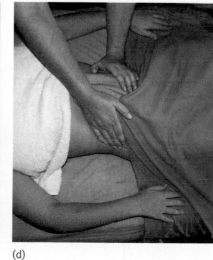
(d)

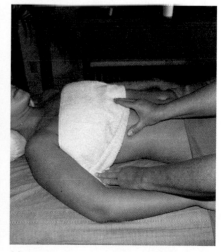
(e)

Figure 4.16

(*a*) Effleurage up arm.
(*b*) Effleurage the length of client's arm, ending at the back of the neck.
(*c*) Acupressure points on palmar surface of hand.
(*d*) Thumb glide on posterior aspect of forearm. (*e*) Thumb glide on anterior aspect of forearm. (*f*) Thumb glide down triceps. (*g*) Shoulder stretch. (*h*) Shoulder traction.

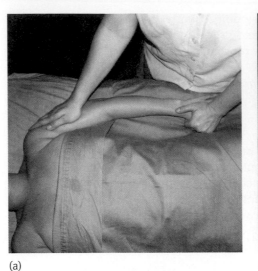

(a)

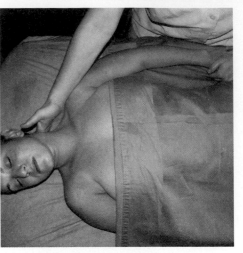

(b)

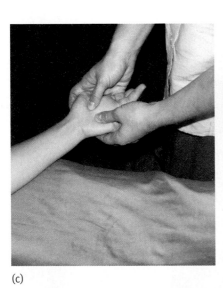

(c)

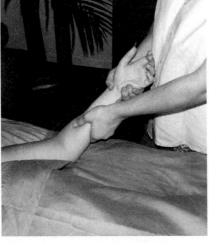

(d)

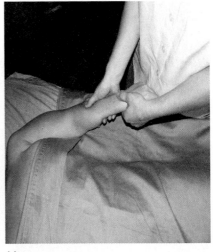

(e)

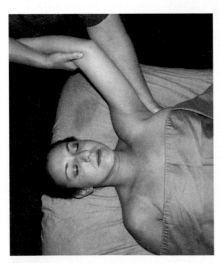

(f)

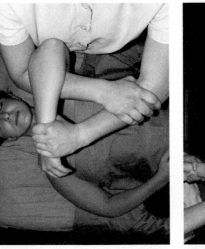

(g)

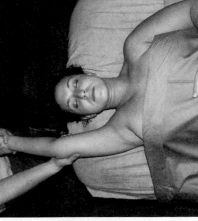

(h)

the hand over: slip your little finger in between the client's middle and ring finger, and your fourth finger between the client's ring and little finger. Slip your other little finger between the client's middle and index finger, and your ring finger between the client's index finger and thumb. Open the palm of the hand and work with thumb glides; hold acupressure points (unlike the foot, these points are held two at a time: hold 1 and 2 at the palm heel, move one thumb's width toward the fingers for 3 and 4, move one thumb's width toward fingers for 5 and 6, and move back down). Release the fingers and hold the hand with one of your hands; draw the forearm up to a 45-degree angle, elbow resting on the table. Use one-handed petrissage on the forearm, alternating hands. Thumb glide and friction the forearm.

Step up next to the client's shoulder.

TECHNIQUE EMPHASIS Place your left knee (the knee closest to the head of the table) on the table under the sheet; lay the client's arm over your leg.

This allows you to use both hands at once to petrissage the upper arm and is actually a very stable position. If you are not comfortable standing on one leg, allow the arm to remain on the table and draw the elbow out slightly; effleurage and petrissage the arm, being careful not to place any pressure over the elbow. Drop your knee off the table, holding the elbow with your right hand. Use your left hand to glide around the deltoid cap. Switch hands, holding the elbow now with your left hand and use your right hand to glide down the triceps. Glide with the palmar surface of your hand down the triceps brachii, teres minor and major, and latissimus dorsi, and back up; gently traction the arm and replace it on the table. Move to the client's left side and perform the same movements.

Chest (Approximately 1 to 2 Minutes)

Figure 4.17 illustrates the sequence for chest. Effleurage the chest (pectoralis) with fingers pointing toward the sternum (not down toward the breasts), out over shoulders, around the back of the upper trapezius, and up the back of the neck. Repeat several times; give the neck a gentle traction as you draw the hands up the neck. Thumb glide from clavicles downward slightly (staying on the pectoral muscle and above the breasts). Work one side of the sternum and then the other. Step to the client's left, lay the right arm out to the side, and glide with your fingertips over the pectoralis from

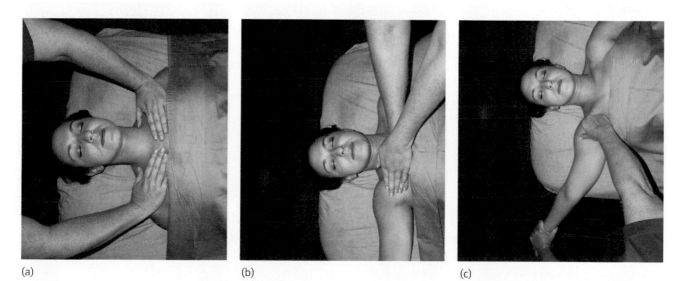

(a) (b) (c)

Figure 4.17
(*a*) Effleurage across pectoralis. (*b*) Finger glide across pectoralis. (*c*) Pectoralis stretch.

sternum to shoulder, changing to a flat hand over the shoulder joint. Maintaining contact with the shoulder, walk around to the other side, slide the hands down the arm to place it back on the table. Repeat the movements on the left side of chest (pectoralis).

Neck and Head (Approximately 10 Minutes)

Figure 4.18 illustrates the sequence for neck and head. Effleurage the shoulders and up the back of the neck several times. Slip your hands and arms under the back as far as you can reach (palms are up, fingers press up, and hands are on either side of the spine). Draw hands up slowly, stopping at the occipital ridge and gliding out laterally. Carefully pick up the client's head and turn to it the left. With the back of the right fist, glide up and down the neck and trapezius (keep the ulnar side of the fist on the table for a guide). Thumb glide. Turn the client's head back to neutral before turning it to the right. Repeat.

With fingertips starting at the superior angle of both scapula, press and hold these points; continue to move medially and up the back of the neck, back of the head, and over the top of the head (switch to the thumbs to press across the top of the head). With thumbs, press two points on the forehead, gliding down to the temples for thumb circles. Repeat two more times. Press under the cheekbones at the nostrils, gliding up to

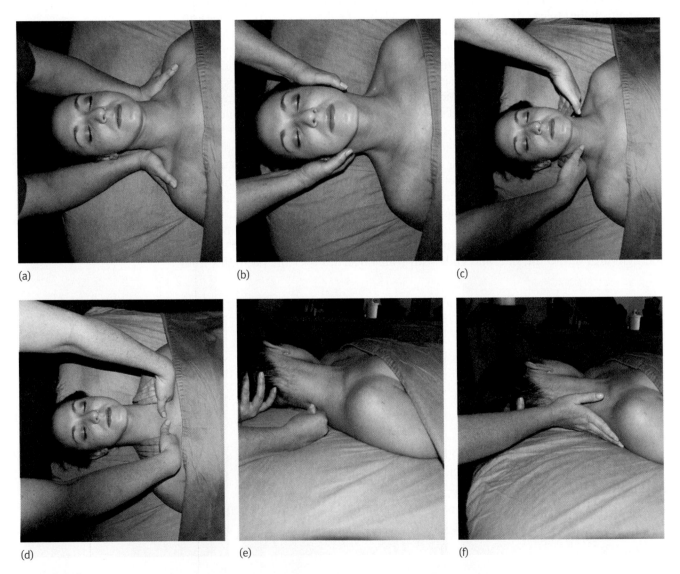

(a) (b) (c)

(d) (e) (f)

Figure 4.18

(*a*) Effleurage across upper trapezius. (*b*) Effleurage up levator scapulae. (*c*) Effleurage scalenes. (*d*) Effleurage over clavicles.
(*e*) Thumb glide on levator scapulae. (*f*) Effleurage levator scapulae and scalenes.

the temples and doing thumb circles; press at the chin and glide up to the temples for thumb circles. Massage all over the scalp with fingertips. Starting in "prayer" position on the forehead (palms together, heels of hands on the client's forehead), open your hands as you glide down the sides of the forehead (figure 4.19). Repeat two more times.

Effleurage across the shoulders and up the back of the neck a few times. Gently slide the client's head laterally with left ear to left shoulder, back to neutral, and right ear to right shoulder (figure 4.20).

TECHNIQUE EMPHASIS For a calming finish, pause for a moment with your hands cupping the client's shoulders.

At this time—depending on your spiritual inclinations—silently say a prayer or ask for healing (figure 4.21). You can repeat the Thai phrase *Na-A Na-Wa Rokha Payati Vina-Santi*, which loosely translates as "May I do no harm and bring healing to this client."

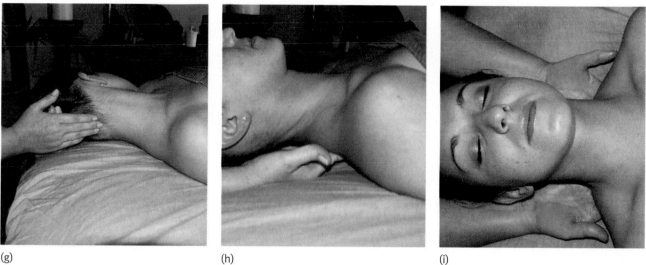

(g)   (h)   (i)

Figure 4.18 (*Continued*)
(*g*) Finger pressure on occipital ridge. (*h*) Acupressure points on upper back. (*i*) Acupressure points up back of neck.

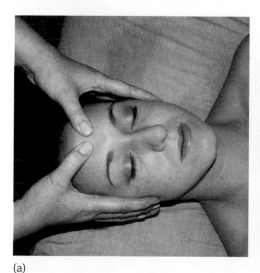
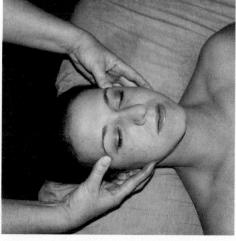

Figure 4.19
(*a*) Acupressure points on forehead. (*b*) Thumb circles at temples.

(a)   (b)

Figure 4.19 (*Continued*)
(*c*) Acupressure points above upper lip. (*d*) Acupressure points on chin. (*e*) Effleurage up sides of face. (*f*) Ear pull. (*g*) Scalp massage.

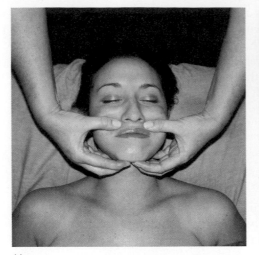
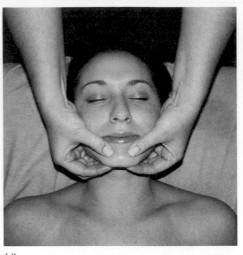

(c)

(d)

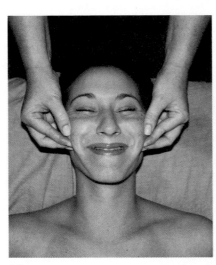
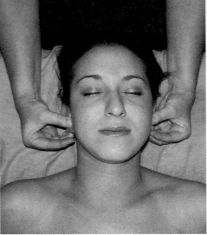
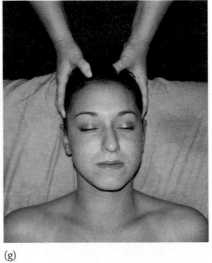

(e)

(f)

(g)

Figure 4.20
(*a*) Neck traction.

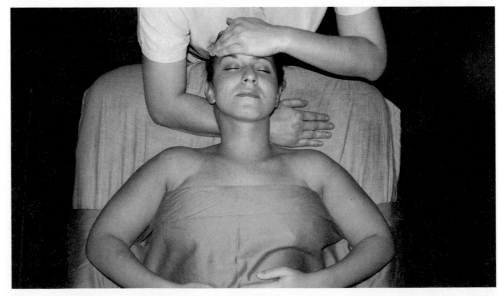

(a)

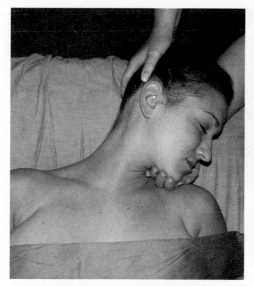

(b)

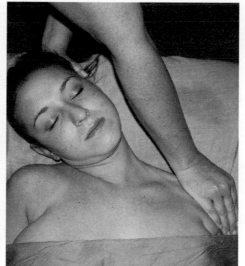

(c)

Figure 4.20 (*Continued*)
(*b*) Lateral neck stretch.
(*c*) Lateral neck stretch with added pressure.

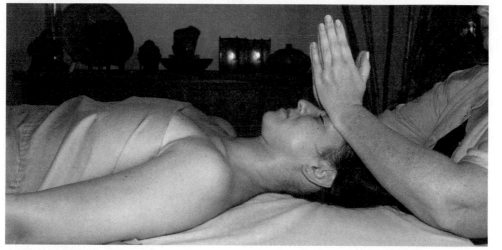

Figure 4.21 "Prayer" on forehead

Chair Massage Sequence

By: Peter Joachim, LMT, NCTMB

Being able to perform a memorable chair massage routine is a great asset to any massage therapist. Many therapists prefer to work with the chair rather than the table and will create an entire one-hour routine all done on the chair. Others use chair massage as a modality because it is versatile and adaptable: it can be delivered in short sessions, performed almost anywhere (office, school, or social gatherings), is done with clothing on, and—although the experience is enhanced with the use of a massage chair—it does not need equipment per se. Chair massage can also be a great marketing tool (see chapter 21).

The basics of a chair massage are depicted in figure 4.22. Your own techniques or movements can easily be added to this 10-minute routine.

The client is placed comfortably on the chair after you have made any necessary adjustments in the seat, chest plate, and face cradle. Care should be taken with seniors or clients who have knee problems; the chairs are not always the easiest to sit on and even more difficult to get up from. Offer the appropriate assistance as needed for the client to get on and off the chair.

As with any other massage routine, begin by rubbing your hands together to warm them and doing some deep breathing to center and focus. Maintain focus throughout the massage, just as you would when working on a client on a table or mat.

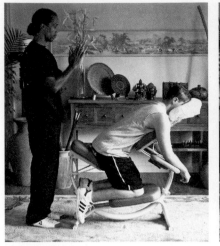
(a)

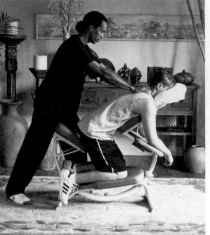
(b)

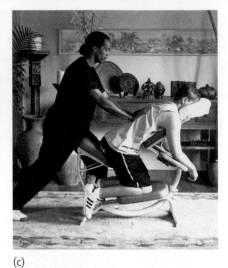
(c)

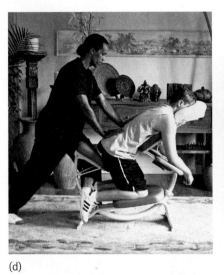
(d)

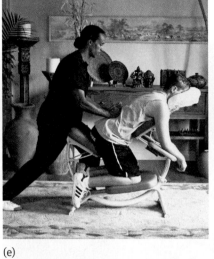
(e)

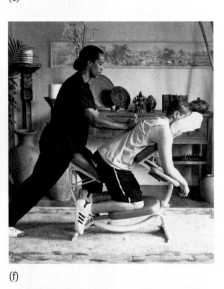
(f)

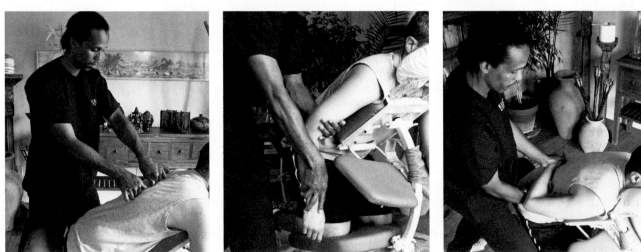
(g)

(h)

(i)

Figure 4.22

(a) Begin with centering and grounding. *(b)* Begin routine with moderate petrissage to upper trapezius. *(c)* Apply palm presses down and up back on both sides of spine. *(d)* Continue applying palm presses. *(e)* Apply presses up paraspinals with lightly closed fists. *(f)* Continue work on paraspinals. *(g)* Thumb friction along paraspinals. *(h)* Draw client's right arm down. *(i)* Place client's hand on low back.

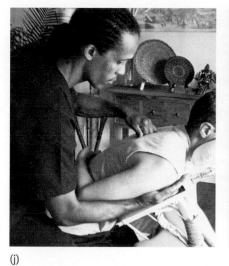

(j)

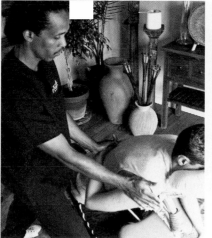

(k)

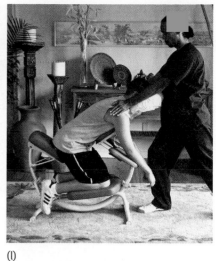

(l)

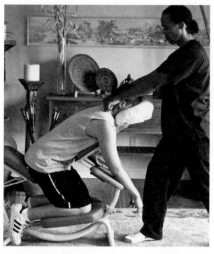

(m)

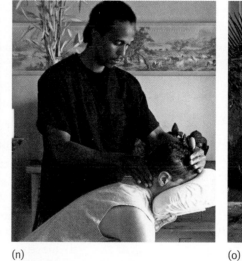

(n)

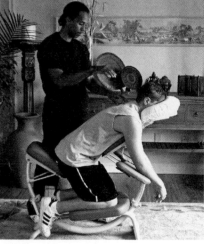

(o)

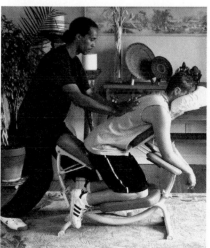
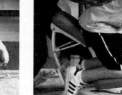

((p(1))

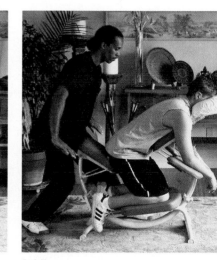

(p(2))

(p(3))

Figure 4.22 (*Continued*)

(*j*) Place left thumb on vertebral border of right scapala. (*k*) Right hand cups client's right shoulder and draws it back onto left thumb. Release arm gently and let it hang. Repeat sequence (to this point) on left side. (*l*) Working from the front, simultaneously apply equal pressure to both shoulders to relax the trapezius. (*m*) Apply pressure to acupressure points laterally along upper trapezius. (*n*) Apply light petrissage to back of neck. (*o*) Apply finger tapping (tapotement) to upper back. (*p*) Conclude routine with gentle nerve strokes down entire back.

Chapter Summary

The profession of massage therapy is both exciting and rewarding. Many therapists report they have a calling to the profession. Whether this calling emanates from within or beyond, it is the driving force that creates the desire to heal and show compassion for others. No matter which discipline within the field of massage you choose, it will be one in which you as the therapist can infuse your core beliefs into your work.

From the very beginning of your training as a massage therapist, you must educate yourself as to the potential benefits and hazards of performing massage on certain clients. Recognizing that grey areas exist—that cut-and-dried answers to massage questions do not always exist—should encourage you to further your studies and help you in developing clinical reasoning.

Applying Your Knowledge

Self-Testing

1. Any stroke that glides along the body is considered a(n) _____ stroke.
   a) Effleurage
   b) Petrissage
   c) Tapotement
   d) Vibration

2. Which is *not* one of the six considerations of massage strokes?
   a) Rhythm
   b) Direction
   c) Frequency
   d) Aura

3. Skin rolling
   a) is a valuable connective tissue technique.
   b) is applied with force.
   c) determines body fat composition.
   d) smoothes out wrinkles.

4. The definition of *prone* is:
   a) face up.
   b) face down.
   c) side-lying.
   d) None of the above is correct.

5. Petrissage is also known as:
   a) kneading.
   b) pulling.
   c) compressing.
   d) a pet massage.

6. The definition of *tapotement* is:
   a) a warming stroke.
   b) a percussion stroke.
   c) a slow, soothing stroke.
   d) a kneading stroke.

7. Frequency as one of the six considerations indicates:
   a) the number of times one gets a massage.
   b) the number of times a particular stroke is done (e.g., effleurage three times).
   c) the total number of times a client is scheduled during treatment.
   d) the setting for electric stimulation known as "E Stim."

8. If it is not a good idea to do a massage, it is called:
   a) indication.
   b) contraindication.
   c) beneficial.
   d) area of endangerment.

9. The term *centripetal* refers to:
   a) away from the heart.
   b) toward the heart.
   c) on the extremities only.
   d) against venous flow.

10. The term *medial* refers to:
    a) toward the head.
    b) toward the feet.
    c) toward the midline of the body.
    d) toward the outside of the body.

Case Studies/Critical Thinking

A. A friend of yours who is in his mid-forties complains of middle- and lower-back pain and asks you to work on him. You are aware that he has an irregular heartbeat for which he sees a cardiologist and takes prescribed medication. Otherwise, he is physically active and in good health. Would you work on him? If so, under what conditions?

B. A 20-year-old client informs you that she tests positive for HIV but has been told by her physician that she does not have AIDS. You do not have any indication that she could be considered as falling into the high-risk category of someone who uses drugs or has multiple sexual partners. Would you work on this client? If so, under what conditions?

References for information in this chapter can be found in Quick Guide C at the end of the book.

CHAPTER 5

Physiological Effects of Therapeutic Massage

LEARNING OUTCOMES

After completing this chapter, you will be able to:

- Identify the principle physiological mechanisms of massage.
- List and understand the physiological effects of massage on various body systems.
- Discuss the reflexive mechanism connection to somatic and visceral disorders.
- Understand the physiological effects of the various strokes and techniques used in massage.
- Discuss the physiological effects of heat and cold application.

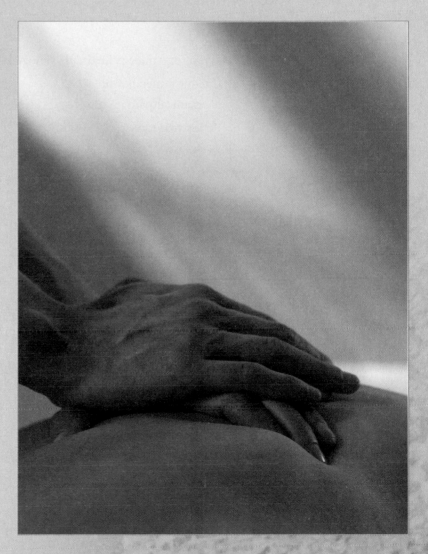

KEY TERMS

autonomic nervous
   system (ANS) *(p. 119)*
baroreceptors *(p. 116)*
central nervous
   system (CNS) *(p. 118)*
hyperemia *(p. 117)*

hypertension (HTN) *(p. 116)*
lymphocytes *(p. 117)*
macrophages *(p. 117)*
mechanoreceptors *(p. 115)*
nociceptors *(p. 115)*
parasympathetic *(p. 119)*

peripheral nervous system (PNS)
   (p. 118)
reflexive response *(p. 115)*
soma *(p. 123)*
sympathetic *(p. 119)*
viscera *(p. 123)*

INTRODUCTION

Many beginning massage therapists have asked themselves, "What does physiology have to do with massage?" Physiology has everything to do with massage. Each time you place your hands on a client, you are affecting the physiology of that client. Remember that physiology is the study of the function of the body and its parts. Understanding and applying this knowledge will help you in developing therapeutic goals and moving your client toward optimal healing and health. This chapter illustrates the physiological effects of massage on various body systems.

Principal Physiological Mechanisms

Massage affects three primary physiological processes in the body:

1. Chemical/metabolism
2. Mechanical/pain perception
3. Reflexive response

Chemical/Metabolism

Metabolism is the sum of all physiological activity in the cell. Any change that affects the body processes—such as pH, nutrient levels, oxygen, water, heat, and pressure—can lead to metabolic dysfunction. Metabolic dysfunction of the cell begins a cumulative effect that will lead to cellular and systemic dysfunction.

Mechanical/Pain perception

Massage produces short-lived analgesia by activating the gate theory mechanism to block painful stimulus. (The gate theory states that there is a mechanism functioning at

---

Think About It	Sensory Receptors

1. Proprioceptors—detection of position and rate of motion
   a. Muscle spindle fibers
   b. Golgi tendon organs
2. Exteroceptors—relay information regarding external environment (senses)
3. Visceroceptors—relay information about internal organs (viscera)
4. Nociceptors—pain receptors
5. Thermoreceptors—detection of temperature changes
6. Chemoreceptors—detection of chemical changes
7. Photoreceptors—detection of light changes (located in the eye)

---

the level of the spinal cord where pain impulses pass through a "gate" to reach the brain. Massage can be a stimulus to suppress the sensation of pain, especially sharp pain, according to the gate theory.) **Mechanoreceptors** (movement receptors) carry impulses more quickly than **nociceptors** (pain receptors), thus blocking the input of pain impulses. In addition, the pain relief and relaxation effects accompanying massage are thought to be the result of the release of systemic hormones such as endorphins and serotonin. Localized hormones, such as enkephalins and dopamine, further modify the perception of pain.

Reflexive Response

> ★ **EXAM POINT** Massage can stimulate or inhibit cutaneous receptors, muscle spindle receptors, proprioceptors, and superficial skeletal muscle.

These structures produce impulses that reach the spinal cord, generating various effects including moderation of the facilitated segment and somatovisceral reflex changes to the viscera (see p. 123 for more information). The body uses these **reflexive responses** as protective mechanisms to prevent present or future injury.

Effects of Massage on Body Systems

By understanding the physiological effects of massage on the body, you will be better able to provide the type of massage treatment that will be of the greatest benefit to your client. The most important point to remember about the physiological effects is that they are not limited to the surface of the skin. Recall the levels of organization of the body: biochemical, cellular, tissue, organ, system, and organism. Treatment to one level of the body ultimately affects the whole organism. Each system of the human body is interdependent. No function or dysfunction is isolated; everything is connected. It is possible, however, to identify and treat what is believed to be the primary cause or dysfunction, thus allowing the body to heal and repair.

Cardiovascular System

One of the most integrated systems of the body—the cardiovascular system—is responsible for the transport of blood and its constituents, and the exchange of oxygen, nutrients, and waste products throughout the body. Every other body system depends on the cardiovascular system; without blood flow, cells die. The body monitors cardiovascular health by evaluating the amount of blood and oxygen traveling through the blood stream.

> ★ **EXAM POINT** Massage therapy is used to increase venous blood flow and therefore increase the exchange of nutrients and waste.

Blood flow is evaluated by measuring a person's blood pressure and heart rate.

Blood pressure depends on the amount of space within the interior of the vessel (diameter of the blood vessel interior) and the amount of blood present (volume.) When the vessel diameter increases, opening up the space, the blood volume decreases and blood pressure drops. Therefore, blood vessel diameter is inversely related to blood volume, which is directly related to blood pressure (figure 5.1).

> **TECHNIQUE EMPHASIS** The diameter of the blood vessels is regulated by the sympathetic and parasympathetic divisions of the autonomic nervous system.

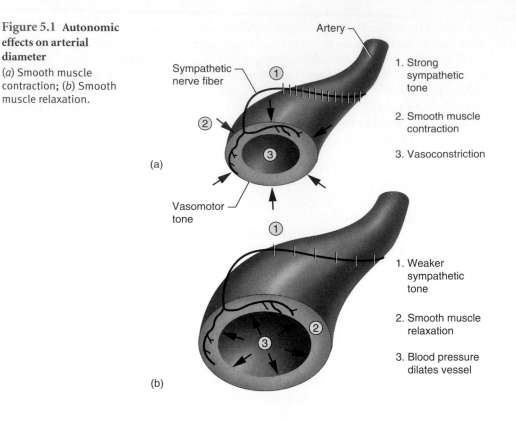

Figure 5.1 Autonomic effects on arterial diameter

(*a*) Smooth muscle contraction; (*b*) Smooth muscle relaxation.

In **hypertension (HTN)**, blood pressure and blood flow are affected by changes to the vessels. Essential hypertension, high blood pressure not due to any underlying pathology (disease or condition), occurs when the diameter of the blood vessel decreases, resulting in increased blood volume. An increase in sympathetic tone produces a tightening or constriction in the arterioles (arteriolar vasoconstriction) with a subsequent relative increase in blood volume. With time and repeated episodes of increased blood pressure due to increased sympathetic tone, the body resets special receptors—called **baroreceptors**—and the elevation of arterial blood pressure or hypertension becomes sustained as the new normal perceived by the body. Many individuals are prescribed diuretics to control blood volume. The thought is that if blood volume is reduced, then blood pressure will decrease. This creates a conflict with the idea that hydration is key in promoting physiological and metabolic clearing. Hydration is still important, but the effects of decreasing vessel diameter still apply, and improving blood flow is still necessary.

EXAM POINT   The goal for the massage therapist is to relax the client by decreasing sympathetic input and promoting a widening of the lumen in the blood vessel called vasodilation, resulting in decreased volume and a lower (decreased) blood pressure.

When providing massage to a client with cardiovascular disease, remember that the best therapy goals are made through clinical reasoning and understanding of the condition.

 TECHNICAL EMPHASIS   Apply the knowledge that massage helps open blood vessels and improves the rate of blood flow, allowing for increased cellular respiration and removal of waste.

But, if contraindications apply, communicate and collaborate with the client's physician to determine the best approach for treatment.

The Inflammation Response

When inflammation in the body occurs, many changes also occur to the vascular parts of the cardiovascular system. Localized swelling, redness of tissue, heat, and pain are produced when tissue becomes inflamed. The redness is the result of vessel dilation and the increase of blood flow and volume within the affected area. This condition is called **hyperemia**, which means an excess of red blood cells is congesting the tissues.

As the body tries to repair itself by the inflammation response, this congestion of red blood cells forces fluid through the capillary walls and into the surrounding tissue spaces (causing the response known as edema). Fibroblasts arrive to form fibers around the affected area and enclose the inflamed tissues in a sac of connective tissues. This response helps contain the tissue fluids, known as exudates, from spreading or further weakening the area.

The heat aspect of an inflamed area comes from the excess blood that is deep in the tissues. Pain receptors are activated by the swelling and heat. This deep-tissue blood, which is considerably warmer than the surrounding tissue, rises to spread into the surface area.

The physiological response of inflammation is usually brought about by a pathogen; white blood cells accumulate at the sites to help control the pathogens by phagocytosis. Inflammation can be caused by excessive physical activity or injury as well as blood chemical factors. If a muscle or joint has been injured, phagocytic cells clean up the debris of dead cells left over from the inflammation so new healthy cells can restore the body's function.

Cardiovascular System Effects

Massage affects the cardiovascular system in the following ways:

- Increases local blood supply to soft tissue, muscle, and joints
- Delivers oxygen and nutrients to cells
- Removes toxins and metabolic wastes
- Promotes vascular health and flexibility
- Affects heart rate and blood pressure
- Balances pH levels
- Increases cellular metabolism
- Increases skin temperature and venous blood flow
- Improves overall blood and lymph circulation

Lymphatic System

Closely related to the cardiovascular system, the lymphatic system collects accumulated tissue fluid around the cells and returns it to the blood stream (figure 5.2). The lymphatic system is similar in structure to the venous system: movement is slow and aided by muscle contraction, respiration, and skin and fascial movement. Stagnation of blood or lymph can lead to seepage of lymph into the surrounding interstitial space and cause edema. Massage techniques promote lymph flow back to the cardiovascular system for removal.

The lymphatic system also plays a key role in defending the body. **Macrophages**, located in lymph nodes and tissues, process antigens and release them to **lymphocytes** to help the immune system fight infection. Macrophages also filter worn-out red blood cells and destroy microorganisms. The immune system has many similarities to the nervous system:

- Tremendous sensory and effector capacities
- Influenced by other processes in the body

Figure 5.2
The lymphatic system feeds back into the cardiovascular system to maintain fluid balance and defend against infection.

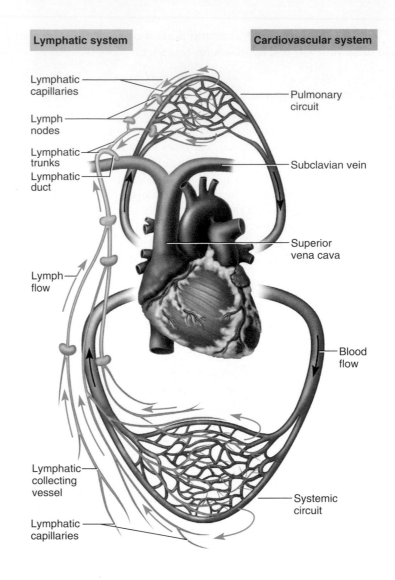

Lymphatic system

- Lymphatic capillaries
- Lymph nodes
- Lymphatic trunks
- Lymphatic duct
- Lymph flow
- Lymphatic collecting vessel
- Lymphatic capillaries

Cardiovascular system

- Pulmonary circuit
- Subclavian vein
- Superior vena cava
- Blood flow
- Systemic circuit

- Responsive to external forces
- Shared chemical signals

By influencing the responsiveness of the immune and nervous systems through massage, the body is better able to fight off disease.

Lymphatic System Effects

Massage has several effects on the lymphatic system:

- Opens lymph channels for better flow
- Increases venous and lymphatic return, augmenting reduction of edema
- Increases drainage and reduction of swelling in soft tissue, muscle, and periarticular (areas surrounding joints) regions
- Increases urine volume and excretion
- Promotes immune function and cellular repair

Nervous System

The nervous system is the control center of the human body. It monitors, coordinates, and controls all activity through its two divisions: the **central nervous system (CNS)** and the **peripheral nervous system (PNS)**.

The ANS is divided into the parasympathetic and sympathetic branches of the nervous systems. The **parasympathetic** branch is dominant in nonstressful situations. You are constantly receiving stimulus, or input, from the outside world; your body and nervous system are interpreting it and responding accordingly.

The **sympathetic** branch (figure 5.3) promotes fight-or-flight responses such as those experienced in stressful situations. We experience stress everyday. How we deal with this stress influences the mechanisms of health and disease. Continued stress leads to a continued sympathetic state of being. Parasympathetic systems (figure 5.4) allow for rest, relaxation, digestion, and healing. Without time to relax and heal, the cumulative effects of stress will manifest as illness and disease. How your body responds or reacts to these stimuli is where the focus of your massage therapy should begin.

The parasympathetic and sympathetic systems display a fine balance between relaxation and excitability. The sympathetic system serves as a protective mechanism during times of danger and prepares your body for fight or flight. The nervous system is able to adapt quickly within a short time, but it is the endocrine system that allows for a longer duration of adaptation. These systems influence each other, causing sustained periods of sympathetic response. In today's stressful culture, we tend to be in sympathetic overload. Our bodies' needs for constant adaptation to stress have led to dangerous physiological changes. Higher incidences of heart disease, immune fatigue, digestive disorders, and pain are just a few negative results.

Some people believe that the body stores a person's memories, experiences, and emotions within its tissues. Negative reactions such as anger or stress cause the body to tense and constrict (see chapters 12 and 17). Positive reactions such as happiness and joy allow the body to move and flow freely. Over time, stress and negative reactions will accumulate and without release will lead to physical, emotional, and mental exhaustion and injury. Somatoemotional releases such as those seen with massage give the body a way of letting go of the negativity to begin healing.

The mind-body connection is important in that the mind or central nervous system is the control center of the body. Two approaches have been used to address the nervous system: psychological mechanisms and mechanical mechanisms. Massage therapists often incorporate a variety of psychophysical techniques, such as guided imagery, into massage treatment (see chapter 17). Mechanical techniques are chosen based on the intended outcome or result of the technique: do you want to relax or stimulate the nervous system?

Think About It   General Principles

- Parasympathetic and sympathetic systems often have antagonistic effects in each organ.
- Sweat glands and most vascular smooth muscles have only sympathetic innervation.
- The ciliary muscle of the eye has only parasympathetic innervation.
- The bronchial smooth muscle has only parasympathetic innervation (constriction) but is sensitive to circulating adrenaline (dilation).
- Parasympathetic and sympathetic systems produce similar, rather than opposite, effects in salivary glands.

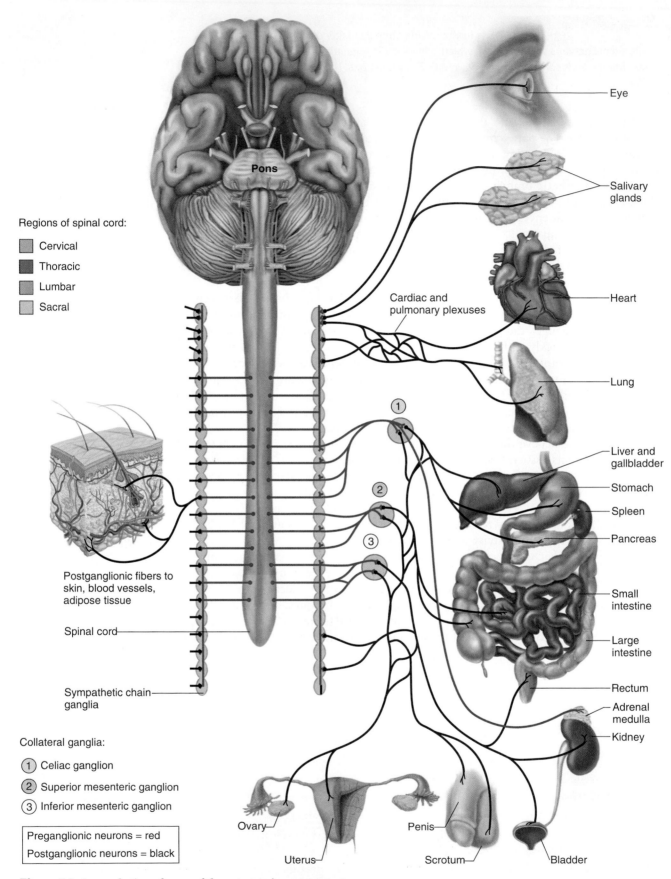

Regions of spinal cord:

- Cervical
- Thoracic
- Lumbar
- Sacral

Pons

Eye

Salivary glands

Cardiac and pulmonary plexuses

Heart

Lung

Liver and gallbladder

Stomach

Spleen

Pancreas

Small intestine

Large intestine

Rectum

Adrenal medulla

Kidney

Postganglionic fibers to skin, blood vessels, adipose tissue

Spinal cord

Sympathetic chain ganglia

Collateral ganglia:

1. Celiac ganglion
2. Superior mesenteric ganglion
3. Inferior mesenteric ganglion

Preganglionic neurons = red
Postganglionic neurons = black

Ovary

Uterus

Penis

Scrotum

Bladder

Figure 5.3 Sympathetic pathways of the autonomic nervous system

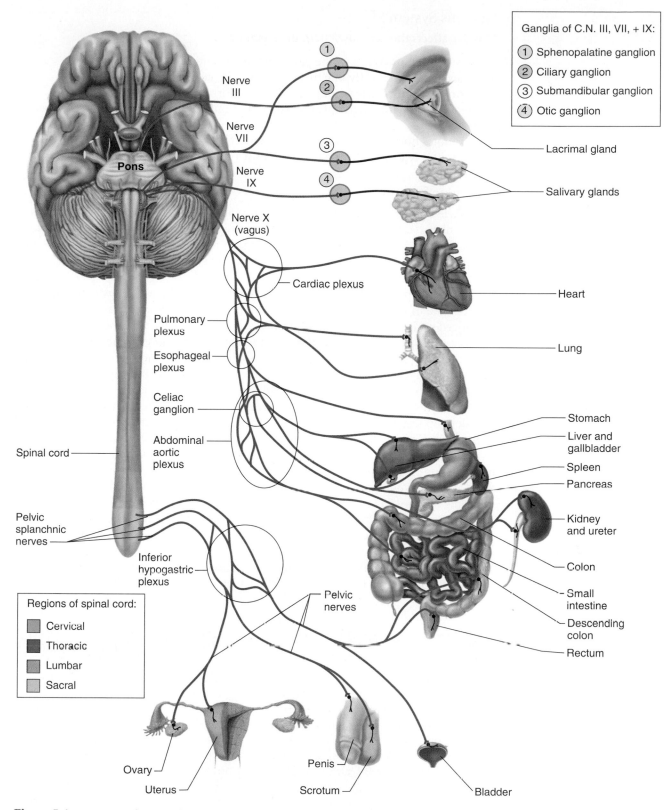

Ganglia of C.N. III, VII, + IX:
1. Sphenopalatine ganglion
2. Ciliary ganglion
3. Submandibular ganglion
4. Otic ganglion

Nerve III

Nerve VII

Pons

Nerve IX

Nerve X (vagus)

Cardiac plexus

Pulmonary plexus

Esophageal plexus

Celiac ganglion

Abdominal aortic plexus

Spinal cord

Pelvic splanchnic nerves

Inferior hypogastric plexus

Pelvic nerves

Lacrimal gland

Salivary glands

Heart

Lung

Stomach

Liver and gallbladder

Spleen

Pancreas

Kidney and ureter

Colon

Small intestine

Descending colon

Rectum

Regions of spinal cord:
- Cervical
- Thoracic
- Lumbar
- Sacral

Ovary

Uterus

Penis

Scrotum

Bladder

Figure 5.4 Parasympathetic pathways of the autonomic nervous system

Nervous System Effects

Massage affects the nervous system in several ways:

- Promotes homeostasis in the parasympathetic and sympathetic systems
- Alleviates pain directly, chemically, and via the nervous response
- Promotes natural release of pain killers (endorphins and enkephalins)
- Reduces pain and interrupts the pain sensation cycle, resulting in increased ease of mobility
- Promotes hormonal release with systemic effects
- Promotes relaxation by the natural release of dopamine and serotonin

Muscular System

Each skeletal muscle is an individual organ made up of hundreds and thousands of muscle fibers (cells), large amount of connective tissue, nerve fibers, and many blood vessels. Demand on the muscle creates change in muscle physiology and its structure. Muscles require nutrients from the cardiovascular system, and muscle tone is determined by the nervous system.

Muscles depend on the cardiovascular system for nutrients to allow for contraction and removal of waste. Muscles that maintain excess tone—or constant contraction for prolonged periods of time—work beyond their capacity. This can produce pain, which may increase spasm, causing further toxin release and possibly an increase in pain—a cycle of pain-spasm-pain. A common cause of muscle dysfunction is fatigue. Fatigue can lead to physiological changes such as low levels of adenosine triphosphate or calcium, depletion of oxygen or glucose, and high levels of lactic acid.

If muscle fatigue occurs, the muscles become undernourished and overworked, and may develop trigger point pain, weakness, increased density in the surrounding ground substance (gelatinous substance), and increased metabolic toxicity. Massage can be used to relieve this cycle by softening the tissue, reducing tone, and flushing out the toxins as new blood is brought to the area. Tense muscles and scars in muscle and connective tissue may restrict joint movement. Massage affects conditions found in the soft tissues surrounding the joint and thereby can aid in maintaining joint range of motion and mobility.

The nervous system provides the innervation or stimulus necessary for a muscle to contract. The muscle contains neuromuscular junction muscle points that provide muscle tonicity for a quick contraction or maintaining posture. Trigger points can be caused by increased activity in the belly of the muscle that leads to localized hyperstates of muscle contraction. Other factors include high levels of stress, which cause the ner-

---

Think About It | Adenosine Triphosphate

Each skeletal muscle is an individual organ made up of hundreds and thousands of muscle fibers (cells), large amounts of connective tissue, nerve fibers, and many blood vessels. Muscles depend on glucose from the breakdown of the food a body consumes. Through a series of three reactions—glycolysis, citric acid cycle, and electron transport chain—the metabolism of glucose provides adenosine triphosphate (ATP), the primary energy component of all living human cells. Figure 5.5 shows how ATP is used by the body. In addition, muscles require calcium to allow for a contraction to occur. Demand on the muscle creates change in muscle physiology and its structure. Muscles depend on the cardiovascular system for nutrients to allow for contraction and removal of waste. Muscles that maintain excess tone—or constant contraction for prolonged periods of time—work beyond their oxidative capacity. This produces pain, which increases tone, causing further toxin release and an increase in pain—a cycle of pain-spasm-pain. A common cause of dysfunction is muscle fatigue, which can lead to physiological changes such as low levels of ATP or calcium, depletion of oxygen or glucose, and high levels of lactic acid.

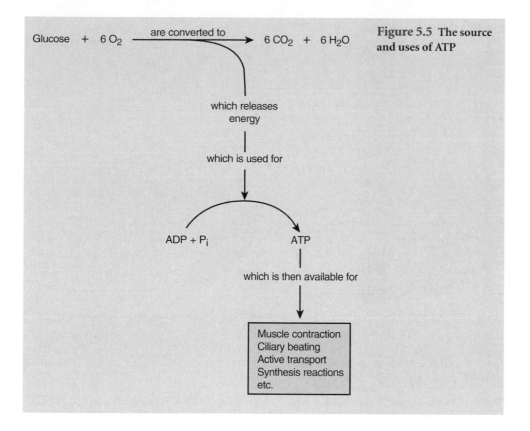

$$Glucose + 6\,O_2 \xrightarrow{\text{are converted to}} 6\,CO_2 + 6\,H_2O$$

which releases energy

which is used for

ADP + P$_i$ ATP

which is then available for

Muscle contraction
Ciliary beating
Active transport
Synthesis reactions
etc.

Figure 5.5 The source and uses of ATP

vous system to experience periods of sustained excitability. This excitability can lead to decreased blood flow and stagnation within the muscle due to hypertonic muscle causing areas of restriction and decreasing vessel diameter.

Muscular System Effects

Massage has several effects on the muscular system:

- Increases muscle relaxation and reduces muscle guarding or holding
- Relieves spasms, cramps, and pain
- Prevents adhesions and fibrotic buildup
- Improves muscle tone
- Decreases tendency toward muscle atrophy during long periods of immobilization or disuse
- Increases flexibility and mobility
- Increases joint range of motion

The human body has two major anatomical and physiological components: soma and viscera.

Reflex Mechanisms of Massage

★ **EXAM POINT** The **soma** includes all the cells and tissues in the body considered collectively, with the exception of germ cells, such as skin, fascia, and muscles. The **viscera** include the internal organs of the body such as those contained within the dorsal and ventral cavities.

The soma provides our ability for movement and interaction with environment, and serves as a protective covering for the viscera. Somatic and visceral structures are wired

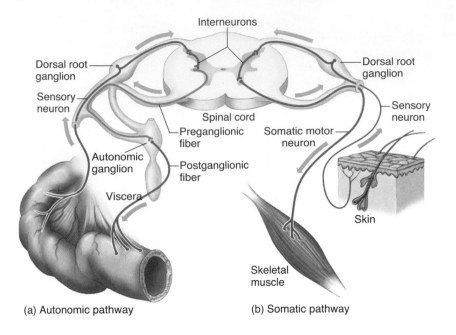

Figure 5.6 Motor pathways
(a) Autonomic pathway has two neurons; (b) somatic pathway has one neuron between the CNS and an effector.

together by the nervous system (figure 5.6). These connections are possible because of four principal reflexes:

Viscerosomatic reflex: This reflex establishes the connection between the inner organ and a particular area of the skin and connective tissue structures (fascia or aponeurosis). This reflex mechanism is better known as a referred pain in that the viscera and somatic structure are innervated by the same spinal segment.

Somatovisceral reflex: This reflex is similar to the viscerosomatic reflex in that it establishes a connection between the affected inner organ and a particular somatic structure. As a result of a chronic somatic or visceral disorder, hypertonic abnormalities (in the form of hypertonicity or trigger points) are formed in the skeletal muscles. These abnormalities are innervated by the same segment of the spinal cord as the originally affected inner organ.

Somasomatic reflex: This reflex establishes cause-effect relations between the different somatic structures located along pathways of the same peripheral nerve. For example, a condition known as "double crush" refers to thoracic outlet syndrome, a chronic compression of the brachial plexus, ultimately causing carpal tunnel syndrome due to the compromised neurological communication to the distal nerve endings.

Viscerovisceral reflex: This reflex establishes a connection between different visceral structures. The autonomic nervous system provides dual innervation to the viscera through its parasympathetic and sympathetic divisions. Sympathetic innervation to the heart, lungs, and main viscera of the gastrointestinal system arises from the medulla, providing a single input and resulting in coordinated response. For example, an increase in heart rate will automatically trigger an increase in the respiratory rate, and vice versa.

The reflex mechanism of massage therapy allows the therapist to dramatically improve the outcome of somatic conditions and to be proactive in the treatment of visceral disorders. These reflex mechanisms are responsible for the formation of localized changes and dysfunction in the areas of soft tissues that are innervated by the same segment of the spinal cord as the original somatic or visceral disorder. The disorders do not form immediately upon clinical presentation of the original disorder. Somatic abnormalities may take an average of two to three weeks. While visceral disorders may be formed after approximately three months.

The purpose of massage is to bring about changes that will aid the body in returning to homeostasis and to achieve normalization of tissue through mechanical mechanisms. These mechanical mechanisms change the structure and facilitate the function of the body and its parts. In the study of therapeutic massage, the student must remain mindful of the basic chemical foundations of life and the dynamic process of change. Each time therapists massage a client, they become part of the stimulus pattern. This pattern is likewise the activation process for chemical reactions and change within the body.

Massage consists of a group of manual techniques that include applying fixed or movable pressure, holding, or causing movement of or to the body. The hands are primarily used to apply the techniques, but therapists sometimes use other areas such as the forearm or elbow. The therapist controls several variables of massage, including environment. Actual application of treatment includes the variables of rhythm, rate, pressure, direction, and duration.

The rhythm of massage strokes also should be regular and cyclic. The rate of application for massage varies with the type of technique. The amount of pressure depends on technique and desired results. Light pressure may produce relaxation and relative sedation and may decrease spasm; breakdown of adhesions and intervention at a deeper tissue level may require heavier pressure. Treatment of edema and stretching of connective tissue generally requires intermediate amounts of pressure. Direction of massage often is centripetal to provide better mobilization of fluids toward the central circulation. The sequence of tissues treated is often performed in centripetal fashion. When muscles are treated, motions generally are kept parallel to muscle fibers. If the treatment goal is to reduce adhesions, shearing forces are circular or at least include cross-fiber components.

Physiologic Effects of Western Massage Techniques

Swedish massage is the basis of Western massage. Also based on modern concepts of anatomy and physiology, Western massage includes a wide variety of manipulative techniques that go beyond the original framework of Swedish massage (see chapter 4).

Swedish Massage

Swedish massage uses a system of long, gliding strokes, kneading, and percussion and tapping techniques on the more superficial layers of muscles. It is designed to promote generalized relaxation and increase circulation, which may improve healing and decrease swelling from an injury.

Neuromuscular Massage

Neuromuscular massage is a comprehensive program of soft-tissue manipulation, trigger point massage, and myotherapy that balances the body's central nervous system with the musculoskeletal system. Using neurological principles that explain how the central nervous system initiates and maintains pain, the goal is to help relieve the pain and dysfunction by identifying and alleviating the underlying cause. Neuromuscular therapy can help individuals who experience biomechanical dysfunction by releasing and uncovering symptoms of a deeper problem. It is also used to locate and release spasms and hypertonic tissues, eliminate trigger points that cause referred pain, rebuild the strength of injured tissues, assist venous and lymphatic flow, and restore postural alignment, proper biomechanics, and flexibility to the tissues.

Deep Tissue Massage

Deep tissue massage is used to release chronic patterns of muscular tension using slow strokes, direct pressure, or friction. Deep tissue/deep muscle massage is administered to affect the sublayer of musculature and fascia that support muscle tissues and loosen bonds between the layers of connective tissues. Often the movements are directed across the grain of the muscles (cross-fiber) using the fingers, thumbs, or elbows. This approach is applied with greater pressure and at deeper layers of the muscle than Swedish massage, which is why it is called deep tissue massage.

Manual Lymph Drainage Massage

The strokes applied in manual lymph drainage massage are intended to stimulate the movement of the lymphatic fluids to assist the body in cleansing. This approach improves the flow of lymph fluid with gentle, rhythmical strokes and is used primarily to alleviate conditions involving poor lymph flow that can lead to stagnation and edema. By improving lymph flow, this technique cleanses the connective tissue of inflammatory materials and toxins, enhances the activity of the immune system, reduces pain, and lowers the activity of the sympathetic nervous system.

Physiological Effects of Eastern Massage Techniques

Eastern methods of massage are based primarily on the principles of Chinese medicine but also include Ayurvedic, Japanese, and Thai techniques. All of the Eastern methods center around the flow of energy (Qi, *prana*, or Ki) through the body's meridians, or energy points. With these massage techniques, strong pressure or very light pressure is applied by finger or thumb tips to predetermined points, concentrating on unblocking the flow of energy and restoring balance in the meridians and organs to promote self-healing. There are over a dozen varieties of Eastern massage and bodywork therapy, but the most common forms are acupressure and shiatsu (see chapter 15).

Acupressure and Shiatsu

Considered similar techniques, acupressure and shiatsu are both based on applying pressure to a pattern of specific points that correspond with the acupuncture points. Pressure is applied with the thumb, finger, and palm rather than using needles. Shiatsu also incorporates stretching and movement to influence the flow of energy. The goal of both shiatsu and acupressure is the efficient and balanced flow of energy through the meridians. It is believed that where tension or stress is held in the body, the flow of energy is impaired through those areas. Blocked energy can lead to chronic problems, not only in the musculature but also in the associated organs.

Effects of Hydrotherapy

Although hydrotherapy is covered in other chapters, we include it here as well because of the definitive physiological effects it causes when used by a massage therapist.

⭐ **EXAM POINT** Hydrotherapy takes advantage of water's unique ability to store and transmit both cold and heat (see chapters 13 and 14 for more information on hydrotherapy).

Cold-based hydrotherapies, such as ice packs and cold compresses, have what is known as a "depressant" effect: Cold decreases normal activity, constricting blood vessels, numbing nerves, and slowing respiration. On the other hand, heat-based hydrotherapies, such as whirlpools and hot compresses, have the opposite effect. As the body attempts to throw off the excess heat and keep body temperature from rising, dilation of blood vessels occurs (figure 5.7), providing increased circulation to the area being treated.

The effects of water, as with all other therapeutic agents, may be either local or general, according to the mode of application. Water is given either internally (such as drinking a glass of water) or externally (taking a steam bath). Many modifying circumstances—such as age, sex, and physical condition—affect the results to a greater or lesser degree.

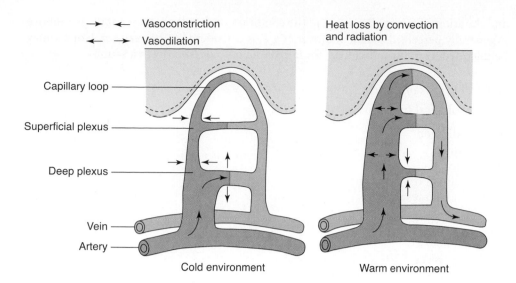

Figure 5.7
Vasoconstriction and vasodilation in response to heat and cold

Vasoconstriction → ←
Vasodilation ← →

Heat loss by convection and radiation

Capillary loop

Superficial plexus

Deep plexus

Vein

Artery

Cold environment   Warm environment

Effects of Cold Applications

Cold applications may be made by means of ice, cold water, or cold air, or by the evaporation of water or other liquids from the surface of the body. Although the applications may vary, the principles and effects remain consistent. The primary or direct effect of cold applications is depressant. This leads to a decrease in function, either locally or systemically, depending on the application. The longer and colder the application, the longer and more intense will be the depressant effect. However, as the body responds to the cold application, there is a return to normal function that may lead to a state of increased activity. This is known as the secondary (or indirect) effect of cold; this effect is also known as the reaction. If the cold application is a short one, the reaction follows quickly, its intensity reflecting the intensity (coldness) of the application.

The secondary effect (or reaction) occurs only when the body has the vitality to respond to the cold, either following the removal of the cold from the body (in such applications as showers, sprays, and baths) or after the body has warmed the application (in such applications as cold compresses or packs). In most cases, the colder the application, the greater the reaction. Many hydrotherapy techniques are directed at producing the reaction to the cold application.

General Effects of Cold

Cold penetrates deeper than heat. All physiological functions decrease:

- Vasoconstriction
- Decreased blood flow
- Decreased respiration
- Decreased metabolism

Effects of Local Cold

- Vasoconstriction
- Decreased pain (analgesia)
- Decreased blood flow
- Decreased muscle spasm

Effects of Heat Applications

Heat may be applied to the body in a variety of ways, including hot packs, fomentations, steam, hot air, baths, and showers. All hot applications produce definite physiological responses that are attempts of the body to eliminate heat to prevent a rise in body temperature. The effects produced by hot applications depend on the mode, temperature, and duration of the application and the condition of the client. Water at 98°F or above is generally perceived as *hot*, and over 104°F, is considered to be *very hot*. Hot air may be tolerated by many individuals for fairly long periods, such as in a sauna.

General Effects of Heat

All physiological functions increase:

- Vasodilation
- Sweating
- Hyperemia
- Increase in oxygen content in blood
- Increase in respiration

Effects of Local Heat

- Vasodilation
- Erythemia
- Decrease in pain (analgesia)
- Decreased muscle spasm

Take precautions with both hot and cold water treatments. Do not use a microwave to heat a compress because the material will get too hot too quickly. Soak the compress in hot water from the tap and test its temperature before applying it to a body. When using ice, do not put the ice or ice pack directly on skin. Wrap it in a slightly damp towel and then apply. Hydrotherapy that uses extreme temperatures is not recommended for pregnant women or people who have a heart condition, circulation disorder, high blood pressure, or diabetes.

Chapter Summary

In this chapter, we looked at how massage affects the physiology of the body. The body has many ways to protect and heal itself, but there comes a time when intervention is needed. Massage therapists have a unique opportunity to facilitate healing in the human body when the body itself is not capable. Massage is a valuable tool in the management of health and personal well-being. However, a massage therapist must understand why and how treatments will affect the client to prevent injury or reinjury to the client. A therapist's goal is to understand the disease process and to help promote healing by using the knowledge gained through study and practice. The education and clinical decision-making skills of the therapist—in conjunction with other members of the health care team—will help in determining the appropriate approach and treatment plan. Knowledge and communication combined with diligence and professionalism will produce positive results for you and your client.

Applying Your Knowledge

Self-Testing

1. What are the three primary mechanisms that massage affects?
   a) Circulatory, digestive, and neurological
   b) Metabolism, pain, and reflexive
   c) Muscular, circulatory, and skin
   d) Metabolism, circulatory, and neurological

2. Metabolism is the sum of all physiological activity in the body.
   a) True
   b) False

3. Which mechanism uses the gate control theory?
   a) Metabolism
   b) Pain
   c) Reflexive
   d) None of the above is correct.

4. Which mechanism uses the sensory and motor pathways associated to the brain and spinal cord?

   a) Metabolism

   b) Pain

   c) Reflexive

   d) None of the above is correct.

5. Which organ system is most integrated within the body?

   a) Cardiovascular

   b) Lymphatic

   c) Muscular

   d) Nervous

6. Which system is most closely related to the cardiovascular system?

   a) Lymphatic

   b) Muscular

   c) Nervous

   d) Respiratory

7. Which system is most dependent on circulation and innervation for proper function?

   a) Cardiovascular

   b) Lymphatic

   c) Muscular

   d) Nervous

8. Massage therapists can promote injury if they do not understand the effects of massage.

   a) True

   b) False

Case Studies/Critical Thinking

A. Jonie's doctor has referred her to your clinic for massage. She has had trouble sleeping since moving to your town. She also has mild anxiety occasionally that appears to be related to the stress of a new job. Since her insomnia and anxiety were diagnosed as mild, her doctor decided that massage could bring about the changes needed and did not prescribe medication for the problems. What massage technique would best address Jonie's concerns? How often should she be massaged? Jonie is also putting in a lot of overtime at the new job and complains of pains in her neck and shoulders. Could trigger point therapy lessen the neck pain? What reflex mechanism may be at play here?

B. Lamarcus has returned to school to begin training for a new career. His frequent headaches, confusion, and dizziness sent him to his physician for a consultation. After his blood pressure and respiration (rate of breathing) were monitored for several weeks, it was discovered that Lamarcus suffers from "situational hypertension," which means the blood pressure rises due to physiological responses to his anxiety over the new classes. He also tends to hyperventilate after he takes a test. It is noted that on the days he does not attend class, his blood pressure and breathing are normal. Would massage therapy techniques help Lamarcus deal with the stress and reduce his blood pressure? If he continues to have episodes of quickly rising blood pressure due to a situation, will he be diagnosed with hypertension and placed on medication? What reflex mechanism is responsible? Would Eastern or Western massage methods be the best type of treatment? What approach would you choose?

References for information in this chapter can be found in Quick Guide C at the end of the book.

PART II

Kinesiology, Anatomy, and Pathophysiology

CHAPTER 6   **Biomechanics of Movement**

CHAPTER 7   **General Overview of the Body and the Skeletal System**

CHAPTER 8   **Muscular System**

CHAPTER 9   **Other Body Systems**

Biomechanics of Movement

LEARNING OUTCOMES

After completing this chapter, you will be able to:

- List the body planes, normal ranges of motion, and the factors that affect them.

- Identify the different joint movements and the associated axes of rotation.

- Describe some of the biomechanical properties of various structures of the musculoskeletal system.

- Discuss the significance of anthropometric measurements and somatotyping.

- List some of the measures recommended for preventing musculoskeletal injuries.

- Discuss how you will apply your knowledge of biomechanics to improve massage techniques.

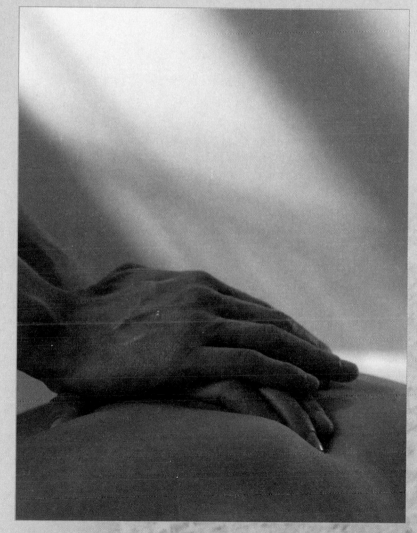

KEY TERMS

abduction *(p. 137)*

adduction *(p. 138)*

agonist *(p. 143)*

amphiarthrotic or cartilaginous
   joints *(p. 144)*

anatomical position *(p. 135)*

antagonist *(p. 143)*

anthropometry *(p. 134)*

axes of motion *(p. 136)*

body's center of gravity *(p. 136)*

circumduction *(p. 139)*

concentric action *(p. 143)*

depression *(p. 140)*

diarthrotic or synovial
   joints *(p. 144)*

dorsiflexion *(p. 140)*

dynamic *(p. 134)*

eccentric action *(p. 143)*

elevation *(p. 140)*

ergonomics *(p. 145)*

eversion *(p. 140)*

extension *(p. 137)*

fast twitch fibers *(p. 143)*

flexion *(p. 137)*

frontal plane *(p. 136)*

horizontal or transverse
   plane *(p. 136)*

hyperextension *(p. 137)*

inversion *(p. 140)*

isometric action *(p. 143)*

kinematics *(p. 134)*

kinesiology *(p. 134)*

kinetics *(p. 134)*

lateral bending or lateral flexion
   (p. 140)

lateral rotation *(p. 140)*

medial rotation *(p. 140)*

parallel muscles *(p. 143)*

pennate muscles *(p. 143)*

plane *(p. 135)*

plantar flexion *(p. 140)*

posture *(p. 146)*

pronation *(p. 140)*

protraction *(p. 139)*

retraction *(p. 139)*

sagittal plane *(p. 136)*

slow twitch fibers *(p. 143)*

somatotyping *(p. 145)*

stabilizer or fixator *(p. 143)*

static *(p. 134)*

supination *(p. 140)*

synarthrotic or fibrous joints
   (p. 144)

thixotropic *(p. 143)*

INTRODUCTION

Biomechanics is the mechanical analysis of living organisms. It involves *describing* the action of forces on a body part that is either in a **static** (not moving) phase or in a **dynamic** (acceleration) phase. Biomechanics includes **kinematics** (describing the appearance of motion relative to space and time) and **kinetics** (describing the forces causing the motion). Biomechanical assessments are usually qualitative (descriptive) or quantitative (a number-assigned value). Both types of assessments are important to evaluating the performance of the musculoskeletal system.

The elements that will make understanding biomechanics more meaningful include:

- The study of the anatomical and mechanical bases of human movement (otherwise known as **kinesiology**)
- The ability to identify body planes
- The bony landmarks (see chapter 7)
- The various types of joints and their ranges of motions
- The muscles' attachments and direction, and types of muscle fibers (see chapter 8)
- The relationship between the nervous and musculoskeletal systems and their physiologic functions (see chapter 5)

The ability to assess anthropometric measurements is important. The science of **anthropometry** involves measuring the body, including the size, shape, and weight of body segments, to render a thorough biomechanical analysis. The ability of any given body part to produce the amount of force necessary to accomplish a desired movement is determined by these variables of size, shape, and weight. The practical application of such knowledge will enhance the massage therapist's ability to assess the musculoskeletal system. Being familiar with biomechanics will also help the therapist to develop any necessary recommendations for clients to prevent injury during daily activities and in various static and dynamic postures.

Terminology and Basic Concepts

Using biomechanics in evaluating human performance is a valuable tool for a massage therapist. It involves studying and analyzing the action of force on living organisms during a standing-still position (static) and during motion with acceleration (dynamic). Learning about certain anatomical and functional aspects of the body is fundamental to successfully and effectively evaluating performance techniques or forms (kinematics). It will also help in determining if muscles used during the action generate the necessary amount of force required to perfect the technique (kinetics).

When a person moves, a complex series of movements usually occur in different planes around different axes to accommodate and facilitate the movement. To assess such motion, it is necessary to know how to describe, measure, and reference these movements using the correct terms. The basic forms of motion occur along a line (linear movement), in a curved path (angular movement, or rotation), or in a combination of both. Identifying specifics of movement requires knowledge of anatomical reference positions, body planes, axes, and joint movement terminologies.

Anatomical Reference Position

EXAM POINT The starting position for human segment movements is **anatomical position**, or standing erect with the feet slightly separated, the arms hanging relaxed at the sides, and the palms of the hands facing forward (figure 6.1).

Functional position differs from anatomical position in that the palms face the body (figure 6.2).

The Anatomical Reference Planes

EXAM POINT There are three imaginary reference planes: sagittal, frontal, and transverse. A **plane** is a two-dimensional flat surface that divides the body in half by mass or weight (figure 6.3).

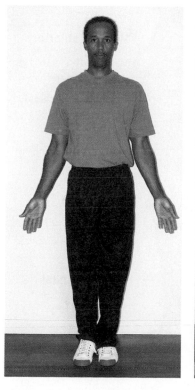

Figure 6.1 Anatomical position

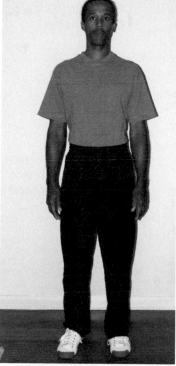

Figure 6.2 Functional position

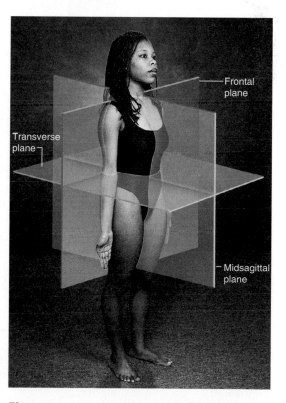

Figure 6.3 Anatomical planes of reference

The **sagittal plane** (also known as the median plane) divides the body vertically into right and left halves. The midsagittal plane divides the body into equal right and left halves. The **frontal plane** (also known as the coronal plane) splits the body vertically into front and back halves of equal weight. The **horizontal or transverse plane** divides the body into equal-weight top and bottom halves. The point at which the three planes intersect is known as the **body's center of gravity.**

The Anatomic Reference Axes

> ★ **EXAM POINT** Movements of body segments occur around imaginary axes.

The three main reference axes that describe human motion are the transverse, antero-posterior (or front to back), and longitudinal axes.

The **axes of motion** are perpendicular, or at a right angle, to the planes of motion. For instance, the transverse axis (otherwise known as the frontal axis) is perpendicular to the sagittal plane. Rotation around the transverse axis allows movement in the sagittal plane.

Directional Terms

Directional terms describe how body parts relate to other body parts. It is essential that you, as a massage therapist, are familiar with these terms so that you can properly describe different areas of the body. Figure 6.4 illustrates these locations.

- Superior (cranial): Nearer to head
- Inferior (caudal): Nearer to feet

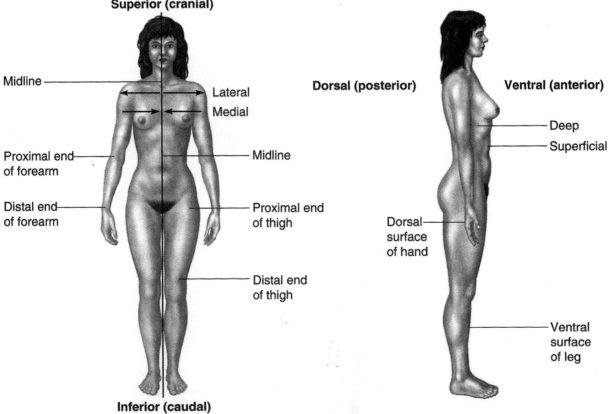

Figure 6.4
Directional terms provide mapping instructions for locating organs and body parts.

- Anterior (ventral): Nearer to front
- Posterior (dorsal): Nearer to back
- Medial: Nearer to median plane or midline of the body
- Lateral: Farther from median plane or toward the outside of the body
- Proximal: Nearer to trunk or torso
- Distal: Farther from trunk or torso
- Superficial: Nearer to surface
- Deep: Farther from surface

⭐ **EXAM POINT**   Movements occurring from the anatomical position in the sagittal plane are flexion, extension, and hyperextension.

Body Movements and Ranges of Motion

In anatomical position, the shoulders, elbows, wrists, and hips and knees joints are all 180 degrees to the sagittal plane.

Flexion is the act that decreases the angle between the bones, forming a joint. Shoulder, elbow, wrist, and hip flexions are movements that reduce the angles present at these joints. (Normal degree of flexion is 180 degrees at the shoulder, 135 degrees at the elbow, 80 degrees at the wrist, 120 degrees at the hip, and about 135 degrees at the knee.) See figure 6.5.

Extension is the movement of returning the body segment back to the anatomical position from flexion. (The normal degree of extension is 45 degrees at the shoulder, 0–5 degrees at the elbow, 70 degrees at the wrist, 30 degrees at the hip, and 0 degrees at the knee.)

Hyperextension occurs when a body segment is moved in extension beyond the anatomical position. The movements of flexion, extension, and hyperextension are demonstrated in figures 6.6 and 6.7.

Abduction is movement of a body part away from the body or away from the midsagittal line (180 degrees at the shoulder, 45 degrees at the hip).

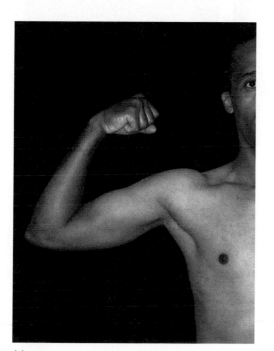

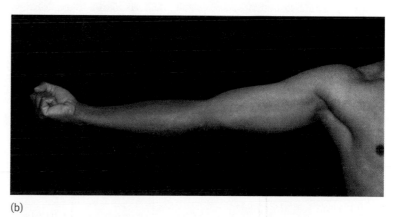

(a)   (b)

Figure 6.5
(*a*) Flexion of the elbow. (*b*) Extension of the elbow.

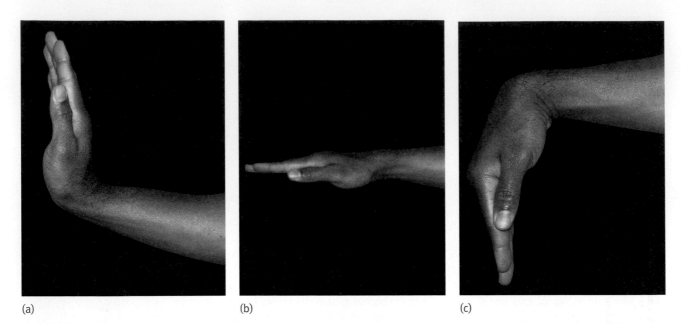

Figure 6.6
(*a*) Hyperextension of the wrist. (*b*) Extension of the wrist. (*c*) Flexion of the wrist.

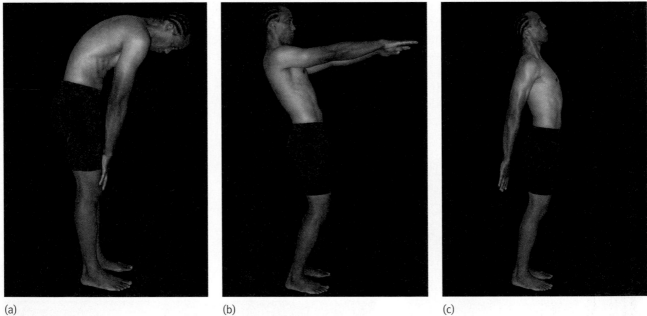

Figure 6.7
(*a*) Flexion of the spine. (*b*) Extension of the spine and flexion of the shoulder. (*c*) Hyperextension of the shoulder.

Adduction is movement of a body part toward the body or toward the midsagittal line (40 degrees at the shoulder, 20 degrees at the hip).

⭐ **EXAM POINT** Movements occurring from anatomical position in the frontal plane are abduction and adduction.

Other movements in the frontal plane include spinal lateral flexion, elevating or depressing the shoulders, and moving the hand toward the thumb side (radial deviation) or toward the little finger side (ulnar deviation).

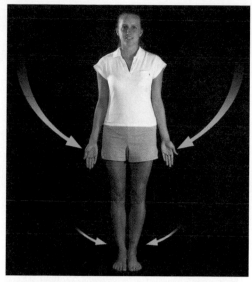
(a)

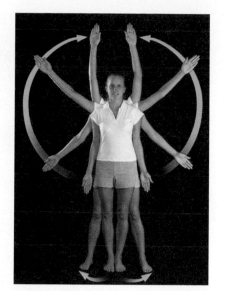
(b)

Figure 6.8

(*a*) Adduction of the limbs. (*b*) Abduction of the limbs.

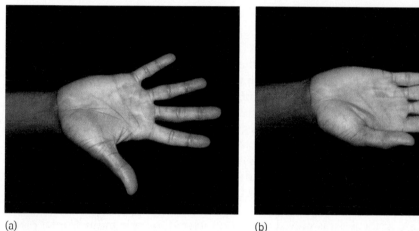
(a)   (b)

Figure 6.9

(*a*) Abduction of the fingers. (*b*) Adduction of the fingers.

If an arm or thigh is flexed to 90 degrees, then moved in the transverse plane away from the midline, the movement is referred to as horizontal abduction. If the movement happens toward the midline, it is called horizontal adduction. Figures 6.8 and 6.9 illustrate abduction and adduction.

Protraction is movement of a body part forward (anteriorly) in the horizontal plane, while **retraction** is movement of a body part backward (posteriorly) in the horizontal plane.

The sideways movements performed by the jaw are referred to as medial and lateral excursions.

Circumduction is a circular movement that combines flexion, extension, abduction, and adduction at a joint. An example of this would be using one finger to draw a circle in the air without moving the rest of the hand.

Movements in the transverse plane are rotational movements around the longitudinal axis. These movements include moving the head, neck, or trunk in left or right rotation, and moving the arms or legs in medial (inward) or lateral (outward) rotation

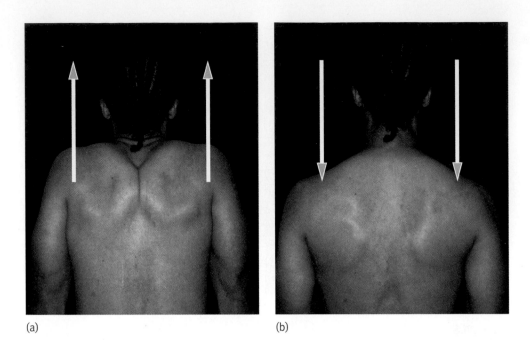

(a)   (b)

Figure 6.10

(*a*) Elevation of the scapulae. (*b*) Depression of the scapulae.

from the midline. Other movements include supination (palm up) and pronation (palm down) of the forearm, and inversion (inward rotation of the sole of the foot) and eversion (outward rotation of the sole of the foot).

Opposition is movement of the thumb with the thumb touching the other fingers, and reposition is the returning of the thumb back to anatomical position.

Lateral bending or lateral flexion involves sideways movement of the neck or the trunk in the frontal plane (about 20-45 degrees at the cervical spine, 20-40 degrees at the thoracic spine, and 25 degrees at the lumbar spine).

Movement of the shoulder in the superior direction is called **elevation** (figure 6.10). Moving the shoulder inferiorly is called **depression**. (Protraction of the shoulder is movement of the shoulder forward, while retraction of the shoulder is backward or posterior movement in the horizontal plane.)

If the hand at the wrist is moved to the thumb (radius) side in the frontal plane, this is radial deviation (20 degrees). If the hand is moved to the little finger (ulnar) side, this movement is described as ulnar deviation (30 degrees).

The ankle movements include **plantar flexion** (when the toes point down, 50 degrees) (figure 6.11) and **dorsiflexion** (when the toes are raised, 20 degrees).

⭐ **EXAM POINT** Transverse plane movements include all rotational movements.

These movements occur along a longitudinal axis. The head, neck, and trunk can rotate either to the right in right rotation or to the left in left rotation (70–90 degrees at the cervical spine, 45 degrees at the thoracic spine) (figures 6.12 and 6.13). If the arms or legs are moved as a unit in the transverse plane toward the midline, this is called **medial rotation** (figure 6.14). If the movement is away from the midline, it is called **lateral rotation**. **Supination** is the outward rotation of the forearm, or palm facing up (90 degrees) (figure 6.15). The inward rotation of the forearm is known as **pronation**, or palm facing down (90 degrees). When the sole of the foot is rotated outward, this is called **eversion** (20 degrees) (figure 6.16); inward foot rotation is called **inversion** (40 degrees).

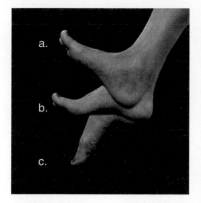

Figure 6.11
(*a*) Dorsiflexion; (*b*) extension;
(*c*) plantar flexion.

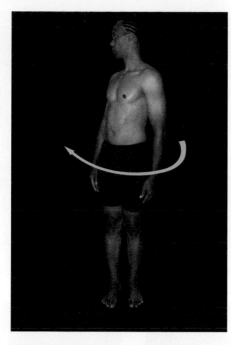

Figure 6.12 Rotation of the spine

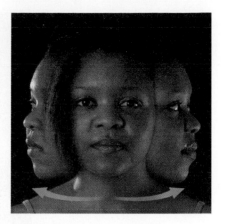

Figure 6.13 Rotation of the neck

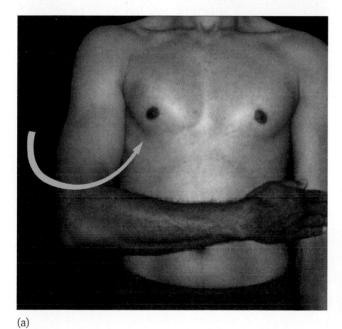

(a)

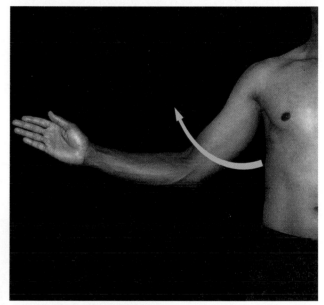

(b)

Figure 6.14
(*a*) Medial rotation of the humerus. (*b*) Lateral rotation of the humerus.

Certain movements transect more than one plane and are listed as general motion. A person drawing an imaginary circle in the air using an extremity (such as an arm or leg) actually uses the combined movements of flexion, extension, adduction, and abduction; this is described as circumduction (figure 6.17).

Figure 6.15
(a) Supination of the forearm.
(b) Pronation of the forearm.

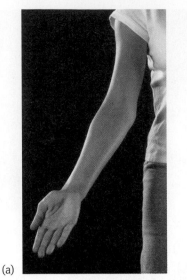

(a)

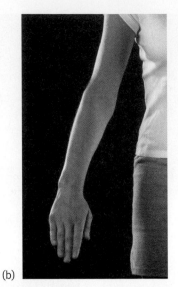

(b)

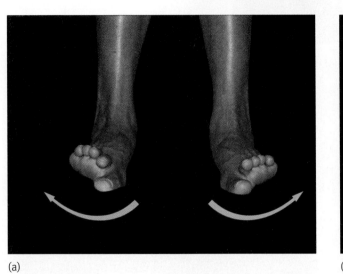

(a)

(b)

Figure 6.16
(a) Eversion. (b) Inversion.

Figure 6.17 Circumduction of the upper limb

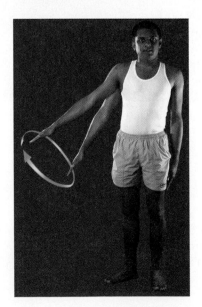

A good understanding of the biomechanics of the musculoskeletal system is important in ensuring the massage therapist's effectiveness and techniques.

 EXAM POINT The human body is made up of four basic types of tissue: muscle, nerve, epithelium, and connective tissue.

Biomechanics of Connective Tissue

The connective tissue contains cells, connective tissue fibers, and ground substance. Connective tissue fibers include collagen (tensile), elastin, and reticulin (the latter two considered to be elastic).

EXAM POINT The ground substance is the medium that contains the cells and holds together the fibers of the connective tissue.

This ground substance is **thixotropic** in nature, meaning it moves from a gel-like state to a more liquefied state when worked or massaged and then returns to the gel-like state afterward. From a biomechanical prospective, the connective tissue has both viscous (permanent) and elastic (temporary) deformation characteristics.

Biomechanics of Muscle

Muscle fibers can be categorized into fast twitch or slow twitch fibers. The **fast twitch fibers** support activities that require strength, while the **slow twitch fibers** support activities requiring endurance.

These characteristics and the arrangement of fibers within a muscle influence the strength of muscle contraction and the range of motion that it can generate. **Pennate muscles** (the fibers lie at an angle to the longitudinal axis of the muscle) contain more fibers compared to **parallel muscles** (the fibers are parallel to the muscle's longitudinal axis) of similar size and can produce more force.

EXAM POINT Parallel muscles can generate larger ranges of motion than pennate muscles of equal size.

Other properties that influence the functionality of muscle tissue include extensibility (the ability to stretch and increase its length), elasticity (the ability of the muscle to return to its normal length after being stretched), irritability (the muscle ability to respond to a stimulus), and ability to develop tension. Tension develops during contraction of a skeletal muscle due to the muscle's pull of its points of attachments (tendinoskeletal attachment) on the bone toward the muscle's center. If muscle shortening causes a change in an angle at joint, the muscle action is referred to as **concentric action**. If the muscle develops tension without changing its length, the muscle action is referred to as an **isometric action**. If the muscle lengthens as it develops tension, the muscle action is referred to as **eccentric action**. A muscle can act as an **agonist**, or prime mover, if its role is to cause movement by concentric action. A muscle functions as an **antagonist**, or opposing muscle, when it opposes movement at a joint by eccentric action. A muscle serves as a **stabilizer or fixator** when its role is to stabilize a body part against a particular force. A muscle acts as a neutralizer if it prevents unwanted actions produced by an agonist.

Some of these mechanical factors that are considered in evaluating the muscle's ability to generate force include the location of the muscle attachments, the number and types of joints the muscle crosses, the muscle shortening velocity, the muscle length at activation, and the duration of the muscle activation.

The biomechanical forces and stresses generated by muscle contractions force the connective tissue within the muscle to "remodel" to accommodate for any needed tissue changes. The muscle connection to the tendon (musculotendinous junction) allows the transfer of forces through the connective tissue insertion into the bone, where force is dissipated. These areas are considered weak and subject to injury. Greater forces are generated by muscle contraction at the tendon-bone (tendinoskeletal) junction than at the sites of ligament and joint capsule-bone junction.

Biomechanical Properties of Joints

The human body has three types of joints: synarthrotic (fibrous), amphiarthrotic (cartilaginous), and diarthrotic (synovial). These joints are categorized by their makeup and function.

Synarthrotic Joints

Synarthrotic or fibrous joints unite two bones by fibrous tissue with no joint cavity in between and with almost no movement. The types of fibrous joints include sutures between the bones of the skull.

Amphiarthrotic Joints

There are two types of **amphiarthrotic or cartilaginous joints:** synchondroses and symphyses. Synchondroses are cartilaginous joints joining two bones by hyaline cartilage. Minimal movement is allowed between the bones in these joints. An example is the epiphyseal plates of growing bones. Symphyses are fibrocartilage joints uniting two bones together. The pubic symphysis is an example of this type of cartilaginous joint.

Diarthrotic Joints

Diarthrotic or synovial joints are more complex in design and allow more movement. All synovial joints have the following features in common: a capsule that is composed of two layers and encloses the joint cavity; synovial tissue that lines the inner surface of the capsule and is covered with a film of synovial fluid; and hyaline cartilage that covers the surfaces of the enclosed contiguous bones.

> **EXAM POINT** There are six types of diarthrotic or synovial joints: plane or gliding, saddle, hinge, pivot, ball-and-socket, and ellipsoid or condyloid joints. Examples of each are: plane or gliding (clavicle and rib), saddle (thumb), hinge (elbow), pivot (atlas-axis), ball-and-socket (hip), ellipsoid or condyloid (wrist).

The biomechanical properties of each type are determined by the shape of the joint's articular surfaces and can be described according to the following criteria:

- Uniaxial joints allow motion in only one of the planes of the body around a single axis and are described as having one degree of freedom joint motion (e.g., hinge and pivot joints).
- Biaxial joints have two degrees of freedom in which the bony components are free to move in two planes around two axes (e.g., saddle joints).
- Triaxial joints enjoy three degrees of freedom with the bony components able to move freely in three planes around three axes (e.g., plane and ball-and-socket joints).

> **EXAM POINT** Different types of joints connect about 200 bones in the human body.

Joints with a simple design have a primary function of providing stability, while joints with a more complex design provide mobility. Most joints in the human body serve dual mobility-stability functions; this means that they function together to provide dynamic stability.

Anthropometry

Human body measurements are an important factor in studying biomechanics and will be important to those students who wish to participate in cross-discipline studies (such as physical therapy and athletic training). Anthropometry is a science that deals with body measurements. Obtaining accurate, standardized anthropometric measurements is useful in assessing a person's body image, sports performance, health, and body composition. These measurements are also useful in determining an appropriate workplace design.

Standard sites in the body are used to take the measurements of skin folds, girths, heights, and breadths. Anthropometric measurements can be used to compare a person's body part sizes (mass) or height to other functions or to compare a person's measurements to those of other human beings. The study of comparative sizing is referred to as allometry.

Somatotyping is used to describe the body type of an individual. This typing is likewise a tool for analyzing body image and assessing body changes during the different phases of growth and aging, and in comparing athletes at various levels of training and competition. Somatotyping is expressed in three values that are always presented in the same order. The first value indicates the relative fatness (endomorphy), the second value indicates the relative musculoskeletal robustness (mesomorphy), and the third value indicates the relative linearity of the body (ectomorphy). Estimating body fat and obtaining the anthropometric measurements help in categorizing an individual's somatotype and are biomechanically significant in kinetics studies.

These measurements can be used in creating computer-generated three-dimensional body images to provide a realistic representation of the body form. Such measurements help you to determine how much of a change is needed in areas of concern and to evaluate improvements.

Biomechanics and Ergonomics

The successful design of objects used during work and other daily activities requires good knowledge of a person's biomechanical characteristics.

Ergonomics is the study of the anatomical, physiological, and psychological aspects of humans in the work environment. Evaluation of a person's anthropometric measurements and biomechanics are used in making recommendations of products (generally furniture and office equipment) that are specifically designed to reduce potential stresses against the musculoskeletal system.

Kinesiology and Movements

Accurately analyzing the performance of movement requires knowledge of kinematics (the study of the musculoskeletal system) and kinetics (the study of forces with movement). These two elements together give an idea of the efficiency of movement as well as stress on the body.

Basic Biomechanical Concepts

Biomechanics analysis for the evaluation of the performance of the musculoskeletal system involves kinematics and kinetics. Kinematics describes the appearance of motion and involves studying the basic elements of motion, which are linear kinematics (linear motion with respect to time) and angular kinematics (rotational motions around axes).

Most of the human body's motions involve the rotation of bones around imaginary axes of rotation passing through the joint centers; such motions can be described as angular. Several instruments can be used for direct measurement of joint angles on a human subject. These instruments are called goniometers (figure 6.18). Kinetics is the study of the forces associated with motion.

Figure 6.18
A goniometer is used to measure joint angles.

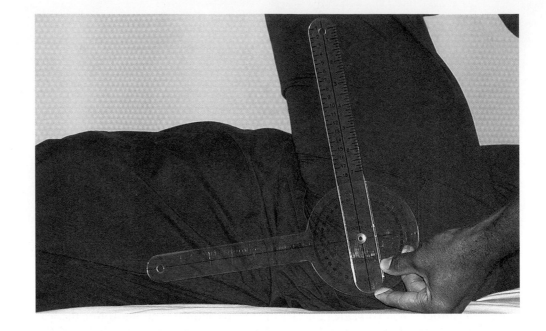

Analyzing the involved forces provides answers to why the movement occurred, how to predict its occurrence, or what to do if there is a need to modify it. The physical laws formulated by Sir Isaac Newton govern most of the basic kinetic quantities and can be used to determine how forces initiate and impact motion. The first law—law of inertia—states that a body will maintain a state of rest or constant velocity unless acted on by an external force that changes the state. The second law—law of acceleration—states that a force applied to a body causes an acceleration of that body of a magnitude proportional to the force, in direction of the force, and inversely proportional to the body's mass. The third law—law of reaction—states that when a body exerts a force on a second, the second body exerts a reaction force that is equal in magnitude and opposite in direction on the first body.

Posture and Equilibrium

Posture reflects the ability of a person to maintain balance and muscular coordination with the least amount of energy expenditure. Studying posture requires reviewing the body during both static and dynamic postures.

A simple instrument used to evaluate static posture is a plumb line, which represents the line of gravity. During the evaluation, you should view the body from the back, front, and side. Look for and make note of any muscular asymmetries (see chapter 3, p. 63).

Equilibrium is influenced by the location of the body's center of gravity (the point around which the body's weight is equally balanced in all directions) against force. Mass and the location of the base of support are all considered factors that influence a body's stability.

Examination of Active Movements and Gait

You will be able to evaluate active movements by observing the entire spine. It is recommended that you observe combined motions such as forward bending, side bending, and rotation to the same side to assess the flexibility of the myofascial planes on the opposite side of the movement. It is also important to observe backward bending. If you notice that your client experiences restrictions or pains, tell the client to consult a qualified medical professional for further evaluation.

In evaluating the normal gait, the gait should have a smooth-flowing pattern with the arm swings in tandem with the opposite leg to produce a balanced gait. A normal gait includes two phases: the stance phase (heel strike, foot flat, midstance, and toe-off)

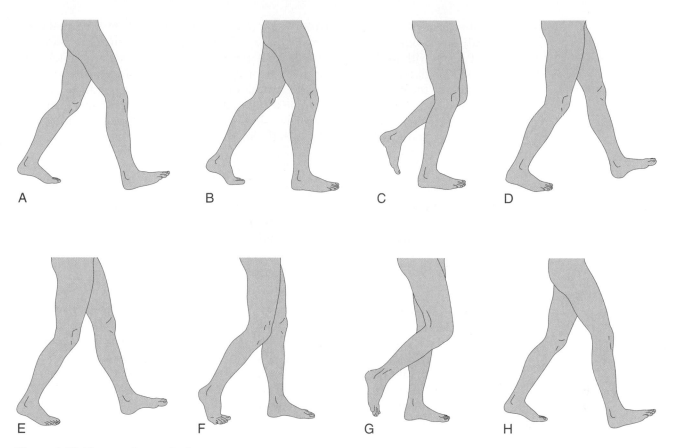

Figure 6.19 The two phases of gait

(*a*) through (*d*) show the movements of the stance phase; (*e*) through (*h*) show the movements of the swing phase: (*a*) right heel strike, (*b*) flat right foot, (*c*) midstance, (*d*) push off with right foot, (*e*) right foot poised, (*f*) left heel strike, (*g*) midswing, (*h*) right heel strike.

and the swing phase (acceleration, midswing, and deceleration). Figure 6.19 pictures the stance and swing phases. In the stance phase, pain due to a heel spur usually results in the person avoiding the heel strike; persons with an unstable knee (due to weak anterior thigh muscles) may attempt to support it by using their hand to push it in extension. Persons with weak dorsiflexors may slap their foot down instead of landing it smoothly during foot flat. During the midstance, the foot should provide even weight distribution to the surface. Individuals with flat feet suffer from discomfort—and sometimes pain—during the midstance. A weak gluteus muscle may result in a lurch toward the involved side that is observed during the midstance, while a weak gluteus maximus results in thrusting the thorax posteriorly. Healthy toes are needed to support the push-off. Acceleration and midswing of a healthy swing phase of the gait cycle depend on normal, dorsiflexsors and knee and hip motions. A successful deceleration depends mainly on normal, healthy hamstring muscles.

Other Examples of Abnormal Findings During Observation of a Gait

The massage therapist needs to be well versed in muscle action to correctly identify those muscles that may be causing the problem and how to best address them.

Some of the most common causes of pathologic gait pattern include pain as well as central nervous system or musculoskeletal disorders. Pain usually causes the person to avoid weight bearing on the affected limb. This usually results in a gait pattern called antalgic gait. Neurological or musculoskeletal disorders may produce altered gaits. People affected by cerebrovascular accidents, Parkinson's disease, or cerebral palsy may show abnormal gait patterns. Such patterns include stiff-legged gait, scissor gait, and hurried small-step gait. Musculoskeletal disorders can result in a wide variety of abnormal gaits, mostly due to limited muscle strength, or excessive or limited joint range of motion.

Persons with weakness of the anterior leg muscles may have a drop foot gait. Weakness of the gluteus muscles causes abductor lurch. A flat foot gait can be caused by weakness of the posterior leg muscles. Anterior thigh muscle weakness causes the person to walk with back knee gait. People with instability widen their gait base. Torn knee collateral ligaments or menisci can cause the knee to buckle. A stepping gait may indicate weak foot dorsiflexors. Again, such findings require further evaluations by a qualified medical professional.

Prevention of Musculoskeletal Injuries

Avoiding physical stresses is the best preventative measure against musculoskeletal injuries. The suggestions given below are just some of the measures that may help you and your clients avoid the damaging effects of physical stresses on the musculoskeletal system.

Maintain Good Posture (at Work and at Home)

As a general rule, sitting, standing, or walking with a balanced posture improves your chances of avoiding muscle fatigue. Shift body positions frequently, and be sure to properly stretch the muscles that are used the most during activities. Strengthening muscle groups that are used the least should help the body's musculoskeletal system stay healthy and decrease the chances for injuries. Balanced sitting posture—ears over shoulders over hips with straight back and relaxed shoulders with the elbows, hips, and knees maintained approximately at a 90 degrees angle with the feet flat on the floor or elevated with a slight incline—is advisable. Avoid slouching, twisting in a chair, or sitting with crossed legs for long periods.

Use Proper Lifting Techniques

Lifting injuries could lead to diminished quality of life. The following are good practices that reduce the chance for injuries:

- Think and plan the best way to move the object before lifting.
- Keep heavy objects close to the body's center of gravity.
- Widen the base of support by spreading the feet apart, stick out the chest, tuck in the chin, tighten the abdominal muscles, and keep the back upright.
- Bend at the knees, not at the hips.
- Keep the shoulders parallel to the floor as much as possible.
- When carrying a load over for a long distance or for a long time, shift the load occasionally from one side to the other and change its position, or put the load down and stretch the arms over the head, breathing in deeply.
- Avoid lifting and twisting at the same time.
- Avoid leaning forward without bending at the knees and lifting objects above the level of the shoulders (figures 6.20 and 6.21).

Improve Your Sleeping Habits

A good position for the spine during sleep is lying on the side or on the back with the knees and hips slightly flexed. Placing a pillow high enough under the head should keep the head and neck in alignment with the rest of the spine. Placing a pillow between the knees or under one knee will take pressure off of the sciatic nerve (make sure the thigh is lower than the hip). It is advisable to avoid sleeping face down as this position may cause abnormal curvatures in both the low back and the neck. It is also advisable to roll on the side—curling up in a ball—to stretch the spine when in bed and to uncurl and stretch out the arms and legs. Gently squeeze the neck muscles with the fingers while breathing deeply several times. Lie flat on your back and relax for a few moments before sleeping.

Other sensible practices include avoiding bringing work to bed, going to bed when feeling tired, and using a comfortable bed with a good-quality mattress.

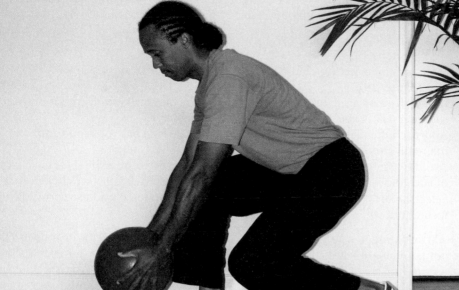

Figure 6.20 **Proper lifting technique**

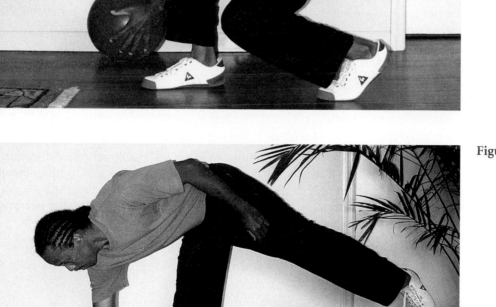

Figure 6.21 **Golfer's pickup**

Massage therapy manipulates the soft tissues of the body, resulting in a soothing effect on the nervous and muscular systems. Massage works to enhance local and general circulation of the blood and lymphatic fluids. The rhythmic, stroking actions produce deep, penetrating forces that act tangentially to the body for deep soothing, while percussive massage stimulates nerve endings, which allows muscles in spasm to relax.

Having a good knowledge of the basic concepts of biomechanics and applying those concepts during a massage session can benefit you as the massage therapist by protecting your own body from fatigue and injuries while producing the best effect on

Biomechanics and Massage

the person receiving the massage (see figure 4.9). The following measures should help you to maximize your use of biomechanics:

- Maintain good muscle strength through a regular exercise program (see chapter 19).
- Stretch using basic stretching techniques before the massage session (see chapter 19).
- Adjust the massage table height to minimize the biomechanical stresses on your shoulders, neck, and upper extremities (see chapter 4).
- Approach the massage table with a stance using a wide base of support to maintain good balance (see chapter 4).
- Avoid twisting movements of the trunk to minimize the possible shearing effects of such movement on the spine, especially the lower back area (see chapter 4).
- Select a massage table that can be moved around with ease, and use correct lifting techniques when handling it (see chapter 2).

Participating in a stretching program (with a qualified instructor or trainer if you are not familiar with stretching) will give you a good grasp of how your clients should feel when you are stretching them. Further, observing the simple measures recommended above will most likely contribute to a productive practice with fewer chances of injuries to your musculoskeletal system.

Chapter Summary

The study of the anatomical and mechanical bases of human movement, the various types of joints and their ranges of motions, the muscles' attachments and direction and types of muscle fiber, and the relationship between the nervous and musculoskeletal systems and their physiological functions is integral to understanding the body. An understanding of such principles will enhance the massage therapist's ability to assess the musculoskeletal system and to avoid injury of both the client and the therapist.

Applying Your Knowledge

Self-Testing

1. Biomechanics, or the study of actions, is divided into statics and _____ .
   a) motion
   b) action
   c) dynamics
   d) acceleration

2. Basic forms of movement are categorized as linear and _____ .
   a) lateral
   b) transverse
   c) angular
   d) horizontal

3. What is the point at which the body's planes meet called?
   a) Center of gravity
   b) Rotational point
   c) Center point
   d) Axis point

4. What is the study of the body in motion known as?
   a) Kinemotion
   b) Statics
   c) Kinematics
   d) Propriomatics

5. What percent of body weight is connective tissue?
   a) 3%
   b) 11%
   c) 16%
   d) 20%

6. What is the anatomical position?
   a) Standing erect, palms facing forward
   b) Standing erect, palms facing the sides of the body
   c) Standing in a symmetrical position
   d) Standing erect, arms out to the sides and level with shoulders

7. What is the instrument that measures amount of movement in the joint?
    a) Sphygmomanometer
    b) EKG
    c) Goniometer
    d) Pedometer

8. In what plane does abduction and adduction occur?
    a) Frontal
    b) Transverse
    c) Coronal
    d) Horizontal

9. Somatotyping assesses body changes _____ .
    a) during movement
    b) at rest
    c) during growth
    d) None of the above is correct.

10. Ergonomics is the study of the _____ aspects in the working environment.
    a) anatomical
    b) physiological
    c) psychological
    d) All of the above are correct.

Case Studies/Critical Thinking

A. Describe the movements necessary and the planes in which they occur to turn a doorknob to the left with the right hand, to the right with the right hand, to the left with the left hand, and to the right with the left hand.

B. You have a client who suffers from back pain and has been told by her physician that she has sciatica. She has trouble sleeping comfortably and asks you for advice on a sleeping position that will not further inflame the sciatic nerve. What would you advise for her?

References for information in this chapter can be found in Quick Guide C at the end of the book.

CHAPTER 7

General Overview of the Body and the Skeletal System

LEARNING OUTCOMES

After completing this chapter, you will be able to:

- Understand body positions in relationship with the organs of the body.
- Describe the substances that make up cells.
- Understand the overall structure of the skeleton.
- Understand gender and age differences in the skeleton.
- Name the bones of the axial and the appendicular skeleton.
- Identify the function of the skeletal system.
- Understand the formation and growth of bones.
- Define the classifications of the bones of the body.
- Describe and give examples of bony markings.
- Acquire a practical understanding of palpation techniques.
- Define common pathologies of the skeletal structure.

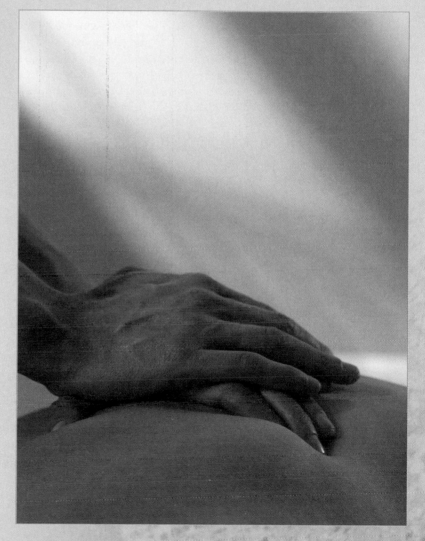

KEY TERMS

anatomy *(p. 154)*

amphiarthrotic joints *(p. 173)*

appendicular bones *(p. 166)*

articulation *(p. 173)*

axial bones *(p. 166)*

cell *(p. 158)*

diaphysis *(p. 169)*

diarthrotic joints *(p. 174)*

endochondral ossification *(p. 168)*

epiphyseal plate
 (or epiphysis) *(p. 169)*

epithelial tissue *(p. 163)*

fontanels *(p. 166)*

fossae *(p. 172)*

intramembranous
 ossification *(p. 168)*

medullary cavity *(p. 171)*

meiosis *(p. 162)*

metacarpals *(p. 181)*

mitosis *(p. 161)*

muscle tissue *(p. 163)*

nerve tissue *(p. 163)*

organs *(p. 158)*

ossifies *(p. 166)*

osteoblasts *(p. 168)*

osteoclasts *(p. 168)*

osteocytes *(p. 168)*

palpation *(p. 171)*

periosteum *(p. 171)*

physiology *(p. 154)*

synarthrotic joints *(p. 173)*

INTRODUCTION

Anatomy is the structure of the body of any living thing and the study of that structure. This science is largely based on dissection, from which it gets its name: The word *anatomy* is derived from two Greek words that mean "a cutting up." The science of human anatomy can be traced to ancient Egyptian times. Leonardo da Vinci (1452–1519) is most often credited with leading the way to refining and revolutionizing the science of human anatomy. Da Vinci was fascinated by the way things worked. His drawings of the principle bones and muscles of the body and his analytical study of the eye inspired others to follow his path. Andrea Vesalius, a Flemish scientist and Da Vinci's successor, published the first accurate and comprehensive anatomical text in 1543, *De Humani Corpus Fabrica* (figure 7.1). In the centuries since, the medical knowledge of human anatomy has been greatly expanded and continues to advance. Anatomy, together with the science of **physiology** (the functioning of the body), forms the foundation of all medicine and allied health studies.

Figure 7.1 Illustration from *De Humani Corporus Fabrica*

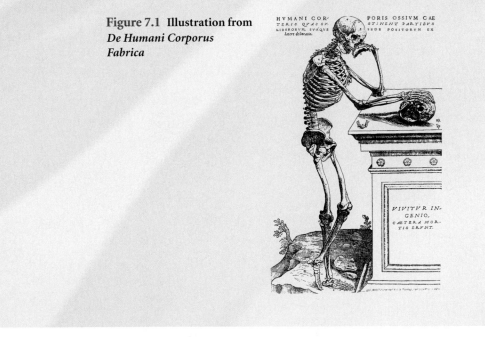

Terminology and Basic Concepts

Anatomical Positioning

A number of terms are used in anatomical positioning to delineate areas of the body. These terms utilize a consistent language for positioning that allows the massage therapist to better communicate and document areas of treatment or physical conditions (figure 7.2).

Because communication with other health care professionals must always meet a clinical standard, documentation for records given to physicians or referrals of your own must contain highly detailed and accurate information. Without accurate documentation at the time of the visit, insurance companies will not pay for your services, and your business or profession will suffer.

In this section, we will begin to explain anatomical landmarks and the structural layout of the body. You should carefully study the diagrams in this section to gain a working knowledge of anatomical structure, and the body planes and cavities.

Directional Terms

Since basic anatomical structure is the same for all humans, massage client intake forms include a blank anatomical chart for marking conditions and observations. Areas of treatment can also be marked so that when the client returns, there is a quick visual record of where the client felt discomfort and what type of treatment was applied. This simple diagram usually contains the spinal column, which forms the central axis, but has little detail. Massage therapists use their knowledge of the body's organization to enable them to correctly record the treatment session.

The organization map of the body begins with the transverse plane (figure 7.3). This plane is a horizontal imaginary line that divides the body into a top half and a bottom half. Body parts in the upper half are considered superior. Body parts below the line are considered inferior. For instance, the calf area of the legs is in the inferior portion of the body. However, the terms *superior* and *inferior* may refer to the location relationship between two body parts and not just the sides of the transverse plane. An example of this is a reference to the knee being superior to the heel or the heel being inferior to the knee. Two other directional terms related to the transverse plane are *cranial*, which means in the location close to or toward the head, and *caudal*, which refers to the direction close to the sacral region at the base of the spine.

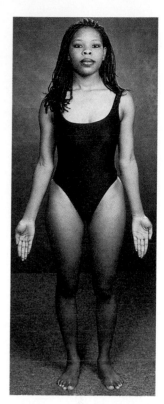

Figure 7.2 Anatomical position

The feet are flat on the floor and close together, arms are downward, and supine and the head is forward.

Figure 7.3 Anatomical planes

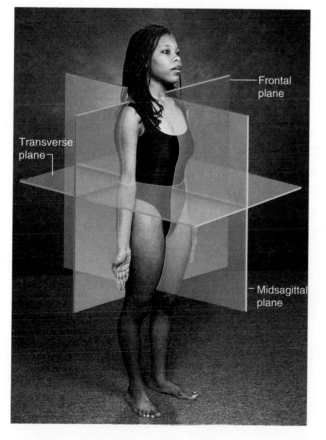

Frontal plane

Transverse plane

Midsagittal plane

The sagittal, or median, plane divides the body into right and left parts. *Midsagittal* refers to the plane that divides the body into right and left halves. Body parts close to the midline are called medial, and body parts away from the midline of the body are called lateral. The frontal or coronal plane divides the body into a front section and a back section. Body parts in the front of the plane, or on the front of the body, are called ventral or anterior. Body parts on the back of the body are called dorsal or posterior.

The directional terms *proximal* and *distal* are used to describe the location of the extremities (arms and legs, sometimes referred to as apppendicular) in relation to the main trunk of the body. Generally, this location is measured from a point of reference. Body parts close to the point of reference are called proximal, and body parts distant from the point of reference are called distal. For example, in describing the relationship of the wrist to the shoulder (point of reference), the wrist is distal.

Body Cavities

Body cavities (figure 7.4) are spaces within the body that contain vital organs (viscera). There are two main body cavities: the dorsal or posterior cavity and the ventral or anterior cavity.

The dorsal cavity (table 7.1) is divided into two sections: the cranial cavity, which contains the brain and related structures, and the spinal cavity, which contains the spinal cord. The posterior surface of the torso (trunk of body) is also divided into the vertebral, or spinal, regions. Each region is named for the section of the spine it includes (see table 7.2).

The ventral cavities are larger than the dorsal and are separated into two distinct sections by a dome-shaped muscle called the diaphragm. The thoracic cavity is located in the chest and contains the esophagus, trachea, bronchi, lungs, heart, and large blood vessels. The abdominal or abdominopelvic cavity is divided into two parts. The upper abdominal cavity contains the stomach, small intestine, most of the large intestine, appendix, liver, gallbladder, pancreas, and spleen. The lower abdominal or pelvic cavity contains the urinary bladder, the reproductive organs, and the last part of the large intestine.

Three small cavities are the orbital cavity (eyes and related structures), nasal cavity (nose and related structures), and the buccal cavity (mouth, teeth, and tongue).

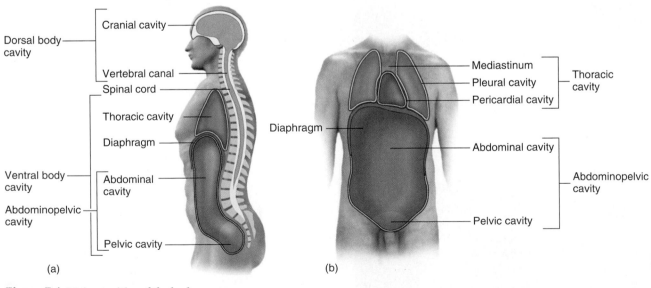

Figure 7.4 Major cavities of the body
(*a*) Left lateral; (*b*) anterior view of the ventral body.

Table 7.1	Body Cavities and Membranes	
Name of Cavity	**Associated Viscera**	**Membranous Lining**
Dorsal body cavity		
Cranial cavity	Brain	Meninges
Vertebral canal	Spinal cord	Meninges
Ventral body cavity		
Thoracic cavity		
Pleural cavities (2)	Lungs	Pleurae
Pericardial cavity	Heart	Pericardium
Abdominopelvic cavity		
Abdominal cavity	Digestive organs, spleen, kidneys	Peritoneum
Pelvic cavity	Bladder, rectum, reproductive organs	Peritoneum

Table 7.2	Spinal/Vertebral Regions
Cervical region	7 cervical vertebrae (neck)
Thoracic region	12 thoracic vertebrae (chest and ribs)
Lumbar region	5 lumbar vertebrae (loin)
Sacral region	5 sacral vertebrae (sacrum) (fused into 1 bone as we age)
Coccyx	4 coccygeal vertebrae (tailbone) (fused into 1 bone as we age)

Abdominal Regions

The abdominal cavity is divided using two methods. It can be divided into quadrants, meaning four sections (figure 7.5). This division produces the right upper quadrant (RUQ), the left upper quadrant (LUQ), the right lower quadrant (RLQ), and the left lower quadrant (LLQ) (figure 7.6).

EXAM POINT The method of division used by most physicians divides the abdominal region into nine regions: (top row, from the right) right hypochondriac region, epigastric region, left hypochondriac region; (middle row) right lumbar region, umbilical region, left lumbar region; and (bottom row) right iliac region, hypogastric region, left iliac region (figure 7.7).

The 9 region method is used most often for locating pain on or in the body trunk.

The human body is a highly organized and complex machine (figure 7.8). To understand the way the body was designed to work, you must first understand the cellular structure of the body and how these cells come together to make organs and systems. All living things begin with minute particles that combine to make atoms. These atoms combine to make a molecule, which is the smallest particle of a substance that carries all the properties of the substance. The molecules are grouped together to form compounds, and the compounds form matter. This matter in living things is protoplasm, the basic substance of life.

Basic Structure and Systems of the Human Body

Figure 7.5 External division of the body into four quadrants

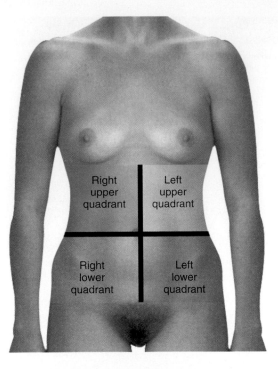

Figure 7.6 Internal anatomy associated with the four quadrants

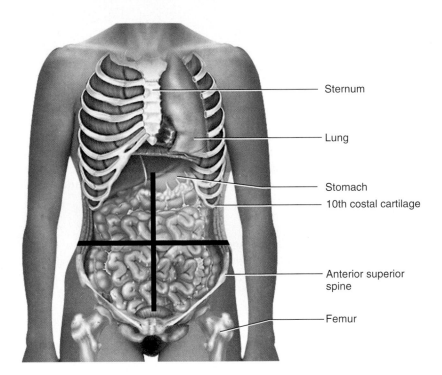

Protoplasm contains common elements such as carbon, hydrogen, nitrogen, oxygen, phosphorus, and sulfur. Within the human body, the basic unit of structure and function is the **cell**. The cells come together to form groups called tissues. The tissues are able to form structures that perform specific activities. The structures formed from tissue become **organs**. The organs are two or more types of tissue that have joined together to perform a certain bodily function, such as a heart or stomach. When organs and other body parts join together to create a unit, specific to a vital function, such as providing oxygen to the blood or digesting food, you have a body system.

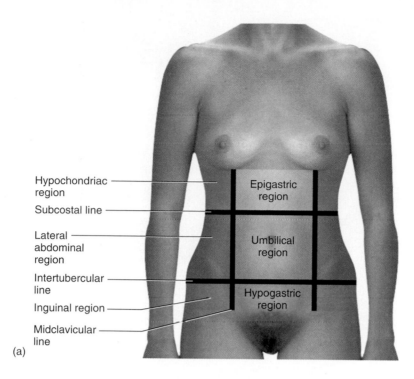

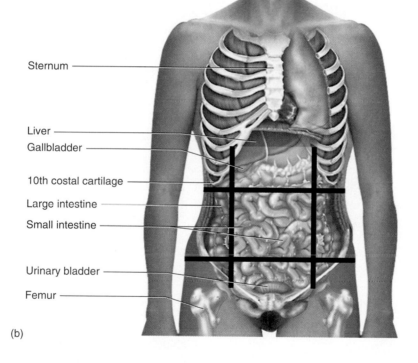

Figure 7.7
(*a*) External division of the body into nine regions. (*b*) Internal anatomy associated with the nine regions

Cells: The Basis of Life

As was stated before, the basic unit of structure and function in the human body is the cell. Body cells are so small that they must be viewed through a microscopic lens, but they carry on the functions of life. They use oxygen and food. They produce energy, and some cells move around within the body to remove toxins and help maintain immunity. Refer to figure 7.9 to see the basic cell structure.

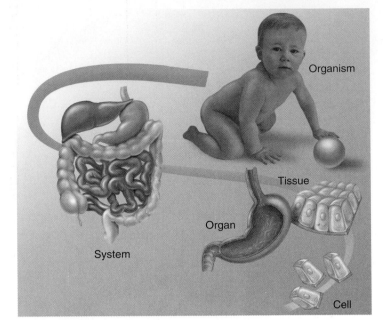

Figure 7.8 The body's structural path

Organism

Tissue

Organ

System

Cell

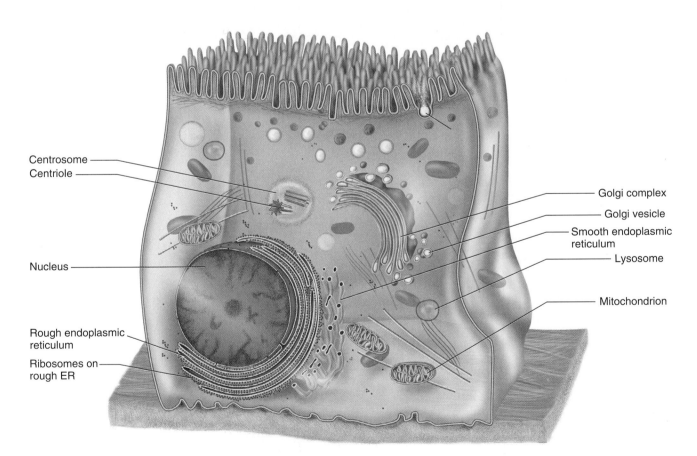

Centrosome

Centriole

Nucleus

Rough endoplasmic reticulum

Ribosomes on rough ER

Golgi complex

Golgi vesicle

Smooth endoplasmic reticulum

Lysosome

Mitochondrion

Figure 7.9 Basic cell structure

Cell Structure

- *Cell membrane*—semipermeable, outer protective covering of the cell. Another name for cell membrane is plasma membrane.
- *Centrosome*—found in the cytoplasm near the nucleus. It is the site of cell division; when the two centrioles (tubular structures) separate, cytoplasmic spindle fibers form between the centrioles and attach to the chromosomes. This creates an even division of the chromosomes in the two new cells.
- *Chromatin*—made up of deoxyribonucleic acid (DNA) and protein. When a cell begins to split, the chromatin compacts to form chromosomes.
- *Cytoplasm*—fluid inside the cell that contains water, protein, fats (lipids), carbohydrates, minerals, and salts. All of the cell's chemical activity is done within the cytoplasm.
- *Endoplasmic reticulum*—located in the cytoplasm, these tubelike structures transport materials into and away from the nucleus. They also produce protein in the ribosomes and store raw materials. The smooth endoplasmic reticulum does not contain ribosomes and produces cholesterol, maintains fat metabolism, and detoxifies drugs at the cellular level.
- *Golgi apparatus*—membrane layers located within the cytoplasm that store, produce, and combine secretions for removal from the cell. Large numbers of Golgi apparatus cells are found in the gastric, salivary, and pancreatic glands.
- *Lysosomes*—found within the cytoplasm, these structures contain enzymes that digest old cells, bacteria, and foreign bodies. Lysosomes are very important to the body's immune system.
- *Mitochondria*—rod-shaped organelles located throughout cytoplasm. They break down carbohydrates, proteins, and fats to produce adenosine triphosphate (ATP), which is the energy source of the cell.
- *Nucleolus*—located inside the nucleus and important in cell reproduction. The ribosomes, which are made of ribonucleic acid (RNA) and protein, are made by them. The nucleolus move from within the nucleus to the cytoplasm, or they can be attached to the endoplasmic reticulum.
- *Nucleus*—the "brain" of the cell. It controls all cellular activity and cellular reproduction.
- *Organelles*—the name for the cellular bodies located within the cytoplasm. They are the nucleus, mitochondria, ribosomes, lysosomes, centrioles, Golgi apparatus, and endoplasmic reticulum.
- *Pinocytic vesicles*—folds in the cell membrane that allow molecules of matter, such as protein or fats, to enter the cell. When molecules come into contact with the cell membrane, these folds cover the matter, which is then absorbed into the cell.

Cell Division

Cell division and reproduction occurs in the body in two forms: mitosis and meiosis. **Mitosis** is a form of division that is asexual reproduction, which is where the cell divides into two identical cells with equal parts. Blood-forming cells, skin cells, and cells that line the intestines reproduce continuously. The cells of muscles only reproduce every few years. That is why proper treatment of muscle injury is so important. Cells such as nerve cells in the brain and spinal cord do not reproduce after they are formed before birth. So if these cells are destroyed, others will not be created to replace them.

Before mitosis begins, chromatin in the nucleus tightens and compacts itself to form chromosomes, and then each chromosome is duplicated. The two pairs of the same chromosome are called chromatids and are joined together by a centromere. The cell begins to divide, and the centrioles in the centrosome move to opposite ends of the cell. The nuclear membrane dissolves, and the pairs of chromosomes attach to spindles at the center of the cell. They then split, form halves, and move to the opposite ends of the cell. Each cell half will have 23 identical pairs of chromosomes. The cytoplasm divides, and two new and identical cells form cell membranes.

With **meiosis**, the form of cell division that produces ovum and sperm, each cell contains 23 chromosomes. The ovum and sperm combine to become 46 chromosomes and form a zygote. The zygote has 23 pairs of chromosomes. Most cells contain the same basic parts, but they can form variations of shape, size, and function. When cells that are of the same type join together toward a single purpose, they form a tissue.

Tissues of the Body

Tissue is of great importance to the massage therapist.

⭐ **EXAM POINT** As part of massage treatment, you work directly with the four primary types of body tissue: connective tissue (fat and cartilage), epithelial tissue (skin), muscle tissue, and nerve tissue.

Table 7.3 defines the four main classes of tissue. In addition to body tissue, there is a fifth tissue, liquid tissue. Tissue is embedded in a substance called the matrix. The matrix is different with each type of tissue, that is, how the tissue moves and how much support a particular tissue needs.

⭐ **EXAM POINT** Connective tissue is the most widely distributed tissue within the human body.

This tissue supports and holds together the body and its many parts. It is also responsible for transport of materials through the body, and some of the connective tissue components are specialized to aid in ridding the body of foreign substances.

There are two main types of connective tissue: soft and hard. Soft tissue includes adipose or fatty tissue, which stores fat, insulates the body from heat and cold, and cushions the ligaments and tendons to protect them from damage. The hard type of con-

Table 7.3	*The Four Primary Tissue Classes*	
Type	**Definition**	**Representative Locations**
Epithelial	Tissue composed of layers of closely spaced cells that cover organ surfaces, form glands, and serve for protection, secretion, and absorption	Epidermis Inner lining of digestive tract Liver and other glands
Connective	Tissue with more matrix than cell volume, often specialized to support, bind together, and protect organs	Tendons and ligaments Cartilage and bone Blood
Nervous	Tissue containing excitable cells specialized for rapid transmission of coded information to other cells	Brain Spinal cord Nerves
Muscular	Tissue composed of elongated, excitable cells specialized for contraction	Skeletal muscles Heart (cardiac muscle) Walls of viscera (smooth muscle)

nective tissue is used as bone and cartilage. Cartilage is found on the ears and nose, between the bones of the spine, and at the ends of long bones, where it helps to cushion joints. Sometimes physicians refer to bone as osseous tissue because of the calcium content. Without bone, our bodies would not have an upright and rigid structure.

Blood and lymph are liquid connective tissue, which is sometimes referred to as vascular tissue. Blood carries nutrients and oxygen to all the cells of the body. It also carries waste products away from the cells. Lymph tissue transports proteins, fats, and immune system components from the tissues to the circulatory system.

Epithelial tissue is the main tissue of the skin. This type of tissue is also found lining the intestines, respiratory tracts, urinary tracts, and other body cavities. The glands of our bodies are formed of highly specialized epithelial tissue, and they produce and secrete substances that help to maintain homeostasis.

Nerve tissue cells are called neurons. Neurons transmit messages throughout the body and make up the brain, nerves, and spinal cord. These neurons as sensory nerves in the skin and organs of hearing, taste, smell, and sight are constantly giving brain cells feedback in response to stimuli. Other neurons form neural pathways to relay touch, pain, heat, and cold messages to the brain.

Muscle tissue makes up muscle fibers that control movement by contraction. The three types of muscle tissue are cardiac, skeletal/voluntary, and smooth (visceral). Cardiac muscle contracts and relaxes to allow the heart to beat. Skeletal muscle is attached to bones and allows for the movement of the body. Smooth muscle tissue is found in the hollow organs of the stomach, small intestines, urinary bladder, colon, and blood vessels. Smooth muscle tissue is nonstriated and allows for the movement of food through the digestive tract. It also provides the constriction needed to empty the bladder and the force that allows blood to flow through the blood vessels.

Organs

When tissues join together to perform a certain function, they form an organ. The heart, lungs, kidneys, and spleen are examples of organs. When these organs and other body parts join together to perform a specific bodily function, the joined parts are called a system.

How Systems Work Together

The human body is a complex organization of systems that work together to maintain homeostasis—the ability to maintain internal stability—within the body as a unit. Homeostasis results from the body's ability to detect change and activate mechanisms to control the effects of the change on the internal conditions that keep the body stable, such as temperature, hydration, and pH balance.

Even when an organ is not involved in a function, the very act of its uninvolvement is part of the function. The body is programmed to work as a whole, and if one body part fails to meet its demands, then the entire body can suffer. This also can be said as, "If a part of the body is made to be healthier, then the body as a whole will benefit." It is crucial for a massage therapist to understand the body's structure and function in order to evaluate and plan sessions for treatment that will bring the optimum result in the client. We begin the study of systems with the skeletal system, which includes all of the bones of the body and their associated cartilage, tendons, and ligaments.

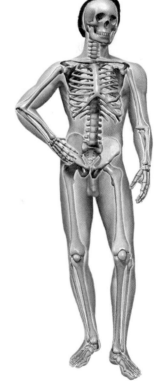

Figure 7.10 Skeletal system
Principal organs: Bones, cartilages, ligaments.

The skeleton is the framework of the human anatomy that supports the body and protects its internal organs (figure 7.10). Every movement we make involves the skeletal system. Even sitting still and breathing would not be possible without the skeletal structure. This system includes all of the bones and their associated cartilage, tendons, and ligaments.

Skeletal System

Table 7.4 details the bones contained in the human body. Most of these bones are connected to other bones at flexible joints, which lend the framework a high degree of flexibility. Before you can study muscles and their actions, you need to understand how bones are formed and classified, as well as the characteristics that they possess (called markings or landmarks).

Table 7.4	Bones of the Adult Skeletal System		
Axial Skeleton			
Skull	Total: 22	*Auditory ossicles*	Total: 6
Cranial bones		Malleus (2)	
Frontal bone (1)		Incus (2)	
Parietal bone (2)		Stapes (2)	
Occipital bone (1)		*Hyoid bone* (1)	Total: 1
Temporal bone (2)		*Vertebral column*	Total: 26
Sphenoid bone (1)		Cervical vertebrae (7)	
Ethmoid bone (1)		Thoracic vertebrae (12)	
Facial bones		Lumbar vertebrae (5)	
Maxilla (2)		Sacrum (1)	
Palatine bone (2)		Coccyx (1)	
Zygomatic bone (2)		*Thoracic cage*	Total: 25
Lacrimal bone (2)		Ribs (24)	
Nasal bone (2)		Sternum (1)	
Vomer (1)			
Inferior nasal concha (2)			
Mandible (1)			
Appendicular Skeleton			
Pectoral girdle	Total: 4	*Pelvic girdle*	Total: 2
Scapula (2)		Os coxae (2)	
Clavicle (2)		*Lower limb*	Total: 60
Upper limb	Total: 60	Femur (2)	
Humerus (2)		Patella (2)	
Radius (2)		Tibia (2)	
Ulna (2)		Fibula (2)	
Carpals (16)		Tarsals (14)	
Metacarpals (10)		Metatarsals (10)	
Phalanges (28)		Phalanges (28)	
			Grand total: 206

An Overview of the Skeleton

The bones of the skull form a strong protective case that surrounds the brain and other major sense organs, and acts as a sentry to guard the entrances to the digestive and respiratory systems (figure 7.11). The skull sits atop the spine, which is composed of 33 small, irregularly shaped bones called vertebrae. The five vertebrae of the sacrum and the four coccygeal vertebrae are fixed, meaning they do not move separately of one another, so they are counted as one bone each. The spine is in every sense the backbone of the body. It directly or indirectly anchors all other bones. Each bone of the body has a special size and shape, depending on the work it does and its location in the body. Twelve pairs of ribs are held in place by the spine. The bony case formed by the ribs protects the major organs. They are strong, yet flexible, swinging upward and outward as the lungs take in air.

The arms and their surrounding bones form one of the most exquisite feats of engineering known. The complex articulations in the hand, elbow, and shoulder allow a wide range of movement from large, sweeping motions to minute manipulations. Together with the 27 bones of the hand, the versatile arm is well-suited to the varied manipulations and motions required in such activities as ballet dancing, watchmaking, and boxing.

The pelvis is the bony structure at the base of the spine. It connects the legs to the rest of the skeleton. The leg bones are the body's support system. They are much larger and stronger than the arm bones.

> ★ **EXAM POINT** The thigh bone, or femur, is the largest bone in the body.

Each foot is made up of 26 bones. These bones allow a wide array of flexibility while being able to withstand incredible amounts of stress. It is estimated that each stride of an adult places over 900 pounds per square inch on the bottom of the foot. When a person stands, the weight is distributed evenly along the foot. Half of the weight is funneled to the calcaneus (heel bone), while the other half is channeled into the tarsal bones that make up the arch of the foot. Bones are well designed for the work they do.

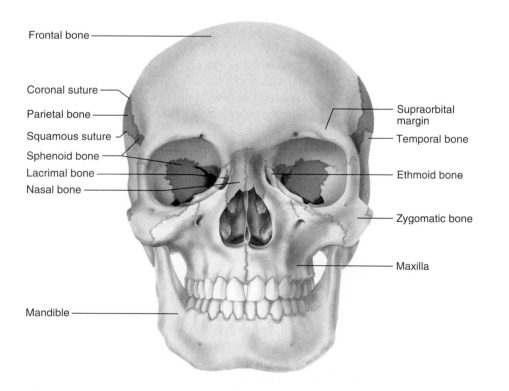

Figure 7.11 **The skull, anterior view**

Labels: Frontal bone, Coronal suture, Parietal bone, Squamous suture, Sphenoid bone, Lacrimal bone, Nasal bone, Mandible, Supraorbital margin, Temporal bone, Ethmoid bone, Zygomatic bone, Maxilla

Gender and Age Differences

This particular difference makes childbirth easier.

At birth, babies have about 350 individual bones. Many of these bones fuse together as they grow. By the time they are adults, they have 206 bones. The skull bones begin as 26 separate bones. In babies, these bones are connected by flexible cartilaginous membranes called **fontanels**. This membrane **ossifies** over time, forming the rigid sutures of the adult skull.

Axial and Appendicular Skeleton

Two basic classification methods exist to categorize the bones of the body. These two classification systems are based on anatomical location (axial or appendicular) and shape (long, short, flat, irregular, and sesamoid) (figure 7.13).

The shape classifications include long bones such as the radius, humerus, and femur, short bones such as the carpals, tarsals, and manual and pedal phalanges, flat bones such as the sternum, skull bones, and scapulae, and irregular bones such as the vertebrae.

Function of the Skeleton

Bones can provide strength and support because the cells of these organs surround themselves with hardened, mineral material, such as calcium phosphate. Understanding the structure and function of the skeletal system will help you understand the workings of other bodily systems. Just as a strong, weight-bearing framework that functions

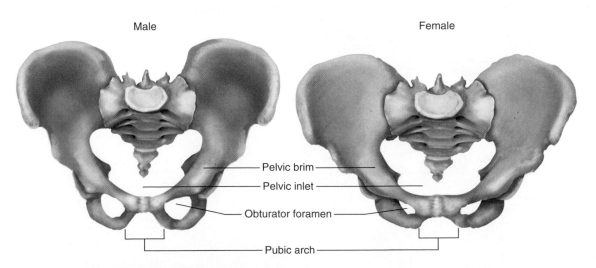

Male   Female

Pelvic brim
Pelvic inlet
Obturator foramen
Pubic arch

Figure 7.12 Comparison of the male and female pelvis

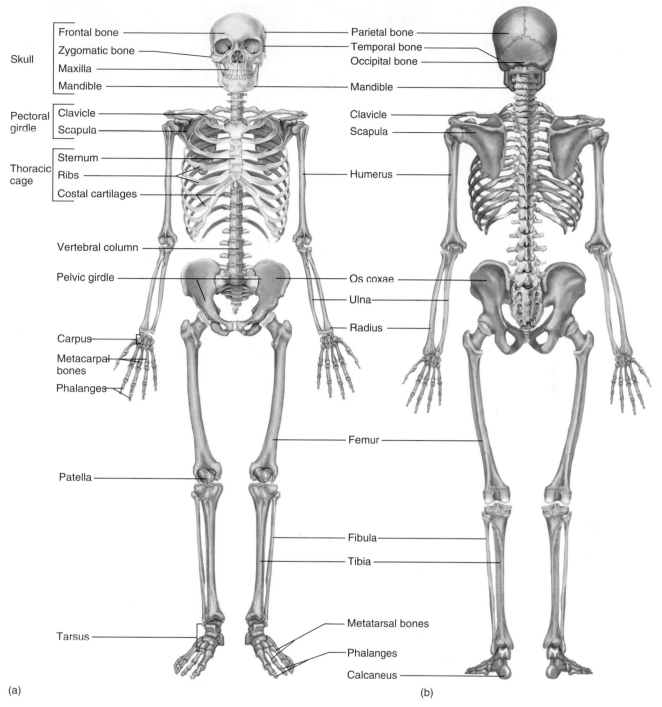

Figure 7.13 The adult skeleton

(*a*) Anterior view, (*b*) posterior view. The appendicular skeleton is colored blue; the remainder is axial skeleton.

with certain flexibility makes a house safe and livable, the skeleton determines how the body will function as a whole.

★ **EXAM POINT** Six main functions are associated with the skeletal system: support, protection, movement, storage, hemopoiesis, and sound conduction.

The skeletal system:

- Supports and stabilizes muscles, blood vessels, nerves, fat, and skin.
- Protects vital, internal organs of the body, such as the heart, lungs, liver, brain, and spinal cord.
- Allows for movement by providing sites of attachment for muscles.
- Stores minerals, such as calcium and phosphorus, and fats.
- Is the site of hemopoiesis (manufacturing of blood cells), primarily in the red bone marrow.
- Conducts sound in the bones of the inner ear.

Bone Formation and Growth

The Greek word for skeleton means "dried"; however, the bones of the body are very much alive. The bones are made from living tissues that are capable of growth, can detect pain and other stimuli, change when under stress, and make repairs when they are injured. Bones, sometimes called osseous material, are connective tissues. The parts of the bones outside of its cells make up most of their characteristics.

When we are merely a fetus within the womb, we have a complete skeletal framework formed by the end of the first trimester of our mother's pregnancy. This tiny, still-growing skeleton is formed of cartilage. As we continue to grow and change, the cartilage begins the process of **endochondral ossification,** which turns the soft, flexible cartilage into the harder bone. This is done by osteoblasts invading the cell and building bone.

There are two types of ossification: **intramembranous ossification,** in which connective tissue membranes are replaced by calcium deposits and form bone, and endochondral ossification, in which cartilage is the environment in which bone cells develop. In the intramembranous form, the membrane becomes the periosteum of the bone, with a spongy center (figure 7.14). The bones of the cranium or skull are formed by this process. Ossification does not complete until several months after birth. The "soft spot" or fontanels on the baby's skull are an example of this. If the baby's skull were fully formed and hardened before traveling through the birth canal, the baby could sustain fractures and injury.

In endochondral ossification, the osteoblasts are surrounded by the bone matrix, and the cells become mature bone cells or osteocytes. Regardless of which method is used by the body, the bones that are formed become compact tissue.

In the formation of bone, the body utilizes three types of bone cells: osteoblasts, osteoclasts, and osteocytes. Bone develops from cells called **osteoblasts** that begin from undifferentiated bone cells, called osteoprogenitor cells. Osteoblasts are formed beneath the membrane that covers a bone, which is called the periosteum (figure 7.15). Osteoblasts are also found in the endosteum, which lines the bone marrow cavity. The amount of bone formed is controlled by the amount of pressure on the particular bone. The heel and femur are large and strong with a high amount of solid bone because they carry so much weight within the body. This process of bone formation accounts for why children who sit all day and do not run and play will not develop a strong bone structure and may be candidates for easy fractures in the future. This process happens in reverse when someone is paralyzed, in a cast, or is simply sedentary (also known as a couch potato), making the bones weak.

Osteoclasts are cells that come into play when a break occurs within a bone. These cells are stimulated by secretions from **osteocytes,** which are mature osteoblasts, and

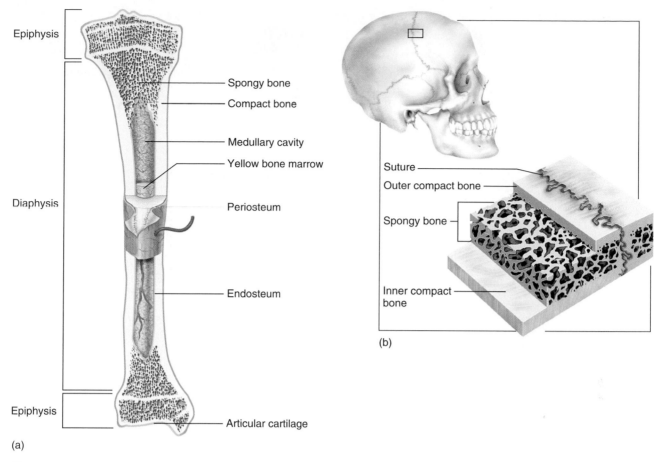

(a)

Figure 7.14
(a) Long bones; (b) flat bone of cranium.

are responsible for the reabsorption of bone. The large-celled osteoclasts break down the inner side of bones and actually reconstruct or remodel the shape of the bone. When a brace is applied to curved or weakened bones (providing stress or pressure), the osteocytes deposit new bone material and the osteoclasts remove old bone. By working together, they function to change the bone structure and shape.

Classification of Bones

The bones of the human body are divided into five classifications for easier study. These classifications are defined by shape and are categorized as long, short, flat, irregular, and sesamoid (figure 7.16).

Structure of Long Bones

Long bones are defined as bones that have a length that exceeds their width and consist of a long, usually central shaft called a **diaphysis,** which is composed of mostly compact bone material. The **epiphyseal plate (or epiphysis)** is where the growth of the bone occurs and is sometimes called the "growth plate." The bone is thicker toward the middle, where it is not supported as well, and is curved to help carry the weight of the attached muscles.

The surface of the bone, where one bone meets another bone is covered with a layer of material called articular cartilage. This cartilage allows bone to move freely when rubbed against another bone and cushions the bone surface from wear. The articular cartilage has a limited supply of blood and depends on synovial fluid for nourishment.

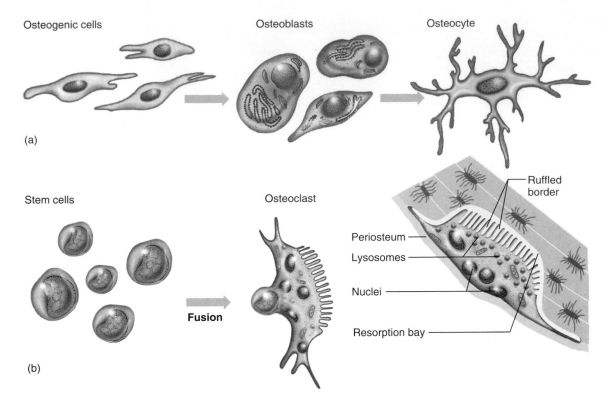

(a)

(b)

Figure 7.15 The development of bone cells

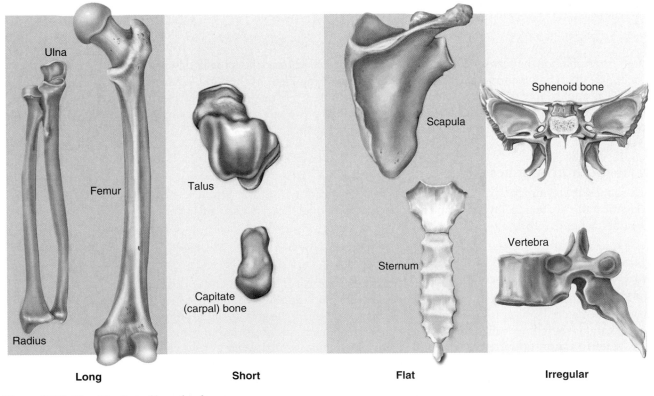

Long   **Short**   **Flat**   **Irregular**

Figure 7.16 Classification of bone by shape

Small subsynovial blood vessels also provide nourishment to the fluid, which in turn supplies the cartilage.

The outside or external surface of the bone is called the **periosteum**. This fibrous layer is made from collagen and bone-forming cells. Some of the periosteum fibers continue into tendons that anchor muscle to bone, and some of the fibers penetrate the bone matrix. The periosteum is important in providing strong attachment from muscle to tendon to bone. The inside or internal surface of a bone is lined with endosteum. This is a layer of connective tissue and osteogenic cells that will become other types of bone cells.

The interior of the shaft is the **medullary cavity**. This cavity is filled with the yellow bone marrow, which consists primarily of fat cells. The epiphyses are broad and reaching so they can articulate with other bones and provide a large surface for attachment of muscle.

Examples of long bones are the 2 clavicles, 2 humerus, 2 radius, 2 ulna, 2 femur, 2 tibia, 2 fibula, 10 metacarpals of the hand, 10 metatarsals of the foot, and 56 phalanges of the fingers and toes.

Structure of Short Bones

Short bones do not have a long shaft. They have a thin layer of compact bone tissue over a large amount of spongy bone. Examples of short bones are the 16 carpal bones of the wrists and 14 tarsal bones of the feet.

Structure of Flat Bones

The flat bones provide a large area for extensive muscle attachment. They protect soft, vital organs within the body. They are curved and consist of flat plates of compact tissue that cover spongy or cancellous bone. Red bone marrow fills the spaces within the cancellous bone. The function of the red bone marrow is hematopoiesis, or the formation of red and white blood cells and blood components such as platelets. Blood cells in several stages of development can be found within the red bone marrow at the same time. Examples of flat bones are the sternum, ribs, scapula, parts of the pelvic bones, and some of the bones found in the skull. The flat bones are 6 cranial bones, 2 scapula, 24 ribs, and 1 sternum.

Structure of Irregular Bones

Irregular bones consist primarily of spongy bone enclosed by layers of compact bone tissue. Spongy or cancellous bone has many open spaces that are filled with bone marrow. Compact or dense bone is strong and solid. These bones are called irregular because of their uneven and different shapes. Examples of irregular bones are 1 cranial, 14 facial bones, 6 ossicles, 1 hyoid, 26 vertebrae, and 2 pelvic bones.

Structure of Sesamoid Bones

The sesamoid bones are rounded and very small. These bones are enclosed in tendon and fascial tissue and are always located next to or within joints. Examples of sesamoid bones are the two patella. Some of the bones within the wrist are classified as short bones but work with the muscles and joints as a sesamoid bone would function.

Palpation and Bony Landmarks

Excellent **palpation** skills can be the key to distinguishing a massage therapist as a valued professional within the allied health field. The ability to locate anatomical landmarks and examine tissue by feel or touch, and know what normal tissue feels like, when it is dysfunctional, and what techniques to use to normalize dysfunctional tissue is the foundation for providing profound results through massage (see Procedure 7.1).

PROCEDURE 7.1 Palpation Exercises

1. Have a partner stand in front of you and open and close his or her mouth while you palpate the temporomandibular joints bilaterally.

2. Place a gloved index finger gently into the ear and have the partner open and close his or her mouth to also feel the temporomandibular joints.

3. Place your fingertips on the partner's face just below his or her ears. Have your partner clench his or her teeth. Feel the muscles of the lower jaw tighten.

4. Palpate the angle of the jawline (mandible) while moving your fingers anteriorly along the inferior margin of the mandible and stop at the mental protuberance.

5. Have your partner lie on a massage table or mat on the floor. Inspect and palpate the clavicle from the acromioclavicular joint to the sternoclavicular joint. Reverse and palpate the clavicle from the sternoclavicular joint toward the acromioclavicular joint.

6. Palpate the olecranon process at the elbow.

7. Palpate the lateral supracondylar ridge and the lateral epicondyle of the humerus.

8. Palpate the iliac crests before palpation of the greater trochanter of the femur.

9. Palpate the head of the fibula.

10. Palpate the tibial tubercle and the anterior tibial crest.

11. Palpate the lateral and medial malleolus.

12. Palpate the iliac crests.

13. Palpate the medial longitudinal arch of the foot.

14. Have your partner recline on the massage table. Make sure his or her hips are even or level. Place your partner's ankles together laterally. Have your partner flex his or her feet and check to see if one leg appears longer than the other.

Each bone has several landmarks designed specifically to serve as muscular attachments. Some landmarks are easy to palpate, while others are impossible to examine by touch due to their location deep within the structures of the musculoskeletal system and their coverings of tissue layers. It is essential that the massage therapist have an in-depth knowledge of these landmarks to be able to isolate specific musculotendon units.

Bony Markings and Landmarks

The outer surface of a bone has certain projections called processes or bony processes, and indentions and depressions called **fossae**. These markings help line up the bones to one another, provide an area for attachments of muscles, or serve as a passageway through the bone for nerves and blood vessels. You will need to know and be able to palpate all of the landmarks in order to find the muscles to massage.

The following is a list of bony landmarks and their definitions:

Bony Landmarks

Condyle—a rounded or knobby prominence usually found at the point of articulation with another bone (e.g., lateral and medial condyles of the femur, located at the distal end and palpable just superior to the knee. Both medially and laterally, these serve as attachments for the gastrocnemius, popliteus, and plantaris muscles)

Tubercle—a small, round process (e.g., the lesser tubercle of the humerus)

Trochlea—a process shaped like a pulley (e.g., the trochlea of the humerus, located at the proximal end of the humerus. Also serves as an attachment for the rotator cuff muscles)

Trochanter—a large projection (e.g., the greater and lesser trochanter of the femur)

Crest—a narrow ridge of bone (e.g., the iliac crest of the pelvis)

Line—a less prominent ridge of a bone

Head—a terminal enlargement (e.g., the head of the femur)

Neck—a part of a bone that connects the head to the rest of the bone (e.g., the neck of the femur)

Spine—a sharp, slender projection (e.g., the spinous process of a vertebra)

Styloid process—a needlelike pointed projection (e.g., the styloid process of the vertebrae)

Suture—a narrow junction (e.g., the sutures of the skull bones)

Foramen—an opening through which blood vessels, nerves, and ligaments pass (e.g., the foramen magnum of the occipital bone)

Meatus or canal—a long tunnel-like passage (e.g., the auditory meatus)

Sinus or antrum—a cavity within a bone (e.g., the nasal sinuses)

Sulcus—a furrow or groove (e.g., the intertubercular sulcus or groove of the humerus) (figure 7.17)

Joints and Articulations

As mentioned in chapter 6, there are three classifications of joints: synarthrotic, amphiarthrotic, and diarthrotic. Diarthrotic joints are further broken down into six types: saddle, ball-and-socket, hinge, plane or gliding, ellipsoid or condyloid, and pivot. Please review the section on joints in chapter 6.

An **articulation** is the site where the union between two or more bones occurs, regardless of how or what degree of movement is involved. Vertebrae articulate with each other by articular facets located on the superior and inferior portions of the bone. The action of this joint, known as a zygapophyseal or intraarticular facet joint, is of a gliding joint so flexibility can be allowed. The joint between the first cervical vertebra (atlas) and the second vertebra (axis) is a pivot joint to allow for head rotation.

> **EXAM POINT** Only one bone, the hyoid bone, is not directly connected to another bone in such an articulation. It anchors the tongue and is attached to the styloid processes of the skull by ligaments.

Joint Classifications

As we think of the joints of the body, it is easy to forget that some joints do not move. Joints are classified or divided into three major groups according to their function (the degree of movement they allow) and their structure (the type of tissue or material that holds them together).

Synarthrotic Joints

Synarthrotic joints are characterized by unions between bones that allow little or no movement. There are three types of these synarthroses (figure 7.18):

> **EXAM POINT** Suture, where bones are united by a layer of fibrous tissue, as in the skull

Syndesmosis, in which the bones are joined by ligaments, such as where the radius articulates with the ulna

Gomphosis, in which a process fits into a socket and is held in place by ligaments, such as teeth

Amphiarthrotic Joints

Amphiarthrotic joints are characterized as joints that allow only slight movement. There are two types of these amphiarthroses:

Figure 7.17 Surface features of bones
(*a*) Skull; (*b*) scapula; (*c*) femur; (*d*) humerus.

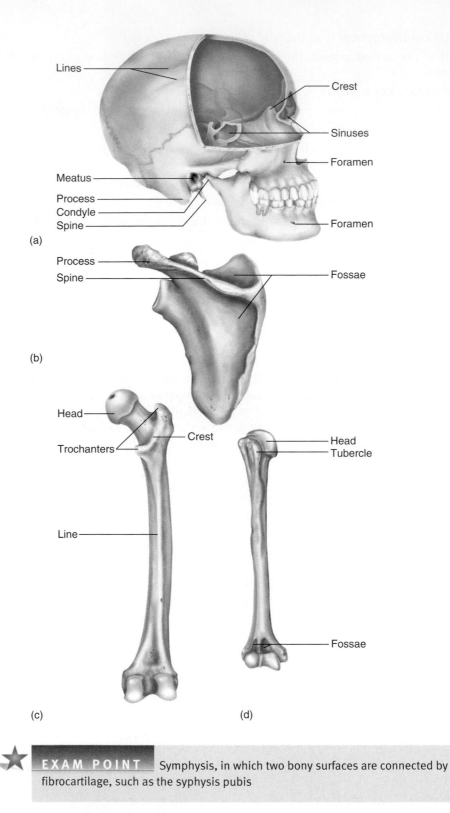

Lines

Crest

Sinuses

Foramen

Meatus
Process
Condyle
Spine

Foramen

(a)

Process
Spine

Fossae

(b)

Head

Trochanters

Crest

Line

Head
Tubercle

Fossae

(c)

(d)

★ **EXAM POINT** Symphysis, in which two bony surfaces are connected by fibrocartilage, such as the syphysis pubis

Synchondrosis, in which two bony surfaces are connected by hyaline cartilage. The cartilage is replaced by permanent bone later in life, such as in the epiphysis and diaphysis of a long bone (growth plate).

Diarthrotic Joints

Diarthrotic joints, sometimes called synovial joints, are allowed to move freely and are divided into six types: saddle, ball-and-socket, hinge, gliding or plane, condyloid or el-

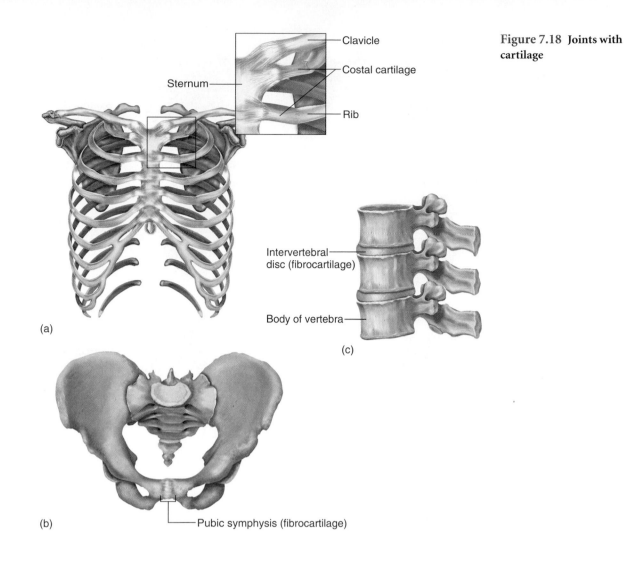

Clavicle

Costal cartilage

Sternum

Rib

Figure 7.18 **Joints with cartilage**

Intervertebral disc (fibrocartilage)

Body of vertebra

(a)

(c)

(b)

Pubic symphysis (fibrocartilage)

lipsoid, and pivot (figure 7.19). They are characterized by a cavity that is enclosed within a capsule. The cavity itself is enclosed by fibrous articular cartilage with reinforcing ligaments. The capsule is lined on the inside with synovial membrane that supplies synovial fluid to the joint capsule and lubricates the joint for easier movement. Synovial or diarthrotic joints have a number of functions. They bear weight and allow movement; they are made up of ligaments, tendons, and articular cartilage to provide stability and control of movement; and they provide fluid to lubricate the joint and nourish the cartilage.

Diarthrotic Joint Structure

The following properties exist in the various types of diarthrotic joints:

- Joint capsule—surrounds the articular surfaces of bones (at the joint)
- Synovial membrane—lines the inside of the joint capsule and secretes synovial fluid to lubricate the joint
- Articular surface—cartilage-covered ends of bones
- Joint cavity—inner space of joint capsule
- Ligaments—dense, fibrous tissues that connect bones to other bones
- Bursae—synovial fluid-filled sacs found between tendons and bones that allow for friction-free movement
- Menisci—fibrous discs that allow for shock absorption and distribute force (found in knee and jaw)

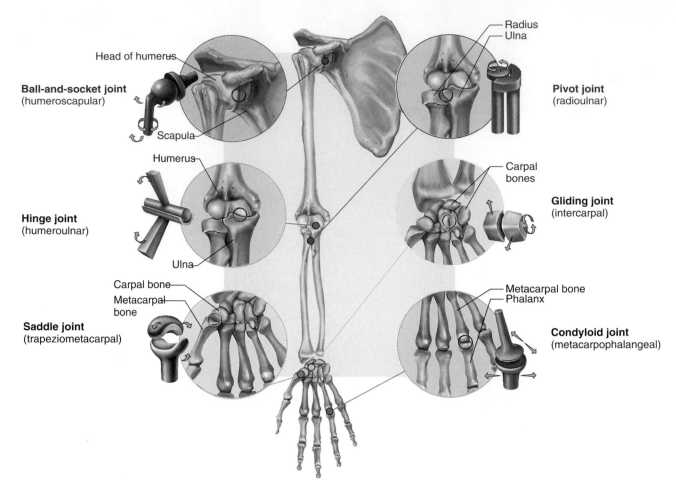

Figure 7.19 **The six types of synovial joints**

Cartilage Classification and Properties

Joints and articulations depend on ligamentous or cartilage attachments. There are three classes of cartilage:

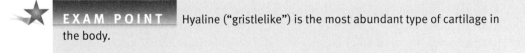

EXAM POINT Hyaline ("gristlelike") is the most abundant type of cartilage in the body.

- It is found in long bone articulations.
- Fibrocartilage (white fibrous) is strong and rigid, found between intervertebral discs, vertebrae, and symphysis pubis.
- Elastic cartilage has strength and maintains shape. It forms the external ear, ear canals, and epiglottis.

A Detailed Look at Skeletal Components

This section outlines skeletal components: the skull, sinuses, shoulder girdle, bones of the arms and hands, ribcage, spine, pelvis, legs, and feet.

Skull Structure

The skull is one of the principle groups of bones in the human anatomy. The skull consists of 26 bones: 8 bones that form the cranium, which houses the brain and ear ossicles;

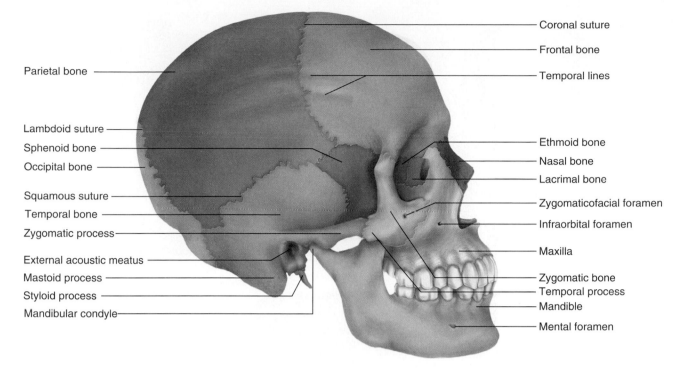

Figure 7.20 The skull, right lateral view

14 facial bones that form the front of the face, jaw, nose, orbits, and the roof of the mouth; 3 bones that make up the inner ear ossicles; and 1 hyoid bone, which is in the neck and is attached to the temporal bone by ligaments and anchors the tongue (figure 7.20).

The skull also contains teeth, which are not bones, though they do share some of the characteristics of bone tissue.

★ **EXAM POINT** Children may grow 20 deciduous (nonpermanent) teeth that will eventually fall out and be replaced by the 32 permanent teeth.

Skull Divisions

The bones of the skull include the frontal bone, which makes up the forehead and roof of the orbits; the occipital bone, which forms the back and base of the skull; two parietal bones, which form the roof and upper sides of the skull; and two temporal bones, which form the lower sides of the skull and house the inner ear ossicles. The lower rearmost part of each temporal bone is called the mastoid process, but because it is separated from the temporal bones by a suture, it is sometimes considered a separate bone. The sphenoid bone forms the central base of the skull and spans the skull from side to side, the greater wings forming side plates of the skull.

The sections of the ethmoid bone are positioned between the orbits, forming the walls and roof of the nasal cavity, while the three middle ear ossicles—stapes, malleus, and incus—are located within the temporal bones on each side of the skull. The U-shaped hyoid bone is found in the neck and is attached by ligaments to the temporal bones.

In the face, the two maxillary bones form much of the orbits, nose, upper jaw, and roof of the mouth, while the malar or zygomatic bones form the cheeks. The lacrimal bones are located on the inner sides of the orbits and are attached to the ethmoid and maxillary bones. Within the nasal cavity, the vomer is located in the low center and forms the thin flat bone of the nasal septum, while two inferior turbinates form the

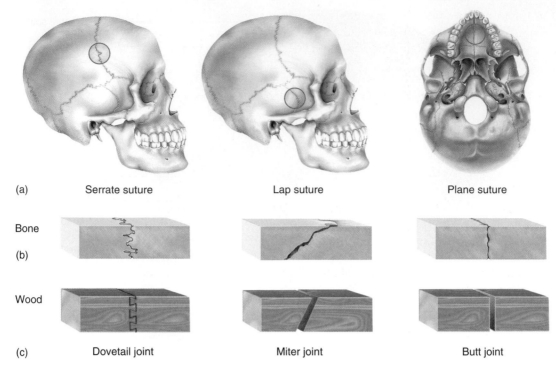

| (a) | Serrate suture | Lap suture | Plane suture |

| Bone (b) | | | |

| Wood (c) | Dovetail joint | Miter joint | Butt joint |

Figure 7.21 Types of sutures
(*a*) Examples; (*b*) structure of adjoining bones; (*c*) comparison to common wood joints.

lower sides of the cavity, and two palate bones form the floor of the nasal cavity as well as the roof of the mouth. The mandible is the only movable part of the skull, forming the lower jaw and mounting the teeth.

Skull Sutures

The bones of the skull—with the exception of the mandible—are held together by very thin sutures, or seams, in which the periosteum of the individual bones interweave with each other (figure 7.21) and are cemented by a fibrous, connective tissue. In the newborn, these sutures are not yet developed, with the bones being attached by cartilage that ossifies over time as the bones of the skull fuse together. The most evident external sutures of the cranium include the coronal suture (joining the frontal and parietal bones), the sagittal suture (joining the parietal bones to each side), the lambdoid suture (joining the occipital and parietal bones), and the squamosal suture (joining the temporal and the sphenoid bones to the parietal bone on each side of the skull). The pterion is the short segment of the suture joining the sphenoid and parietal bones.

Sinuses

The bones of the skull also feature a number of sinuses, which are cavities between bones, and foramina (plural of *foramen*), meaning hole or opening. Four pairs of sinuses flank the nasal cavity and are called paranasal sinuses. Two are found in the maxillary bone and are called maxillary sinuses. The sphenoid bone forms two paranasal sinuses called the sphenoids, and the ethmoid bone forms the two paranasal sinuses called ethmoids. Additionally, the frontal sinuses are located in the frontal bone just behind the roof of each orbit.

The foramen magnum is a large, round opening in the base of the skull that admits the spinal cord. At the base of each temporal bone is the external auditory meatus, which serves as the auditory canal. Just above each orbit in the frontal bone is a small notch or hole, called a supraorbital foramen, and just below each orbit, in the maxillary bone, is an infraorbital foramen. Two more openings, one on each side of the skull, can be found in the frontal processes of the malar/zygomatic bones and are called zygomatofacial foramina. On each side of the mandible, just below the lower canines (teeth), are the mental foramina. These facial foramina serve to admit blood vessels and nerves through and into the bone.

The teeth are mounted in the maxillary bone and the mandible, and are brought together for chewing by the hingelike motion of the mandible (lower jawbone).

★ EXAM POINT Tooth enamel (dentin) is the hardest material in the body.

Pectoral Girdle

The pectoral or shoulder girdle consists of two bones. The clavicle (collarbone) is on the anterior of the body, and the scapula (shoulder blade) (figure 7.22) is on the posterior side of the body. The clavicle is a long, slightly curving bone that forms the frontal part of each shoulder. Located just above the first rib on each side of the ribcage, clavicles attach to the sternum in the middle of the chest and laterally to the acromion process of the scapula, forming the acromioclavicular joint (ac joint) (figure 7.23).

Bones of the Arms and Hands

The arm and its bones form complex articulations in the hand, elbow, and shoulder (figure 7.24). These articulations allow a wide range of motion, from waving our arms over our head to picking up grains of sand with our fingers. The structure of the arm is made up of the humerus (upper arm), and the radius and the ulna (lower arm). The proximal "hook" of the ulna (elbow) is known as the olecranon process. The head of the humerus articulates with the glenoid fossa of the scapula to form the glenohumeral joint (shoulder), while the radius and ulna articulate with the carpal bones of the wrist.

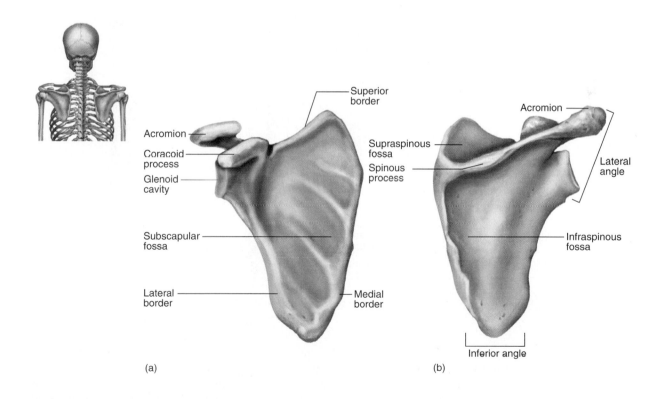

Figure 7.22 The right scapula
(*a*) Anterior view; (*b*) posterior view.

Figure 7.23
Humeroscapular (shoulder) joint, anterior view

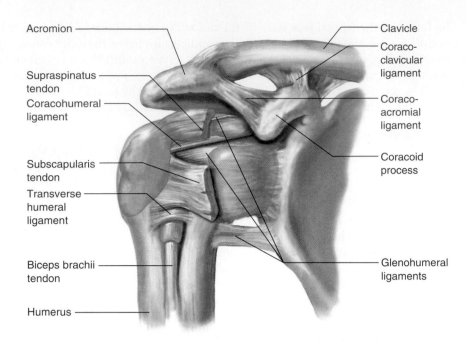

Acromion

Supraspinatus tendon

Coracohumeral ligament

Subscapularis tendon

Transverse humeral ligament

Biceps brachii tendon

Humerus

Clavicle

Coraco-clavicular ligament

Coraco-acromial ligament

Coracoid process

Glenohumeral ligaments

Figure 7.24 Right humerus

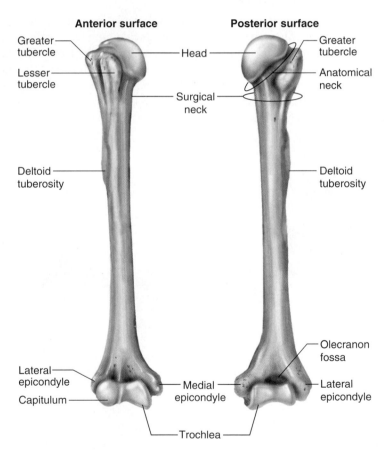

Anterior surface

Greater tubercle

Lesser tubercle

Deltoid tuberosity

Lateral epicondyle

Capitulum

Head

Surgical neck

Medial epicondyle

Trochlea

Posterior surface

Greater tubercle

Anatomical neck

Deltoid tuberosity

Olecranon fossa

Lateral epicondyle

By using the hands, the versatile arm can perform the varied manipulations and motions that are required of a massage therapist, watchmaker, or carpenter.

The humerus, radius, and ulna join to form the elbow joint. This joint features a number of complex points that are attachment sites of ligaments and muscles (figure 7.25). These attachments control the hyperextension (adduction) of the bones of the elbow. The articulation of the elbow is called a hinge joint because it acts like a hinge on a door.

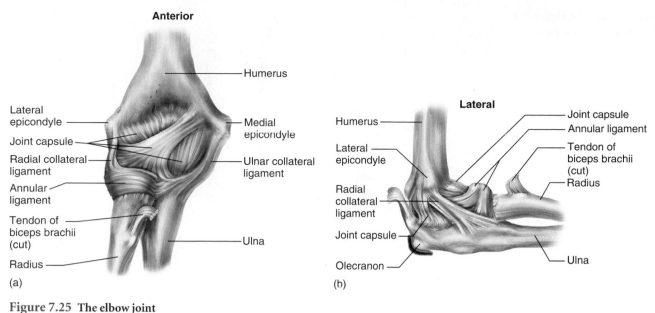

Figure 7.25 The elbow joint
(*a*) Anterior view; (*b*) lateral view.

 EXAM POINT   The elbow joint only permits flexion on one plane (see chapter 6).

Carpals (Bones of the Hand)

Each hand is comprised of 27 bones that form the wrist, back of the hand, and fingers. These bones are articularly specialized, allowing a wide range of flexibility. Eight of the bones form the wrist or carpus. These carpal bones include the scaphoid (navicular), the lunate, the pisiform, the capitate, the trapezium, the trapezoid, the hamate, and the triquetrum.

EXAM POINT   These carpal bones are arranged in two rows, the proximal (toward the body) and the distal (near the fingers). The distal carpals articulate with the five metacarpals.

The long **metacarpals** form the broad structure of the hand, as seen in the dorsal or palmate (palm side) views. These in turn articulate with the end section of the fingers, called the phalanges.

EXAM POINT   The thumb is different in structure in that it does not have a middle phalanx (figure 7.26).

Ribcage

The ribcage is composed of 12 pairs of ribs that articulate with the vertebrae of the spinal column and the sternum to create the thoracic cavity. The ribs themselves are flat, curved bones, all of which articulate posteriorly with the vertebrae at the costal facets.

EXAM POINT   The upper seven pairs of ribs also articulate anteriorly with the sternum and are called true ribs. The eighth, ninth, and tenth pairs are attached by costal cartilage to the seventh pair and are called false ribs, while the eleventh and twelfth pairs are not attached anteriorly at all and are often called floating ribs.

Figure 7.26 The right wrist and hand, anterior view

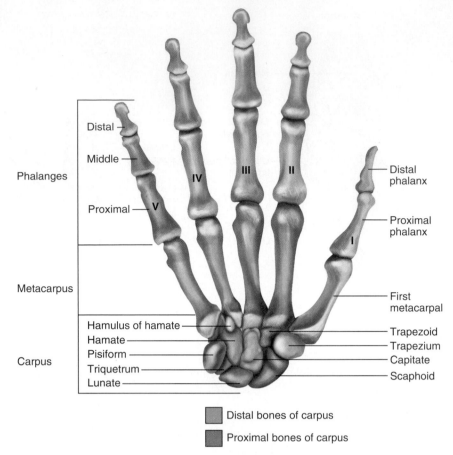

Phalanges
- Distal
- Middle
- Proximal

IV III II

- Distal phalanx
- Proximal phalanx

V

I

Metacarpus

- First metacarpal

Carpus

- Hamulus of hamate
- Hamate
- Pisiform
- Triquetrum
- Lunate

- Trapezoid
- Trapezium
- Capitate
- Scaphoid

Distal bones of carpus

Proximal bones of carpus

The ribcage provides a sturdy support of the thorax—protecting the heart, lungs, and internal organs. The arrangement of the ribs allows the expansion of the ribcage when we breathe. A large number of muscles and ligaments attach to the ribs, which, along with the flexibility of the ribcage, allow the thorax to be flexible and strong.

Spine

The spinal or vertebral column is one of the primary support structures for the human skeleton. Made up of separate and fused vertebrae, the spine features multiple articulations. Such articulations provide support and allow movement of the skull and flexion of the neck and back, and anchor the ribs.

EXAM POINT These articulations support and protect the spinal cord (figure 7.27). The spinal or vertebral column is composed of 7 cervical vertebrae (which form the neck), 12 thoracic vertebrae (which form the upper back), and 5 lumbar vertebrae (which form the lower back). Also part of the vertebral column is the sacrum (a bone made of 5 fused vertebrae).

The sacrum anchors the spine to the pelvic girdle. Finally, the coccyx (tailbone), a semiflexible series of 4 or fewer vertebrae, helps to protect the lower digestive organs. The sacral and coccygeal vertebrae fuse as we reach adulthood and are traditionally counted as one bone each, making the number of vertebrae in the vertebral column represented as 26.

Vertebrae

Between each vertebra is an intervertebral disc made of fibrocartilage, which acts as a shock absorber to cushion the vertebral column from trauma. The spine is held to-

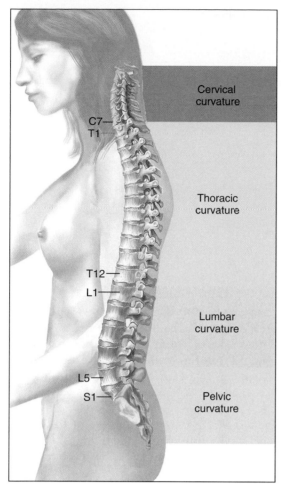

Figure 7.27 Normal curvature of the adult vertebral column

Cervical curvature

C7
T1

Thoracic curvature

T12
L1

Lumbar curvature

L5
S1

Pelvic curvature

gether by a series of ligaments, including the intertransverse ligaments that run the length of the spine, attached to the transverse processes of each vertebra. The spinal cord, which serves as the primary nerve pathway to and from the brain, proceeds down a canal in the center of the spinal column.

Each vertebra is a complex entity (figure 7.28). Following is a list of terms describing the individual parts of each vertebra:

- *C1 atlas and C2 axis*—The axis contains the odontoid process (dens) that forms a pivot point with the atlas; this allows you to shake your head no.
- *Vertebral foramen*—the hole that the spinal cord goes through
- *Spinous process*—posterior point of the vertebra
- *Transverse process*—the lateral, winged projections on each side of the spinous process
- *Transverse foramen*—the holes that go through the transverse process of cervical vertebrae only for the vertebral artery
- *Lamina*—the portion of bone that connects the spinous process to each transverse process
- *Body of the vertebrae*—the large, solid portion of the bone
- *Pedicle*—the portion of bone that connects each transverse process to the body
- *Superior and inferior articulating facets*—form a gliding joint between vertebrae
- *Intervertebral foramen*—the lateral holes formed by the joining of two vertebrae that allow for passage of spinal nerves
- *Anterior and posterior sacral foramen*—the holes in the sacrum that allow for passage of sacral nerves
- *Median crest (sacral crest)*—vertical ridge of bumps that bear the remains of spinous process

Figure 7.28
Anatomy of the representative vertebra

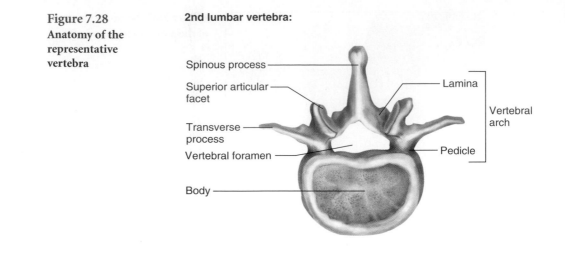

2nd lumbar vertebra:

Spinous process

Superior articular facet

Transverse process

Vertebral foramen

Body

Lamina

Vertebral arch

Pedicle

Pelvis

The pelvis creates the basin of the lower abdominal cavity. It is divided into three separate bones that become fused: the illium, the ischium, and the pubis. The illium is the broad, winglike segment that features the wide, slightly concave surfaces of the back and sides of the pelvic girdle. The ischium forms the smaller, lower portion that bears the weight of the body while sitting. The pubis creates an archway in the front of the basin that allows the urethra, blood vessels, and nerves to pass through the pelvic girdle to the external genitalia and lower body. The pelvis articulates with the sacrum in the posterior portion to form the sacroiliac joint and connects to the rest of the vertebral column. The legs are connected to the sacrum through the ball-and-socket joint formed by the two acetabula of the pelvis and the head of each femur. This is commonly called the hip but is clinically referred to as the coxae (innominate).

Legs

The skeleton of the leg is composed of the femur (thigh bone), tibia and fibula (calf bones), and the patella (kneecap) (figure 7.29).

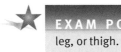 **EXAM POINT** The femur is the longest bone in the body and composes the upper leg, or thigh.

The greater and lesser trochanter, rough prominences at the upper part of the femur, serve as a site for muscle attachments. The tibia is the robust, primary bone of the two in the lower leg and is also sometimes called the shinbone; the tibia bears most of the weight exerted on the leg. The tibia's head, or proximal end, articulates with the parallel fibula and the femur at the knee joint (figure 7.30), while the distal end articulates with the fibula and the talus of the ankle. The large, protruding points at the lower end are called the medial malleolus on the tibia and the lateral malleolus on the fibula.

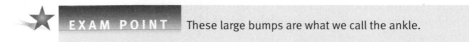 **EXAM POINT** These large bumps are what we call the ankle.

The fibula is the smaller of the two bones of the lower leg. It articulates at each end with the parallel tibia; at its head, it articulates with the femur below the knee joint and, at its lower end, with the bones of the ankle or tarsus.

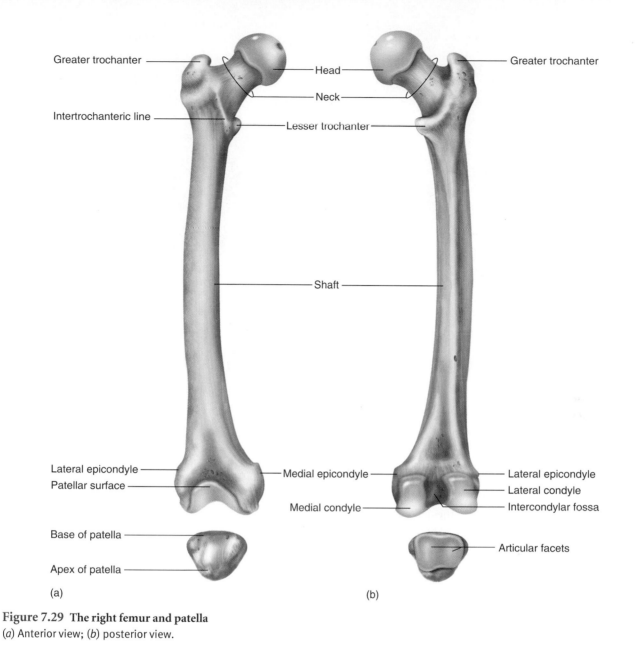

Figure 7.29 The right femur and patella
(*a*) Anterior view; (*b*) posterior view.

The following bones have three primary sites of articulation: the hip joint, formed by the head of the femur and the acetabulum of the pelvis; the knee joint, formed by the joining of the lower end of the femur, the patella, and the superior end of the tibia and fibula; and the ankle, formed by the articulation between the tibia, fibula, and tarsus. The legs are responsible for bearing a great deal of weight and are subjected to intense vertical and lateral stresses, especially at the knee joint. Consequently, the bones of the leg are often cracked or broken, and the knee, hip, and ankle joint are particularly susceptible to fracture, strain, sprain, and dislocation.

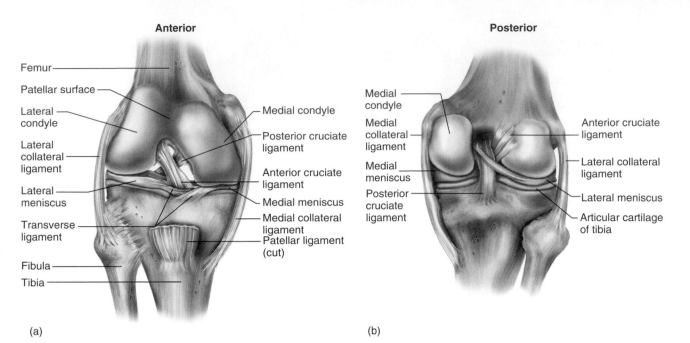

Anterior

Femur

Patellar surface

Lateral condyle

Lateral collateral ligament

Lateral meniscus

Transverse ligament

Fibula

Tibia

Medial condyle

Posterior cruciate ligament

Anterior cruciate ligament

Medial meniscus

Medial collateral ligament

Patellar ligament (cut)

(a)

Posterior

Medial condyle

Medial collateral ligament

Medial meniscus

Posterior cruciate ligament

Anterior cruciate ligament

Lateral collateral ligament

Lateral meniscus

Articular cartilage of tibia

(b)

Figure 7.30 The tibiofemoral joint (knee)
(*a*) Anterior view; (*b*) posterior view.

Knee

The knee is a hingelike joint formed by the lower end of the femur, the upper ends of the tibia and fibula, and the patella (kneecap). The patella is connected to the joint by the medial and patellar retinaculum ligaments and to the tuberosity of the tibia by the patellar ligament. It is not visible in the posterior view and is removed in the anterior view to show the articulation and connective tissues of the bones beneath.

The knee is a joint that is subjected to tremendous lateral (side-to-side) stress during normal activity and is guarded by a number of transverse and cruciate ligaments to help lend it support. Even so, when increased stress is placed on this joint during extreme sports activity that requires the athlete to alter direction rapidly, the knee often bears the brunt of intolerable shearing force. Such incidences often result in torn ligaments within the knee that require surgery.

Within the knee joint is a fibrocartilage padding that helps cushion the femur and the tibia from the stresses placed on them. This cartilage forms two depressions, each of which accepts a condyle of the articular surface of the femur. The lateral meniscus is the slightly concave cavity on the outer side of the joint upon which rests the lateral condyle, and the medial meniscus is a similar depression that articulates with the medial condyle of the femur. This is a common site of sports injury. A torn meniscus can require very aggressive treatment. Athletic participation may be significantly limited as a result of such an injury.

Tarsal (Bones of the Feet)

Each foot is made up of 26 bones that form the ankle, top and bottom of the foot, and toes (figure 7.31). Seven bones form the compact arrangement of the ankle, or tarsus, and the heel. These tarsal bones include the navicular, the three cuneiform, the cuboid, the talus, and the **calcaneus (heel).**

 EXAM POINT   These tarsal bones are arranged in two rows, the proximal row and the distal row. The distal tarsals articulate with the five metatarsals.

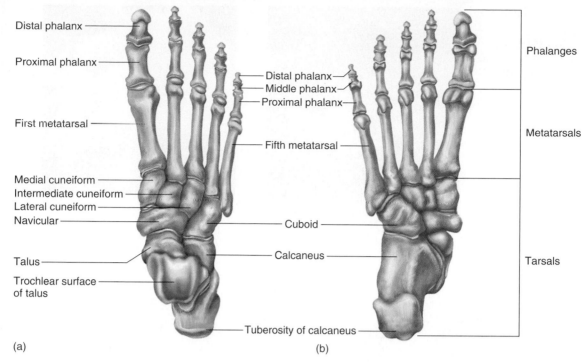

Distal phalanx

Proximal phalanx

First metatarsal

Medial cuneiform
Intermediate cuneiform
Lateral cuneiform
Navicular

Talus

Trochlear surface
of talus

Distal phalanx
Middle phalanx
Proximal phalanx

Fifth metatarsal

Cuboid

Calcaneus

Tuberosity of calcaneus

Phalanges

Metatarsals

Tarsals

(a)   (b)

Figure 7.31 **The right foot**
(*a*) Superior view; (*b*) inferior view.

The long metatarsals form the broad structure of the foot, as seen in the superior view. These articulate with the proximal phalanges (toes). The proximal phalanges join with the middle phalanges, which articulate with the end sections of the toes, called the distal phalanges.

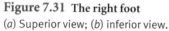 **EXAM POINT**   The large toe, or great toe, is the exception, as it lacks a middle phalanx.

Ligaments connect the bones of the foot together and allow muscles of the calf to remotely direct the toes.

Common Clinical Pathology of the Skeletal System

As a massage therapist, you will likely encounter clients who have pathologies affecting the skeletal system. Such pathologies include:

- *Gout*—an accumulation of uric acid crystals in the joints
- *Osteoporosis*—destructive loss of bone mass
- *Osteoarthritis*—degenerative joint disease, erosion of articular cartilage
- *Pes planus*—"flat feet"; failure of the feet to form an arch
- *Bunions*—localized swelling at the medial or dorsal aspect of the first metatarsophalangeal joint caused by an inflammatory bursa
- *Rheumatoid arthritis*—autoimmune disease of the synovial membrane (figure 7.32)
- *Fracture*—break in a bone. Figure 7.33 illustrates types of bone fractures.
- *Rickets*—Bone softening in children due to lack of vitamin D
- *Kyphosis*—exaggerated thoracic curve, "humpback"
- *Lordosis*—exaggerated lumbar curve, "swayback"
- *Scoliosis*—Lateral curvature of the spine. Figure 7.34 illustrates scoliosis, kyphosis, and lordosis (see also chapter 6).

Figure 7.32 Rheumatoid
arthritis

**Figure 7.32 Rheumatoid
arthritis**
(*a*) Severe case of ankylosis
of the joints; (*b*) x-ray of hand
with rheumatoid arthritis.

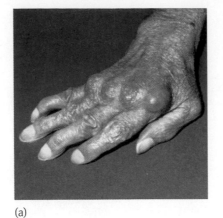

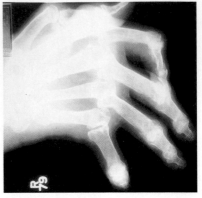

(a)

(b)

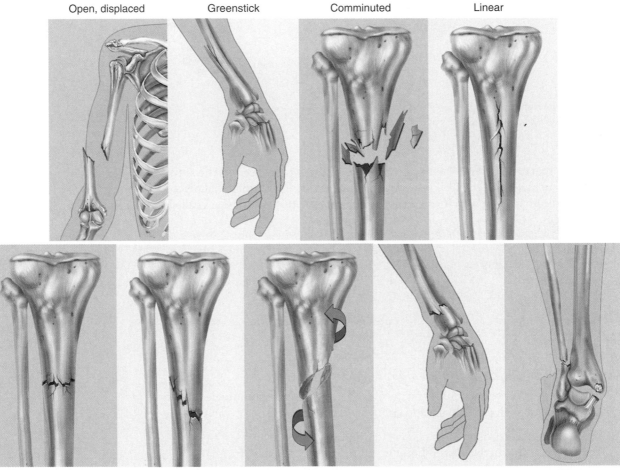

Open, displaced   Greenstick   Comminuted   Linear

Transverse, nondisplaced   Oblique, nondisplaced   Spiral   Colles   Pott

Figure 7.33 Some types of bone fractures

- *Arthritis*—inflammatory condition that affects synovial joints and damages articular cartilage
- *Sprain*—results from damage to the ligaments that occurs when the ligament is stretched beyond its normal limits, tearing collagen fibers
- *Synovitis*—inflamed synovial membrane with swelling and fluid retention

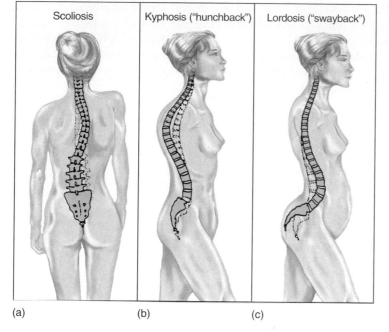

Figure 7.34 Abnormal spinal curvatures
(*a*) Scoliosis, an abnormal lateral deviation.
(*b*) Kyphosis, an exaggerated thoracic curvature.
(*c*) Lordosis, an exaggerated lumbar curvature.

Scoliosis | Kyphosis ("hunchback") | Lordosis ("swayback")

(a)　　　　　(b)　　　　　(c)

- *Temporomandibular joint dysfunction syndrome*—muscle pain and tenderness when chewing, clicking, or popping noises within the joint, and restricted movement
- *Ankylosing spondylitis*—calcification and stiffening of the spine with progressive loss of movement of the vertebra
- *Prolapsed disc*— a condition wherein the disc slipped from the vertebral space and usually presents with neurologic pain as well as restricted movement
- *Whiplash*—the common term for an acute injury of the cervical spine when the neck is suddenly thrown forward, backward, or laterally
- *Bursitis*—pain and inflammation in the bursae
- *Cubital tunnel syndrome*—constriction of the aponeurosis of the flexor carpi ulnaris on the medial aspect of the elbow, resulting in pressure on the ulnar nerve; commonly called tennis elbow
- *Myositis ossificans*—condition in which there is calcification in a muscle
- *Olecranon bursitis*—commonly called miner's elbow, an inflammation of the olecranon bursa usually from repetitious motion
- *Carpal tunnel syndrome*—inflammation and swelling in the structure passing through the carpal tunnel causing compression on the median nerve (see chapter 23)
- *Hip dislocation*—occurs when the flexed hip is forced posteriorly; can lead to fracture or tears in the ligaments
- *Trochanteric bursitis*—a condition that results in pain in the hip that radiates to the knee
- *Housemaid's or roofer's knee*—a condition of an abnormal enlargement of the prepatellar bursa and resultant inflammation, usually caused by pressure and repetitive kneeling
- *Shin splints*—a term used for several conditions involving the lower leg; usually refers to the inflammation caused by repeated stress on the musculotendinous structures arising from the lower part of the tibia

Chapter Summary

As a massage therapist, it is extremely important for you to be knowledgeable about the organization of the body and how the skeleton provides its structural framework. Knowing the framework of the body can help you in understanding the origin, insertion, and action of the muscles, and where the organs and systems are located in relation to each other. This understanding will also help you to realize how the musculoskeletal system is really one system of movement that guides the body in performing many of its necessary functions. Knowing the bony landmarks shown in this chapter can help you develop the palpation skills to complete basic orthopedic assessment and address your client's chief complaint.

Applying Your Knowledge

Self-Testing

1. Cells are composed of which of the following four compounds?
   a) Carbohydrates, fats, proteins, nucleic acids
   b) Cholesterol, fats, proteins, nucleic acids
   c) Carbohydrates, fats, fruits, vegetables
   d) None of the above is correct.

2. Another name for cell membrane is:
   a) cytoplasm.
   b) phospholipid.
   c) organelle.
   d) plasma membrane.

3. In anatomical directions, proximal refers to:
   a) away from the trunk.
   b) toward the head.
   c) toward the trunk.
   d) approximate to body.

4. What is the largest part of the cell, and what is it known as?
   a) Nucleus, "brain"
   b) Nucleus, "power plant"
   c) Golgi apparatus, "carbo factories"
   d) Mitochondria, "control center"

5. To locate pain, how is the abdominopelvic cavity divided?
   a) Using the "rule of nines"
   b) Using the nine regions
   c) Using the four quadrants
   d) Using the eight organelles

6. Which is not one of the seven types of connective tissue?
   a) Hematopoietic, blood, adipose
   b) Ribosomes, mitochondria, centrioles
   c) Cartilage, bone, dense fibrous material
   d) Blood, bone, adipose

7. Which listing has examples of *flat* bones?
   a) Clavicle, humerus, femur, tibia
   b) Hip bone, hyoid, facial, cranial
   c) Cranial, scapula, ribs, sternum
   d) Carpals, tarsals, metacarpals, metatarsals

8. In what part of the body is the foramen magnum located?
   a) Shoulder
   b) Chest
   c) Hip
   d) Skull

9. The "winged projections" of each vertebra are called:
   a) spinous process.
   b) transverse facet.
   c) transverse process.
   d) wing tips.

10. Of the lists below, which contains four of the six functions of the skeleton?
    a) Support, movement, protection, sound conduction
    b) Adipose, cartilage, dense fibrous, areolar
    c) Temperature regulation, sense organ, synthesis, fat storage
    d) Transport, defend, protect, clotting

11. Cranial sutures are which class of joint?
    a) Diarthrotic
    b) Amphiarthrotic
    c) Synarthrotic
    d) Gliding

12. What type of cartilage connects the ribs to the sternum?
    a) Fibro
    b) Hyaline
    c) Articular
    d) Costal

13. *Endochondral ossification* is a description of
    a) formation of bone from blood.
    b) formation of bone from cartilage.
    c) infection of the ossicles.
    d) formation of epicondyles.

14. What type of bone cell is known as a "bone builder?"
    a) Osteopath
    b) Osteoporosis
    c) Osteoclast
    d) Osteoblast

15. Which list gives examples of *long* bone?
    a) Humerus, femur, clavicle, tibia
    b) Carpals, tarsals, ribs, sternum

c) Cranial, facial, ossicles, vertebrae

d) Patella, popliteal, ribs, sternum

16. What are the head, neck, and torso referred to as?

    a) Axial skeleton

    b) Appendicular skeleton

    c) Atlas skeleton

    d) Axon skeleton

17. What are the three divisions of the pelvic girdle?

    a) Ilium, ischium, pubis

    b) Manubrium, body, typhoid process

    c) Iliacus, iliopsoas, pecs

    d) Illiad, idiom, publix

18. The elbow and knee are two examples of this *type* of joint.

    a) Synarthrotic

    b) Amphiarthrotic

    c) Hinge

    d) Saddle

19. What is another name for the hip?

    a) Coxae (innominate)

    b) Coccyx

    c) Mandible

    d) Manubrium

20. Where is the medullary cavity found?

    a) Within the diaphysis

    b) Within the abdominal cavity

    c) Within the cranium

    d) Within the thoracic cavity

21. What is the definition of a foramen?

    a) Depression

    b) Hollow

    c) Hole through a bone

    d) Four men gathered together

22. The malleolus is formed by what two bones?

    a) Tibia and fibula

    b) Femur and tibia

    c) Humerus and ulna

    d) Femur and fibula

23. The thumb is an example of this type of joint.

    a) Hinge

    b) Saddle

    c) Pivot

    d) Ball-and-socket

24. The appendicular skeleton consists of which parts of the body?

    a) Head, neck, upper arms

    b) Head, torso, legs

c) Upper and lower extremities

d) Lower torso and legs

25. Sixteen of which wrist bones are stacked in a proximal and distal row?

    a) Carpals

    b) Tarsal

    c) Fingers

    d) Toes

26. Which suture lies between the frontal and parietal bones?

    a) Skewmous

    b) Sagittarius

    c) Corona

    d) Coronal

27. What is the only bone in the body that *does not* articulate with another bone?

    a) Patella

    b) Ribs

    c) Sternum

    d) Hyoid

28. What is a rough, raised area on a bone called?

    a) Tuberosity

    b) Tubercle

    c) Condyle

    d) Styloid

29. What is the portion of the vertebrae that is between (or connects) the transverse process to the spinous process called?

    a) Cartilage

    b) Vertebral body

    c) Lamina

    d) Lambdoid

30. What is a shallow ditch or depression on a bone called?

    a) Tuberosity

    b) Tubercle

    c) Fossa

    d) Foramen

31. What is osteoporosis?

    a) A loss of bone mass

    b) A blood disease

    c) A bone builder

    d) A spinous process

32. What is the covering of a bone (except at articular surfaces) called?

    a) Endosteum

    b) Epiphysis

    c) Periphysis

    d) Periosteum

33. What is the superior depression above the spine of the scapula called?
    a) Spinous process
    b) Supraspinous fossa
    c) Supraspinous process
    d) Supraspinous foramen

34. What are the smallest bones in the body?
    a) Teeth
    b) Ossicles
    c) Toes
    d) Fingers

35. Which of these is an example of an irregular bone?
    a) Clavicle
    b) Sternum
    c) Patella
    d) Vertebrae

36. What type of joint allows you to shake your head no?
    a) Pivot
    b) Hinge
    c) Saddle
    d) Ball-and-socket

37. Which is the correct list of five *classifications* of bone?
    a) Long, short, flat, irregular, sesamoid
    b) Long, short, round, regular, circular
    c) Tall, small, squamous, saddle, perpendicular
    d) None of the above is correct.

38. What is the roughened area on the upper arm where the deltoid attaches called?
    a) Deltoid tuberosity
    b) Deltoid tubercle
    c) Deltoid process
    d) Deltoid fossa

39. The greater and lesser trochanter are found only on what bone?
    a) Femur
    b) Sternum
    c) Fibula
    d) All bones

40. What is a visible difference between the male and female skeleton?
    a) Width of the pelvis
    b) Tilt of the pelvis
    c) a and b
    d) There is no difference.

41. What is the proximal "hook" on the ulna?
    a) Olecranon process
    b) Olecranon fossa
    c) Olecranon foramen
    d) Ulnanon process

42. Which of these is an autoimmune disease that affects the joints?
    a) Rheumatoid arthritis
    b) Osteoarthritis
    c) AIDS
    d) Rickets

Case Studies/Critical Thinking

A. Michael is a recent graduate of a massage school and has started working in a geriatric assisted living facility. He uses his massage therapy skills to help the residents who have arthritis, Alzheimer's, and minor circulation problems achieve healthier bodies. Today, Michael is seeing Naomi. She is complaining of foot pain and trouble wearing her shoes. When taking a history on Naomi, Michael makes a notation stating that Naomi worked as a bank teller for 25 years. She was required to stand on hard floors for long hours and wore pointed, high-heel shoes. Upon physical assessment, Michael notes that there is a "knot" on the medial side of the metatarsal-phalangeal joint of the great toe, which appears to be a bony misalignment in which the proximal phalanx of the great toe is laterally deviated. The area of the "knot" is red, hot to touch, and painful. What is this condition commonly called? Should massage be contraindicated? Why?

B. On Tuesday, a 12-year-old boy came to see a massage therapist working at an orthopedic clinic. His doctor had referred him to the therapist for massage due to stress on the muscles of his upper left arm caused by a heavy cast on a recent fracture. The doctor had diagnosed a Colles fracture at the distal end of his left radius. Where should the cast be located on the young man's arm to support the area of the fracture? What muscles in his upper arm are affected by the weight of the cast? What might the doctor prescribe to take some of the pulling weight away? Will the inactive muscles of his lower arm be affected in any way while he is healing? Why did the doctor only order massage to the upper arm muscles?

C. Mari is interviewing a new client who complains of back pain and tightness in his lower back muscles. As she notes the history, the client tells her that he has been diagnosed with spondylosis. Mari knows that spondylosis is a general term for any degenerative condition of the vertebrae that can cause pain in the lower back and sometimes the neck. It is often called osteoarthritis of the spine. She also knows that thinning discs in the spine may no longer be elastic or resilient. The damaged discs may be unable to bear weight and can become easily herniated if there is pressure or forced movement in the affected area. How should Mari proceed? Should she ask for more information from his doctor? Should she explain the condition and make recommendations to the client? Can areas not affected by the osteoarthritis be massaged?

References for information in this chapter can be found in Quick Guide C at the end of the book.

CHAPTER 8

Muscular System

LEARNING OUTCOMES

After completing this chapter, you will be able to:

- Explain the primary functions of skeletal, cardiac, and smooth muscle.

- Understand the relationship of the muscular system to other body systems.

- Understand the causes of muscle contraction: neuroelectrical, chemical, and energy sources.

- Explain the structure and function of a motor unit.

- Understand common pathologies of the muscular system.

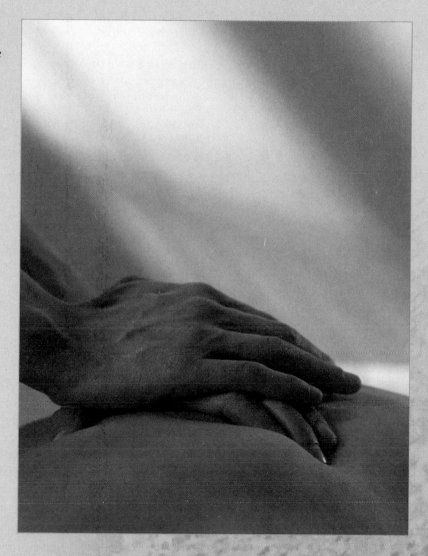

KEY TERMS

actin *(p. 196)*

atrophy *(p. 198)*

cardiac muscle *(p. 194)*

contraction *(p. 197)*

cross-striations *(p. 196)*

endomysium *(p. 196)*

epimysium *(p. 196)*

fascia *(p. 196)*

fasciculi *(p. 196)*

fatigue *(p. 200)*

hypertrophy *(p. 198)*

isokinetic contraction *(p. 198)*

isometric contraction *(p. 198)*

isotonic contraction *(p. 198)*

motor unit *(p. 197)*

perimysium *(p. 196)*

points of attachment *(p. 200)*

sarcolemma *(p. 196)*

skeletal muscle *(p. 194)*

striations *(p. 194)*

tendons *(p. 201)*

tetanic contraction *(p. 198)*

tonic contraction *(p. 198)*

visceral or smooth muscle *(p. 194)*

INTRODUCTION

Many Americans will experience some type of myofascial pain, or chronic pain of a musculoskeletal nature, during their lifetime. As medical care becomes less involved with "touching," people in pain may very likely turn to massage therapists trained in myofascial or musculoskeletal treatment for relief. Many people experiencing injuries (sports-related and otherwise), as well as those seeking relaxation, continue to select massage therapy as their treatment of choice for myofascial and musculoskeletal conditions. As the number of massage therapy clients increases, so does the need for therapists to understand a more diverse list of conditions and symptoms that can be helped by massage. Having a thorough understanding of the muscular system's anatomy (and applying that understanding) will contribute considerably to your ability to excel as a massage therapist.

The human body contains more than 650 individual muscles anchored to the skeleton (figure 8.1). These muscles work together to provide pulling or leveraging power so your body can move, grasp, and turn. In the healthy adult, they make up about 40% of total body weight. Three types of muscles make up the muscular system:

1. Skeletal muscle (figure 8.2) pulls on bones, using them as levers to move the body (see chapter 6).

2. Cardiac muscle (figure 8.3) contracts the heart to move blood through the body.

★ **EXAM POINT**   Cardiac muscle is found only in the heart.

3. Visceral or smooth muscle (figure 8.4) moves fluids, waste, and other products through the organs of the body.

Anatomy and Physiology of Muscle Tissue

The three types of muscle tissue—skeletal, cardiac, and visceral or smooth—have specific characteristics that lend themselves to the functions of the muscle system. Skeletal muscles are striated and voluntary (meaning that we can control the muscle's movement). When viewed under the microscope, skeletal muscle cells are multinucleated and have extraordinary length and thickness. Skeletal muscle cells are called muscle fibers, or myofibrils. The alternating light and dark bands, or **striations,** make up the structure of this type of muscle tissue.

Cardiac muscle is also striated but is uninucleated and found only in the heart. This type of muscle tissue is considered involuntary, which means it is not usually under conscious, deliberate control. Involuntary muscles are never attached to bone.

Visceral or smooth muscle tissue is nonstriated, uninucleated, and involuntary. It is found in the digestive tract and among other internal organs of the body. The visceral muscles are responsible for the peristalsis effect, which enables food to pass through the alimentary canal.

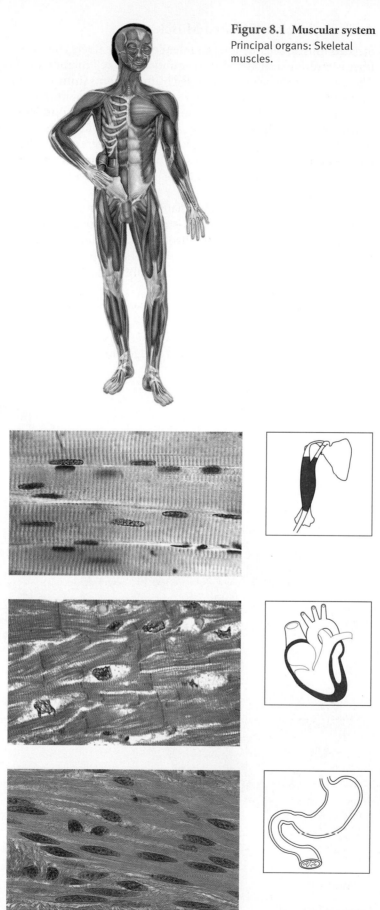

Figure 8.1 Muscular system
Principal organs: Skeletal muscles.

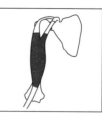

Figure 8.2 Skeletal muscle
Long, cylindrical fibers.

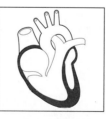

Figure 8.3 Cardiac muscle
Short, branched cells.

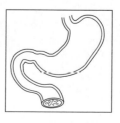

Figure 8.4 Smooth muscle
Short, layered cells.

A Closer Look at Striated Muscle

Striated muscle cells are long and slender muscle fibers (figure 8.5). Each muscle cell or fiber is multinucleated and is surrounded by a cell membrane called the **sarcolemma**. The sarcolemma itself is surrounded by the **endomysium,** one of the three types of connective tissue within the muscular system. The skeletal muscle cells then form bundles, called **fasciculi**. Each bundle is surrounded by the second layer of connective tissue, called the **perimysium**. This layer can be seen without the use of a microscope. The perimysium connects with a rougher, coarser layer of connective tissue called the **epimysium**. These connective tissues hold all of the muscle cells and bundles together like glue. Areolar tissue surrounds the bundles by covering the epimysium and is called the **fascia**.

If you view skeletal muscle striations under a microscope, you will see alternating dark and light bands called **cross-striations**. These striations are due to overlapping dark and light proteins on the myofibrils. The bands that are dark are made of the thicker filaments of the protein myosin. They appear dark because of their thickness and are called A bands. The lighter bands are made up of thinner filaments of a protein called **actin** and are called I bands.

A narrow line of dark staining cells that appears in the center of the I band and resembles the letter *z* is called the Z line. The slightly darker region in the midsection of the A band is called the H band or H zone. This is where the myosin filaments are the thickest and where there are no cross bridges on the myosin filaments.

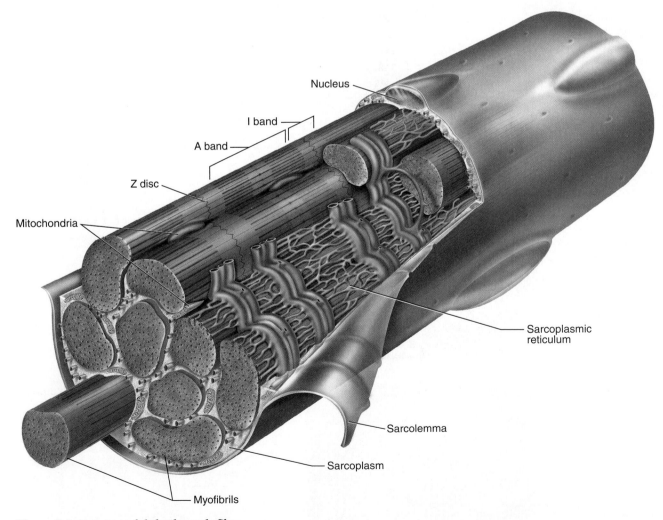

Figure 8.5 Structure of skeletal muscle fiber.

The area between two Z lines is called the sarcomere. It is in the sarcomere that the contraction process begins, making the sarcomere the functional unit of muscle.

Primary Functions of Muscles

Movement is an activity essential to our survival. Without our muscles contracting and relaxing, most of our bodily functions would not be possible. To make movement possible, our muscles perform three primary functions. First, they allow movement of the body by pulling on the bones, using them as levers. The body further relies on the integration of the bones, joints, ligaments, tendons, and fascia to act with muscles to aid in motion. Cardiac muscle performs a vital act by contracting to move blood through the body, and smooth muscle helps move nutrients through the hollow organs and waste products out of the body. Second, our muscles help stabilize and maintain our posture. Third, muscle movement produces heat and helps to regulate bodily temperature.

Properties of Muscle Cells

Four properties are associated with muscle cells: conductivity, contractility, excitability, and elasticity. Muscle cells are excited by a stimulus in the form of a nerve cell. All material within the cell possesses the property of conductivity and allows a response to stimuli to travel throughout the cell. In muscle cells, this conductivity stimulation is called a **contraction**. The elastic property of the cell then allows the cell to return to its original size and shape after the contraction is over. Muscle contraction is caused in three ways: by neuroelectrical factors, by chemical interactions, and by other energy sources.

Contraction

Muscle cells possess special properties that allow for contraction and extension. The muscle cells are innervated by one motor neuron unit called a **motor unit** because when excitement occurs, all of the cells are excited and contract together. Stimulation of this single motor unit causes a weaker but steadier contraction in a large area of the muscle, instead of one stronger contraction at only one small point.

Think About It

A helpful way to remember the primary functions of muscles is to memorize the phrase "miles per hour," where *miles* represents "movement"; *per*, "posture"; and *hour*, "heat."

Muscles control large and small movements of the body. The eye, for instance, has a very small number of muscle fibers in a motor unit. It takes only 10 muscle cells to move the eye from side to side. When you raise your arm, as many as 200 muscle cells can be used.

Muscle Movement Terminology

To understand muscle movement, you must first familiarize yourself with movement terminology. The most common terms relating to muscle movement are:

- *Origin*: the most stationary point of attachment of the muscle
- *Insertion*: the point of attachment of the muscle that is more mobile and moves with the bone
- *Action*: the changes produced in the joint by muscle contraction
- *Prime mover/agonist*: the main muscle that produces a particular movement
- *Antagonist*: the main muscle to oppose a particular movement
- *Synergist*: muscle that assists a prime mover/agonist with movement
- *Fixator/Stabilizer*: muscle that stabilizes the origin of the prime mover to increase its efficiency

When muscles acting in groups move, there is always a prime mover (agonist), a synergist to assist the prime mover, an antagonist that opposes the prime mover, and a fixator that stabilizes the origin of the prime mover and holds the bone of origin in place.

 EXAM POINT As a general rule, only the bone of insertion should be moved.

Naming Muscles

By understanding medical terminology, you will be better able to remember the names of the muscles and their location or characteristics of movement. For example, *longus*, which means "long," lets you know that you are looking for a long muscle; *levator* (lifts) and *scapulae* (scapula) indicate the muscle that lifts the scapula. Table 8.1 lists words that are often used to describe muscles.

Muscle Contractions

Types of Muscle Contraction

There are five types of muscle contractions: tonic, isotonic, isometric, isokinetic, and tetanic. **Tonic contraction** is the continuous partial contraction that does not create movement. **Isotonic contraction** occurs when muscle shortens and produces movement. This is the usual movement associated with walking and lifting. **Isometric contraction** is when a muscle does not shorten and no movement is produced, such as when pushing against a wall. **Isokinetic contraction** occurs when the movement of a joint is kept at a constant velocity. When the speed of the contraction is constant, it results in a maximized muscle-turning effect, known as torsion (torque). **Tetanic contraction** is a sustained contraction that results from repeated stimuli without any rest. A person experiencing lockjaw, for instance, has this condition. A twitch contraction is a rapid, jerky response from a single stimuli—as in a single isotonic contraction.

Effects of Muscle Contraction

The three effects of muscle contractions are hypertrophy, atrophy, and fatigue. **Hypertrophy** occurs when the muscle size is increased by an increase in the size of the muscle fibers. **Atrophy** occurs when there is a decrease in muscle size caused by a de-

Table 8.1 **Words Commonly Used to Name Muscles**

Criterion	Term and Meaning	Examples
Size	Major (large)	Pectoralis major
	Maximus (largest)	Gluteus maximus
	Minor (small)	Pectoralis minor
	Minimus (smallest)	Gluteus minimus
	Longus (long)	Abductor pollicis longus
	Brevis (short)	Extensor pollicis brevis
Shape	Rhomboideus (rhomboidal)	Rhomboideus major
	Trapezius (trapezoidal)	Trapezius
	Teres (round, cylindrical)	Pronator teres
	Deltoid (triangular)	Deltoid
Location	Capitis (of the head)	Slenius capitis
	Cervicis (of the neck)	Semispinalis cervicis
	Pectoralis (of the chest)	Pectoralis major
	Thoracis (of the thorax)	Spinalis thoracis
	Intercostal (between the ribs)	External intercostalis
	Abdominis (of the abdomen)	Rectus abdominis
	Lumborum (of the lower back)	Quadratus lumborum
	Femoris (of the femur, or thigh)	Quadriceps femoris
	Peroneus (of the fibula)	Peroneus longus
	Brachii (of the arm)	Biceps brachii
	Carpi (of the wrist)	Flexor carpi ulnaris
	Digiti (of a finger or toe, singular)	Extensor digiti minimi
	Digitorum (of the fingers or toes, plural)	Flexor digitorum profundus
	Pollicis (of the thumb)	Opponens pollicis
	Indicis (of the index finger)	Extensor indicis
	Hallucis (of the great toe)	Abductor hallucis
	Superficialis (superficial)	Flexor digitorum superficialis
	Profundus (deep)	Flexor digitorum profundus
Number of heads	Biceps (two heads)	Biceps femoris
	Triceps (three heads)	Triceps brachii
	Quadriceps (four heads)	Quadriceps femoris
Orientation	Rectus (straight)	Rectus abdominis
	Transversus (transverse)	Transversus abdominis
	Oblique (slanted)	External abdominal oblique
Action	Adductor (adducts a body part)	Adductor pollicis
	Abductor (abducts a body part)	Abductor digiti minimi
	Flexor (flexes a joint)	Flexor carpi radialis
	Pronator (pronates forearm)	Pronator teres
	Supinator (supinates forearm)	Supinator
	Levator (elevates a body part)	Levator scapulae
	Depressor (depresses a body part)	Depressor anguli oris

crease in the size of the muscle fibers. This condition usually results from disuse. When muscle contractions grow weak from repeated stimulization, the muscle becomes fatigued, which is caused by the depletion of adenosine triphosphate (ATP) (see chapter 5, p. 122). When **fatigue** occurs, there is often a buildup of lactic acid resulting from an oxygen debt. Muscles need oxygen to remove the lactic acid buildup and restore the muscle to a resting state.

Fast Twitch and Slow Twitch Muscle Contractions

Fast Twitch Muscles

Fast twitch muscles provide rapid movement for short periods of time. Fast twitch muscles do not use oxygen; they use glycogen for energy. Reactions using glycogen require anaerobic enzymes to produce power. Glycogen is stored in the muscles and liver, and is synthesized by the body using carbohydrates. There are two types of fast twitch muscles, and they will function during moderate and maximum muscular effort. Fast twitch muscles provide strength and speed.

Slow Twitch Muscles

As their name indicates, slow twitch muscles have a slower contraction time. Slow twitch muscles use oxygen for power and have a predominance of aerobic enzymes. These types of muscles are large muscles found in the leg, thigh, trunk, back, and hip areas of the body and are used for holding posture.

Adenosine triphosphate (ATP) is the main source of energy for all muscle contraction. Several chemical reactions take place to produce ATP. When a muscle is used, a chemical reaction breaks down ATP to produce energy:

$$ATP + actin + myosin \rightarrow actomyosin + phosphate + adenosine\ diphosphate = energy$$

There is only enough ATP stored in the muscle cell for two or three slow twitch contractions (or one burst of power from a fast twitch contraction), so more ATP must then be created.

Three enzyme systems can create more ATP. The enzyme system that is used depends on whether the type of muscle is fast twitch or slow twitch and whether the muscle is used for strength, burst power, or endurance.

Fast twitch muscle—15% of the muscles of the body
- Rapid and forceful contractions
- Large motor units
- Fatigues quickly
- Anaerobic (glycogen)

Slow twitch muscle—50% of the muscles of the body
- Slow and less-intense contractions
- Smaller motor units
- Slower fatigue—holds for longer periods (postural)
- Aerobic (oxygen)

Intermediate—35% of the muscles of the body
- Muscles of the limbs

Attachments

The muscles' **points of attachment** to bones or other muscles are designated as origin or insertion.

Muscles are attached by the tough fibrous structures called **tendons**. Keep in mind that a ligament is a sheet of fibrous connective tissue that connects two or more bones. The attachments bridge one or more joints, and the result of muscle contraction is movement of these joints. The body is moved primarily by muscle groups, not by individual muscles. The groups of muscles power all actions ranging from the threading of a needle to the lifting of heavy weights (figure 8.6).

Muscles of the Face and Head

About 30 muscles associated with facial expression control the eyes, face surface, mouth, and ears (figure 8.7). These muscles take their origin from the bones of the facial skeleton and attach to the soft tissues of the facial skin, such as the eyelids, nose, cheeks, and lips. They aid the body with mastication (chewing) and deglutition (swallowing).

There are 17 smiling muscles (figure 8.8). Some muscles open the facial orifices wide; others narrow or close them. All the muscles of the face are supplied by branches of two main nerves—the right and the left facial nerves—which arise from the brain stem. These branches of the facial nerves control the muscle movements of the face.

The main mover of the muscles of the lateral group is easily found on the anterior and lateral sides of the neck. When only one sternocleidomastoid muscle contracts, it allows for the rotation of the head.

Other muscles in the neck move food around the mouth, aid speech, and allow for swallowing. The muscles and accompanying structures include the hyoid muscles, soft palate, pharynx, and larynx. A series of constriction and relaxation movements by the pharyngeal elevators and the pharyngeal constrictors force food into the esophagus as we swallow.

Muscles of the Torso

The muscles of the torso extend in several directions. They include those that move the vertebral column, those that form the thoracic and abdominal walls, and those that cover the pelvic outlet. The muscles of the thoracic wall are primarily involved in the process of breathing. The abdominal wall consists of four muscle pairs, arranged in layers, and the fascia that envelopes them. The back is crisscrossed by broad bands of muscle. The muscles in the lower back provide support for upright posture. The muscles at the top of the back move the shoulders and arms, and help you to breathe. See table 8.2.

Those in the central group steady the spine and enable you to bend forward and backward and to twist from side to side. The deeper muscles form an overlapping sheet that joins this central region to the scapula and pelvis. Other muscles link these bones

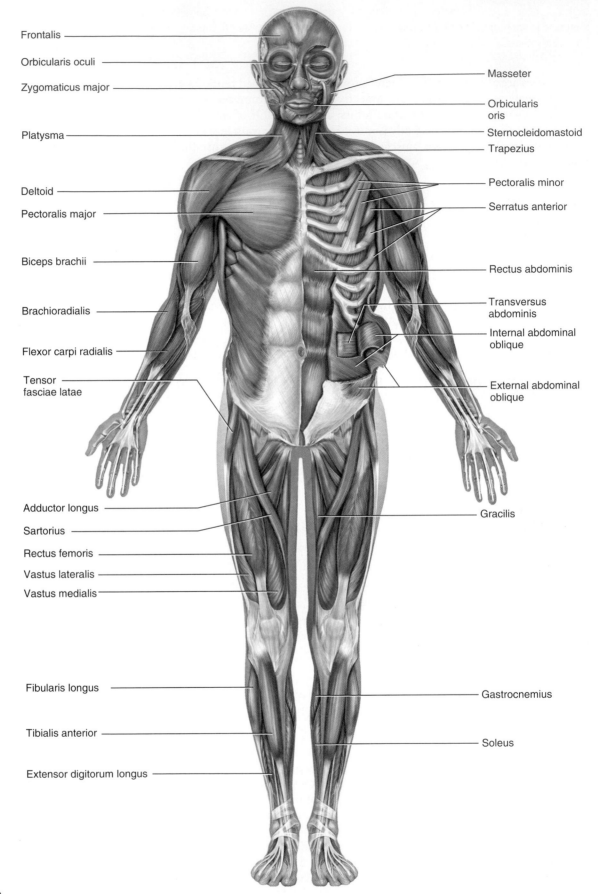

Frontalis

Orbicularis oculi

Zygomaticus major

Platysma

Deltoid

Pectoralis major

Biceps brachii

Brachioradialis

Flexor carpi radialis

Tensor
fasciae latae

Adductor longus

Sartorius

Rectus femoris

Vastus lateralis

Vastus medialis

Fibularis longus

Tibialis anterior

Extensor digitorum longus

Masseter

Orbicularis
oris

Sternocleidomastoid

Trapezius

Pectoralis minor

Serratus anterior

Rectus abdominis

Transversus
abdominis

Internal abdominal
oblique

External abdominal
oblique

Gracilis

Gastrocnemius

Soleus

(a)

Figure 8.6 The muscular system

(a) Anterior aspect. Major superficial muscles on right, deeper muscles on left.

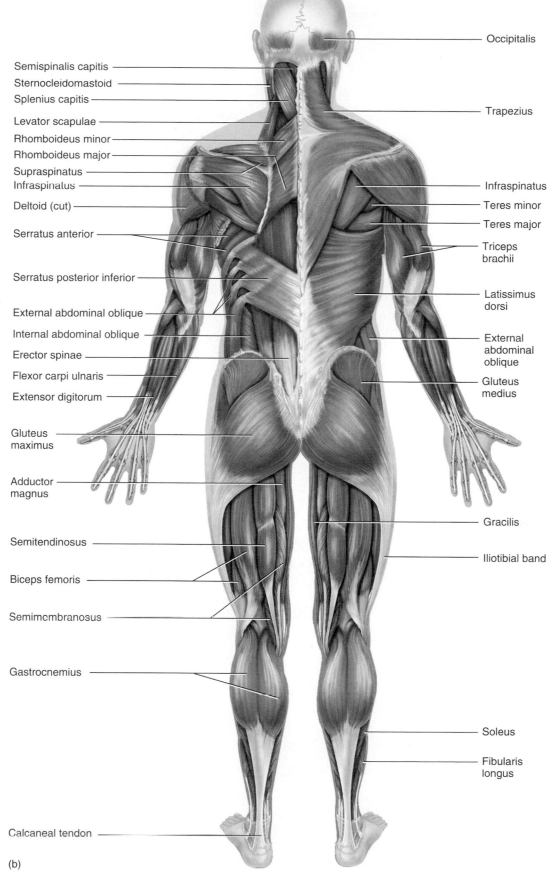

Occipitalis

Semispinalis capitis

Sternocleidomastoid

Splenius capitis

Levator scapulae

Rhomboideus minor

Rhomboideus major

Supraspinatus

Infraspinatus

Deltoid (cut)

Serratus anterior

Serratus posterior inferior

External abdominal oblique

Internal abdominal oblique

Erector spinae

Flexor carpi ulnaris

Extensor digitorum

Gluteus maximus

Adductor magnus

Semitendinosus

Biceps femoris

Semimembranosus

Gastrocnemius

Calcaneal tendon

Trapezius

Infraspinatus

Teres minor

Teres major

Triceps brachii

Latissimus dorsi

External abdominal oblique

Gluteus medius

Gracilis

Iliotibial band

Soleus

Fibularis longus

(b)

Figure 8.6 (continued)

(b) Posterior aspect. Superficial muscles on right, deeper muscles on left.

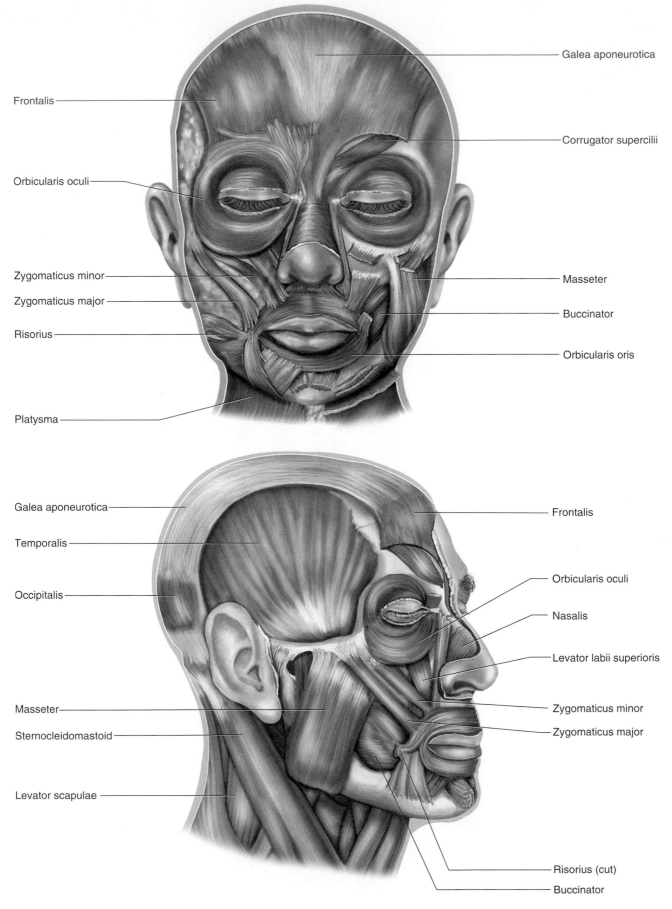

Figure 8.7 Muscles of facial expression

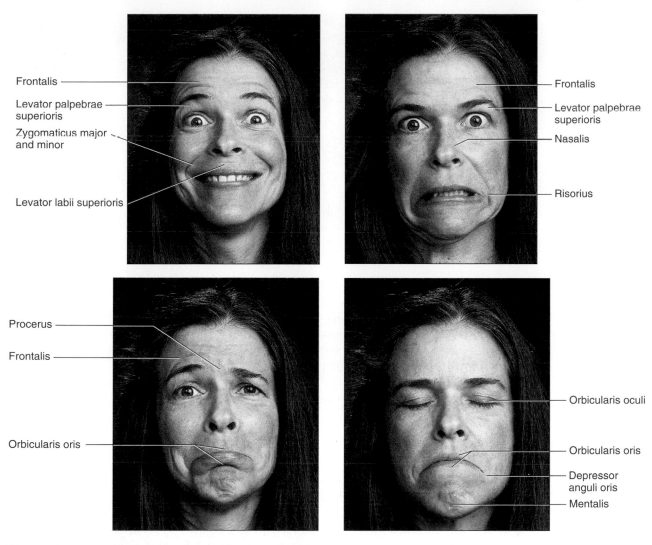

Figure 8.8 Major muscles used for facial expressions

Table 8.2	*Muscles of Respiration*

Diaphram (DY-uh-fram)

Prime mover of inspiration; compresses abdominal viscera to aid in such processes as defecation, urination, and childbirth

External intercostals (IN-tur-COSS-tulz)

When scalenes fix rib 1, external intercostals draw ribs 2–12 upward and outward to expand thoracic cavity and inflate lungs.

Internal intercostals

When quadratus lumborum and other muscles fix rib 12, internal intercostals draw ribs downward and inward to compress thoracic cavity and force air from lungs; not needed for relaxed expiration.

Table 8.3	*Muscles of the Abdomen*

Rectus abdominis (ab-DOM-ih-niss)

Supports the organs of the abdomen, allows the waist to flex; depresses ribs; gives stabilization to the pelvis during leg movement such as walking; increases internal abdominal compression for urination, defecation, and childbirth

External abdominal oblique

Flexes waist as in sit-ups; flexes and rotates vertebral column

Internal abdominal oblique

Movement similar to the external oblique

Transversus abdominus

Compresses abdomen, allows flexion of the vertebral column

to the arms and legs. Many of the muscles that give strength to the back of the upper torso are near the surface of the skin (figure 8.9). See table 8.3.

A deep layer of muscles— some of which are interwoven with the ribs and others linked to the spinal column—provides flexibility and added stability to the back. The muscles of the torso work together in groups, contracting and relaxing to support and move the torso (figure 8.10). See table 8.4.

These muscles also help maintain posture and aid the spinal muscles when bending and twisting, and in a wide range of other movements (such as breathing, coughing, sneezing, and laughing).

Muscles of the Arm

The arm has a wide range of movements; it can swing backward and forward in walking and running, and it can be folded across the chest or raised above the head (figure 8.11). The shoulder forms a base for the arm with most of the upper arm muscles originating from this area (figure 8.12). In the upper arm, the biceps and triceps are arranged to give the forearm power to thrust and bend. The two muscles join at the elbow and allow you to bend and straighten your arm and rotate your wrist and hand. The forearm muscles transmit strength to the wrist, hands, and fingers. A group of flexors and extensors controls the movements of the wrist, acting in conjunction with other muscles of the fingers, thumb, radius, and ulna (figure 8.13). These sets of muscles allow the arm and wrist to bend (flexion) and straighten (extension) as well as move outward away from the body (abduction) and inward toward the body (adduction). Some of these muscles participate in more than one type of movement. The brachioradialis muscle is known as the "handshake" muscle.

Muscles of the Hip and Femur

Included in the muscles associated with the lower limbs are the muscles located in the hips, thigh, legs, and feet. Most of the hip muscles originate at the coax and insert onto the femur (figure 8.14). See table 8.5.

These muscles flex the hip and tense the gluteal muscles and tensor fascia latae to stabilize movement of the femur on the tibia when you are standing. The gluteus maximus (buttock) extends the hip and abducts and laterally rotates the thigh. The gluteus medias abducts and medially rotates the thigh (figure 8.15).

Some of the hip muscles also attach to the coxa and cause the movement of the thigh. They are part of three groups of thigh muscles: the anterior thigh muscles, which flex the hips; the posterior thigh muscles, which extend the hips; and the medial thigh muscles, which adduct the thigh.

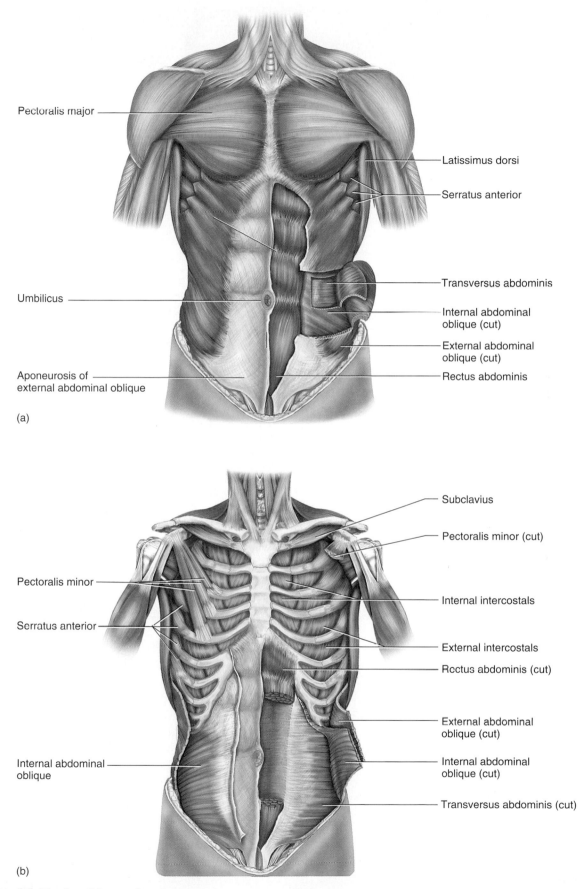

Pectoralis major

Latissimus dorsi

Serratus anterior

Transversus abdominis

Umbilicus

Internal abdominal oblique (cut)

External abdominal oblique (cut)

Aponeurosis of external abdominal oblique

Rectus abdominis

(a)

Subclavius

Pectoralis minor (cut)

Pectoralis minor

Internal intercostals

Serratus anterior

External intercostals

Rectus abdominis (cut)

External abdominal oblique (cut)

Internal abdominal oblique

Internal abdominal oblique (cut)

Transversus abdominis (cut)

(b)

Figure 8.9 Muscles of the trunk

Figure 8.10 Muscles acting on the vertebral column

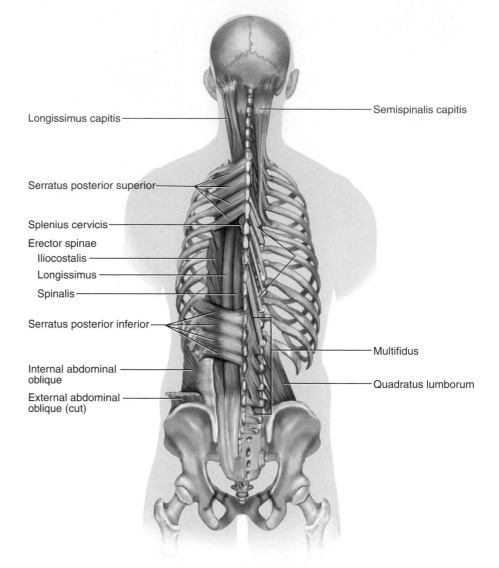

Longissimus capitis

Semispinalis capitis

Serratus posterior superior

Splenius cervicis

Erector spinae
  Iliocostalis
  Longissimus
  Spinalis

Serratus posterior inferior

Multifidus

Internal abdominal oblique

Quadratus lumborum

External abdominal oblique (cut)

Table 8.4	*Muscles of the Back*

Superficial Group—Erector Spinae (ee-RECK-tur SPY-nee)

Iliocostalis cervicis (ILL-ee-oh-coss-TAH-liss SIR-vih-sis), **iliocostalis thoracis** (tho-RA-sis), **and iliocostalis lumborum** (lum-BORE-um)
Extend and laterally flex vertebral column; thoracis and lumborum muscles rotate ribs during inspiration of air.

Longissimus (lawn-JISS-ih-muss) **cervicis and longissimus thoracis**
Extend and laterally flex the vertebral column

Spinalis (spy-NAY-liss) **cervicis and spinalis thoracis**
Extend vertebral column

Superficial Group—Serratus Posterior Muscles

Serratus (she-RAY-tus) **posterior superior**
Elevates ribs 2–5 during inspiration

Serratus posterior inferior
Depresses ribs 9–12 during inspiration

Table 8.4	*Muscles of the Back (Continued)*

Deep Group

Simispinalis cervicis (SEM-ee-spy-NAY-liss SUR-vih-sis) **and semispinalis thoracis** (tho-RA-sis)
Extend neck; extend and rotate the vertebral column

Quadratus lumborum (quad-RAY-tus lum-BORE-um)
Laterally flexes vertebral column; depresses rib 12

Multifidus (mul-TIFF-ih-dus)
Extends and rotates vertebral column

The pelvis is a circle of bone that is held in place by muscles. The muscles of the pelvic floor open and close the openings of the anus, urinary tract, and the reproductive tract. Several of these muscles help regulate urination and defecation. Pelvic floor muscles also contribute greatly to the birthing process in females.

Muscles of the Legs

The muscles and joints of the legs provide strength and stability for the body. The muscles serve to transmit the weight of the body and provide power for such common activities as walking, running, jumping, and lifting. Leg muscles absorb the impact of those activities (figure 8.16). The leg bones are girded on all sides by sets of powerful muscles that allow the legs to bend (flexion) and straighten (extension) as well as move outward from the body (abduction) and inward (adduction) (figure 8.17). Some of these muscles are relatively long and participate in more than one type of movement (figure 8.18).

The posterior thigh muscles, commonly known as the hamstring muscles, are responsible for the flexing of the knee and are a common site for athletic injuries. The anterior thigh muscles are the quadriceps femoris and the sartorius. The quadriceps femoris are the primary extensors of the knee. They are four muscles that have a common insertion point, which is the patellar tendon.

EXAM POINT   The sartorius muscle is the longest muscle in the body.

It flexes the hip and allows for the rotation of the thigh laterally when we sit cross-legged.

The gastrocnemius muscle and the soleus form the calf in the posterior portion of the lower leg. They join to form the calcaneal tendon, commonly known as the Achilles tendon. The 13 muscles of the legs are divided into three groups: anterior, lateral, and posterior. Refer to figure 8.19 for an illustration of these muscles.

Muscles of the Feet

The feet and toes (figure 8.20) are essential elements in body movement. They bear and propel the weight of the body during walking and help to maintain balance during changes in the body's position. See Procedure 8.1 for palpation exercises. The foot can adapt itself to different surfaces and absorb biomechanical shocks. Each foot has about 33 muscles, some of which are attached to the lower leg. There are four plantar (sole of the foot) muscle layers. The first layer includes the adductor hallucis, the flexor digitorum brevis, and the abductor digiti minimi. The second layer consists of the lumbricals, and the third layer includes the flexor hallucis brevis, the adductor hallucis, and the flexor digiti minimi brevis. The fourth layer is composed of the interossei muscles.

Figure 8.11 Muscles of the forearm
(a) Anterior view;
(b) posterior view.

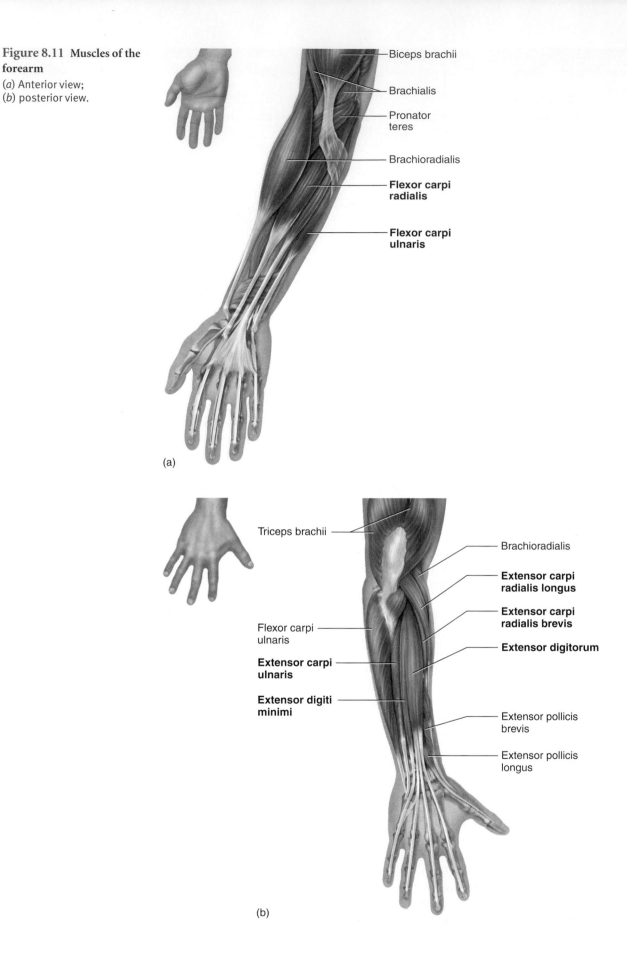

Biceps brachii

Brachialis

Pronator teres

Brachioradialis

Flexor carpi radialis

Flexor carpi ulnaris

(a)

Triceps brachii

Brachioradialis

Extensor carpi radialis longus

Extensor carpi radialis brevis

Flexor carpi ulnaris

Extensor carpi ulnaris

Extensor digiti minimi

Extensor digitorum

Extensor pollicis brevis

Extensor pollicis longus

(b)

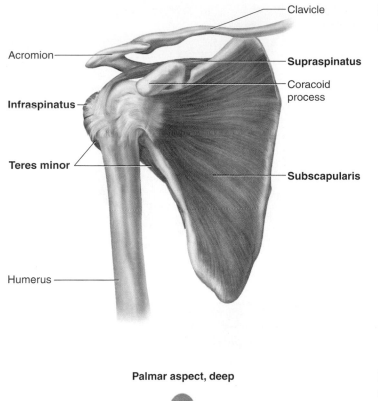

Figure 8.12 Muscles of the rotator cuff

Clavicle

Acromion

Supraspinatus

Coracoid process

Infraspinatus

Teres minor

Subscapularis

Humerus

Palmar aspect, deep

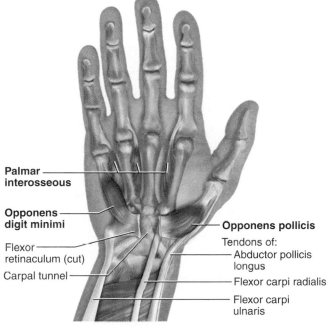

Figure 8.13 Deep palmar aspect

Palmar interosseous

Opponens digit minimi

Opponens pollicis

Flexor retinaculum (cut)

Tendons of:
Abductor pollicis longus

Carpal tunnel

Flexor carpi radialis

Flexor carpi ulnaris

Figure 8.14 Hip joint, anterior view

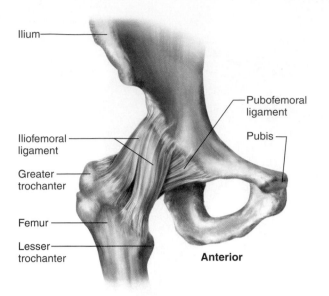

Ilium

Pubofemoral ligament

Iliofemoral ligament

Pubis

Greater trochanter

Femur

Lesser trochanter

Anterior

Table 8.5	*Muscles Acting on the Hip and Femur*

Anterior Muscles of the Hip (Iliopsoas)

Iliacus (ih-LY-uh-cus)
Flexes hip joint; medially rotates femur

Psoas (SO-ass) **major**
Flexes hip joint; medially rotates femur

Lateral and Posterior Muscles of the Hip

Tensor fasciae latae (TEN-sor FASH-ee-ee LAY-tee)
Flexes hip joint; abducts and medially rotates femur; tenses fascia lata and braces knee when opposite foot is lifted from the ground

Gluteus maximus
Extends hip joint; abducts and laterally rotates femur; important in the backswing of the stride

Gluteus medius and gluteus minimus
Abduct and medially rotate the femur; maintain balance by shifting body weight during walking

Lateral Rotators

Gemellus (jeh-MEL-us) **superior and gemellus inferior**
Laterally rotate femur

Obturator (OB-too-RAY-tur) **externus**
Laterally rotates the femur

Obturator internus
Abducts and laterally rotates femur

Piriformis (PIR-ih-FOR-miss)
Abducts and laterally rotates femur

Quadratus femoris (quad-RAY-tus FEM-oh-riss)
Adducts and laterally rotates femur

Medial (Adductor) Compartment of the Thigh

Adductor longus and adductor brevis
Adduct and laterally rotate the femur; flex hip joints

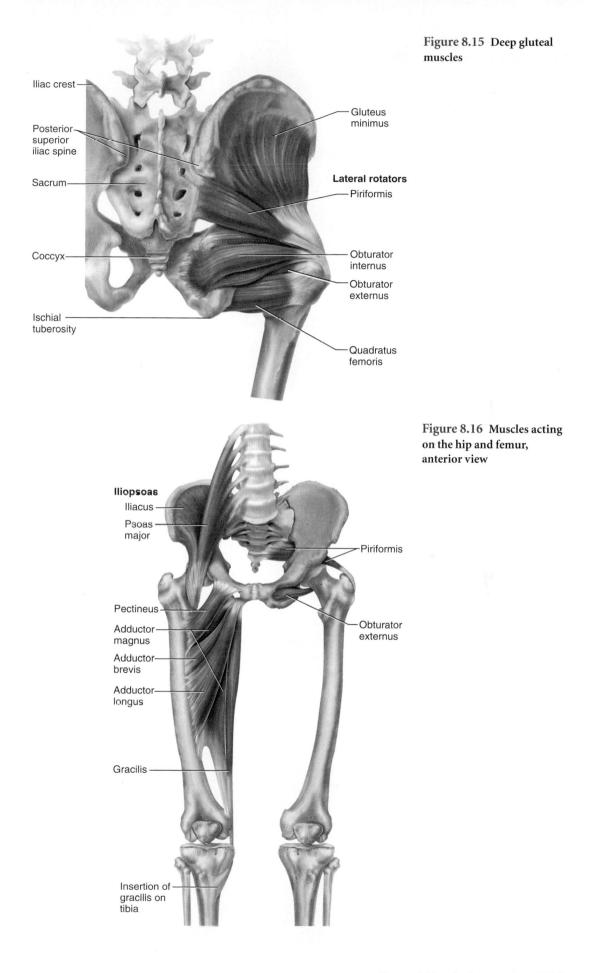

Figure 8.15 Deep gluteal muscles

Iliac crest

Posterior superior iliac spine

Sacrum

Coccyx

Ischial tuberosity

Gluteus minimus

Lateral rotators

Piriformis

Obturator internus

Obturator externus

Quadratus femoris

Figure 8.16 Muscles acting on the hip and femur, anterior view

Iliopsoas

Iliacus

Psoas major

Pectineus

Adductor magnus

Adductor brevis

Adductor longus

Gracilis

Insertion of gracilis on tibia

Piriformis

Obturator externus

Figure 8.17 Gluteal and thigh muscles, posterior view

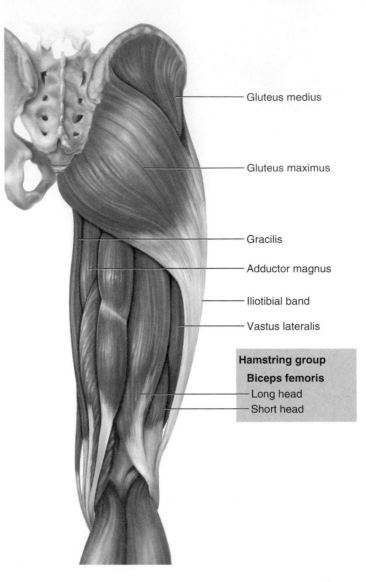

Gluteus medius

Gluteus maximus

Gracilis

Adductor magnus

Iliotibial band

Vastus lateralis

Hamstring group

Biceps femoris

Long head

Short head

Common Pathologies of the Muscular System

The muscular system contributes in a number of ways to help maintain optimal performance of the body. Not only do muscles allow movement, but they also create strength in the limbs and add stability to the spine. They generate between 20% to 25% more energy than needed to perform movement; the excess energy converts to heat to help release toxins, speed up and deepen breaths to reoxygenate tissue, and stabilize metabolism. Injury and disease processes can greatly affect movement, spine stability, and heat production and release.

The body's skeletal muscles cannot function without stimulation by nerves. When nerves are damaged, then the muscle associated with that nerve cannot perform effectively and may atrophy or fatigue. Atrophy and fatigue can also be caused by injury or disease processes. Another cause of muscle disease can be from the motor-neuron response from the improper transmission of contraction impulses or from the brain being unable to decipher the neural codes.

Listed here are a few of the common diseases, conditions, and injuries of the muscular system:

- *Muscular dystrophy:* the most common debilitating disease; muscles show weakness and delayed motor response. This disease can affect all of the skeletal muscles of the body.

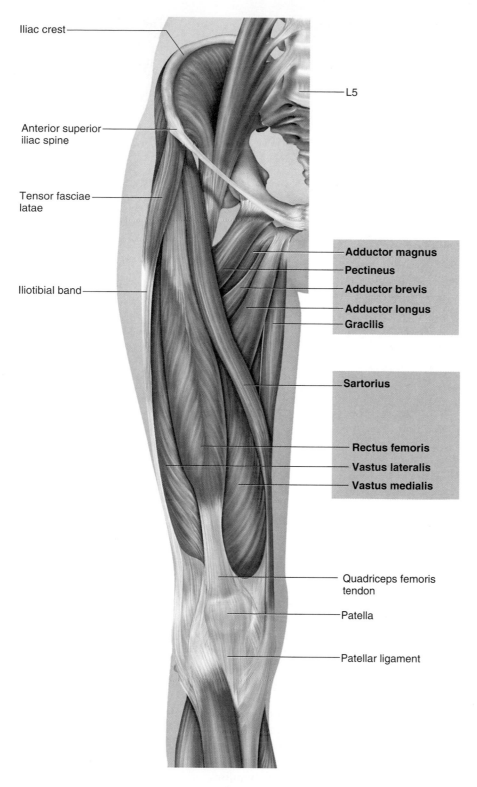

Iliac crest

Anterior superior
iliac spine

Tensor fasciae
latae

Iliotibial band

L5

Adductor magnus
Pectineus
Adductor brevis
Adductor longus
Gracilis

Sartorius

Rectus femoris
Vastus lateralis
Vastus medialis

Quadriceps femoris
tendon

Patella

Patellar ligament

**Figure 8.18 Muscles of the
thigh, anterior view**

- *Myasthenia gravis:* an autoimmune disease that causes the body to attack its own myoneural junctions. A resulting condition caused by the failure in transmission of the contraction impulse from the nerves to the muscles leads to muscle weakness and a lack of control of muscles. The disease affects women more often than men.
- *Rhabdomyosarcoma:* a malignant tumor that can occur in skeletal muscle. This tumor requires surgical removal. After removal, the surrounding muscle may have dysfunction due to scar tissue and surgical nerve damage.

Figure 8.19 Muscles of the leg

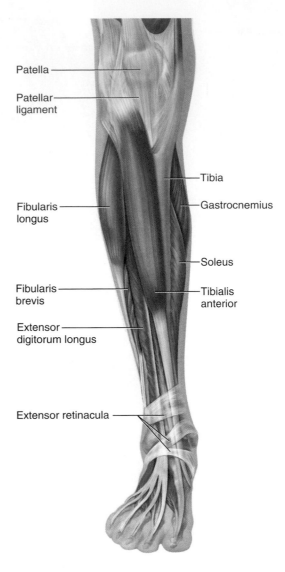

Patella
Patellar ligament
Fibularis longus
Fibularis brevis
Extensor digitorum longus
Extensor retinacula
Tibia
Gastrocnemius
Soleus
Tibialis anterior

- *Osteomalacia:* a condition that can result in muscular weakness and atrophy, and affects the entire skeletal muscle system.
- *Muscular rheumatism:* a very painful form of fribrositis that affects the connective tissue associated with the joints and muscles
- *Multiple sclerosis:* a disease marked by hardened tissue in the brain and spinal cord, which leads to jerky, uncontrolled movement
- *Myalgia:* muscle pain
- *Myositis:* an inflammation of the muscular tissue
- *Parkinson's disease:* a chronic, progressive nerve disease that is linked to decreased dopamine production and results in tremor and weakness of resting muscles and a shuffling gait
- *Tendinitis:* an inflammation of a tendon
- *Contracture:* a condition in which a muscle shortens its length in the resting state; usually happens to bedridden or wheelchair-bound persons
- *Cramps:* spastic and painful contractions of muscles that occur because of an irritation within the muscle such as inflammation of connective tissue or lactic acid buildup
- *Tetanus:* a bacterial infection that makes motor neurons hypersensitive to stimulus. The associated disease is commonly known as lockjaw because the

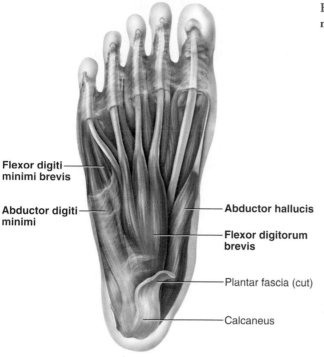

Figure 8.20 The first layer of muscles of the foot

Flexor digiti minimi brevis

Abductor digiti minimi

Abductor hallucis

Flexor digitorum brevis

Plantar fascia (cut)

Calcaneus

P R O C E D U R E 8.1 Palpation Exercises

1. Have your partner lie prone on a massage table. Palpate the medial longitudinal arch of both feet. Are the arches the same height and length in each foot? Which muscle of the leg helps support the medial longitudinal arch of the foot?

2. Inspect and palpate the posterior leg muscles. What are the major actions of the muscles of the posterior compartment of the leg?

3. Movement exercises:
   a. Elevate the shoulders together, then separately.
   b. Flex both arms separately.
   c. Deviate the wrist in the ulnar direction, then deviate it in the radial direction.
   d. Oppose the thumb and the little finger, then each finger in turn.

4. Have your partner sit in a chair facing you. Inspect and palpate the lateral supracondylar ridge and lateral epicondyle of the humerus. What are the three major actions of the muscles that originate from this area?

---

muscles of the jaw eventually clench. Tetanus has a high rate of death but can be easily avoided by having a tetanus immunization.

- *Botulism:* a bacterial form of food poisoning that can cause the paralysis of the muscles involved in respiration and lead to death
- *Fibromyalgia:* a common medical condition characterized by pain and tenderness in the soft tissues of the body (see chapter 21). Recent studies suggest that this is not a muscular condition but a central nervous system pain perception syndrome.
- *Muscle tears:* occur when a muscle is stretched suddenly, too much, or without proper warmup. Scar tissue can form if the tear is inadequately healed, resulting in pain and a decrease of muscle performance.
- *Hernia:* a condition that occurs when one of the three layers of muscle lining the abdomen weaken from pressure from lifting, trapping intestines and organs inside

the weaker area, usually in the groin or the umbilicus section, and cutting off blood and fluid flow.

- *Uterine prolapse:* occurs when the perineal muscles are weakened so that the pelvic organs may descend or protrude outside of the body, such as the uterus descending into the vaginal canal
- *Rotator cuff injury:* a condition usually occurring in athletes or persons who use repetitive motions and resulting in the tearing or inflammation of the muscles and tendons that surround the head of the humerus
- *Hip sprain:* occurs when the anterior iliofemoral ligament causes flexor spasm of the hip
- *Fasciculation:* an involuntary twitch of the muscles of a motor unit, usually of short duration
- *Fibrillation:* an abnormal contraction in which individual muscle fibers contract in an unsynchronized pattern, such as when the heart muscles fibrillate when the electrical impulses that regulate heart rhythm are stopped during a heart attack

Think About It

Rigor mortis occurs a few hours after death when the calcium from the sarcoplasmic reticulum leaks into the sarcoplasm and causes actin-myosin interaction. Forensic scientists use the amount of rigor and the temperature of the liver to establish the time of death if decomposition has not yet occurred.

Chapter Summary

Since all of our body's movement is the result of muscle and muscle-bone-joint interaction, it is easy to see how important an optimally functioning muscular system is to our lives. When this system becomes diseased or debilitated from injury or lack of proper nutrition and exercise, we experience pain and loss of movement. Massage therapists and bodyworkers play a key role in helping their clients to maintain the health and performance of this system. The greater your knowledge of the anatomy, physiology, and pathophysiology of the muscular system (and the response of muscles to the strokes and methods of massage therapy), the better you will be in helping your clients achieve the highest level of physical performance and well-being.

Applying Your Knowledge

Self-Testing

1. Myofilaments are arranged in compartments called:
   a) Myofibrils
   b) Agonists
   c) Visceral
   d) Sarcomeres

2. What is the *longest* muscle in the body?
   a) Latissimus dorsi
   b) Quadriceps
   c) Sartorius
   d) IT band

3. What muscle is the "*handshake*" muscle?
   a) Brachioradialis
   b) Brachioulnarius
   c) Brachialis
   d) Biceps brachii

4. What is another name for the prime mover muscle?
   a) Agonist
   b) Protagonist
   c) Synergist
   d) Antagonist

5. Which are the three gluteal muscles?
   a) Minimus, medialis, lateralis
   b) Minimus, maximus, intermedius

c) Minimus, mediumis, intermedius

d) Minimus, medius, maximus

6. What is the site where muscle attaches to the stationary bone?

a) Origin

b) Insertion

c) Attaching point

d) Insertion point

7. Which is the *correct* listing of contractions?

a) Tonic, isotetanic, titanic

b) Tonic, isotonic, twitch

c) Tonic, metric, tetric

d) Titanic, isotitanic, metrotanic

8. What two movements does the piriformis perform?

a) Abduction and lateral rotation

b) Adduction and medial rotation

c) Flexion of the hip

d) Extension of the hip

9. What are the three erector spinae muscles?

a) QLs, lats, traps

b) Iliocostalis, latissimus, scalenes

c) Supraspinous, infraspinous, erectoralis

d) Ilicostalis, longissimus, spinalis

10. What are the most *superficial* muscles in the back?

a) Trapezius

b) Latissimus dorsi

c) Psoas

d) Erector spinae

11. Which muscle opposes the agonist?

a) Prime mover

b) Synergist

c) Fixator

d) Antagonist

12. What are the three functions of the muscular system?

a) Movement, posture, homeostasis

b) Movement, protection, hemopoisis

c) Movement, posture, heat production

d) None of the above is correct.

13. Which muscle assists the agonist?

a) Synergist

b) Antagonist

c) Protagonist

d) Androgenist

14. What is the point where a muscle attaches to the movable bone?

a) Origin

b) Insertion

c) Lever point

d) Point of attachment

15. Which muscle is the *best* trunk flexor?

a) Rectus abdominus

b) Rectus femoris

c) Rectus flexorus

d) None of the above is correct.

16. What is the *strongest* hip flexor?

a) Rectus abdominus

b) Rectus femorus

c) Bicep femoris

d) Iliopsoas

17. Which grouping contains muscles with multiple attachments?

a) Quadriceps

b) Hamstrings

c) Bicep brachii, bicep femoris, triceps

d) None of the above is correct.

18. What is the definition of *mastication*?

a) Swallowing

b) Chewing

c) Sneezing

d) Blinking

19. Which muscle initiates ambulation?

a) Iliopsoas

b) Quadriceps

c) Hamstrings

d) None of the above is correct.

20. What is the definition of *deglutition*?

a) Swallowing

b) Chewing

c) Urination

d) Defecation

21. What muscle is the prime mover of respiration?

a) Diaphragm

b) Rectus abdominus

c) Intercostals

d) Serratus anterior

22. APT (Adenosine Triphosphate) is the main souce of energy for which types of muscle contractions?

a) All muscles contractions

b) Muscle of Mastication

c) Muscles of the thorax

d) Isometric and Tonic only

23. Adduction is what kind of movement?

a) Lateral

b) Toward the midsaggital plane

c) Toward the superior

d) Toward the distal

24. Anterior muscles usually perform what action?
    a) Extension and supination
    b) Flexion and pronation
    c) Extension and pronation
    d) Flexion and supination

25. Which muscle depresses the ribs?
    a) External intercostals
    b) Serratus anterior
    c) Serratus posterior
    d) Pectoralis major

26. Which two muscles rotate the trunk to the right?
    a) Right external oblique and left internal oblique
    b) Left external oblique and right internal oblique
    c) Rectus abdominus and iliopsoas
    d) Psoas and iliacus

27. What is the name of a malignant tumor that can occur in skeletal muscle?
    a) Tendinitis
    b) Myasthenia Gravis
    c) Multiple Sclerosis
    d) Rhabdomyosarcoma

28. When turning the door handle to the right with the right hand, what action does the wrist perform?
    a) Supination
    b) Pronation
    c) Rotation
    d) Retraction

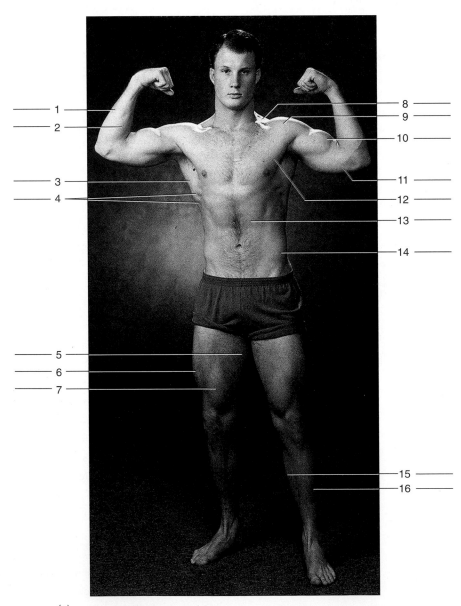

(a)

29. What are muscles named by?
    a) Term and meaning
    b) Location or characteristics of movement
    c) Length and strength
    d) Size and strength

30. Label each of the 30 muscles on the figures using the list of muscles below. Some of these names will be used more than once, since the same muscle may be shown from different perspectives, and some of these names will not be used at all.

a. biceps brachii
b. brachioradialis
c. deltoid
d. erector spinae
e. external abdominal oblique
f. flexor carpi ulnaris
g. gastrocnemius
h. gracilis
i. hamstrings
j. infraspinatus
k. latissimus dorsi
l. pectineus
m. pectoralis major
n. rectus abdominis
o. rectus femoris
p. serratus anterior
q. soleus
r. splenius capitis
s. sternocleidomastoid
t. subscapularis
u. teres major
v. tibialis anterior
w. tranversus abdominis
x. trapezius
y. triceps brachii
z. vastus lateralis

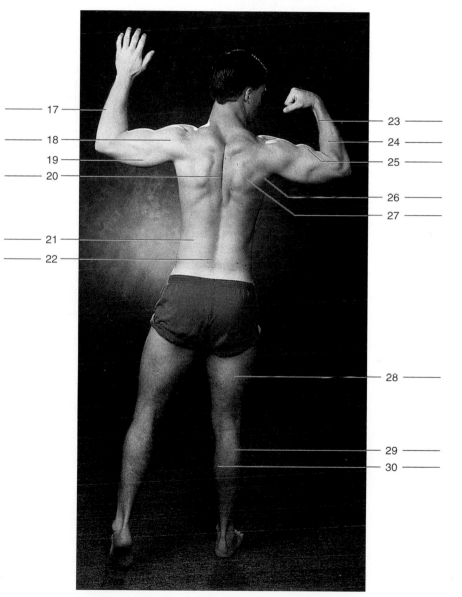

(b)

Case Studies / Critical Thinking

A. Jim Jackson has been a marathon runner for three years. Over the last few months, he has been feeling pain and burning on the bottoms of his feet. The pain has worsened to the point that he has lower leg cramps and begins limping after he runs a short distance or walks up and down stairs at his office. His doctor has referred him to Debby, a massage therapist who works primarily with athletes. Upon palpation of the feet, Debby is told by Jackson that the bottoms of his feet feel bruised, and he has sharp pains usually at the deep arch, heel area, and sometimes even along the length of the foot. His doctor has diagnosed plantar fasciitis. Does Jackson have symptoms of this condition? Is massage indicated? Will massage of the deep calf muscles release tension that can put a strain on the plantar fascia?

B. Hugo Gonzales has been to Kenya's clinic for a massage three times. It is his fourth visit, and she notices that when he lies on his left side, with his right arm above his head, he complains of tingling and loss of sensation in his right arm. He tells her that he often wakes at night with his arm "asleep" and unable to move for several minutes. Kenya recently attended a seminar for Continuing Education credits that discussed thoracic outlet syndrome (TOS). In the seminar, it was explained that TOS is neurovascular entrapment, a condition in which the nerves of the brachial plexus or the blood vessels running to or from the arm are impinged at the thoracic outlet (the area behind the clavicle between the insertions of the trapezius and the sternocleidomastoid). Kenya knows that many conditions may cause pain, muscle weakness, and tingling in that area. Should she continue the massage? Should she stop the massage and refer Gonzales for tests to diagnosis the problem? Which type of health care provider would be effective in determining the cause?

C. A new client has arrived for his appointment with Lisa Liu, a massage therapist who owns the China Lotus Day Spa. He filled out a questionnaire about his health before the massage, and when Lisa checked his answers, she saw nothing that would contraindicate a Swedish massage. However, while holding a drape for him to turn over, he winced and pointed to a large "lump" bulging at the right inguinal area. She stopped the massage and asked if he was aware that he might have a hernia. The client told her that he was scheduled for out-patient surgery the next week. Should she continue the session but avoid the area of the protrusion? What muscles may be involved in relationship to the hernia? How long after surgery should she wait to massage the area? Is massage indicated over a healed inguinal hernia or any healed herniated muscle?

References for information in this chapter can be found in Quick Guide C at the end of the book.

CHAPTER 9

Other Body Systems

LEARNING OUTCOMES

After completing this chapter, you will be able to:

- Understand the purpose and function of each system of organs within the body.

- Describe the mechanisms of breathing, digestion, blood transportation, and disease defense mechanisms.

- List common diseases of each system.

- Apply appropriate terminology to major organs and systems of the human body.

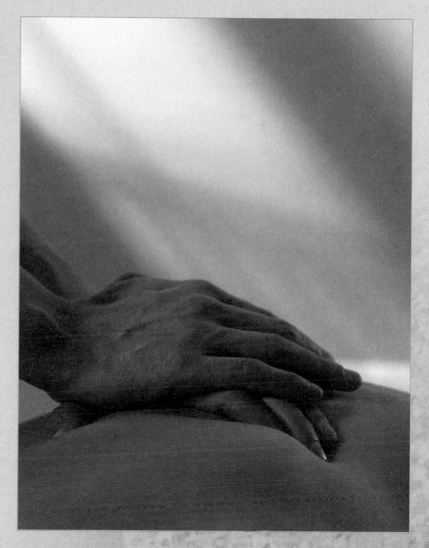

KEY TERMS

arrector pili *(p. 254)*
artery *(p. 224)*
atrium, (plural, atria) *(p. 227)*
autonomic nervous system
   (ANS) *(p. 232)*
blood pressure *(p. 230)*
capillaries *(p. 224)*
central nervous system
   (CNS) *(p. 232)*
contact dermatitis *(p. 244)*

deglutition *(p. 245)*
endocardium *(p. 227)*
epicardium *(p. 227)*
erythrocytes (red blood cells,
   RBCs) *(p. 225)*
leukocytes (white blood cells,
   WBCs) *(p. 225)*
mastication *(p. 245)*
myocardium *(p. 227)*
pericardium *(p. 227)*

peripheral nervous system (PNS)
   (p. 232)
pituitary gland *(p. 237)*
referred pain *(p. 260)*
respiration *(p. 249)*
rugae *(p. 246)*
sphygmomanometer *(p. 230)*
veins *(p. 224)*
ventricle *(p. 227)*

INTRODUCTION

Chapter 9 is devoted to the study of the organ systems that make up the body, how they function, as well as their common disease processes. The anatomy and physiology of each system are defined and explained, as well as how these systems function together to provide homeostasis to the body as a whole. Chapter 5 will help you to understand the role massage plays regarding these systems and the contribution you can make to your client's health and well-being.

Cardiovascular System ★

EXAM POINT The cardiovascular system is commonly called the circulatory system and is comprised of the heart, blood vessels, and blood.

For your body to stay alive, each of its cells must receive a continuous supply of nutrients, such as food, water, and oxygen. At the same time, carbon dioxide and other materials produced by the cells must be picked up for removal from the body. This is a passive process called diffusion, which is extremely important to our health and well-being. When the blood reaches the tissue, nutrients move from inside the blood vessels into the interstitial fluid by diffusion. The opposite also occurs by diffusion. Waste products from the cell move into the blood. Similarly, carbon dioxide and oxygen move by diffusion between the air and blood. The rate of diffusion depends on the distance that separates the two solutions involved.

The circulatory system (figure 9.1) is a network of vessels that enables the heart to pump blood through your body. Blood vessels are small tubes that are responsible for carrying blood to and from all parts of your body. The human circulatory system is composed of three types of blood vessels: arteries, veins, and capillaries. An **artery** (figure 9.2) is a large blood vessel that carries blood away from the heart to the cells and tissues of the body.

★ **EXAM POINT** The **veins** are vessels that carry blood and waste products toward the heart.

Veins have one-way valves. **Capillaries** are microscopic in size. They link the arteries and veins to the tissues of the body. The exchange of oxygen and carbon dioxide takes place across the thin walls of the capillaries.

Arteries transport blood under high pressure and, therefore, have walls that are much more elastic and thicker than those of veins (figure 9.3). The blood flow in the ar-

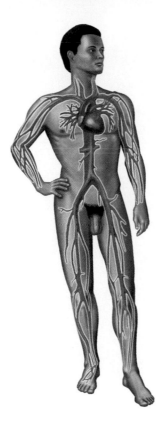

Figure 9.1 Circulatory system
Principal organs: Heart, blood vessels.

tery pulsates. It constantly increases and decreases as a result of the heart pumping a new volume of blood into the arteries 70 times per minute. The effect is what causes the pulse you can feel by placing your fingertips over the arteries in your wrist and neck.

Blood supplies oxygen and transports nutrients, waste, and hormonal messengers to each of the 60 billion cells in your body (figure 9.4). Blood has four main components: red blood cells, white blood cells, platelets, and liquid plasma. **Erythrocytes (red blood cells, RBCs)** carry 99% of the oxygen the body needs. Plasma carries the other 1%. Erythrocytes are the most abundant cells in the body, constituting about 45% of the blood. Their main function is to carry oxygen to the tissue and remove carbon dioxide waste. Erythrocytes contain hemoglobin, a protein that binds with the oxygen for transport. Hemoglobin, which is mainly composed of iron, gives the blood its red color. **Leukocytes (white blood cells, WBCs)** are a part of your body's immune system. Their main function is to provide a defense against infectious agents (figure 9.5).

Platelets are tiny specialized cell fragments that are activated whenever blood clotting or repair to a vessel is necessary. When a blood vessel is cut, platelets rush to the vessel and swell into odd, irregular shapes, grow sticky and clog at the cut, creating a plug. If the cut is too large for the platelets, they send out signals to initiate clotting by releasing a hormone called serotonin, which stimulates blood vessels to contract, thus reducing the flow of blood. Blood plasma, which is the clear liquid portion of the blood in which the cells and platelets are suspended, transforms into insoluble, threadlike strands of protein that mesh around the blood cells, forming a solid clot and creating a scaffold on which the body can build new tissue. Other functions of plasma include transporting nutrients, gases, and vitamins; helping to regulate fluid and electrolyte balance; and maintaining a balanced pH. Albumin, globulin, and fibrinogen are proteins found in plasma. Fibrinogen is the largest of the proteins found in plasma and functions in the coagulation of blood.

Throughout your body, thousands of miles of blood vessels run to every living organ and tissue. The functioning of your body depends on a constant supply of blood and its components.

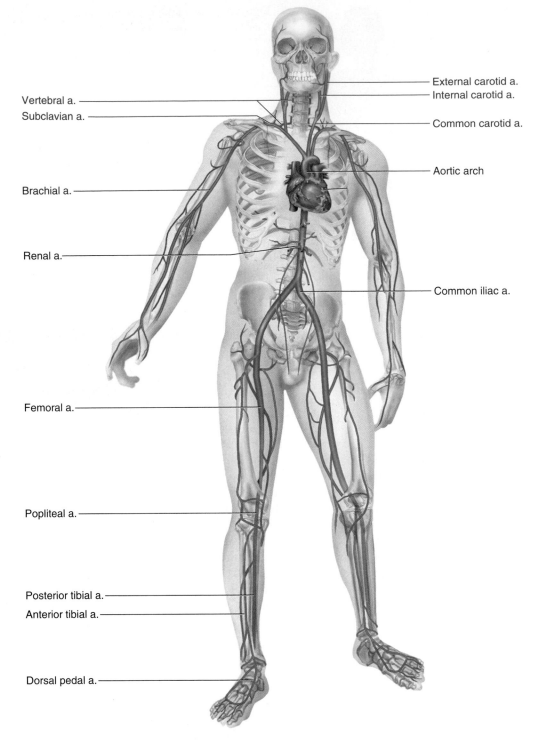

Vertebral a.

Subclavian a.

Brachial a.

Renal a.

Femoral a.

Popliteal a.

Posterior tibial a.

Anterior tibial a.

Dorsal pedal a.

External carotid a.

Internal carotid a.

Common carotid a.

Aortic arch

Common iliac a.

Figure 9.2 Arteries of the human body

The Heart

The heart is a hollow, fist-shaped muscular organ placed between the lungs in the middle of the chest that pumps blood through the body, supplying cells with oxygen and nutrients. It is attached to the breastbone by special connective tissues called ligaments. The apex (blunt point of the lower edge of the heart) lies on the diaphragm, pointing toward the left (figure 9.6).

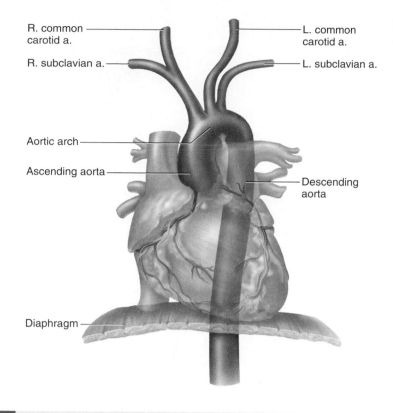

R. common carotid a.

L. common carotid a.

R. subclavian a.

L. subclavian a.

Aortic arch

Ascending aorta

Descending aorta

Diaphragm

Figure 9.3 **Arteries connecting to the heart**

EXAM POINT   Two-thirds of the heart is to the left of the midsternum and one-third to the right.

The apex pulses with every beat of the heart. This is the sensation you feel when you hold your hand against your chest (figure 9.7). The heart is surrounded by the **pericardium,** a sac of serous membrane, which secrets a lubricating fluid that prevents friction from the movement of the heart. The pericardium also maintains the location of the heart within the thoracic cavity.

The **myocardium** is the heart muscle that generates the contractions. The outer membrane of the heart is called the **epicardium** (figure 9.8). The **endocardium** is the smooth, thin inner lining of the heart. The blood actually slides along the endocardium as it flows through the heart.

The heart has four cavities, called chambers: a small upper cavity (**atrium;** one on each side) and a large lower cavity (**ventricle;** one on each side). The thick walls of the atria are separated by the interatrial septum. The ventricles are separated by the inter-ventricular septum, and the atria and ventricles are separated by a fibrous structure called the heart skeleton.

The heart has four sets of valves that open and close to regulate the flow of blood through the heart. Atrioventricular valves allow blood to flow into the ventricles but close to keep it from going into the atria (figure 9.9). Strings of connective tissue known as chordae tendineae cordis connect between the ventricle wall and the valves to help close the valve without letting it collapse into the atria. The bicuspid or mitral valve is located between the left atrium and the left ventricle; the tricuspid valve is located be-tween the right atrium and the right ventricle.

Semilunar valves control the blood flow out of the ventricles into the aorta and the pulmonary arteries, and prevent any back-flow of blood into the ventricles. The aortic valve is between the left ventricle and the aorta, and the pulmonary valve is between the pulmonary artery and the right ventricle. These valves open in response to pressure generated when the blood leaves the ventricle. They close when blood pools in small pockets of the cusps of the valves and pushes the valves closed.

Figure 9.4 The major veins

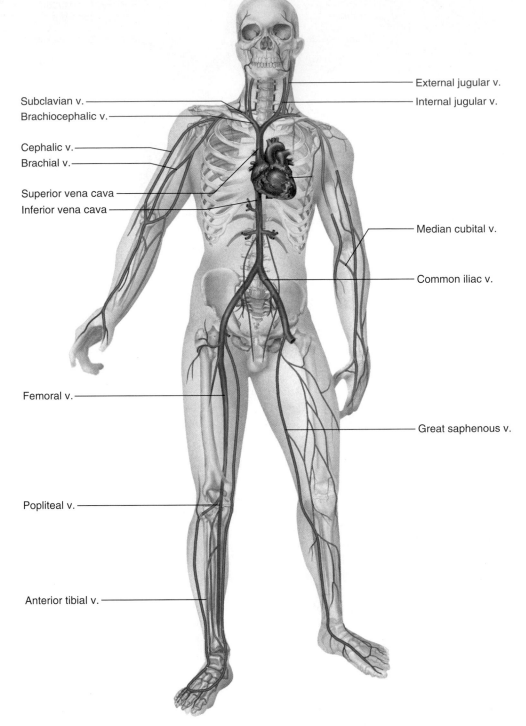

External jugular v.

Internal jugular v.

Subclavian v.

Brachiocephalic v.

Cephalic v.

Brachial v.

Superior vena cava

Inferior vena cava

Median cubital v.

Common iliac v.

Femoral v.

Great saphenous v.

Popliteal v.

Anterior tibial v.

The adult human heart is approximately the size of a fist. In an average adult, it is about 5 inches long and 3.5 inches across at its broadest part, and weighs less than a pound.

As blood travels through the body delivering oxygen and nutrients to the tissue, it also picks up carbon dioxide and other waste materials produced by the cells. This blood that is low in oxygen and rich in carbon dioxide enters the right atrium of the heart through the inferior and superior vena cavae. From the right atrium, the blood flows over the tricuspid valve into the right ventricle. When the right ventricle contracts, blood is forced over the pulmonary valve into a large artery called the pulmonary

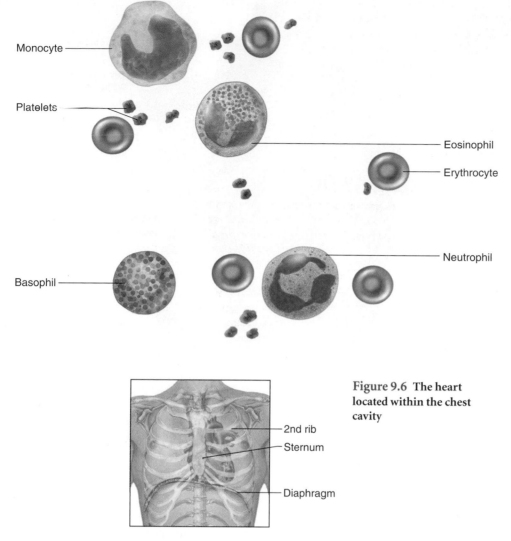

Figure 9.5 The elements of blood

Red blood cells, white blood cells, and platelets.

Monocyte

Platelets

Eosinophil

Erythrocyte

Neutrophil

Basophil

Figure 9.6 The heart located within the chest cavity

2nd rib

Sternum

Diaphragm

trunk. The pulmonary trunk branches into the pulmonary arteries, which carry blood to the lungs. In the lungs, blood picks up oxygen and gets rid of carbon dioxide. Blood rich in oxygen and low in carbon dioxide then returns to the heart through four veins called the pulmonary veins. The pulmonary veins empty the blood into the left atrium. From the left atrium, blood flows over the bicuspid valve, also called the mitral valve into the left ventricle. When the left ventricle contracts, blood is forced over the aortic valve and into the aorta. The aorta distributes blood into its branches and throughout the body. Veins of the body pick up the oxygen-poor blood and empty it into the vena cavae, and the whole process starts over. It is important to remember that arteries carry blood away from the heart and veins carry blood to the heart, and that the right side of the heart delivers blood to the lungs and the left side of the heart delivers blood to all of the other body parts.

Arteries of Importance to Massage Therapy

There are four main arteries of importance to a massage therapist: axillary artery, brachial artery, common carotid artery, and deep femoral artery.

The subclavian artery becomes the axillary artery and is located under the armpit. This artery continues to descend to the tendon of the teres major muscle and becomes the brachial artery. The artery then divides into three parts around the pectoralis minor muscle and brings oxygenated blood to the upper arm and chest area.

Figure 9.7 External anatomy of the heart

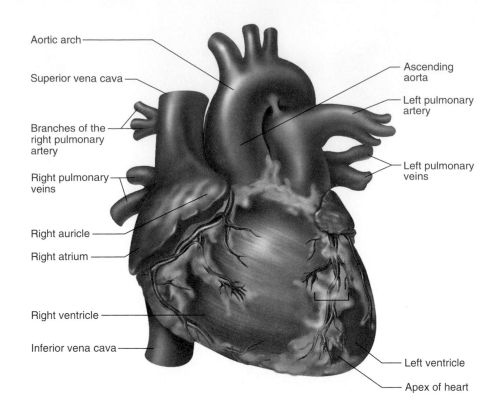

Aortic arch

Superior vena cava

Branches of the right pulmonary artery

Right pulmonary veins

Right auricle

Right atrium

Right ventricle

Inferior vena cava

Ascending aorta

Left pulmonary artery

Left pulmonary veins

Left ventricle

Apex of heart

The brachial artery extends toward the elbow joint and then branches into the radial and ulnar arteries. Your pulse can be felt at the bend of the elbow at the inner rim of the biceps muscle.

The common carotid artery provides oxygenated blood to the head and neck and is divided into left and right branches. These branches travel along the neck and into the head. The artery further branches and sends blood to the parts of the brain, sinuses, and eyes through the internal carotid. The pulse that is taken during cardiopulmonary resuscitation (CPR) is taken at the side of the neck on the carotid artery.

The deep femoral arteries are branches of the iliac arteries and continue down the front and inner part of the thighs, from the groin to the knee, where they become the popliteal arteries. The femoral arteries supply oxygenated blood to the larger part of the legs.

Blood Pressure, Pulse Rate, and Baroreceptors

The force of blood that is exerted against the walls of blood vessels is called **blood pressure**. This pressure is measured as highest in the arteries and lowest in the veins. When blood pressure is measured using a **sphygmomanometer** (commonly called a blood pressure cuff) and a stethoscope, it is the arterial blood pressure that is recorded. The arterial blood pressure is stronger when the heart ventricles contract and less strong when the ventricles relax. This greater pressure is called the systolic pressure. The lesser pressure, measured when the ventricles relax, is the diastolic pressure. This number is usually recorded as systolic over the diastolic. An example would be a systolic of 140 over the diastolic of 80, written as 140/80.

Normal blood pressure for an adult is considered as between 90 and 120 for a systolic reading, and 60 and 80 for a diastolic reading. Currently, readings of 120 to 139 as systolic and 80 to 89 diastolic are considered prehypertensive and bear watching. Blood pressure can be controlled by a number of factors, such as amount of liquid in the blood, strength of muscles in the heart, and certain medications. The amount of blood pumped from the heart is the major control factor.

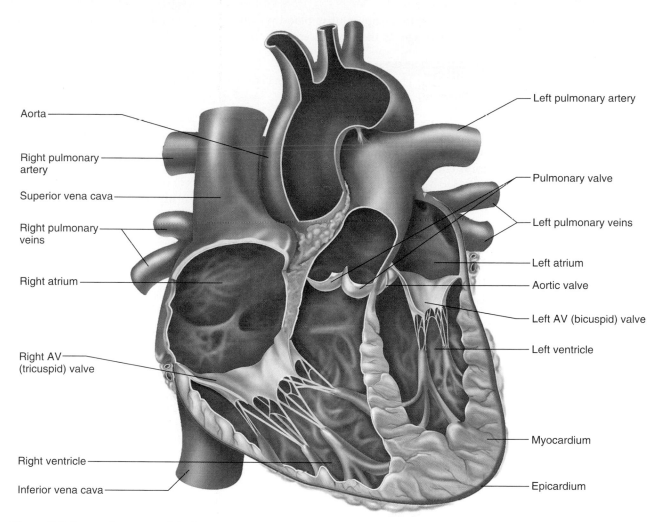

Figure 9.8 Internal anatomy of the heart

Aorta

Right pulmonary artery

Superior vena cava

Right pulmonary veins

Right atrium

Right AV (tricuspid) valve

Right ventricle

Inferior vena cava

Left pulmonary artery

Pulmonary valve

Left pulmonary veins

Left atrium

Aortic valve

Left AV (bicuspid) valve

Left ventricle

Myocardium

Epicardium

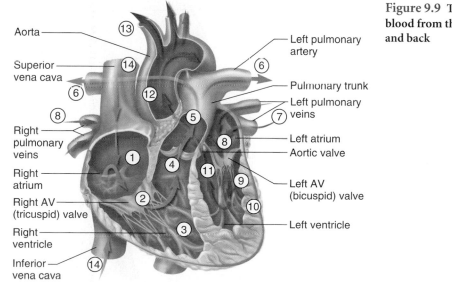

Figure 9.9 The pathway of blood from the right atrium and back

Aorta

Superior vena cava

Right pulmonary veins

Right atrium

Right AV (tricuspid) valve

Right ventricle

Inferior vena cava

Left pulmonary artery

Pulmonary trunk

Left pulmonary veins

Left atrium

Aortic valve

Left AV (bicuspid) valve

Left ventricle

Baroreceptors help regulate blood pressure by registering the blood pressure and sending messages to the cardiac center of the brain.

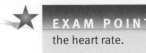 **EXAM POINT** The cardiac center in the medulla oblongata increases or decreases the heart rate.

Increasing heart rate will increase blood pressure, and decreasing heart rate will lower blood pressure. These baroreceptors are located in the aorta and the carotid arteries. The average adult heart rate should be between 60 and 100 beats. The heart rate is affected by the amount of activity in which the body is or has recently engaged. Therefore, a resting rate should always be lower than a rate during strenuous exercise.

Nervous System

The nervous system of the human anatomy is responsible for sending, receiving, and processing nerve impulses (figure 9.10). All of the body's muscles and organs rely on these nerve impulses to function. Three systems work together to carry out the mission of the nervous system: the central, the peripheral, and the autonomic nervous systems. The **central nervous system (CNS)** is responsible for issuing nerve impulses and analyzing sensory data, and includes the brain and spinal cord (figure 9.11). The **peripheral nervous system (PNS)** is responsible for carrying nerve impulses to and from the body's many structures, and includes the many craniospinal nerves that branch off the brain and spinal cord.

The **autonomic nervous system (ANS)** (figures 9.12 and 9.13) is a branch of the peripheral nervous system and is composed of the sympathetic and parasympathetic systems. These systems are responsible for regulating and coordinating the functions of vital structures in the body. Of all of the components of the nervous system, the brain

Figure 9.10 Nervous system
Principal organs: Brain, spinal cord, nerves, ganglia.

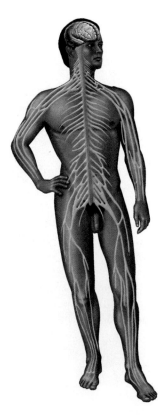

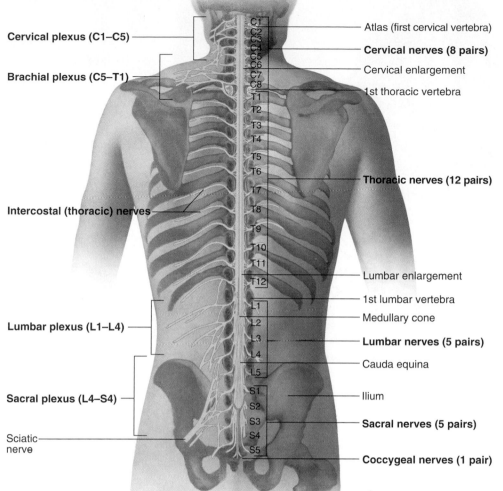

Figure 9.11 Spinal nerves, dorsal view

Cervical plexus (C1–C5)

Brachial plexus (C5–T1)

Intercostal (thoracic) nerves

Lumbar plexus (L1–L4)

Sacral plexus (L4–S4)

Sciatic nerve

Atlas (first cervical vertebra)

Cervical nerves (8 pairs)

Cervical enlargement

1st thoracic vertebra

Thoracic nerves (12 pairs)

Lumbar enlargement

1st lumbar vertebra

Medullary cone

Lumbar nerves (5 pairs)

Cauda equina

Ilium

Sacral nerves (5 pairs)

Coccygeal nerves (1 pair)

is the primary one, occupying the cranial cavity. Without its outermost protective membrane, the dura mater, the brain weighs an average of 3 pounds and comprises 92% of the entire nervous system. It is connected to the upper end of the spinal cord and is responsible for issuing nerve impulses, processing nerve impulse data, and engaging in higher-thought processes.

The spinal cord serves as a sort of telegraph cable that allows signals to be sent from the brain to the structures of the body and received from them in turn. The spinal cord is about a fourth of an inch in diameter and slightly flattened. It passes through the vertebral canal, created by the vertebral arches of the spinal column, and sends out roots and branches much like a tree. These structures contain bundles of nerve fibers that extend all the way down the body, innervating even the skin of the tips of the toes. A single nerve fiber consists of a chain of neurons. Neurons are the basic cells of the nervous system. They are responsible for receiving and transmitting nerve impulses, and forming long fibers by linking together. They consist of a cell body, which contains a nucleus, with one or more axons and dendrites extending from the body. The dendrites are the multibranched portions that receive impulses, while the axons are the elongated structures that carry impulses away from the body of the cell. Billions of neurons are located in the body's nervous system. They are so efficient that a nerve impulse, such as a pain impulse, can be transmitted from the hand to the brain and back again to allow a reflex movement in a fraction of a second.

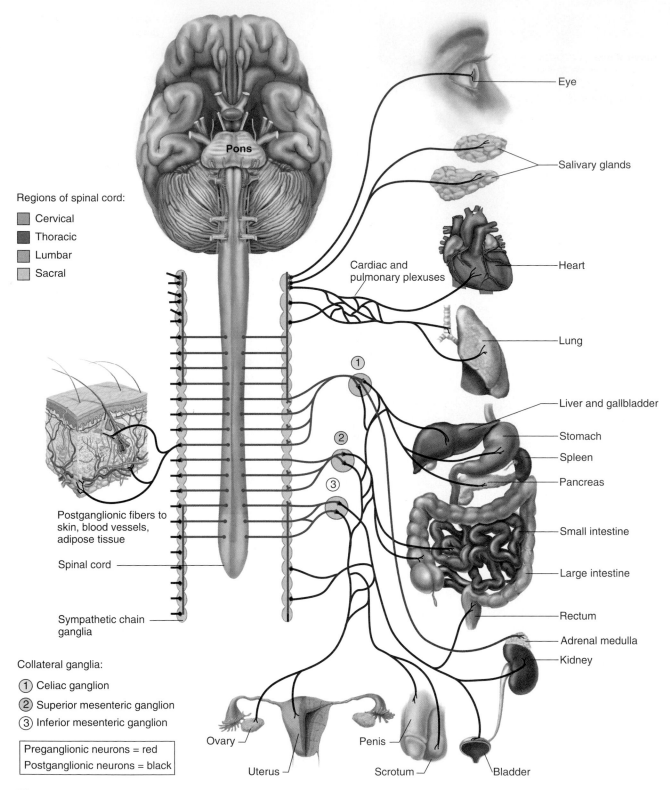

Regions of spinal cord:

- Cervical
- Thoracic
- Lumbar
- Sacral

Pons

Postganglionic fibers to skin, blood vessels, adipose tissue

Spinal cord

Sympathetic chain ganglia

Collateral ganglia:

1. Celiac ganglion
2. Superior mesenteric ganglion
3. Inferior mesenteric ganglion

Preganglionic neurons = red
Postganglionic neurons = black

Cardiac and pulmonary plexuses

Eye
Salivary glands
Heart
Lung
Liver and gallbladder
Stomach
Spleen
Pancreas
Small intestine
Large intestine
Rectum
Adrenal medulla
Kidney
Ovary
Uterus
Penis
Scrotum
Bladder

Figure 9.12 Sympathetic pathways

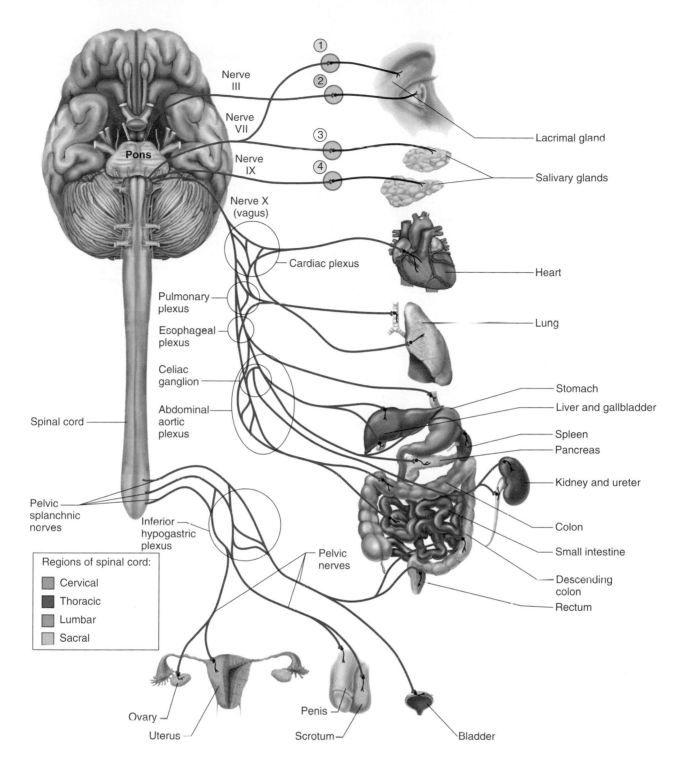

Figure 9.13 **Parasympathetic pathways**

The following labels appear in the figure:

Nerve III
Nerve VII
Pons
Nerve IX
Nerve X (vagus)
Cardiac plexus
Pulmonary plexus
Esophageal plexus
Celiac ganglion
Spinal cord
Abdominal aortic plexus
Pelvic splanchnic nerves
Inferior hypogastric plexus
Pelvic nerves

Regions of spinal cord:
Cervical
Thoracic
Lumbar
Sacral

Lacrimal gland
Salivary glands
Heart
Lung
Stomach
Liver and gallbladder
Spleen
Pancreas
Kidney and ureter
Colon
Small intestine
Descending colon
Rectum

Ovary
Uterus
Penis
Scrotum
Bladder

Cranial Nerves

Twelve pairs of cranial nerves send impulses between the brain and the structure of the head, neck, and upper thoracic area (figure 9.14). The 12 cranial nerves and the structure they innervate are listed in table 9.1.

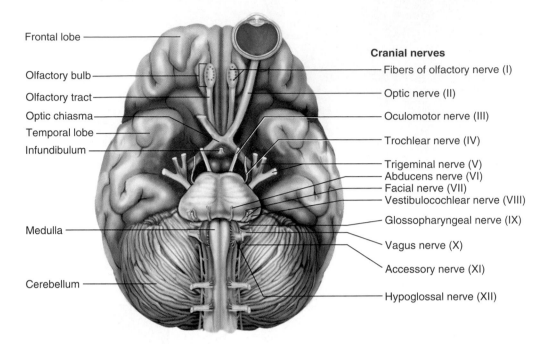

Frontal lobe

Olfactory bulb

Olfactory tract

Optic chiasma

Temporal lobe

Infundibulum

Medulla

Cerebellum

Cranial nerves

Fibers of olfactory nerve (I)

Optic nerve (II)

Oculomotor nerve (III)

Trochlear nerve (IV)

Trigeminal nerve (V)

Abducens nerve (VI)

Facial nerve (VII)

Vestibulocochlear nerve (VIII)

Glossopharyngeal nerve (IX)

Vagus nerve (X)

Accessory nerve (XI)

Hypoglossal nerve (XII)

Figure 9.14 Cranial nerves

Table 9.1	*Cranial Nerves*	
Nerve	**Structure**	**Sensory, Motor, or Both**
I. Olfactory	Nose	Sensory
II. Optic	Eye (vision)	Sensory
III. Occulomotor	Eye (movement)	Motor
IV. Trochlear	Eye (movement)	Motor
V. Trigeminal	Head and teeth	Both
VI. Abduceus	Eye (movement)	Motor
VII. Facial	Face and tongue	Both
VIII. Acoustic	Ear	Sensory
IX. Glossopharyngeal	Tongue, throat	Both salivary glands
X. Vagus	Thoracic and abdominal	Both cavities
XI. Spinal accessory	Shoulder and neck	Motor
XII. Hypoglossal	Tongue (movement)	Motor

Think About It

To remember the 12 pairs of cranial nerves, use this mnemonic: "Oh, Oh, Oh To Touch A Friend And Give Very Special Hugs."

Spinal Nerves

Thirty-one pairs of spinal nerves make up sensory/afferent nerves that send messages *from* sensory receptors to the central nervous system and motor/efferent nerves that send messages from the central nervous system *to* muscles and glands. The motor/efferent nerves are made up of somatic (voluntary) nerves that control the skeletal muscles. Autonomic (involuntary) nerves control cardiac and smooth muscle and the glands. Of the autonomic/involuntary nerves, the sympathetic nerves are the fight-or-flight nerves that use energy, and the parasympathetic nerves regulate and conserve energy.

A reflex is a rapid, automatic response to a stimulus. Reflex arcs are pathways for a reflex. The reflex begins with a stimulus that sets off a sensory nerve fiber to create an impulse. The impulse reaches the spinal cord and is sent to a motor neuron that in turn creates the reflex or action.

A plexus is a network of interlaced nerves. Plexuses are of great importance to massage therapists, especially if a plexus is damaged, resulting in an inability of certain corresponding muscle groups to respond to stimuli. The plexuses are as follows:

1. *Cervical plexus (C1-C5)*—nerves that extend from the vertebrae and affect the skin and muscles of the head, neck, and shoulder

2. *Brachial plexus (C5-T1)*—nerves that extend from the vertebrae and affect the shoulder and upper limbs. An injury to the radial nerve can result in the inability to extend the hand. Median nerve damage can lead to an inability to pronate the forearm and perform flexion. Ulnar nerve damage can cause an inability to adduct or abduct the fingers.

3. *Lumbar plexus (L1-L4)*—nerves that extend from the vertebrae and affect the abdominal wall, genitals, and lower limbs. Femoral nerve damage can lead to an inability to extend the leg.

4. *Sacral plexus (L4-S5)*—nerves that extend from the vertebrae and affect the buttocks and lower limbs. Sciatic nerve damage causes pain radiating down the posterior leg.

The Brain

The brain comprises about 92% of the central nervous system. It is connected to the upper end of the spinal cord through the foramen magnum of the skull and is responsible for issuing nerve impulses, processing nerve impulse data, and engaging in higher-order thought processing. The brain is divided into four parts: cerebrum, cerebellum, diencephalon, and brainstem. The large cerebrum controls speech, sensation, memory, and reasoning. It is often called the "seat of intelligence" and contains two cerebral hemispheres. The smaller cerebellum regulates balance and voluntary movement. The diencephalon houses the pineal gland (which is also the portion of the brain that includes the thalamus and the hypothalamus). The brainstem leads to the spinal cord. The brainstem is also descriptively divided into the medulla oblongata, which regulates breathing, heartbeat, swallowing, and the function of the blood vessels; the midbrain, which regulates auditory and visual senses; and the pons, which connects the spinal cord and brain, and regulates respiration. The brain stem also houses the limbic system, which regulates emotions.

Endocrine System

The endocrine system (figure 9.15) is the chemically controlled plan that involves growth, maturity, metabolism, reproduction, and human behavior. This system works closely with the nervous system. The hypothalamus of the brain sends directions through chemical signals to the **pituitary gland,** known as the master gland of the body, which then stimulates the other glands to secrete hormones to maintain homeostasis. The endocrine

Figure 9.15 The endocrine system
Principal organs: glands of the body.

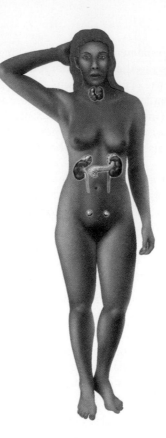

glands are ductless glands that secrete their hormones into the bloodstream. These secretions travel the circulatory system to target organs, in response to the signals, and give the organs instructions to respond in a specific manner. Exocrine glands, which have ducts, secrete directly into an organ; for example, sweat glands secrete to the surface of the body, and salivary glands secrete directly into the mouth (figure 9.16).

Hormone Messengers

The hormones that are secreted control the body from the cellular level up to the organ level. They control cellular respiration, growth, and reproduction, and they control the fluids within the body (such as water). They balance electrolytes and control the secretions of other hormones. It is easy to see that if you have a hormonal imbalance, you can very quickly become ill.

Hormonal systems work much like a thermostat. A normal state within the cells or organ is "set," and when that normal is too high or too low, hormones are sent as messengers to make adjustments. When the adjustment is made and homeostasis resumes, a hormonal messenger is sent to "turn off" the process. This process is happening, within our bodies, every moment that we are living.

Types of Hormones

There are three classifications, or chemical categories, of hormones. The group of the most simplistic form is the hormones that are made up of modified amino acids. These are the hormones secreted by the adrenal medulla—epinephrine and norepinephrine; and the hormones secreted by the posterior pituitary gland—oxytocin and vasopressin. A second category is made up of the protein hormones—insulin, gonad-stimulating hormones, and growth hormones from the anterior pituitary gland. Hormones of the first two categories bind with cell membranes of the target organs and change to a form that regulates cellular activity.

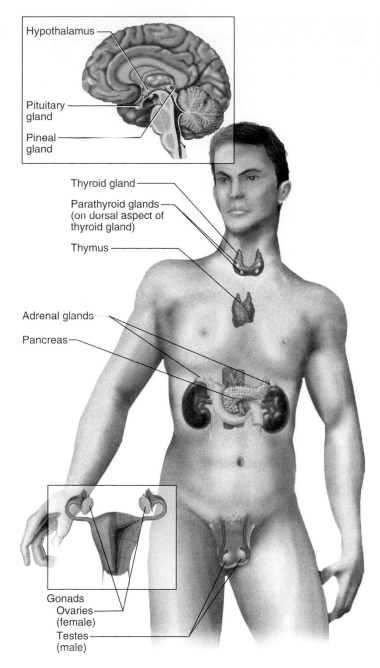

Hypothalamus

Pituitary gland

Pineal gland

Thyroid gland

Parathyroid glands (on dorsal aspect of thyroid gland)

Thymus

Adrenal glands

Pancreas

Gonads
Ovaries (female)
Testes (male)

The third category of hormones includes the steroid hormones, which are made up of substances resembling lipids. These hormones penetrate the target organ cells directly to transmit the message. Examples of these hormones are cortisol, estrogen, and testosterone (table 9.2).

The Main Endocrine Glands

The pituitary gland is about the size of a small pea and is commonly called the "master gland" because it controls all the other glands (refer to figure 9.29). It sits in a shallow depression of the sphenoid bone below the hypothalamus of the brain. It is divided into two sections: the anterior pituitary lobe and the posterior pituitary lobe.

The thyroid gland also consists of two lobes connected by a small band. The lobes are situated on the right and left sides of the trachea, just beneath the larynx. This gland

Table 9.2	Names and Abbreviations for Hormones	
Abbreviation	**Name**	**Source**
ACTH	Adrenocorticotropic hormone (conticotropin)	Anterior pituitary
ADH	Antidiuretic hormone (vasopressin)	Posterior pituitary
ANP	Atrial natriuretic peptide	Heart
CRH	Corticotropin-releasing hormone	Hypothalamus
DHEA	Dehydroepiandrosterone	Adrenal cortex
EPO	Erythropoietin	Kidney, liver
FSH	Follicle-stimulating hormone	Anterior pituitary
GH	Growth hormone (somatotropin)	Anterior pituitary
GHRH	Growth hormone-releasing hormone	Hypothalamus
GnRH	Gonadotropin-releasing hormone	Hypothalamus
IGFs	Insulin-line growth factors (somatomedins)	Liver, other tissues
LH	Luteinizing hormone	Anterior pituitary
NE	Norepinephrine	Adrenal medulla
OT	Oxytocin	Posterior pituitary
PIH	Prolactin-inhibiting hormone (dopamine)	Hypothalamus
PRH	Prolactin-releasing hormone	Hypothalamus
PRL	Prolactin	Anterior pituitary
PTH	Parathyroid hormone (parathormone)	Parathyroids
T_3	Triiodothyronine	Thyroid
T_4	Tetraiodothyronine	Thyroid
TH	Thyroid hormone (T_3 and T_4)	Hypothalamus
TRH	Thyotropin-releasing hormone	Hypothalamus
TSH	Thyroid-stimulating hormone	Anterior pituitary

is composed of spheres of follicles enclosed by connective tissue and requires iodine to function properly.

The parathyroid glands are four glands about the size of cherry pits embedded into the posterior surface of the thyroid gland. Two parathyroid glands are attached to each lobe of the thyroid. These glands consist of tightly packed "chief cells" and are located close to capillary transport. They secrete only one hormone, which is responsible for the regulation of vitamin D and calcium absorption.

⭐ **EXAM POINT** The adrenal glands, also known as the suprarenal glands, are small glands located on the top of each kidney.

Their hormones are released upon signals from the sympathetic division of the autonomic nervous system. The "flight or fight" stress hormones are released from the adrenal glands.

The Pancreas

⭐ **EXAM POINT** The pancreas is a part of both the exocrine and endocrine systems.

Type 1 diabetes, also called juvenile diabetes or insulin-dependent diabetes, is usually diagnosed in children, teens, or young adults. This form of diabetes is caused when the beta cells of the pancreas no longer make insulin because the body's immune system has attacked and destroyed them. Treatment for type 1 diabetes includes taking insulin, making wise food choices, exercising regularly, and controlling blood pressure and cholesterol.

Type 2 diabetes, also called adult-onset or noninsulin-dependent diabetes, is the most common form of the disease. It has almost reached epidemic proportions in American society. This form usually begins with insulin resistance, a condition in which fat, muscle, and liver cells do not use insulin properly. At first, the pancreas keeps up with the added demand by producing more insulin. In time, however, it loses the ability to secrete enough insulin in response to meals. Being overweight and inactive increases the chances of developing type 2 diabetes. Treatment includes taking diabetes medications, making wise food choices, exercising regularly, and controlling blood pressure and cholesterol.

Gestational diabetes is a condition that develops during the late stages of pregnancy. Although this form usually goes away after the baby is born, a woman who has had it is more likely to develop type 2 diabetes later in life. Gestational diabetes is caused by the hormones of pregnancy or a shortage of insulin.

It is also a part of both the digestive system because of the pancreatic juices it secretes and the endocrine system because the islets of Langerhans located within it secrete insulin and glucagons. The pancreas is found behind the stomach, and the exocrine system's pancreatic duct connects to the duodenum of the small intestine. This gland is responsible for the regulation of blood sugar levels. Alpha cells secrete the glucagons and beta cells secrete insulin. These two hormones work in a balancing act to keep blood sugar at stable, normal levels.

The thymus gland is a mass of tissue found in the mediastinum of the body, behind the sternum. This gland is at the height of importance in our early lives. It is crucial to the development of our immune system. It is quite large in a newborn but begins to shrink as we age. Infants born without a thymus gland will not develop an immune system capable of fighting infections from microbial organisms.

The pineal gland is located between the two cerebral hemispheres of the brain and is attached to the upper part of the thalamus. It is pinecone-shaped and secretes hormones directly into the cerebrospinal fluid. It regulates circadian rhythms and smooth muscle contractions.

The testes and ovaries are glands that are involved in the reproductive system. The testes are both endocrine and exocrine. They produce male sex hormones as part of the endocrine system and produce sperm when acting as an exocrine gland. The ovaries control the menstrual cycle, pregnancy, and menopause in the female body. The hormones produced by the sex glands are responsible for development of reproductive structures, sexual characteristics such as facial hair and breasts, and muscle and bone development pertaining to male or female structure.

The endocrine system supports, maintains, and controls our body's function. When this process is interrupted by dysfunction, the body becomes severely distressed.

Lymphatic System

The lymphatic system (figure 9.17) consists of lymph, lymphatic vessels, lymph nodes, lymphocytes, tonsils, the spleen, and the thymus gland. This system functions as part of the body's defense mechanism against microorganisms and harmful toxins. It is responsible for the regulation of the fluid level of the body and absorbs certain fats from the digestive tract.

Figure 9.17 Lymphatic system
Principal organs: Lymph nodes,
lymphatic vessels, thymus,
spleen, tonsils.

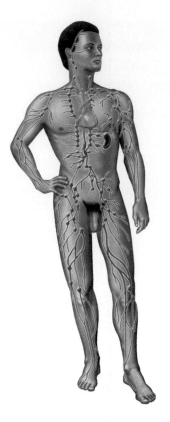

Lymph, which means "spring water," regulates the fluid level from tissue spaces, called the interstitial spaces, by draining the protein-containing fluid that escapes from the blood capillaries. The blood pressure in the cardiovascular system causes a small amount of the blood plasma to go through the capillary walls. This plasma moves into the spaces between tissue cells and is then called interstitial fluid. Some of the fluid will be reabsorbed into the capillary, but the small amount that remains must be drained to prevent the tissue from swelling (edema). The interstitial fluid enters the lymphatic capillaries and becomes lymph (figure 9.18).

EXAM POINT The lymphatic vessels that transport lymph are one-way vessels, meaning they have a closed end. These vessels are not found in the red bone marrow, vascular tissue, central nervous system, and part of the spleen.

The lymphatic capillaries are minute, but they unite with larger vessels with lymph nodes at certain intervals along its path.

EXAM POINT Because of the one-way travel, there is no backflow of the lymph. All of the lymph vessels come together at one of two points: either the thoracic duct or the right lymphatic duct.

Lymph Nodes

The lymph nodes are small, jelly bean-shaped structures found along the path of the lymph vessels. They are also known as the lymph glands. These nodes are grouped together in three regions: groin area, armpits, and sides of the neck. The tissue in the node consists of lymphocytes and other cells. When lymph carrying microorganisms or toxic substances enters the node, an immune response is triggered. This response causes the

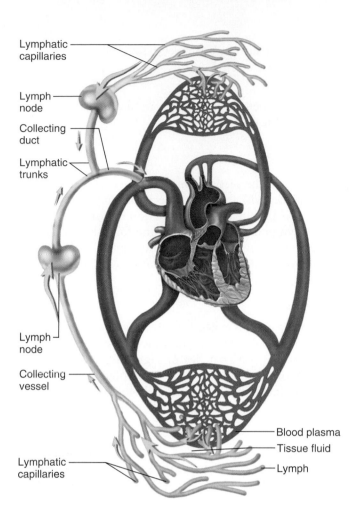

Lymphatic capillaries

Lymph node

Collecting duct

Lymphatic trunks

Lymph node

Collecting vessel

Lymphatic capillaries

Blood plasma

Tissue fluid

Lymph

Figure 9.18 Fluid exchange between the circulatory and lymphatic systems

release of macrophage cells that will remove dead microorganisms, produce antibodies, and destroy foreign substances by phagocytosis.

Tonsils

The tonsils are located at the top of the throat, just below the internal nasal cavity opening. They were once removed when chronic swelling occurred but are now most often left alone. The medical community, through extensive research, has come to understand that they are a very valuable part of our immune response because they form a protective wall around microorganisms entering the nasal or oral cavities. They are still removed if they show signs of severe infection or have swollen large enough to restrict breathing.

The Spleen

The spleen is found in the upper left corner of the abdominal cavity. It filters our blood through two vessels: the splenic artery and the splenic vein.

EXAM POINT When blood passes through the spleen, bacteria, worn-out platelets, and old red blood cells are phagocytized.

When the red blood cells are broken down, hemoglobin is released to be recycled.

Blood is stored in the spleen, and if a hemorrhage occurs in the circulation route, the spleen releases stored blood to keep the body functioning.

The Thymus Gland

The thymus gland has been discussed in the section on the endocrine system. This gland disappears as we age and is replaced with fat and connective tissue. It is involved with the body's immunity because it is the site of the production and maturation of lymphocytes. This gland develops T lymphocytes in the fetus and for a short while after birth. The lymphocytes that leave the thymus enter the bloodstream and travel to lymphatic tissue to help protect against microorganism invasion.

The Digestive System and Immunity

In the small intestines, special lymphatic vessels called lacteals function to absorb fats and transport them from the villi of the small intestine to the bloodstream. Also found within the walls of the small intestines are Peyer's patches, or aggregated lymphatic follicles. They are similar to the structure of tonsils and produce macrophages that destroy bacteria that might penetrate the intestinal walls and go into the bloodstream.

Cells of the Lymphatic System

A whole range of cells play a significant part in the lymphatic system's immunity response mechanism: B cells, plasma cells, helper T cells, killer T cells, suppressor cells, memory cells, and macrophages. These cells are highly specialized and perform an important function in maintaining immunity.

The Skin and Immune Response

The skin, although not a true part of the lymphatic system, also performs specific immune response procedures. The mantle or covering of the skin is acidic and thereby inhibits microorganisms, especially bacteria, from growing. The epidermis provides a protective barrier that, when intact, keeps microorganisms at bay, and sebum from the sebaceous glands has both antibacterial and antifungal components. If a harmful microorganism or foreign substance cannot get into our bodies, then the lymphatic battle is never begun.

Diseases of the Lymphatic System

The most common disorder of the lymphatic system is allergies. Over 20 million Americans have allergic reactions on a daily basis. Many of these are simply a hypersensitivity to dust, smoke, and pollutants. When the nose is affected, it is called hay fever or allergic rhinitis. If the lungs are chronically affected, it is referred to as asthma. If a substance is ingested and triggers an allergic/immune response, cramping, vomiting, and diarrhea may result. Even **contact dermatitis** and hives are allergic responses that come into play when we are exposed to a harmful substance and our lymphatic vessels and cells try to stop the invasion.

AIDS, which is discussed in chapter 2, is caused by infection with the human immunodeficiency virus (HIV); AIDS attacks the T cells. The virus invades the cells and causes the T cells to reproduce the virus instead of destroying it. This compromises the entire lymphatic immunity mechanism and leaves the body wide open for any and all opportunistic infections.

Lymphadenitis is an inflammation of lymph nodes. When a lymph node is involved in the destruction of microorganisms, the gland swells and becomes hot. Physicians see the swollen glands and know that an infection process is happening. Lymphangitis is an inflammation of the lymphatic vessels and can produce red streaks that can be seen through the skin.

Lymphoma is a tumor of lymphatic tissue. It is usually malignant and begins to enlarge. There are two forms of lymphomas: Hodgkin's and non-Hodgkin's. Treatment with medication and radiation therapy is usually effective.

Digestive System

The function of our digestive system is vital to our health and well-being (figure 9.19). It is the responsibility of the digestive system to break down food into molecules small enough to be used by the cells and to absorb nutrients into the blood to be used for metabolism.

> **EXAM POINT** The digestive system begins with the mouth and extends in a continuous tube about 30 feet long until it ends at the anus.

This tube is called the gastrointestinal tract or alimentary canal.

> **EXAM POINT** The primary organs of this system include the mouth (oral cavity), pharynx, esophagus, stomach, and the small and large intestines.

The accessory organs for this system are the teeth, tongue, salivary glands, liver, gallbladder, pancreas, and appendix.

> **EXAM POINT** This system processes food with five basic activities: ingestion, peristalsis, digestion, absorption, and defecation.

Ingestion is the process of eating. We put food into our mouths and chew or masticate. During **mastication,** our tongue, lips, and cheeks help to keep the food where the teeth can reach it. The contour of the mouth helps to shape the food for swallowing, and the uvula prevents food from backing up into the nasal cavity. Three pairs of salivary glands (parotid, submandibular, and sublingual) secrete saliva, which is 99.5% water, into the mouth. The saliva begins the process of dissolving foods by using its remaining 0.5% constituents—primarily amylase, which initiates the breakdown of complex carbohydrates into simple sugars. Mucin in the saliva helps to lubricate the food for easier travel down the esophagus. The saliva also contains an enzyme, lysozyme, that destroys bacteria and protects the mucous membrane lining of the mouth and throat from infection and the teeth from tooth decay.

The pharynx is a part of both the digestive system and the respiratory system. It functions in the digestive system to begin the process of **deglutition** or swallowing. Food in the form of a bolus, or small ball, is passed to the esophagus. The esophagus is a tube about 10 inches long that sits behind the trachea and runs down to the stomach. It passes through the mediastinum, continues through the diaphragm at the esophageal hiatus, and ends at the stomach. The purpose of the esophagus is to transport food to the stomach. It also continues to secrete mucus into the food and has a sphincter known as the gastroesophageal sphincter that controls the flow of the bolus as it travels into the stomach. The bolus is moved toward the stomach by smooth muscle contractions, moving in a wavelike sequence called peristalsis.

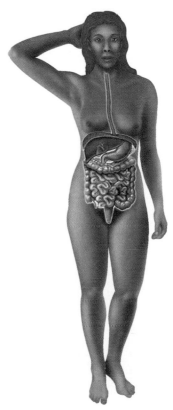

Figure 9.19 Digestive system
Principal organs: Teeth, tongue, salivary glands, esophagus, stomach, small and large intestines, liver, pancreas.

Figure 9.20 Internal anatomy of the stomach

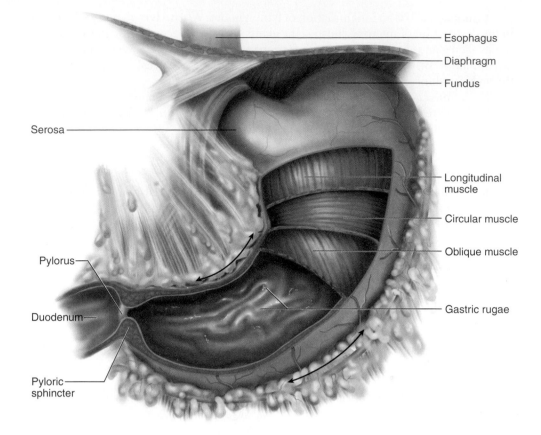

The stomach is an enlarged portion of the gastrointestinal tract. It lies just below the diaphragm in the upper abdominal cavity. It has roughly a J shape and is simply a curved tube that, when empty, has layered folds called **rugae.** The stomach is divided into three parts, the fundus, body, and pylorus. When food enters the stomach, it is divided into complex carbohydrates, protein, and fats. The carbohydrate breakdown occurs the fastest since amylase from the mouth has already begun the process. The gastric enzyme pepsinogen, a precursor to pepsin, mixes with hydrochloric acid to break down proteins, which take the longest time to digest. The stomach is lined with smooth muscle and a thick layer of mucus to protect the stomach lining from digesting itself (figure 9.20). Water and salts are absorbed in the stomach, as well as alcohol and some medications. Fats leave the stomach last and are passed into the small intestine.

The pancreas secretes pancreatic juice composed of digestive enzymes (lipases, carbohydrases, and proteases) that unites with bile as the food moves into the duodenum (figure 9.21).

⭐ **EXAM POINT** The bile is produced by the liver and is stored in the gallbladder until it is needed.

The food then continues to be digested as it moves into the small intestine. Glucagon and insulin are also secreted by cells in the pancreas to regulate the blood sugar level.

The liver is a large organ of the digestive system and is located in the right abdominal quadrant. It performs so many functions for the body that it is impossible to live without this organ. The liver has six main functions:

1. Kupffer's cells of the liver use the process of phagocytosis to destroy certain bacteria, and old white and red blood cells.

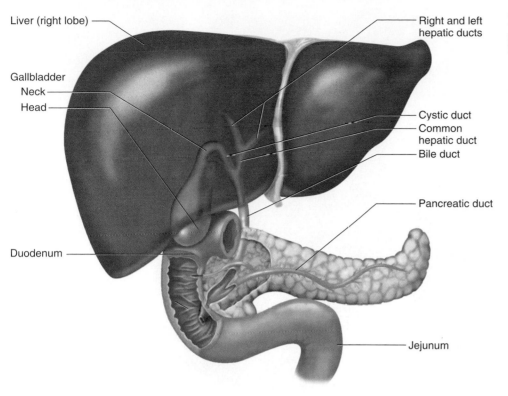

Liver (right lobe)

Gallbladder
Neck
Head

Duodenum

Right and left
hepatic ducts

Cystic duct
Common
hepatic duct
Bile duct

Pancreatic duct

Jejunum

Figure 9.21 Anatomy of the gallbladder, pancreas, and bile passages

2. Liver cells contain enzymes that chemically break down and transform toxins. The liver stores the ones it cannot change to harmless substances that can be excreted by the body.

3. The liver stores excess glucose as glycogen or fat and converts this back to glucose if needed.

4. The liver stores copper, iron, and the vitamins A, D, E, and K.

5. The liver makes heparin, prothrombin, and thrombin, which help with blood clotting.

6. The liver produces bile salts to dissolve fat.

Once the food bolus is in the small intestine, it is mixed with additional digestive enzymes produced by the small intestine, and extra mucus is secreted to change the acidic mixture into an alkaline. The mixture of digested, semi-liquid nutrients is call chyme. It is here that almost all of the absorption of nutrients in the form of amino acids, fatty acids, simple sugars, water, vitamins, and minerals occurs. The small intestine is about 21 feet long and is lined with a network of special folds that function as villi and project into the material for faster absorption. The small intestine is divided into three parts, the duodenum, jejunum, and ileum. A network of capillaries within each villus picks up nutrients and transports them to a small artery. The nutrients connect with the lacteals of the endocrine system to gain fats and are then transported to the rest of the cells of the body.

The function of the large intestine is to absorb water, manufacture and absorb vitamin K, biotin, B5, and form feces (waste material that is not digestible) for expulsion. The large intestine is around 5 feet long and is commonly referred to as the bowel (figure 9.22). It begins at the ileocecal valve, where it connects to the small intestine. Also attached to this conjuncture is the appendix, a small tube about 3 inches long.

★ **EXAM POINT** The colon continues and is divided into several parts: the ascending colon, the hepatic flexure, the transverse colon, the splenic flexure, and the descending colon.

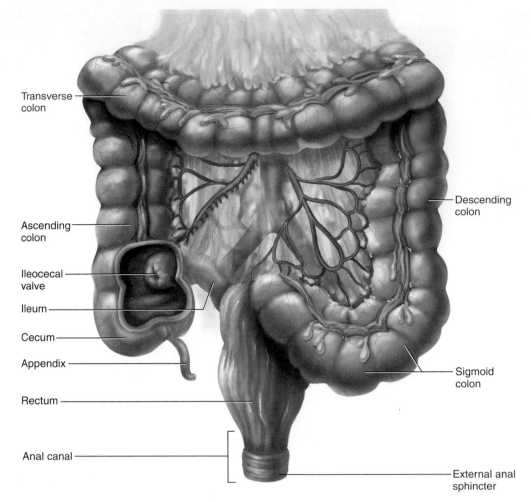

Transverse colon

Ascending colon

Ileocecal valve

Ileum

Cecum

Appendix

Rectum

Anal canal

Descending colon

Sigmoid colon

External anal sphincter

Figure 9.22 **Anatomy of the large intestine**

The last part of the colon, the sigmoid portion, joins the rectum. Waste travels through the colon by three types of churning and peristalsis motions until it reaches the anus and is expelled.

Diseases and Disorders of the Digestive System

The digestive system is a large and intricate machine. Every organ has a special function, and the secretions and chemical involvement must be timed perfectly. It is no wonder that a digestive system illness can literally stop us in our tracks. Besides processing food for energy and nutrients, our stomach often acts as an emotional buffer by responding to anxiety. We have all had that gut feeling when our stomach contracts as the first response to fear or test anxiety that involves a night of illness before the final test. Due to stress, overwork, poor eating habits, and other social problems of today's society, you will probably have a number of clients who may suffer digestive tract distress.

Respiratory System

The respiratory system shares the responsibility of supplying oxygen and eliminating carbon dioxide with the cardiovascular system. Without these two systems working to provide oxygen to our cells, we would die. We have already discussed the cardiovascular system, so let us proceed to the respiratory system and its organs (figure 9.23).

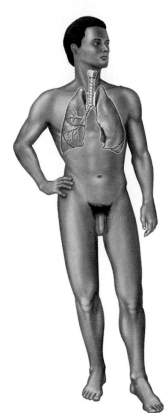

These organs work to take in and transport gases between the air we breathe and the blood. The blood then takes the oxygen and moves it to all the cells (figure 9.24). The term **respiration** refers to the overall exchange of gases between the air, the blood, and the cells.

The respiratory system is often divided into two parts: the upper respiratory tract, which consists of the nose, pharynx (throat), and larynx (voice box), and the lower respiratory tract, which includes the trachea (windpipe), bronchi, and lungs. The nose has a cartilage and bone framework covered with skin and lined internally with mucous membranes. The top of the nose, often referred to as the bridge, is formed by nasal bones. Internal cavities are called the nasal cavities, and the hard palate separates the oral cavity from the nasal.

The pharynx is posterior to the nasal cavity. The four paranasal sinuses (sphenoid, ethmoid, maxillary, and frontal) connect to the nasal cavity, and the lacrimal (or tear sacs) empty into the nose. (See the section on skeletal structure in chapter 7.) The larynx is a short passageway that is connected to the pharynx and the trachea. The trachea is surrounded by cartilage that protects the thyroid gland and forms the Adam's apple. This thyroid cartilage is the largest portion of cartilage in our bodies and moves up and down as we swallow or speak. Skeletal muscles attach the larynx and the rigid rows of vocal cords that vibrate from air and produce sounds. The larynx and pharynx work to-

Figure 9.23 Respiratory system

Principal organs: Nose, pharynx, larynx, trachea, bronchi, lungs.

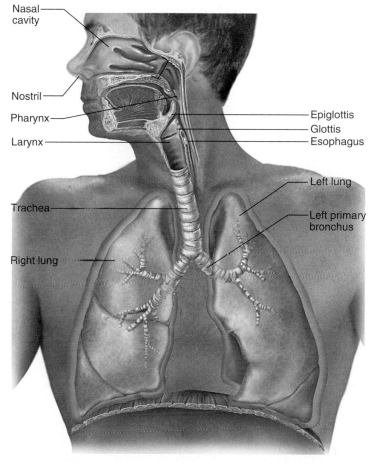

Figure 9.24 The respiratory system

Figure 9.25 Pulmonary alveoli

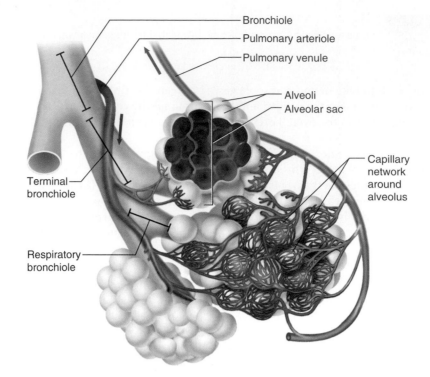

Bronchiole
Pulmonary arteriole
Pulmonary venule
Alveoli
Alveolar sac
Capillary network around alveolus
Terminal bronchiole
Respiratory bronchiole

gether to keep food from going into the lungs, and they work, along with the mouth and nasal cavities acting as resonance chambers, to produce speech by helping to shape the sounds into language.

The trachea is a long tube that allows for the passage of air. It is anterior to the esophagus and extends from the cartilage of the larynx to the fifth thoracic vertebrae. It then makes a lateral divide and becomes the left and right bronchi. The trachea consists of smooth muscle and elastic connective tissue that is encircled by 16 to 20 hyaline rings. These rings are open and resemble the letter *c*. The open section of the *c* faces the esophagus and allows it to expand into the trachea when you swallow. The bronchi also contain hyaline cartilage. When the bronchi enter their respective lungs, they form smaller bronchi called secondary bronchi. These branches reach into the lungs. There is a secondary bronchi for each lobe of the lungs; three lobes for the right and two lobes for the left. The bronchi divide again and become bronchioles. The cartilage disappears, and the smooth muscle increases and further divides to become alveolar. Around each alveolar duct are the alveoli. These alveoli are minute sacs where the exchange of gases occurs between the lungs and blood by diffusion across the alveoli and the capillary walls surrounding them (figure 9.25).

Respiration involves three basic processes. The first process is ventilation, which is movement of air between air outside the body and the lungs. This is referred to as inhalation or inspiration as air comes in and exhalation or expiration as air moves out. The second and third processes involve the exchange within the body. External respiration is the exchange between the lungs and the blood. Internal respiration—the third process—is the exchange of gases between the blood and the body cells.

Urinary System ★

EXAM POINT The urinary system consists of the kidneys, ureters, urinary bladder, and urethra.

The main function of this system is to filter the blood by removing waste products (figure 9.26). However, the kidneys provide other valuable processes such as vitamin D production when they convert vitamin D into calciferol; they also regulate blood pres-

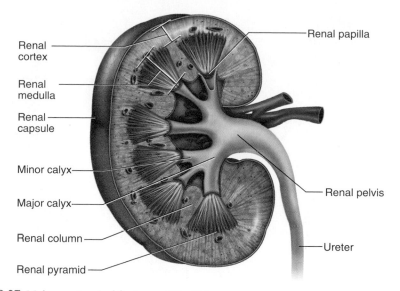

Renal cortex
Renal medulla
Renal capsule
Minor calyx
Major calyx
Renal column
Renal pyramid
Renal papilla
Renal pelvis
Ureter

Figure 9.27 Major anatomical features of the kidney

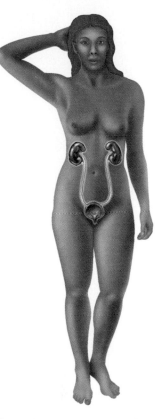

Figure 9.26 Urinary system
Principal organs: Kidneys, ureters, urinary bladder, urethra.

sure by secreting an enzyme called renin and produce erythropoietin (a hormone that stimulates red blood cell production within red bone marrow). The urinary system also maintains electrolyte, pH, and fluid balance, which is essential to a healthy body.

Waste is produced when the body metabolizes food, cells form carbon dioxide waste, and especially when the breakdown of proteins into amino acids produces nitrous wastes, such as ammonia. The liver takes the ammonia and changes it into urea, which is less harmful to the body.

The main organ of the urinary system is the kidney (figure 9.27). The body has two kidneys located on the right and left upper quadrants, with the left kidney being slightly higher than the right.

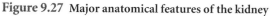

EXAM POINT Within the kidney are nephrons, known as the functional units of the kidney.

Nephrons serve to remove the urea and other waste products from the blood. This filtration process is controlled by the sympathetic nervous system, and the volume and pressure of the blood. The resulting filtration product, called urine, is mostly water with urea, uric acid, and other components such as any medications or drugs you may be taking. The kidney holds this product in collection tubules. The cleansed blood returns through the renal veins to reenter the blood stream. The urine flows through the ureters, one for each kidney, toward the bladder. The urine is held in the bladder until contractions of the smooth muscles send the urine out of the body through the urethra.

Reproductive System

The main function of the reproductive system is to provide for the survival of the human species. The primary organs of the male reproductive system are the testes or gonads, which produce sperm (figure 9.28). They also produce the male sex hormones. Accessory structures include the scrotum that surrounds and supports the gonads, and the many interior components that store the sperm. Accessory glands add secretions to the seminal fluid, and the penis is used as an organ of transport.

In the female reproductive system, ovaries or female gonads produce eggs (figure 9.29). There are two ovaries that are located just above the uterus. They are held in position by suspension ligaments. The egg (ovum) develops in a follicle, and

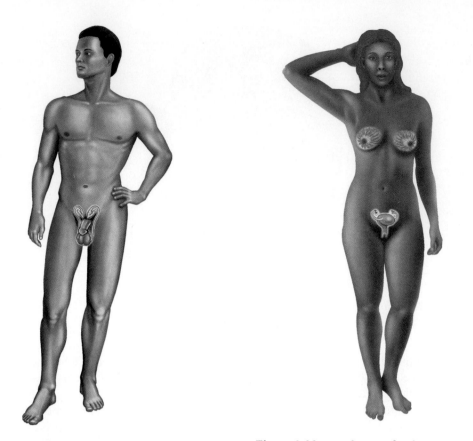

Figure 9.28 Male reproductive system
Principal organs: Testes, epididymides, spermatic ducts, seminal vesicles, prostate gland, bulbourethral glands, penis.

Figure 9.29 Female reproductive system
Principal organs: Ovaries, uterine tubes, uterus, vagina, vulva, mammary glands.

when mature, it is released into the fallopian tubes and travels to the uterus. When the ovum is about to be released, the ovaries produce estrogen, a hormone. The same follicles produce progesterone when the ovum is released to stimulate the uterus into preparing a place for the ovum to attach. If the ovum is fertilized, progesterone continues to be produced, the uterine walls thicken, and a fetus begins to grow. If the ovum is not fertilized, the uterine wall is shed. This cycle, also known as the menstrual cycle, varies in length, usually taking between 24 and 35 days.

At the base of the uterus is the cervix. When a child is born, the baby passes through the dilated cervix and travels through the vagina. The external reproductive organs are the labia majora, labia minora, and the clitoris. The mammary glands within the female breasts are considered accessory organs. The mammary glands are triggered by hormones during pregnancy and produce milk when the child is born. The milk is made by the alveolar glands. The hormone oxytocin induces the ducts to deliver milk through an opening in the nipples.

The health of the individuals contributing the sperm and ovum to be fertilized can play a big role in the development of a healthy child. Many mothers turn to massage for stress relief when trying to become pregnant and continue massage during pregnancy (chapter 10).

Integumentary System ★ **EXAM POINT** The integumentary system is made up of skin, the largest organ in our bodies, and its accessary components: sweat and oil glands, nails, and hair.

The integumentary system gives us our outward appearance (figure 9.30). This system can indicate any nutritional imbalances or pathological conditions that the body may be experiencing and gives massage therapists information into the health of an individual without invasive testing that is beyond their scope of practice.

People of our society are more concerned than ever with their appearance and spend millions of dollars a year to have attractive, vibrant, and healthy-looking skin. They also purchase numerous products for hygiene, such as deodorants, lotions, creams, shampoos, and skin treatments. This trend in society—along with the fact that a massage therapist touches or manipulates the skin with every stroke—makes it imperative that the massage therapist understands every aspect of the integumentary system.

Functions of the Integumentary System

The integumentary system has many valuable functions, besides the general appearance of the body. They are:

Protection against ultraviolet (UV) light and the invasion of the body by microorganisms. The skin also protects against dehydration by reducing water loss.

Temperature regulation by controlling the blood flow through the skin and the sweat gland activity

Sensation from sensory receptors that detect touch, pressure, pain, heat, cold, and moisture levels

Synthesis of vitamin D: Cholesterol in the skin cells is synthesized into vitamin D when struck by UV light.

Fat storage under the dermal layer.

Excretion of waste products through the skin, and glandular excretions.

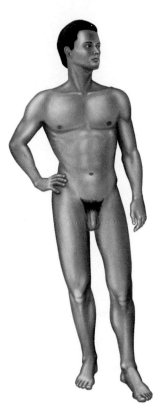

Figure 9.30 Integumentary system
Principal organs: Skin, hair, nails, cutaneous glands.

The Skin

★ **EXAM POINT** The skin consists primarily of two layers, the epidermis and the dermis, and sits on the hypodermis, a foundation of tissue that attaches the skin to the bone and muscle (figure 9.31). The hypodermis is also where blood vessels and nerves are located and is often called the subcutaneous layer or tissue.

This subcutaneous layer is a loose connective tissue that contains stored fat that acts to cushion and insulate the body from heat or cold. The distribution of this layer depends on age, gender, and diet.

The Dermis

The dermis is a dense connective tissue that contains fibroblasts, fat cells, and macrophages. It has fewer fat cells and smaller blood vessels than the hypodermis. Nerve endings, smooth muscles, hair follicles, and lymphatic vessels extend into and through the dermis. The dermal papillae that form the fingerprints, the sudoriferous glands that secret fluid commonly called "sweat," and the sebaceous glands that secrete sebum (or oil) are also found in the dermis. The skin's structural strength is maintained by dermal collagen and elastic fibers. The orientation of these fibers allows the skin to stretch, and their direction produces lines of tension. Scar tissue forms if the skin is

Think About It

The phrase "Please Tell Stephen Something Funny Everyday" should help you to remember the functions of the integumentary system.

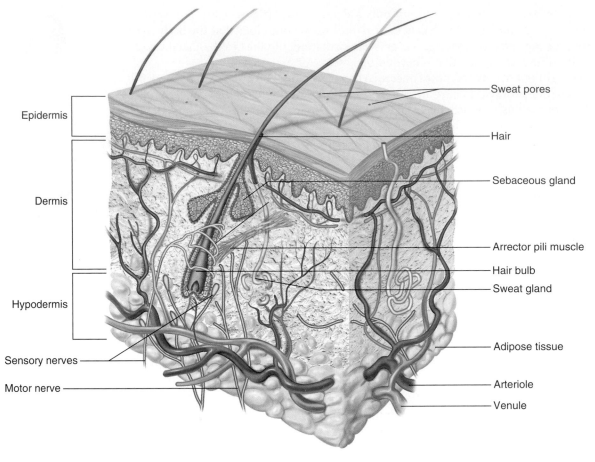

Figure 9.31 Structure of the skin

overstretched, such as with a pregnancy or rapid weight gain. The skin will form a gap and protrude when cut in a nonparallel manner, as in surgery or injury.

The **arrector pili** is a smooth muscle associated with each hair follicle. The muscle contracts, causing the hair to stand perpendicular to your skin's surface when you are cold or frightened. This reaction gives the skin the appearance of goose bumps or goose flesh.

The Epidermis

The epidermis consists of stratified squamous epithelium. These cells are produced by mitosis, and as newer cells are formed, older cells are pushed to the surface. Once on the surface, they flake off. The outer layer of cells protects the deeper, forming cells and contains keratin—a protein that becomes hardened into a barrier that resists scrapes and invasion of microorganisms. The epidermis is divided into three layers:

1. Stratum germinativum, which is where the new cells are produced. It takes about 40 to 56 days for the cells to reach the surface.

2. Pigment layer, which consists of the cells called melanocytes that produce melanin in the presence of UV rays and protects against UV penetration

3. Stratum corneum, which is the outer layer and contains keratin

The Senses ★ **EXAM POINT** Our senses—smell, taste, vision, hearing, balance, and touch—give us information about the world around us.

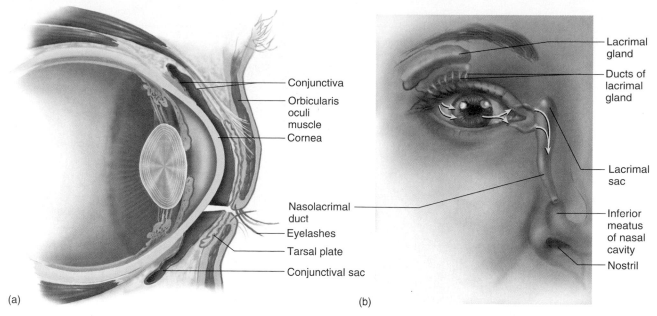

Figure 9.32 Structures of the eye
(*a*) Section of the eye and orbit; (*b*) lacrimal gland.

They are made up of specialized sensory receptors in the eyes, ears, nose, tongue, and skin.

Eyes

Eyes are the organs used in sight. They are protected by bony sections of the skull called orbits and are further protected from dust and foreign bodies by the eyebrows, eyelashes, and tears. The eye is spherically shaped and filled with two fluids: the aqueous humor, a watery fluid anterior to the lens, and the vitreous humor, a jellylike fluid posterior to the lens (figure 9.32).

The eye has three layers. The sclera is the outermost layer, or what we commonly call the white of the eye. It is composed of connective tissue. The cornea is a transparent part of this layer and permits light to enter the eye. The choroid contains the blood vessels and pigment cells and is the second layer. The colored iris is found in this layer. The third layer is the retina. It is usually ashen in color and contains the light-sensitive cells known as the rods and cones. The rods are receptors for night vision and sense black and white, and the cones are receptors for day vision and sense color.

The Ear

The ear is divided into three sections: the external, the inner, and the middle ear (figure 9.33). It is here that we find the organs of balance and hearing. The part of the ear that extends from the outside of the head to the tympanic membrane (eardrum) is called the external ear. The air-filled canal that contains the auditory ossicles—the malleus (hammer), incus (anvil), and stapes (stirrups)—is called the middle ear. The inner ear is a made up of fluid-filled chambers that lie within the temporal bone. It contains the cochlea, which is part of hearing, and also the vestibule and semicircular canals, which maintain balance. The vestibule works to keep the body balanced in regard to how the head lines up with gravity, and the semicircular canals determine the changes need in regard to movements that rotate the head.

The Tongue

Our sense of taste comes from the taste buds located on the papillae, which are elevations found on the surface of the tongue. They are also found on the palate of the

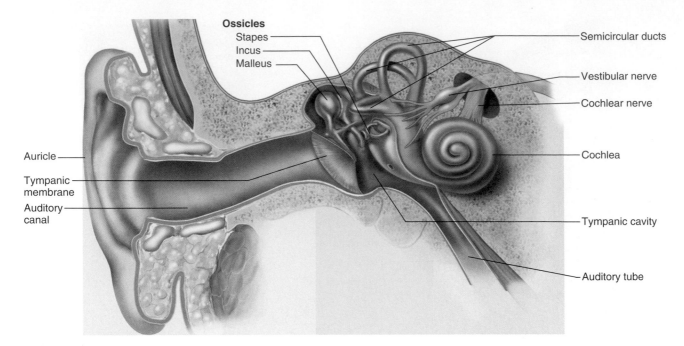

Figure 9.33 Internal anatomy of the ear

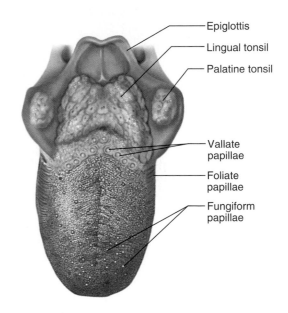

Figure 9.34 The tongue

mouth, the pharynx, and the inside of the cheeks. Taste buds are composed of special receptor cells. Saliva dissolves the chemicals to be tasted, and the cranial nerves VIII, IX, and X transmit the sensations of taste to the brain. In the brain, the gustatory cortex of the cerebrum interprets the taste and categorizes it. There are four types of sensations: sweet, sour, salty, and bitter. The sense of smell adds to the ability to taste (figure 9.34).

The Nose

Our olfactory sense, or sense of smell, comes into play when molecules in the air enter the nasal cavity and become dissolved by mucus. Figure 9.35 illustrates structures of the nasal receptors. The chemical component comes in contact with the olfactory neurons and they respond. The odor molecules then bind to receptor sites along the dendrites, and the neurons transmit the impulse to the olfactory cortex, which is found in the tem-

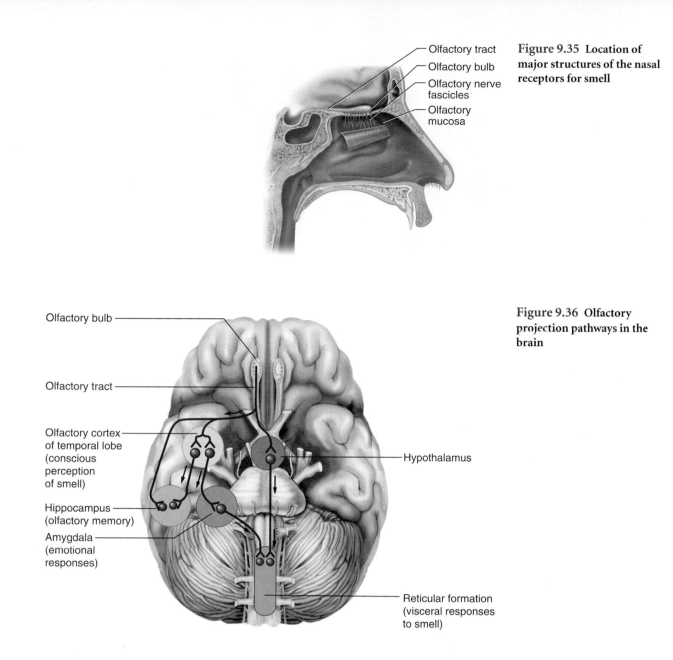

Figure 9.35 Location of major structures of the nasal receptors for smell

- Olfactory tract
- Olfactory bulb
- Olfactory nerve fascicles
- Olfactory mucosa

Figure 9.36 Olfactory projection pathways in the brain

- Olfactory bulb
- Olfactory tract
- Olfactory cortex of temporal lobe (conscious perception of smell)
- Hippocampus (olfactory memory)
- Amygdala (emotional responses)
- Hypothalamus
- Reticular formation (visceral responses to smell)

poral and frontal lobes of the cerebrum (figure 9.36). Sense of smell varies from person to person and is closely related to the sense of taste. We have all experienced feelings or memories when certain scents are present, and many studies are being conducted to understand the roles that smell plays in the brain.

Touch

The touch receptors, found within our skin and the deeper structures (such as tendons, ligaments, and muscles), are very complex. The simplest of these receptors are the free nerve endings that sense pain and crude touch. They are distributed throughout almost all of our body. Some of the free nerve endings respond to pain, others to temperature, and some to movement.

The more complex receptors are enclosed in capsules. Meissner's corpuscles are deep within the epidermis and localize fine touch and vibration. Ruffini's corpuscles sense touch and continuous pressure. The deepest receptors are associated with joints and tendons and are called Pacinian corpuscles. They sense and relay information concerning deep pressure, vibration, and proprioception.

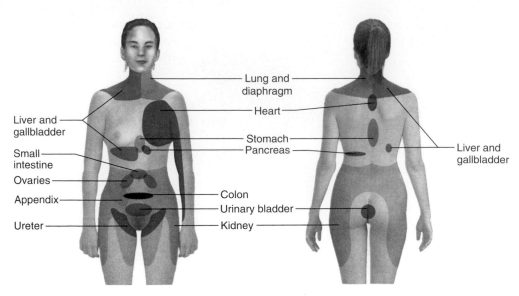

Figure 9.37 Referred pain
Pain from the viscera is often felt in specific areas of the skin.

Referred pain is a painlike sensation that originates in a region of the body that is not the source of the pain stimulus. Referred pain is often sensed in the skin but involves a deeper structure or internal organ that is damaged, diseased, or inflamed (figure 9.37).

Chapter Summary

The body is a very complex machine that works in a highly synchronized manner to maintain homeostasis. It can be easily disrupted and begin to give in to disease and decay that shortens our life and limits our lifestyle. By understanding all of our bodily processes and how our systems work together to maintain our health, we can make choices that will enable us (as well as our clients) to secure a long and healthy future.

Applying Your Knowledge

Self-Testing

1. What is the primary function of skin?
   a) Odor release
   b) Protection
   c) Tanning
   d) Identification

2. In which cavity is the heart located?
   a) Abdominal
   b) Dorsal
   c) Mediastinum
   d) Pelvic

3. What are the heart actions of contraction and relaxation called?
   a) Contract and relax reflex
   b) Systole and diastole
   c) Systemic and pulmonary
   d) Specific and nonspecific

4. What happens to the blood in the lungs?
   a) It drops off oxygen and picks up carbon dioxide.
   b) It drops off carbon dioxide and picks up oxygen.
   c) It picks up both carbon dioxide and oxygen.
   d) It drops off both carbon dioxide and oxygen.

5. What structure is known as the "functional unit" of the cardiovascular system?
   a) Heart
   b) Arteries
   c) Veins
   d) Capillaries

6. Which has stronger, thicker walls?
   a) Arteries
   b) Veins
   c) Capillaries
   d) All are the same.

7. Which is the largest organ in the lymphatic system?
   a) Tonsils
   b) Thymus
   c) Spleen
   d) Pancreas

8. Of what are the approximately 16 to 20 *c* shaped rings of the trachea made?
   a) Bone
   b) Muscle
   c) Cartilage
   d) Ligament

9. What is the function of the kidney?
   a) To store urine
   b) To make urine
   c) To excrete urine
   d) To pass urine

10. What two systems are involved in gas exchange?
   a) Respiratory and digestive
   b) Respiratory and cardiovascular
   c) Digestive and coronary
   d) Digestive and urinary

11. Which structure is also known as the voice box?
   a) Larynx
   b) Pharynx
   c) Trachea
   d) Mouth

12. What is the hollow space in the food tube called?
   a) Esophagus
   b) Eustachian
   c) Lumen
   d) Serosa

13. What are the elevations on the tongue where taste buds are found?
   a) Papillae
   b) Erector pilli
   c) Frenulum
   d) Polyps

14. What are the wavelike, rhythmical contractions that push food through the gastrointestinal tract called?
   a) Peritoneum
   b) Deglutition
   c) Peristalsis
   d) Mastication

15. What are the three divisions of the stomach?
   a) Fundus, body, pylorus
   b) Appendix, small intestine, large intestine
   c) Duodenum, jejunum, ileum
   d) Appendix, gallbladder, pancreas

16. Where does carbohydrate digestion begin?
   a) Mouth
   b) Esophagus
   c) Stomach
   d) Intestines

17. What are the three parts of the small intestine?
   a) Cecum, transverse colon, rectum
   b) Fundus, body, pylorus
   c) Duodenum, jejunum, ileum
   d) Incisors, canines, premolars, molars

18. What is the mixture of food and gastric juices called?
   a) Fecal matter
   b) Bile
   c) Lumen
   d) Chyme

19. What is the ring of muscle that acts like a valve called?
   a) Sphincter
   b) Papillae
   c) Plicae
   d) Uvula

20. What are the folds that make up the inner lining of the stomach called?
   a) Chyme
   b) Rugae
   c) Plicae
   d) Fat

21. What are the folds in the small intestine called?
   a) Chyme
   b) Rugae
   c) Plicae
   d) Pilli

22. B and K vitamins are made in which organ?
   a) Large intestine
   b) Stomach
   c) Gallbladder
   d) Liver

23. The ovaries are paired _____ located in the upper pelvic cavity on each side of the uterus.
   a) intestines
   b) glands
   c) appendages
   d) ducts

24. The simplest nerve receptors _____:
   a) are found throughout the stomach tissue.
   b) are free nerve endings that sense touch and pain.
   c) die very easily if you are dehydrated.
   d) also carry blood to organs.

25. The liver makes _____ to help with blood clotting.

 a) heparin, prothrombin, thrombin

 b) leukocytes and eosinophils

 c) vitamin K

 d) thyroxin and thyrosine

Case Studies/Critical Thinking

A. Charles Rester is a regular weekly client for a full-body massage. He is 52-years-old, in very good health, and plays golf at least twice a week. Three days before his massage appointment, Rester slipped on wet grass and fell down a small hill. He landed in the middle of a small ditch after hitting his left calf area on a drainage pipe. During his massage session today, you notice bruises (ecchymosis) that are purplish to black in color on the back of his lower leg. Would you feel the area to see if it is hot to the touch? Should you apply heat and cold alternately at the site of the bruise to encourage macrophage activity to clean up the area? Is doing anything to the bruised area within your scope of practice? Can you proceed with the rest of the massage while avoiding the area of the bruise?

B. Angela has called to tell you she is not feeling well and will reschedule her appointment. After asking her a few questions, you find out that she has nasal discharge, a sore throat, a slight fever, and a headache. She seems to have all the symptoms of a common cold. Should you tell her to come on in because a massage would make her feel better, or do you ask her to reschedule for at least five days out? If you were to proceed with a massage, would you use circulatory massage techniques? Would a massage during the acute stage of the infection spread the cold virus more quickly through Angela's body?

C. Ola Mae Stetson is a resident of an elderly care facility. She has Alzheimer's and has been receiving massage weekly for the past three months. She usually hums and smiles during the massage, but today she is confused about getting on the table and rocks back and forth with a frown on her face. Because she has Alzheimer's, she cannot communicate with words. Is she trying to tell you there has been a change in how she perceives massage? Do you think she will be comfortable while on the table and being touched? Could her condition have changed since her appointment last week? What should you do?

References for information in this chapter can be found in Quick Guide C at the end of the book.

PART III

Beyond the Basic Curriculum

CHAPTER 10   **Maternity, Infant, and Pediatric Massage**

CHAPTER 11   **Massage for Special Populations (Children with Special Needs, Geriatric, Hospice & Palliative Care)**

CHAPTER 12   **Massage for Survivors of Abuse**

CHAPTER 13   **Sports Massage: For Amateur and Professional Athletes**

CHAPTER 14   **Spa Therapy: Peace, Beauty, and Massage**

Maternity, Infant, and Pediatric Massage

LEARNING OUTCOMES

After completing this chapter, you will be able to:

- Recognize proper massage techniques and procedures for pregnancy and postpartum massage.

- Recognize the physiological changes of pregnancy and how massage impacts these changes.

- Explain the importance of touch during pregnancy.

- Recognize indications and contraindications for pregnancy massage.

- Explain the importance of touch during infancy and childhood.

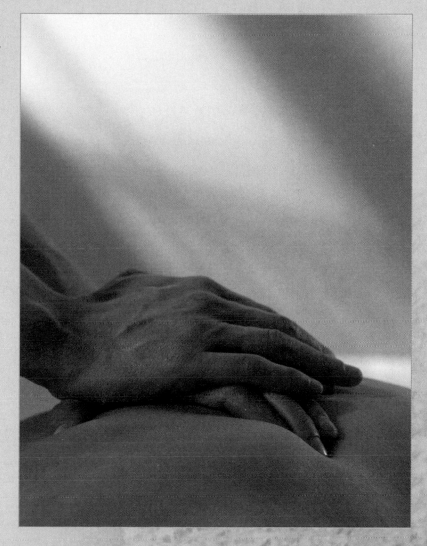

KEY TERMS

bonding *(p. 280)*
estrogen *(p. 274)*
femoral vein *(p. 275)*
fibrinolysis *(p. 275)*
Field, Tiffany *(p. 280)*
human chorionic gonadotropin
   (HCG) *(p. 274)*

inferior vena cava *(p. 275)*
maternity massage *(p. 266)*
progesterone *(p. 274)*
relaxin *(p. 274)*
shea or cocoa butter *(p. 274)*

supine hypotensive
   syndrome *(p. 272)*
touch relaxation *(p. 285)*
Touch Research Institute *(p. 268)*

INTRODUCTION

While all work in the massage field is deeply rewarding, many massage therapists find working with mothers and children to be especially meaningful. Helping a woman cope with the challenges and changes of pregnancy—both physical and emotional—can be quite rewarding for the therapist. Introducing a newborn to massage and playing a role in strengthening the mother-child bond are gifts in themselves. Massage further offers a means for parents to stay connected to their children as they grow.

    This chapter includes sections called "Applications of Theory and Practice." These sections offer additional content for those who want to study these massage specialties in greater depth.

Prenatal, Labor, and Postpartum Massage

By Carla DiMauro, BBA, LMT

Maternity massage (including prenatal, during labor, and postpartum) offers an opportunity for the massage therapist to provide physical and emotional support for clients during pregnancy, childbirth, and during the postpartum period.

    One of the greatest miracles of life is the process of gestation and childbirth. It is a transitional time in a woman's life that requires special attention; to share in this phenomenon unites us as human beings. Massage therapy is an effective form of complementary health care providing many benefits to the woman and baby, as well as great rewards to the therapist. This connection exemplifies the ancient Chinese philosophy that regards humans and the universe as one undifferentiated and integrated whole.

    While massage therapy is never intended to replace appropriate prenatal care, it does supplement such care by providing women with both physical and emotional benefits. This assertion contradicts the teachings that most massage therapists have had over the years; indeed, some massage schools still teach that pregnancy is a contraindication to massage. It is important to understand, however, that pregnancy is a time of major physiological, psychological, spiritual, and social changes. Many of these changes produce discomforts and concerns, all of which can be addressed with appropriate massage therapy.

    Studies have shown that the more a pregnant woman learns about and understands her changing body and the process of childbirth, the more her satisfaction and participation increase and the need for pain medication decreases. Learning what is normal in her body can relieve her worries, allowing for a positive and deeply satisfying experience, rather than one filled with fear and anxiety. The same holds true for the massage practitioner; the more that can be learned and understood about a pregnant woman's physiological and emotional changes, the less apprehensive a therapist will be in using massage.

    With the advent of alternative health care practices, interest in natural childbirth has increased. Mother-baby-centered birthing options including water-birthing, home deliveries, and birthing centers with midwife and doula assistance are growing in popularity. Massage therapists can take an active role in supporting the mother-to-be and her team of natural childbirth professionals in providing her with the nurturing and support her body needs through this natural process.

Physiological Changes

Every pregnant woman is aware of the many discomforts of pregnancy. As blood flow increases, more oxygen is required, leaving many women to experience hot flashes. These women may become irritable, depressed, and fearful. The baby's increasing weight strains muscles from the neck all the way down to the feet. The mother's body continues to stretch more and more to accommodate the uterus.

In addition to these physical changes are psychological pressures. While this is a blessed event for most, there are also mothers-to-be who are overworked, stressed, or experiencing tension and pressures in the home. The pregnancy experience is not as joyful for some women as for others. Unfortunately, too much stress can lead to toxic buildup in the body and this is unhealthy.

EXAM POINT Historically, massage during pregnancy was contraindicated because it was thought to release toxins into the system and harm the baby. Today, it is considered an indication as an important part of pregnancy to assist the lymphatic system in the removal of toxins from the cells.

Fortunately, massage can safely, comfortably, and effectively relieve much of the increased stress and physical discomforts that women encounter during pregnancy.

EXAM POINT Stress activates the sympathetic branch of the autonomic nervous system (the unconscious branch). High levels of stress can have a negative impact during pregnancy, childbirth and in babies' early development.

EXAM POINT Relaxation activates the parasympathetic branch of the autonomic nervous system, which positively affects physiological changes that promote health. This is essential to maximize uterine blood flow, which carries much needed nutrients and oxygen to the baby and ensures efficient removal of waste.

Muscle tension and stress decrease nutrient absorption and toxin elimination for healthy cells. Research reveals the following effects of stress on pregnancy:

- Increase in heart rate, blood pressure, nausea, and toxemia
- Reduced blood supply to the uterus
- Weakening of the immune system
- Increase in maternal complications, miscarriages, premature births, and prolonged labor
- Increase in postpartum complications
- Problems with fetal nervous system development, fetal distress, and low birth weight

Research now shows that the increased levels of stress hormones in the pregnant woman's body can be passed to the unborn baby which can negatively affect their development. This could be a possible cause of infant depression and other disorders such as ADHD which are so prevalent in our society today.

Massage promotes deep relaxation. It is during this state that a pregnant woman's circulation improves, more nutrients are absorbed and the lymphatic system works more efficiently to remove toxins.

A reduction in stress can have the following positive results:

- Increased parasympathetic response and endorphin levels
- Increased systemic and local blood circulation
- Decreased anxiety and depression
- Decreased stress hormones, cortisol, and norepinephrine
- Decreased heart rate and blood pressure

Why Massage During Pregnancy?

⭐ **EXAM POINT** Relaxation activates the parasympathetic branch of the autonomic nervous system which helps the body reduce stress and promote health and well-being.

This helps the pregnant woman's body find balance and adjust to the necessary changes taking place. During the first trimester, massage can help relieve headaches, alleviate morning sickness and nausea, and reduce fatigue. The benefits will shift in the second trimester to alleviating backaches, leg cramps, and sciaticlike pain. For many women, this pain begins in the second trimester as the pelvis extends, especially at the joint of the sacrum and pelvic bone on both sides. The resulting sensation is a burning feeling as if the sciatic nerve is inflamed, referring pain down the leg or just in the calf. Massage of the back and legs helps to relax the muscles around the joints and reduce the burning sensation. Benefits during the last trimester include reducing swelling and helping to alleviate insomnia.

Massage will benefit pregnancy in relieving overall muscle soreness due to exercise or sitting too much by releasing the lactic acid that builds up in muscle tissues. Pressure is also created in the sciatic nerve area by sitting too much, thus causing strain and soreness in the legs as the baby gains weight. Massage will not only help alleviate the stress caused by excessive sitting, but it will also work those inactive muscles by toning them.

Massage will aid in overall muscle tone and elasticity. This is especially important as the baby grows and the woman's body must change to accommodate this growth.

⭐ **EXAM POINT** The obvious changes that a pregnant woman's body goes through is evidence enough to clearly support the need for frequent massage therapy. The skin of the abdomen, breasts and surrounding tissue are stretched to the extreme. With the increase in breast size and while the uterus enlarges, her upper, mid and lower back are strained as her center of gravity shifts. Her legs and feet also experience tension, cramps and spasm as they must bear the additional weight.

Massage is known for its ability to maintain the flexibility in muscles, ligaments, tendons, and joints as the baby grows. Furthermore, massage reduces the stress on the weight-bearing joints and related musculofascial structures, and relieves muscle spasms, cramps, and myofascial pain, especially in the back, neck, hips, and legs.

Studies have shown that emotional support and nurturing touch are important benefits of massage for the pregnant woman. It provides her with the positive experience of nuturing touch, so that she may in turn provide this for her baby. The outcome of labor is improved in many ways in women who have received massage throughout their pregnancy. Massage also promotes postpartum recovery—both physically and emotionally—and provides support for the woman experiencing the stresses of new motherhood.

The **Touch Research Institute** conducted the most recent and specific study of massage for laboring women. Mothers receiving massage from their partners during labor experienced decreased levels of anxiety and pain. They needed less medication, and their labors were shorter than those of the control group receiving only routine obstetrical care. Massage therapy techniques are as effective during labor as they are during the prenatal period. Benefits include reducing stress and promoting relaxation, relieving muscle tension and cramping, and providing support for physical and emotional needs that arise during labor and delivery.

Hydrotherapy

> ★ **EXAM POINT** Cold applications may be used to reduce discomfort and pose no harm to the expectant mother or baby. Hot packs should be used sparingly and limited to applications of less than 20 minutes at a very mild temperature.

Anything that rapidly raises the pregnant woman's body temperature, even one degree, is dangerous for the baby. Prolonged heat applications should be avoided altogether in the first 20 weeks, as this could interfere with the development of the fetus. When receiving spa treatments, pregnant women should not use the sauna, whirlpool, hot tub, or steam room. Only body wraps that utilize no heat, produce no temperature increases, and do not produce sweating would be indicated.

Massage Techniques to Reduce Pain

A variety of bodywork techniques can be used to provide relief and reduce back pain during pregnancy and after. Specialized training programs are available for pregnancy massage, and a therapist's increased level of confidence gained by this training can only enhance client feelings of well-being.

The most commonly used techniques are Swedish massage, gentle acupressure (shiatsu), reflexology, passive stretching, assisted-resisted stretches, postural retraining, lymphatic drainage, strain-counterstrain or positional release, skin rolling, lomi lomi, myofascial release, cross-fiber friction, and craniosacral therapy.

Musculoskeletal pain and discomforts should be addressed in sessions with careful and accurate attention to proper positioning. Pain from the massage should never exceed a 7 on a pain threshold scale of 1 to 10, with 10 being the most painful. While every person feels pain differently, a 7 marks the point where increasing pressure begins to change from purely pleasurable to mild discomfort. First and foremost, a prenatal massage must always be gentle and relaxing. This is especially true during the first trimester, when the woman is at highest risk of miscarriage. No one is exactly sure what causes miscarriage during this time; however, experts believe that some dramatic change is responsible. An apprehensive therapist may feel more comfortable in instructing the newly pregnant woman to wait until her thirteenth week to receive massage and allow her body to get used to the changes and new sensations of her first trimester. A capable massage therapist understands that this is the time when the woman is most vulnerable to miscarriage and will avoid anything but the most gentle, relaxing strokes. No abdominal massage should ever be performed in the first trimester, nor any compressions, friction, or deep tissue in the lower back region. Massage can be performed more strongly once the woman enters her third trimester and increase in intensity through labor and delivery.

A more gentle massage during pregnancy is important for other reasons as well. Heart rate and blood pressure rise during massage techniques that may initiate pain. As her circulatory system adjusts to metabolic demands, the woman may already be experiencing these changes naturally. Studies show that the baby needs stable blood pressure and a constant heart rate, which is produced through deeply relaxing massage techniques. Anything else may have a negative impact on the baby. The baby is most comfortable when it feels gentle, rhythmic strokes. A massage therapist should never use any deep tissue or "digging" techniques with the thumb or fingertips directly into

Figure 10.1

The lumbosacral stretch is a passive pelvic tilt used to reduce hip and low back pain.

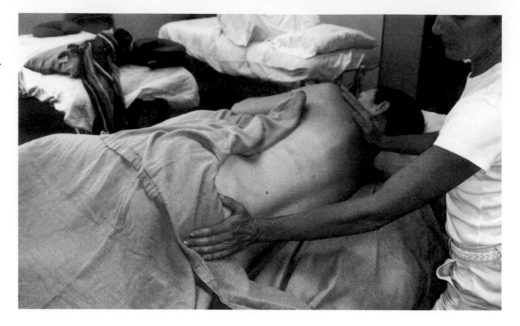

the muscle or tissue. Massage techniques can only be done with the flats of the thumbs and fingers, whole hand, or palm without any potential negative impact on the expectant mother or baby. The lightest pressure is beneficial as it stimulates lymphatic drainage and blood flow. Gentle palmar effleurage effectively reduces inflammation and pain in the sciatic area without further irritation. Myofascial techniques, such as the lumbosacral stretch (figure 10.1), are always most effective when exercised with great patience and control, moving at the slowest pace possible to allow the tissues to release themselves naturally.

TECHNIQUE EMPHASIS Massage during pregnancy is best performed using gentle, slow, nurturing techniques to produce the optimal results.

Contraindications and Precautions

Abdominal Massage

Abdominal massage should be avoided in the first trimester when the risk of miscarriage is the highest. It should only be performed with superficial, gentle effleurage strokes thereafter. Appropriate direction is always clockwise.

Reflex Massage

Reflex massage should be avoided in the first trimester. Release points of acupuncture, which produce uterine contractions, should be avoided throughout the pregnancy until the due date. These points include spleen 6 or "triple yin," where the spleen, kidney, and liver meridians meet (four finger widths' proximal to the malleolus, along the tibia border); kidney 3 (on the superior border and just posterior to the medial malleolus); liver 3 (proximal border of the first and second metatarsal bones); and the large intestine point 4 in the fleshy part between the index finger and the thumb. Overstimulation of these points of expulsion during massage can cause the vagina to relax, the cervix to open, and the embryo to be discharged. During labor, it is precisely these points that are worked on to speed up delivery.

There are several additional release points where only broad, general pressures should be applied: along the neck and collarbone area at gallbladder 21 (halfway between the nape of the neck and the acromion process); around the shoulder blades where it is sensitive at the insertion of the rhomboids; and the areas of the bladder meridians 31–34 near the lower sacrum. Overstimulation of these areas—while less potent—can result in bleeding, spotting, mild contractions, premature labor, and a shift in the position of the baby.

Deep Tissue Techniques

Deep tissue techniques should be restricted to areas of muscular pain and never done in the abdomen or medial portion of the legs (due to clotting and varicose veins). Caution should always be exercised because of the softening results of the relaxin hormone.

Joint Movements

Joint movements should not include rocking during times of nausea. Extreme care should be given to avoid excess movement with pubic symphysis separation to avoid excruciating pain. Extreme range of motion should be limited at all times due to the affects of relaxin.

Swedish Massage

Swedish massage and other techniques that promote venous return should not be performed during the third trimester on pregnant women who have heart disease. The legs of women on bed rest should not be massaged to avoid possible thrombosis.

High-Risk Pregnancies

Women with high-risk pregnancies are oftentimes the ones most in need of massage. However, this should only be done with a doctor's permission. The following conditions are regarded as high risk by the American College of Obstetrics and Gynecology:

- Previous complications in pregnancy
- Multiple pregnancy
- Drug exposure
- Diabetes
- Heart disorder
- Chronic hypertension
- Under 20 or over 35 years of age
- Asthma

Trimester Positioning and Recommendations

The massage table should be placed higher than usual. Since no deep pressure will be used that a lower setting facilitates, it is more convenient for the therapist to work at waist level using proper body mechanics at all times. Working on the client's back in a side-lying position may be a little awkward at first, but with practice, your own style will develop comfortably. You should take extra care to keep your wrists straight in line with the forearms at all times to prevent any muscular strain. The only pressure applied should come as a result of your "rocking" into each compression or stroke. A small stool may be used to help the woman get on and off the table more comfortably.

First Trimester

During the first trimester, studies show that massage can effectively relieve headaches, help alleviate morning sickness and nausea, reduce fatigue, and stimulate blood flow to assist in the prevention of anemia. Caution should be used, as chance of miscarriage is the highest during this period.

Prone and supine positioning are both safe and acceptable. Structural stresses are minimal, but consideration should be given to comfort as the woman's breasts may become enlarged and tender. As her therapist, you should be sensitive to her emotional needs and give her the opportunity to express her feelings about the pregnancy and any concerns that she may have. Listen supportively and refrain from giving advice, referring her to other professionals if she should discuss concerns that are outside the scope of massage practice.

Second Trimester

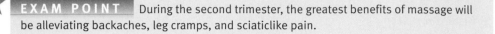

⭐ **EXAM POINT** During the second trimester, the greatest benefits of massage will be alleviating backaches, leg cramps, and sciaticlike pain.

The woman's body begins to experience structural stresses on the lower back, upper spine, and pectoral girdle as the baby begins to "show." Skin stretching, muscle cramping, and uterine ligament strain also begin to occur. Varicose veins may begin to develop. During the second trimester, a pregnant woman can still lie on her back easily and comfortably (figure 10.2). From week 14 to 22, a small pillow should be placed under the right hip in supine position. In side-lying position, the pillow should be placed under the abdomen on the right side (figure 10.3).

⭐ **EXAM POINT** Take all precautions to prevent **supine hypotensive syndrome**, which results from the weight of the uterus on the inferior vena cava and leads to a rapid decrease in blood pressure, causing fainting and dizziness. Fetal blood circulation is also challenged.

Figure 10.2
Semireclining position should be used after 22 weeks to avoid supine hypotension.

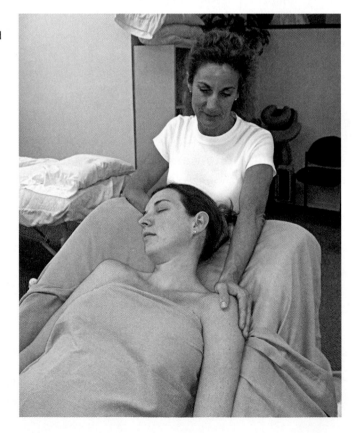

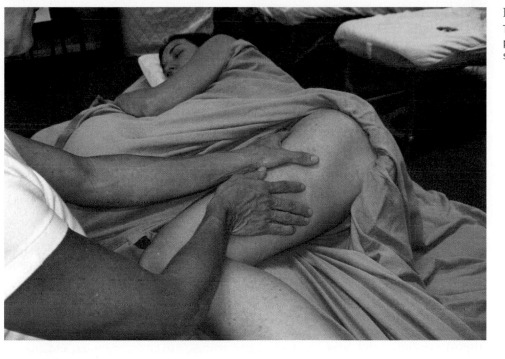

Figure 10.3
The safest position for pregnancy massage is side-lying.

To ensure complete relaxation, the woman's knees should be bent using proper bolstering underneath for low back support. A pillow can be placed under her head, neck, and shoulders to make breathing easier, taking the strain off the diaphragm that is caused by enlarged breasts and expanding belly. If the pregnant client expresses any discomfort in supine position, then side-lying position should be utilized. In a side-lying position, the lower leg should be straight and the upper leg bent so that the lower portion is parallel with the table and the thigh is perpendicular to the table. Pillows or support cushions are placed under the flexed top leg, bringing the knee to a level that is equidistant with the hip. The body cushion support system (see chapter 2) is ideal for side-lying positioning to allow extra space for the shoulder girdle. An additional pillow should be given to her to hug, providing support for the arm superior to the torso. Prone position should be avoided. Tables or support cushions that encourage prone positioning are not recommended because uterine ligaments can be further stretched and lumbar conditions worsened as pressure is placed on the lower back area.

Third Trimester

> **EXAM POINT** Once the client enters the last trimester of her pregnancy, most of the massage will be performed in the side-lying position.

Supine positioning should be done only in a semireclining position. A table with an adjustable back, a medical wedge, and other support cushions are best to support the pregnant woman. The torso should be positioned at a 45-degree angle with a bolster under the knees and low back in correct position, flush to the back support cushions, to avoid excess lumbar curvature.

The most notable benefits of massage relate to reduction of swelling and relief from insomnia. The size of the baby or unusual positioning of the organs can cause numbness and tingling from compression on nerves and continued structural pain and fatigue. Massage can bring considerable relief and is known for its ability to maintain the flexibility in muscles, tendons, ligaments, and joints needed during the final growth stage of the baby in utero.

Applications of
Theory and
Practice for
Massage During
Pregnancy:
Organized by
Body System

System Changes Massage

A pregnant woman's body experiences many changes that are profound on both local and systemic levels. It is important to recognize and understand these changes and how they affect the provision of appropriately supportive massage therapy practices.

Endocrine System

EXAM POINT The endocrine system orchestrates changes such as mood swings and altered metabolic functions. The pituitary, thyroid, and adrenal glands increase in size. The pregnancy hormone **estrogen** stimulates uterine growth and blood supply.

It balances salt, water, and insulin levels as well as increases metabolic efficiency in sugar and carbohydrate utilization. The increased production of estrogen lends itself to many alterations in mood. In one day, a pregnant woman's body produces as much estrogen as a nonpregnant woman does in three years. Most of this production is placental in origin and occurs only with the help of the fetus.

The pregnancy hormone **progesterone** increases energy storage by promoting fat disposition in the pelvic area, quadriceps, hamstrings, and gluteal muscles, and around internal organs. It relaxes smooth muscles in the digestive tract, thus maximizing intestinal absorption time and uptake of iron, calcium, and other nutrients; in the uterine muscles to prevent excessive, premature contractions; and in the vascular walls to maintain a healthy low blood pressure. Decreased peristalsis function is often a side effect of the increased production of progesterone. Shortness of breath—a common complaint during pregnancy—is a corresponding hormonal effect and does not occur just from weight gain alone.

Human chorionic gonadotropin (HCG) prevents the mother's body from rejecting the embryo. Body temperature in the mother increases as a result of an increase in the basal metabolic rate produced by HCG.

Relaxin increases the elasticity in the connective tissue. It softens the ligament of the pelvic joints to increase the capacity of the pelvis, making it more pliable to open for delivery. Massage therapists should avoid extreme range-of-motion techniques as her joints become loose and these techniques may cause discomfort, pain or injury.

Research shows that massage therapy assists the glandular system, stabilizing hormonal levels and lessening the severity of side effects. The thyroid gland often overproduces in pregnancy, causing "hot flashes," irritability, and increased breathing frequency and pulse. Maintaining and balancing this gland through massage can control the negative side effects. The adrenal glands are also believed to be a cause of swelling. Massage is one of the most effective ways for regulating the adrenal gland and reducing edema. Another important gland affected by massage is the thymus gland, which is stimulated by massage to boost the immune system and help fight off infection.

Integumentary System

The fascia, muscles, and skin of the abdomen and breasts are stretching and enlarging by the eighth week of pregnancy. Skin can change color and become dry or oily.

EXAM POINT Lubricants such as **shea or cocoa butter** will help mosturize the overstreached skin and may minimize the apprearance of stretch marks.

Circulatory System

Pregnant women's bodies respond to metabolic demands with many internal changes in the circulatory system. The enlarging uterus compromises circulation.

EXAM POINT The heart enlarges, changes position (moving more upward, anterior and to the left), and increases the volume of strokes up to 32% by the twenty-eighth week.

There is an increase in the number of blood vessels, components, volume, and interstitial fluids. Since red blood cell components increase at lower rates, many pregnant women become anemic. A woman's diet and prolonged sitting or standing can also contribute to edema and varicose veins.

Fibrolynic activity is decreased, which can lead to the development of thrombi. Some discomfort is produced when clots accumulate in the vessels but pose no major threat unless inflammation or infection develops. **Fibrinolysis,** the body's bloodclotting capacity, increases during pregnancy to prevent hemorrhaging. Clots can dislodge five to six times more frequently in pregnancy, which can result in thrombophlebitis or thromboembolism, the highest risk being in the third trimester and postpartum. While most women will develop clots during pregnancy, the less active a woman is, the higher the likelihood of thrombi. Women on bed rest are also at higher risk, as are those who are obese.

The pulse rate increases, and functional changes include heart murmurs and palpitations, which are the result of fatigue, emotional stress, and overexertion. With the additional weight and increased pressure of the uterus on the pelvic veins, many women may develop varicose veins during pregnancy. Increased pressure on the **femoral vein,** the longest and thickest, challenges the integrity *of the valves of the femoral and saphenous veins* already compromised by progesterone's relaxation of the smooth muscle walls.

The discomforts of edema, high blood pressure, and varicose veins can be effectively relieved through massage therapy. Techniques common to Swedish and lymphatic drainage massage—such as effleurage, petrissage, and pumping—promote circulation of blood and lymph, and support healthy circulatory function. Precautions for leg massage must be taken due to the decrease in fibrolynic activity. This includes careful consideration of the "valley of the clots" or medial portion of the leg housing the femoral and saphenous veins. Deep tissue massage and any kind of stripping techniques should be avoided in this area as such techniques could dislodge clots. Leg discomforts indicating possible clotting include edema, heat, redness, and constant achiness. All Swedish massage on the legs should be avoided with women on bed rest.

Considerations for massage would include careful positioning to prevent supine hypotensive syndrome. Supine hypotensive syndrome can occur when the weight of the uterus presses against the **inferior vena cava,** which runs between the spine and the uterus. Symptoms include dizziness or fainting as a result of restricted blood flow back to the heart; after the twenty-third week, the pregnant woman should be placed only in a semireclining position. This can easily be done with pillows or a medical wedge with bolstering under her knees for low back support.

Respiratory System

The expectant mother experiences changes in respiration, both functionally and structurally.

EXAM POINT Elevated levels of progesterone prompt an increase in tidal volume.

Respiratory rate increases along with the volume of air taken with every breath. Increased intake of oxygen improves supply to the fetus, which enables easier transfer of carbon dioxide from the fetal to the maternal blood. As the fetus grows and occupies more space in the abdominal cavity, the mother's breathing relies more on the movement of the ribs than on the diaphragm.

> **★ EXAM POINT** The rib cage elevates and flares with the growing uterus, and the diaphragm elevates as much as 4 cm. Breathing occurs more in the upper lobes of the lung, and the woman has a tendency to rotate the pectoral girdle anteriorly.

With enlarged abdomen and breasts, the mother tends to lean backward for balance, which shifts the upper thoracic region more anteriorly, further aggravating respiration as well as structural integrity. To compensate, her head and neck jut forward.

These compensations strain all of the upper body musculature. Appropriate massage therapy and breathing exercises will promote relaxation, reduce stress, relieve musculoskeletal strain on the neck, chest, and upper back, and improve breathing and respiration. A "sawing" technique, using the side of the hand and flats of the fingertips, can reduce strain in the scalenes and intercostals and help to decrease neck pain. Myofascial release techniques can reduce strain in the pectoralis major and minor, and help to decrease the anterior rounding of the shoulder girdle.

Postural retraining, such as the Alexander technique, will make her more comfortable where the objective is not to be perfect but aware. Instruction in pelvic tilts will help her realign the pelvis to support the weight of the torso. Traditionally, many expectant women are taught pelvic tilts through the tightening of the gluteus maximus and hamstring muscle groups, which tend to hold the pelvis in an unnaturally clenched position. The body then has a tendency to thrust the weight back toward the heels.

> **TECHNIQUE EMPHASIS** A passive tilt is more appropriate for gentle alignment and pelvic support. The massage therapist's focus should be on encouraging the psoas muscle to contract. One way this can be done is by having the woman think about moving into a sitting position but instead of going down, lift the hips forward and up, and keep the spine erect.

Your goal as the massage therapist is to help foster deeper diaphragmatic breathing patterns in the expectant mother.

Gastrointestinal and Urinary Systems

Many of the more noticeable discomforts pregnant women experience are related to the digestive tract. The most common complaints are nausea, heartburn, indigestion, and constipation. Morning sickness generally begins between the second and sixth week and ends by the fourteenth week. Heartburn and indigestion are due in part to the displacement of the digestive organs and the high levels of progesterone, which relaxes smooth muscles and lowers tone in the digestive tract. The expanding uterus pushes the stomach and the intestines up and to the side, causing the valve at the top of the stomach where the esophagus enters to work less efficiently. This shift in position is the probable cause of heartburn, *which is experienced by 75% of all pregnant women.* As food takes longer to move through the stomach and intestines because of the increased smoothness of the muscle, more water is absorbed from the stool, which then tends to harden. Peristaltic activity is also decreased, leading to constipation, *which is experienced by 25% of all pregnant women.*

A few of the urinary dysfunctions and discomforts experienced by the expectant mother include frequency of urination, kidney and bladder infections, and stress incontinence. The enlarged uterus presses down on the bladder, reducing space and slowing urination. Like the digestive tract, the urinary tract is made of smooth muscle, which loses tone as a result of the higher levels of progesterone, and it takes longer for the bladder to empty. This—in addition to the tremendous load on the kidneys to filter waste for both mother and baby—increases the chance of urinary infections. Urinary stress incontinence, which occurs in nearly 50% of all pregnant women, is a result of the strain placed on the pelvic floor muscles by the additional weight gain during pregnancy and possible damage to the pelvic floor during vaginal birth because of weak muscle tissue.

The use of Kegel exercises, the tightening of the pelvic floor muscles, are useful in relieving the symptoms of bladder dysfunction. Massage therapist will do well to remind their pregnant clients to practice "Kegels" on a daily basis. With advanced training, a massage therapist can use reflexive massage in the hands and feet to stimulate peristalsis, reduce nausea, and relieve bladder symptoms. Ohashiatsu, a gentle shiatsu technique developed by Ohashi of the Ohashiatsu Institute in New York, can help restore energy flows throughout meridians in the body to improve digestion and enhance bladder and kidney functions.

No passive joint movement, range of motion, or rocking should be performed with women experiencing nausea as this will aggravate the condition. Pregnant clients should be encouraged to urinate before the session to avoid interrupting the session; however, such interruptions may be unavoidable during the last month when the pressure of the uterus is greatest on the bladder. Allow ample time and patience during the massage session to accommodate these minor inconveniences.

Musculoskeletal System

The additional anterior weight from the growing uterus creates a shift in the woman's natural balance.

⭐ **EXAM POINT** In order to compensate for this imbalance, the muscles of the back, hips and legs become tense and overstressed.

With the increasing anterior weight, she becomes "front heavy" and the pregnant woman will find herself leaning back in order to counterbalance the shift in her center of gravity. This often strains the scalenes in the anterior cervical musculature as well as creating tension in the posterior cervical muscles. Her jaw may become tight as a result of this tension while the chin arches forward. The entire back muscles, from the attachments at the occiput all the way down to the iliac crest, will become tense and in a continuous state of overuse while standing or walking.

As the breasts and abdomen become larger, most pregnant women will begin to experience tension, discomfort and pain in the upper and mid back. As the rib cage flares due to the enlarging uterus, the intercostals muscles tend to stretch and become irritated.

The additional weight and anterior rotation of the pelvis creates pressure in the hips as well as the lower lumbar and sacral regions. As the uterus grows, the hips externally rotate creating tension in the lateral hip rotators. Her legs have to support this additional weight and the hip movers will often become tense with frequent occurrence of spasms, as well as the gastrocnemius muscles and arches of the feet.

The most stressed muscles for the pregnant client can be identified as trapezius, erector spinae, quadratus lumborum, psoas, hip rotators, gluteals, pectoralis major and minor, intercostals, and abdominals. The massage therapy session should address these groups specifically.

The greatest impact from stress on the weight-bearing joints is felt in the intervertebral (semimovable) and facet (gliding) joints, particularly in the lumbar spine, lumbosacral joint, sacroiliac joints, pubic symphysis, and hip joints. This impact is increased in women who exceed the recommended weight gain. As her body produces more of the hormone relaxin, which causes her connective tissue to soften, she may experience soreness and additional discomforts in these weightbearing joints. This is felt not only in the specific joint structure, but also radiates into the surrounding soft tissue of the glutes, lower lumbar and pubic areas.

EXAM POINT Extreme care should be given to pregnant women as they change position during the massage session and as they get on and off the table to prevent any additional pain in these highly stressed joints.

Because of the increased levels of relaxin, caution should be exercised when performing range of motion or any deeper work in the joint areas.

TECHNIQUE EMPHASIS Only gentle compressions should be applied on the left side when relieving pressure in the area of the sacroiliac joint, because this is the side where the placenta is connected to the body; if too much pressure is applied in this area, it could break a weak connection.

Over nine months of pregnancy, the vast expanse of the uterus is suspended by the supportive structures of ligaments that, through continually stretching, refer pain beyond their attachment sites. The two broad ligaments extend laterally and are attached to the internal pelvic walls. The increased strain by the sixth month creates pain that is referred to the low back and buttocks region. This may be misinterpreted by the expectant mother as sciatica and usually disappears around the seventh month. Two round ligaments arise from the anterior, superior surface of the uterus and attach in the connective tissue of the pubic area (mons). Increased strain in the round ligament during the second trimester creates one-sided diagonal groin pain. Sensitivity exists because, whereas ligaments traditionally connect bone to muscle, this connection is soft tissue to soft tissue. The sacrouterine ligaments connect the posterior uterus to the posterior pelvic cavity wall at the anterior surface of the sacrum. Pain may be referred from the sacrouterine ligament as a deep achiness anterior and lateral to the sacrum and occurs more commonly in the third trimester.

Labor and Postpartum

Massage can also be helpful during both labor and postpartum. Most of the massage techniques discussed can be adapted for these stages, and there are a few additional techniques you can use during labor. Massage is just one tool a partner or labor coach may use during labor to facilitate relaxation and help ease discomfort. Studies show that decreased muscle tension decreases labor pain. When massaging a woman in labor, focus on areas that she feels need attention.

For back pain during labor, compressions on the sacrum can bring some welcome relief. A variation of this technique is to compress on the sacrum while she rocks back and forth on her hands and knees. The sides of the hips can also be compressed. This will open the pelvis and give the baby more room to move down the birth canal. To reduce uterine and abdominal pain, apply deep compressions using the knuckles, fingers, or hand on the outside edge of the erector spinae and sacrospinalis muscles next to the spine.

Depending on where she feels muscle tension most, use a combination of compression, firm effleurage, and petrissage on problem areas such as the upper trapezius and shoulders. Apply constant pressure during a contraction; effleurage and petrissage between contractions. Massage techniques may be helpful to relieve stress in her jaw and forehead due to strain and clenching of the teeth. Compress on the side of the jaw during a contraction and perform gentle, circular effleurage between contractions. Massaging the hands and feet will soothe the nervous system and can be very comforting to laboring women throughout the entire process. A useful technique to use during labor is to take the big toe and the next two toes and squeeze them together at the same time. This helps create reflexive relaxation on the inside of the thigh and pelvic floor muscles. Because tightness of the abdominal muscles keeps the baby from moving down the birth canal, gentle effleurage between contractions can be used to soothe and relax abdominal muscles. Muscle cramps can also be relieved between contractions by petrissaging the calf muscles. Work deeply in the area above the ankle, specifically around the *tsubo* point spleen 6 or "triple yin," where the three yin meridians of the lower leg (spleen, liver, and kidney) meet. Massage is an effective way to reduce stress and create relaxation, and relaxation promotes a faster, easier labor.

Postdelivery massage offers continuing benefits to the woman. Emotionally, it provides the support for the new mother experiencing changes in her schedule and lifestyle. She may be lacking support from the extended family and will find massage a time of restoration and a means of tapping into new resources of inner strength. "Baby blues"— postpartum depression—affects nearly 85% of all new mothers to some degree, and massage provides the woman with the extra nurturing she needs to bond with and nurture her baby. Postdelivery massage stimulates glandular activity and stabilizes hormone levels, which reduces depression.

Research shows that, physically, massage promotes restoration of the abdomen and weight-bearing joints, alleviates muscle strain and fatigue caused by labor and delivery, and restores prepregnancy physiological function through enhanced circulation and removal of waste (lymphatic drainage).

Recovery from a cesarean section is much quicker if a woman is receiving regular massage. Continue positioning as you would during her last trimester (side-lying and semireclining). Avoid any deep tissue work; your focus should be on enhanced circulation to promote healing.

Finally, massage is effective in reducing the muscle strain and structural stress of carrying and caring for a newborn. Breast-feeding brings new muscular aches in the midback region, shoulders, and arms from holding the baby in new positions. New muscle strain occurs as the baby gains weight and can be appropriately addressed with massage therapy.

Full-body Swedish massage is most effective postpartum with appropriate combinations of lymphatic drainage, trigger point therapy, myofascial release, neuromuscular reeducation, and stretching exercises. Reflexology and acupressure may also facilitate postpartum relaxation and recovery.

Infant and Pediatric Massage

Infants and children are the focus of infant and pediatric massage. Touch helps the baby's systems to function by providing tactile stimulation and a connection. Massage therapists can encourage emotional bonding between parents and children by working with families to teach them massage techniques.

★ **EXAM POINT** Scientific research shows that tactile stimulation plays an essential role in the development of stronger, more complete nerve connections in the brain.

Nurturing touch to the mother enhances energy flow to the fetus, which strengthens development of the nervous system. Healthy nerve connection patterns established early in a child's life contribute to important facets of growth that affect development in communication, intelligence, and coordination.

Parent-Child Bonding Through Massage

Infant massage is becoming more and more popular among new parents and caregivers in America because of its benefits: deeper sleep patterns, relief from colic and digestive

Chapter 10 Maternity, Infant, and Pediatric Massage

problems, healthy personality development, and stress control. While many massage students relish the idea of working on babies, the therapist's focus should be on instructing parents and caregivers in how to massage their babies. While numerous physiological benefits exist, the greatest benefit is that it enhances bonding. **Bonding** is described as "a unique relationship between two people that is specific and endures through time." In animals, the crucial period for bonding is within minutes or hours after birth and takes place through licking and touching. Similarly, as studies paralleling animal research have shown, there is also a sensitive period of bonding in humans. Affection and tactile stimulation create bonds between caregiver and baby that ensure positive interaction and healthy development throughout their lives.

In his book *Touching*, world-renowned anthropologist Ashley Montague's basic thesis is that touch is a form of social communication that crosses species, cultures, genders, and age groups. As we discussed in the Overview and Introduction, without touch, there may be growth deprivation, communication failures, aggression, and war. According to Montague, "Even though touch is the largest sense organ in the body, it is the one that has been the most neglected. The skin is one of the earliest developed and most fundamental functions of the body. Touch is the first communication a baby receives, and it is the first language of his or her development." It is difficult to understand then why touch has been the most neglected sense. There are many reasons why we may avoid all but the most "necessary" forms of touch. **Tiffany Field,** founder of the Touch Research Institute and leading authority on the subject, explains that "In earlier years, experts were worried we would spoil the child, and today experts are worried that children could be abused if teachers were allowed to touch them. On one side of the world, children in Romanian orphanages are attaining half their expected height because of touch deprivation, and on the other side, American teachers are not allowed to touch children for fear of child abuse accusations." Results from years of research reflect that it is neglect, rather than attention, that damages the child.

The problems and dysfunctions of today's society are reflected in the actions of our children. Statistics report that since the 1990s, there has been a steady increase in juvenile delinquency in our society. Through the process of rehabilitation, psychologists have revealed a lack of connection within the families of these youth. Studies show that prevention starts with the bonding of a family. An important dynamic within the family bonding process is attention given to not only the physical needs but also to the emotional needs of the child. Recognizing problems and finding solutions openly works toward a deepening trust within the family and lays a strong foundation in providing security.

Social and emotional deprivation in infancy is actually more destructive than poor nutrition or neglect with negative behavioral problems reverberating far into an individual's life. Parent-infant bonding through infant massage provides the basic security that enables babies to grow and develop to their full capacity physically, mentally, and spiritually.

Researchers believe that the key to early positive development and intelligence lies in the attention given to babies in-utero through two years of age, with the crucial time before six months. Where social and emotional deprivation may have occurred during this sensitive time, it may be a concern that irreparable damage has been done; however, man should place no limitation on the dynamic makeup of the human body, mind and spirit. We are miraculously designed to heal and transform through the power of touch and the loving support systems around us. Professionals, including massage therapists, can strengthen the attachment bonds of families by skillfully listening to concerns of the parents and by offering tools of intervention such as infant massage that will be helpful, empowering, and welcome.

Harmful Effects of Touch Deprivation

★ **EXAM POINT** Tiffany Field and other professionals agree that touch deprivation is one of the leading causes of aggression and violence in children.

Cross-cultural studies have demonstrated that in societies where infants are held, carried, and breast-fed, adults are less aggressive and violent, and more cooperative and compassionate.

Knowing why affectionate touch is important to the nurturing of babies, massage therapists can share that with parents so it becomes a tool for maintaining a child's health and well-being on many levels. It also empowers parents and caregivers with the security of knowing that they can do something effective and positive for their children and receive a positive response in return.

Tactile stimulation enhances functioning of babies' systems, and touch enhances emotional bonding between parents and children. Massage is particularly beneficial to high-risk babies and their parents as a means of promoting early recovery and emotional bonding, thereby helping to prevent abuse and neglect. Not only is touch deprivation one of the leading causes of aggression and violence in children, it is also a large cause of abuse in the home. Lack of bonding puts families at a much higher risk of abuse.

Infant Massage in Global Practice

Infant massage has been around for thousands and thousands of years. In countries all over the world, infant massage is a common child care practice, and babies are massaged and caressed every day. In many cultures, infant massage is a traditional practice passed down from generation to generation. In America, because it is a relatively new society, some of these ancient cultural traditions have been lost. Some of our basic human instincts were turned aside in the early twentieth century in the interest of progress and consumerism. However, as research shows that the unfolding of human potential depends on a nurturing environment during childhood, the art of infant massage is coming to the forefront.

Massage as a Resource for Family Ties

Psychologists today are very concerned about the family as a unit and have many opinions as to how to raise children. We live in a society where, oftentimes, both parents are working and do not have the quality time or energy to spend with their children. Massage therapists can be a great resource in helping families deepen the connections through touch therapy practices. Parents who regularly frequent massage therapy and have had the opportunity to learn infant massage from a licensed professional often become loyal "family clients." Whole family sessions generally consist of both mother and father receiving hourly massages and the children receiving 15-30 minutes of massage therapy each. Specialized training in infant and child massage instruction is available. The techniques used are based on the teachings of two massage therapists who received their training in India, Amelia Auckett and Vimala Schneider McClure. In the early 1970s, while working in an orphanage in Calcutta, India, McClure realized how important massage was to babies and children. In spite of their obvious disadvantages, these babies and children were given the greatest gift in life—the gift of love and security. She observed how daily massage helped to make the children more compassionate and responsible human beings. After she returned to the United States, her work with parents and babies led her to found the International Association of Infant Massage, which hosts training seminars on the art of infant massage around the world.

Procedure and Technique

Infant massage is a simple early intervention program of family bonding techniques. Professionals need to recognize that today's parents are very busy, so any suggested intervention technique (such as infant massage) should be presented in a straightforward, flexible, and empowering manner. The purpose of infant massage is to encourage parents to touch their children and to bond, communicate, and feel connected with them.

Infant massage presents all of the elements of bonding: direct eye contact, sense of smell, soothing voice, affectionate tactile stimulation, and synchronized breathing. It is

Applications of Theory and Practice for Infant and Pediatric Massage

Orphans: A Special Tribute

In 2002, massage therapist Carla DiMauro volunteered as part of a pediatric health care team in an orphanage in Uzbekistan. The Westerners were brought in to review practices and conduct workshops with orphanage administrators and caregivers on the proper care and handling of children. The previous government had established the facility for children with physical disabilities before Uzbekistan gained independence. For years, the children had been kept in deplorable conditions and suffered from malnutrition, and many had never known a loving touch. Most of the children were far from the expected size for their age and could not speak. Cerebral palsy afflicted nearly 75% of the children, with many extreme cases. These children were in severe permanent contractures because little early intervention had been done, in contrast to the United States, where physical therapies begin as soon as the diagnosis is made.

Handling of the children had often been rough, involving aggressive stretching of the limbs in an attempt to straighten and support blood flow. By going with the direction of muscle shortening to disengage the reflex, DiMauro was able through massage to unwind little bodies that were withered and grossly contorted. Although the results were not permanent, the children experienced greater freedom in their bodies for longer periods of time, increasing circulation, deepening respiration, and improving sleeping patterns and appetite.

Since the health care team's visit, massage therapists continue to be hired, along with caregivers, nurses, teachers, and more, at the orphanage. The facility has been remodeled, and orphanage workers have learned to build physical therapy equipment using local resources. Wheelchairs and other medical supplies donated from America have greatly improved the operations of the orphanage and the quality of life of the children.

Massage for orphans requires a somewhat different interaction than with children who are with their natal families. Special, individualized attention is necessary because of the grief they carry over having been separated from their mothers at birth. Many of the Uzbek orphans began to cry and experience emotional release when massage was performed on the chest region. Emotional energy is carried in this area of the heart, and the body will store trauma and stress. The children began to discharge grief as their bodies responded to the massage strokes done on the chest, down the arms, and on the face.

Orphaned children need special understanding with regard to the tremendous loss they have experienced in infancy and early childhood. Nurturing touch through massage helps them feel safe, secure, and loved. At the end of the team's two weeks at the orphanage, the social interaction observed in the children was greatly improved. Eye contact was more direct, conversation and laughter increased, and the children were much more active in classroom activities and play.

---

quality time that takes as little as 15 minutes, costs nothing, and can be done in the privacy and convenience of the parent or caregiver's home.

As an infant massage instructor, you can hold classes with many parents or caregivers and babies in one location or provide one-on-one instruction during a house call. In a group setting, babies' age should be limited to that of precrawling to avoid distractions other than of verbal expression. Parents or caregivers will learn to massage their babies while following your lead as you perform strokes on a doll. More detailed instruction with an individual may be given by placing your hands over the parent's or caregiver's hands as a guide for a specific stroke. Your focus should not be on massaging the infant but on guiding the parent or caregiver.

Reciprocal Interaction and Massage Routine

The infant massage routine (figure 10.4) is based on reciprocal interaction; that is, each partner, as in the process of bonding, has a role in facilitating each stage. At first, the parent or caregiver stimulates the infant with appropriate cues, which trigger a response in the infant. The infant's cues then trigger further involvement by the parent. These continually reciprocated cues include eye contact, smiling, flowing body movements, speech, and sounds.

The infant massage instruction session begins with the therapist leading a few deep-breathing exercises to relax the parent or caregiver so the baby does not mirror

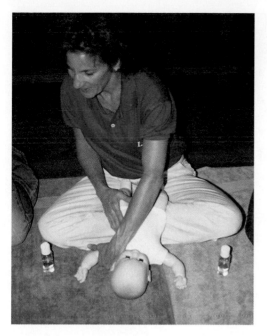

Figure 10.4
The instructor demonstrates infant massage for parents using a doll.

any negative emotions. The initial sounds of deep breathing are also very soothing for the baby. The parent or caregiver begins by warming oil in their hands and making a "swooshing" noise next to the baby's ear. This is the first cue that something good is happening as the baby becomes more familiar with the routine of massage. Next, the parent or caregiver asks "for permission" and waits for a cue from the baby that it is OK to proceed. Baby's affirmative cue might simply be direct eye contact, a smile, or a gurgle. Eyes darting away, flailing of the arms, or any fussing is an indication that the baby is not yet ready for massage. Patience should be encouraged, and the instructing therapist may discuss stages of growth and how massage benefits the baby during these stages. Once the baby is more comfortable and receptive, instruction for the massage routine may continue.

The infant massage routine, as developed in the Western world by McClure, encompasses three traditions: Indian milking, which are strokes away from the heart to encourage waste removal; Swedish massage, utilizing strokes toward the heart to encourage blood flow; and reflexology, which involves simply pressing points all over the hands and feet. It is recommended to begin supine, with the legs (figure 10.5), because this is the least intrusive part on the baby's body and generally well received. Indian milking strokes are done by holding the baby's foot with one hand and stroking from the hip laterally all the way down to the foot with the hand wrapped snugly around the leg. Alternating hands, the stroke is repeated on the medial portion of the leg. Each stroke should be done with rhythm and continuity, and repeated three to six times. This is followed by a "squeeze and twist" stroke in which both hands are wrapped around the baby's upper thigh and proceed to gently squeeze and twist, in a very gentle wringing fashion, down to the ankle. Pressure should be applied using a "gentle strength"—not too light to where it tickles nor too hard that it is uncomfortable for the baby (watch facial expressions and body language), but just enough so that the baby's skin will develop a little more color. Feather strokes are used to say "bye-bye" to each leg. The same order is followed and done on the arms. Massage should never be forced. If an arm is in flexion, the stroke should be performed in the direction the arm is curved, allowing the baby to relax and extend it itself. The chest may be a more sensitive area as the baby feels the need to be protected. Gentle strokes are done from the center with full hands spreading out to the shoulders in an "open a book" move (figure 10.6). Crisscrossing may be done from the side, alternating hands to each shoulder to shape a "butterfly" across the chest. Abdominal strokes are always very

Chapter 10 Maternity, Infant, and Pediatric Massage

Figure 10.5
The instructor (center) uses a doll to demonstrate infant massage strokes.

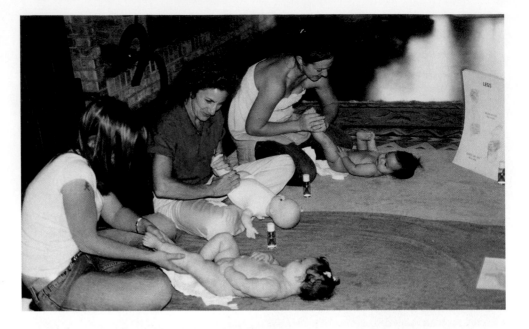

Figure 10.6
Gentle stroking on the chest with alternating hands.

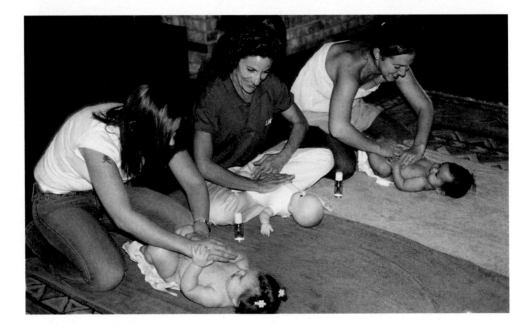

gentle and done in a clockwise direction. Verbal description of each stroke and words of affirmation by the parent or caregiver are always encouraged, as voice is an element of bonding. Telling the baby "you are so beautiful," "oh, how we love you," and "what a good baby" is very effective in the early development of self-esteem for the child. Gentle stroking of the face and head may be done, being careful of the soft cranial plates. Little circles around the jaw, lips, and mouth will prepare the baby for soothing touch to relieve teething pain.

The baby is placed prone (figure 10.7) to massage the back. Using both hands simultaneously, horizontally effleurage the back from the neck to the buttocks. Placing one hand on the buttocks, the other hand "swoops" down the back to end with the other. Little circles are done alongside the spine (figure 10.8), up one side and down the other, but never over the spine as it is sensitive and still developing. Because every baby has a different stimulation threshold, the length of the massage will vary. The first whimper is not always an indication that the baby has had enough, especially if all the

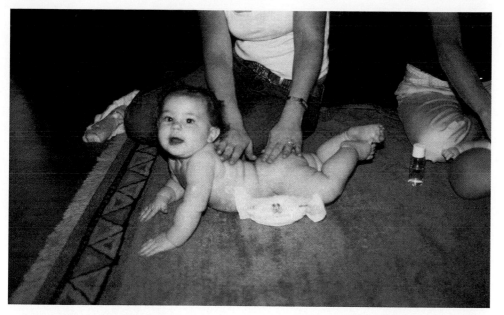

Figure 10.7
Baby is placed prone so work can begin on the back.

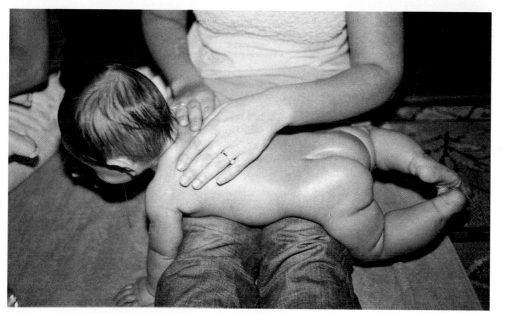

Figure 10.8
Effleurage is performed in a circular motion up one side of the spine and down the other.

basic needs have been met. If they have just been fed, changed, and are well rested, and they still begin to fuss early in the massage, they may just be integrating the new sensations. A technique called **"touch relaxation,"** also developed by McClure, involves the parent or caregiver stopping at a point of tension, taking the body part in their hands and molding to it, then gently bouncing or just holding still and in a calm voice encouraging the baby to "relax and let go." The direct eye contact, calming voice, and soothing, consistent touch will get a favorable response. As soon as relaxation is felt in the baby, the baby should be given positive, encouraging feedback, and the parent or caregiver may then proceed with the routine. It helps the baby associate relaxation with the touch of the parent or caregiver, and children who have learned "touch relaxation" techniques in infancy continue to respond as they age. This technique is proven ideal as children approach the so-called "terrible twos" or stages of independence. If the baby just does not respond after two or three attempts at "touch relaxation," she may very well have developed an appetite, have grown tired, is ready for a bowel movement, or simply has reached her stimulation threshold. Infant massage is best done during a "calm alert" state, when the baby is fully aware yet her body is relaxed. This state fully lends itself to the reciprocal interaction encouraged between parent or caregiver and infant; however, infant massage should be done as often as possible. Bed and bath times are good opportunities. Oil should be all natural and cold-pressed. A good choice is grapeseed oil because it has high nutritive value and is unscented so it will not interfere with the bonding element of smell. No mineral oil-based products should be used, as they are drying and will draw nutrients out of the baby's skin. Cornstarch is also a comfortable and often convenient alternative to oil.

The massage therapist should always keep in mind that infant massage is a playful time between parent or caregiver and baby. You should stay flexible and respect each individual's style. Remember that massage is natural, so each stroke does not have to be done perfectly. Stay nonjudgmental, flexible, and sensitive. Above all, this is a time to have fun, and as the instructing massage therapist, you will surely find great satisfaction in witnessing the deepening of family bonds. Ideally, infant massage teaches a child the difference between healthy and unhealthy touch from an early age. Children massaged from infancy have many advantages over children who have simply been told what the boundaries are regarding healthy and unhealthy touch. They know what healthy touch feels like, and the positive experience will be strengthened and enjoyed as they grow.

Massage for Children

As the child grows, the infant massage strokes will be modified to accommodate the longer legs and arms. If a child between the ages of 1 and 3 has not been massaged from infancy, she will be very busy and may not stay still (figure 10.9). Providing a toy such as a stuffed animal to play with or having the child flop down in front of the TV may lessen the challenge. Sometimes, allowing the child to feel the oil in their own hands and rub it on you can create a positive response. Positioning will be different, and the parent or caregiver may be more comfortable sitting beside the child.

The massage therapist's focus should remain on the instruction of techniques to encourage massage on a regular basis in the home. Some parents, however, will hire a therapist to massage the children before or after the parent's session. A massage table can be used, and children's massage is not much different than a gentle adult Swedish massage. Using the face cradle becomes somewhat of a novelty for the child and may even keep her still for longer periods of time. Generally, 30 minutes is sufficient, unless a child has

Figure 10.9
Massage strokes are modified to accommodate the older child's body.

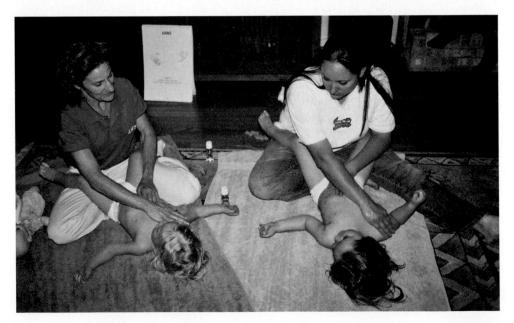

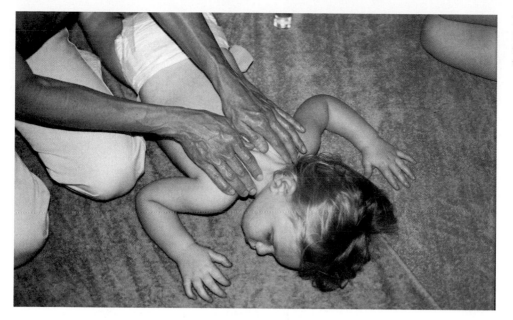

become accustomed to regular massage and would be perfectly comfortable through a full-hour session. Parental or guardian supervision is essential. Undergarments should remain on at all times, and draping should be conservative, with strokes on the leg remaining distal to midthigh. As children tend to be more sensitive, pressure should be light. Use a slow, consistent rhythm with many repetitions. Ask the child for feedback, watch facial expressions, and listen to her body language. Children who are massaged tend to grow up feeling more confident and comfortable with their bodies (figure 10.10). In general, well-touched children tend to be emotionally warmer, less fearful and hyperactive, and more likely to communicate openly with their parents or guardians.

Chapter Summary

Performing massage on expectant mothers as well as their newborns can be quite rewarding. Infants' tactile experiences blossom through the power of touch offered by parents, siblings, extended family members, and other caregivers. Some massage therapists believe they are called to work with this segment of the population almost exclusively, while others find it a rewarding complement to their general practice. Whatever your motivation, you will be rewarded many times over by working with mothers and children.

Applying Your Knowledge

Self-Testing

1. Which hormone stimulates uterine growth?
   a) Human chorionic gonadotropin
   b) Thyroxin
   c) Estrogen
   d) Calcitonin

2. What would be a good choice of lubricants for a pregnant woman?
   a) Shea or cocoa butter
   b) Comfrey oil
   c) Myrrh oil
   d) Crème with cinnamon oil

3. Which of the following circulatory changes take place during pregnancy?
   a) Pulse rate increases
   b) Heart murmurs
   c) Heart palpations
   d) All of the above are correct.

4. From the thirteenth to the twenty-third week of pregnancy, the side-lying position is preferred because of what structure?
   a) Fetal position
   b) Inferior vena cava

c) Bladder

d) Uterus

5. As the pregnancy progresses, breathing becomes more
   a) costal.
   b) diaphragmatic.
   c) nasal.
   d) All of the above are correct.

6. Some of the most stressed muscles during pregnancy are trapezius, erector spinae, quadratus lumborum, and
   a) psoas
   b) gastrocnemius
   c) serratus anterior
   d) rhomboids

7. Reflex massage is indicated during pregnancy.
   a) True
   b) False

8. The infant massage routine developed by McClure encompasses three tradtions: Indian milking, Swedish massage, and
   a) acupressure
   b) stretching
   c) reflexology
   d) aromatherapy

9. In a recent study conducted by the Touch Research Institute, mothers receiving massage during labor experienced decreased levels of _____
   a) anxiety.
   b) pain.
   c) hunger.
   d) a and b

10. Touch deprivation is one of the leading causes of aggression in children.
    a) True
    b) False

Case Studies/Critical Thinking

A. *Your client is in her second trimester of pregnancy. How will you position her for massage? What techniques will you employ? What type of hydrotherapy, if any, will you use? What precautions will you take?*

B. *A pregnant woman who has been told by her doctor that she falls within the high-risk category schedules a massage with you. How will you handle this situation?*

References for information in this chapter can be found in Quick Guide C at the end of the book.

Massage for Special Populations (Children with Special Needs, Geriatric, and Hospice and Palliative Care)

LEARNING OUTCOMES

After completing this chapter, you will be able to:

- Explain the importance of touch during early childhood and childhood.
- Implement massage techniques for children with special needs.
- Recognize the special accommodations necessary for massage of the elderly.
- Detail the massage therapist's role in the hospice and palliative care setting.

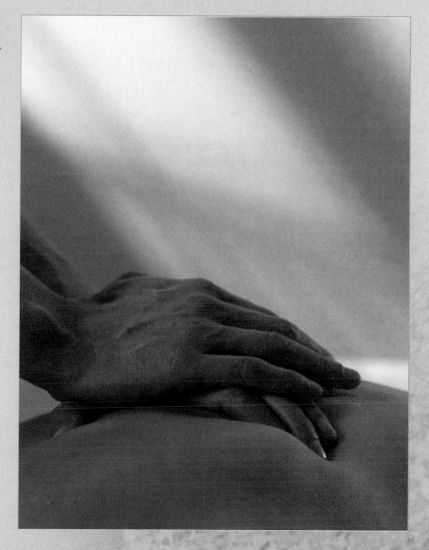

KEY TERMS

acquired immune deficiency
    syndrome (AIDS) *(p. 296)*
asthma *(p. 295)*
attention deficit hyperactivity
    disorder (ADHD) *(p. 294)*

autism *(p. 293)*
cerebral palsy (CP) *(p. 292)*
colic *(p. 290)*
dementia *(p. 297)*

Down's syndrome *(p. 294)*
hospice *(p. 299)*
palliative care *(p. 299)*

INTRODUCTION

Working in any capacity with children is rewarding, but working with children who have special needs is doubly rewarding. As a massage therapist, you will have a profound effect on special needs children by encouraging them to be responsive to their environment through the powers of touch. This massage specialty is truly an art.

At the other end of the age spectrum is an increasingly large group of prospective clients. With improved health care, life expectancy continues to edge upward. Seniors who seek massage therapy have different requirements from infants and toddlers. Unfortunately, some seniors will experience lengthy or terminal illnesses requiring long-term hospice or nursing home care. Still, another group—younger adults and children—may also face end-of-life situations. Both groups can benefit from a trained and compassionate massage therapist.

This chapter includes sections called "Applications of Theory and Practice." These sections offer additional content for those who want to study these massage specialties in greater depth.

Special Needs Children

By Carla DiMauro, BBA, LMT

Modern medical advancements have contributed to saving the lives of many children who used to die in infancy; this has led to a rise in the number of individuals with disabilities in the United States. Massage can benefit special needs children in many ways. Because of their high stress levels, they have a greater need for physical and mental relaxation. Children with special needs tend to be more socially isolated and touched less than other children. Massage can go a long way toward meeting this need for caring, nurturing touch as it also helps supply extra information to the brain about body position, muscle tension, and movement. This extra information is essential to help develop a healthy body image, despite the obvious challenges. Massage also helps relieve the discomfort or pain these children often experience from necessary medical procedures and provides them with something that simply feels good. The bonding process is often challenged in the family with special needs children. The child with developmental, visual, hearing, or other impairments sometimes cannot respond in the "normal" manner to parents' or caregivers' cues. This may lead parents or caregivers to feel inadequate in providing for their special needs child. In addition to physiological benefits, massage can be a wonderful bonding tool to keep the family in touch with each other and open the channels of communication.

Applications of Theory and Practice for Specific Needs Massage

The routines that follow are examples of ways in which massage therapists can help parents and other caregivers cope with various situations and are not meant to replace a physician's advice.

Gas and Colic

Babies with colic will cry for extended periods of time and are obviously experiencing pain (figure 11.1). **Colic** is not completely understood, but experts suggest that it may

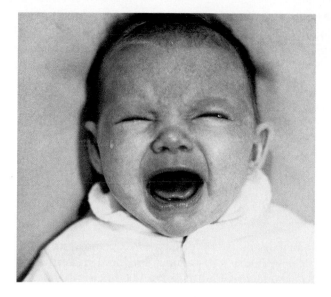

Figure 11.1
Research shows that the "colic relief routine" administered twice daily can relieve symptoms within two weeks.

be due to babies' underdeveloped gastrointestinal or nervous systems. It is not easy to comfort a colicky baby, and the entire household may suffer for weeks on end. Massage therapy has proven to be an effective method of reducing or eliminating the symptoms of colic when done consistently and regularly. Often, results are seen within two weeks. The colic routine should be performed two to three times daily. Listen to the baby's cries respectfully, and stay focused as you work gently and with confidence. This will offer the baby greater feelings of security as she goes through this difficult time. The colic routine is four steps, and the giver should maintain soothing verbal communication at all times to relax the child.

1. With very warm, well-lubricated hands, "paddle" with the side of the palm, hand over hand from the belly button down to the bladder. This effleurage stroke thoroughly prepares the area for deeper strokes and movements. Repeat six times.

2. Gently flex and push the knees in toward the chest and hold for 15 to 20 seconds. Shake the legs out with a rhythmic bouncing, then simultaneously perform effleurage from the hips down to the toes six times.

3. Stroke down the baby's left side, tracing the descending colon line, to encourage release of waste material, then complete with a full clockwise circle around the baby's tummy. Repeat six times.

4. Repeat step 2.

Each baby will respond differently. "Touch relaxation" a technique coined by Vimala McClure, founder of the International Association of Infant Massage and author of *Infant Massage—A Handbook for Loving Parents*, should be used when necessary to lessen the baby's stress or if the baby seems to be overstimulated. It is essential to perform all strokes as slowly and methodically as possible, and the key is consistency. Many families have reported a welcome relief from symptoms of the baby's colic within two weeks.

Preterm Infants

Preterm infants who are massaged experience many benefits. The Touch Research Institute at the University of Miami School of Medicine conducted its first groundbreaking study involving preterm infants in 1984. In that study, 20 preterm neonates received 45 minutes of massage per day (in 15-minute sessions) for 10 days. The results were significant, showing that massaged infants:

- Gained 47% more weight than the nonmassaged control group.
- Were more awake and actively alert than the control group.

- Showed better performance on the Brazelton scale on habituation, orientation, motor activity, and regulation of state behavior.
- Were released from the hospital six days earlier than the control infants, yielding a cost savings of approximately $3,000 per infant.

In addition to the need for massage therapists to instruct parents and caregivers in how to massage their preemie in the hospital or once they get home, there is an increasing need for this work in the neonatal intensive care unit. Because of liability, most touch is limited to that of parents or within the general job responsibilities of the hospital staff. The International Association of Infant Massage is working with nationwide hospital networks to bring infant massage to their hospitals and is promoting certified infant massage instructors through them.

Cerebral Palsy

Cerebral palsy (CP) is a developmental disability that originates when the parts of the brain that control movement are damaged during gestational development, birth, and early infancy (figure 11.2). It affects about three out of every 1,000 newborns in the United States. The damage can result from problems in pregnancy (often due to maternal illness), birth trauma (lack of oxygen), or trauma in early infancy (accidents, "shaken baby syndrome," or infection such as meningitis or encephalitis). Several types of CP have been identified that fall into the categories of hypotonic, hypertonic, or mixed.

Massage provides many benefits to improve the quality of life of children with CP. Positioning is the utmost importance, and the child should be carefully arranged among pillows and bolsters. CP children suffering from respiratory problems should remain in the position that allows easier breathing, whether prone or supine, for the duration of the massage. For the hypertonic child, a combination of light effleurage and gentle shiatsu is most effective to reduce tone. For the hypotonic child, bouncier and swifter strokes help to increase active voluntary movement. Much of the damage for a CP child is manifested in the tightening of the connective tissue wrapped around the muscles, producing involuntary action. These contractures in the musculoskeletal system are merely a symptom of a complication deep within the brain. Massage therapy is most beneficial to help prevent contractures from starting or worsening. Whereas physical therapy focuses on stretching and lengthening skeletal muscles, massage can offset

Figure 11.2 Cerebral palsy
Massage helps normalize muscle tone and prevents contractures from worsening in the cerebral palsy child.

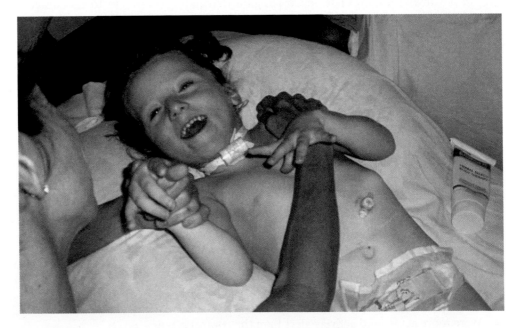

this often-rigorous exercise by indirectly affecting muscle tone through techniques that engage the child's limbs in ways they don't automatically resist. This is done with strokes that go with the direction of muscle shortening in order to disengage the reflex. The therapist will ultimately learn to incorporate many different approaches, including craniosacral work, vibration techniques, myofascial release, rocking, and gentle range of motion, to produce the desired results for the CP child. Whether the condition is mild or severe, regular massage therapy will help to improve circulation, alleviate constipation, normalize muscle tone, encourage deeper breathing, and overall make a significant improvement in the quality of life for the child with cerebral palsy.

Autism and Autistic Spectrum Disorders

Autism is a physical disorder of the brain in which a young child experiences developmental delays and irregular behaviors. These irregular behaviors involve disturbances in communication, failure to "connect" with others socially, and abnormal response to sensory stimulation. Children with autism tend to be compulsive and display repetitive behavior patterns such as tapping and rocking. Specific developmental disorders such as Asperger's syndrome, Rett's disorder, and pervasive developmental delay are specific types of autism each with varying symptoms. Typically, an autistic infant does not cuddle and avoids direct eye contact. Older children may act as if they are in their own world, unresponsive to the moods and expressions of others. Since the 1980s, the prevalence of autism has been increasing at a truly alarming rate. The Cure Autism Now foundation reports that in 2004, one in 166 children was diagnosed with a disorder on the autistic spectrum. Autism and autism-related disorders are two to four times more common in boys than girls.

Massage therapy has proven to be beneficial in helping children with autism become accustomed to touch, relax, and have greater body awareness. As touch in itself is powerful communication, it offers a means to break through their isolation; however, care must be taken not to overstimulate the child with touch or force it on the child. Such children may be sensitive to smells and textures, so the use of sheets and scented oils may be irritating. Allowing the child to lie fully clothed in a prone position on the massage table and working cautiously at his speed (first only on the arms) can prove

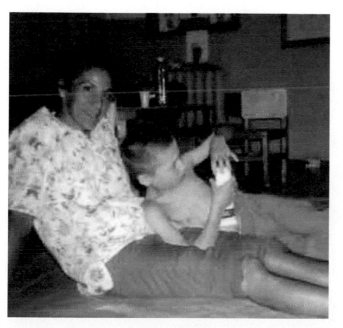

Figure 11.3 Autism
Massage increases body awareness and must be given within the autistic child's tolerance level.

nonthreatening and help him to relax. Gentle, slow effleurage or brushing strokes can be calming on the shoulders, arms, and hands, along with slow, rhythmic compressions along the back and legs. Pay close attention to facial expressions and body language, and use what works best for the child. Sometimes only a few moments may be tolerated, but with repeated sessions (in addition to the parents giving massage once or twice daily), the child's stimulation threshold will be raised and greater connections can be made.

Attention Deficit Hyperactivity Disorder

Attention deficit hyperactivity disorder (ADHD) is the most common of all neurodevelopmental disorders, affecting up to 5% of all children. Statistical data show that the disorder is up to four times more common in boys than girls. Children with ADHD tend to be hyperactive, easily distracted and have difficulties paying attention for extended periods of time. Treatment for these children usually includes family counseling, special school programs, and psychologically stimulating medications such as ritalin. These drugs may have adverse effects, and the long-term impact on personality development is relatively unknown.

A more holistic approach to medication that has proven successful is the combination of the natural herb melissa supreme and massage therapy. Craniosacral therapy as well as myofascial release and acupressure can help release tension and pressure, and facilitate greater balance for the child. While the ADHD child may not have the patience to lie still on a massage table for long, utilizing the face cradle or a face hole will provide an added novelty. Providing the child with a seated chair massage can improve focus for the child, allowing the therapist to work primarily on the back and shoulders for an effective, but brief, period to relieve built-up stress. Massage is proven to lower the stress hormones. Over time, children with ADHD can learn to relax, breathe deeply, and experience the freedom from unnecessary buildup of body tension that a full body massage can offer.

Down's Syndrome

Down's syndrome is a chromosomal disorder that results in mental retardation and physical abnormalities (figure 11.4). Physical and mental developmental delays are experienced by children with Down's. Infants tend to be quiet and passive with hypotonicity of the muscles. Early intervention with educational and other services (including massage therapy) greatly improves the functioning of young children with Down's syndrome.

Figure 11.4 Down's syndrome
Massage increases muscle tone and improves motor functioning for children with Down's syndrome.

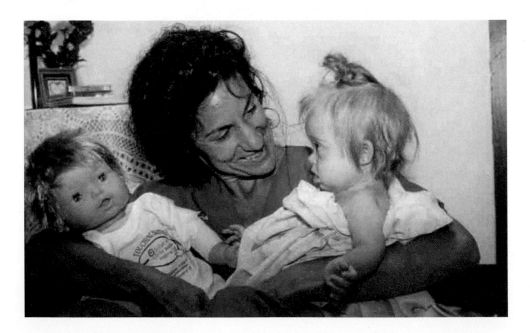

Studies at the Touch Research Institute have shown improvements in fine and gross motor functioning and decreases in hypotonicity from regular massage in Down's syndrome children. Muscle tone also has shown to significantly increase when massage is administered before exercise. Children with Down's syndrome often have cervical vertebral instability, and extreme caution should be used when massaging in the neck area to avoid overstretching. There may be joint limitations, so be sure to check with the child's physical therapist or doctor before administering range-of-motion techniques. Children with Down's syndrome often have heart defects, and many develop thyroid disease. Massage can help to balance hormone levels and promote faster recovery from surgery. As a result of uncoordinated muscle contractions and hypotonicity, constipation is an ongoing problem for children with severe developmental disabilities. Abdominal massage can effectively relieve much of the pain and discomfort, and significantly reduce the problem. Most children with Down's syndrome tend to be affectionate in nature and are responsive to touch. Swedish techniques with long, warming strokes and extra attention to the hands and feet can help to increase body awareness and improve relaxation. Because the hearing of children with Down's syndrome is often challenged and their language skills typically develop slowly, therapists need to be sensitive to each child's tolerance levels.

Visual Impairments

Massage offers blind children many benefits, including a new way to communicate. It helps to improve posture and increase body awareness so important for balance, gait, and movement. Muscle tension commonly associated with visually impaired children can be relieved in the head, neck, face, and upper back with massage. Blind children should be allowed to explore the surface area of the massage table before getting up on it; use of the face cradle is not recommended as it may be too confining. Describing each stroke as you move to different body parts can improve relaxation and comfort levels, and help to build trust. Rubbing the arms and legs against one another can increase spatial awareness and help to develop a distinct body image. A flowing, Swedish massage is most effective with extra attention spent on the head and upper back.

Hearing Impairments

A 1988 pilot program of the New York Education Department in which massage was administered to deaf children for three months showed a 69% improvement in language skills and, for one-third of the children, a 19% increase in sleep time. Massage can also help to increase body awareness and help to redefine their position in time and space. Swedish massage with long, flowing strokes is most effective with extra time spent on the head and face, particularly around the ears. Talking to the deaf child throughout the massage will provide additional sensory stimulation from the vibration of the voice through the hands.

Asthma

Asthma is a chronic disease of the lungs in which the airways narrow in response to certain stimuli (figure 11.5). It is an allergic disorder that is compounded by emotional stress and is reaching epidemic proportions in the United States. Asthma affects 17 to 18 million people, and incidents of acute asthma among children (currently 5 million) have doubled in the past 10 years. Experts believe factors that contribute to pediatric asthma include immune deficiencies, allergies, air pollution, and stress.

Massage is useful during an asthma attack to relieve muscle spasm, help dilate the bronchioles, and encourage deeper breathing. Effleurage and friction strokes should be administered with a gentle strength in the muscles of the shoulders to release tension and in the mid- and low back to encourage respiration. Massage the chest and space between the ribs by using the flats of your fingers to produce a "sawing" motion. This relaxes the intercostal muscles, which allows more freedom of movement in the ribs. Long strokes in the lamina groove next to the spine will help to relieve tightness and should be followed with vibration to soothe overstressed vertebral muscles. As a preventive

Figure 11.5 Asthma
Massage relieves the tension in respiratory muscles caused from the stress of asthma attacks.

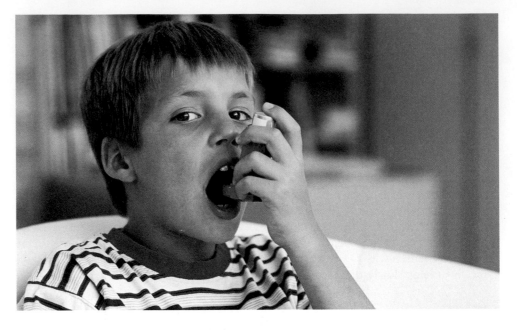

measure, massage is an important part of relaxation training for the child with asthma. Exercises to encourage diaphragmatic breathing are essential. This can also be done while massaging the abdomen. With one hand placed under the low back and the other hand moving slowly across the abdomen in a clockwise direction, have the child breathe deeply and increase the space between your hands. Massage slowly and focus on "lifting" the abdomen with each inhalation.

Acquired Immune Deficiency Syndrome

Numerous animal studies have shown that loving, nurturing touch, especially in early childhood, can stimulate immune function. Massage can benefit the child with **Acquired Immune Deficiency Syndrome (AIDS)** in many ways by boosting the immune system, improving circulation, relieving muscle aches and cramps, and helping to regulate sleep. Many children with AIDS do not have their need for touch met, due to others' fear of contracting the disease. Massage provides them with the touch necessary for growth and development, and serves to greatly improve the quality of their life. Appetite is increased by skin stimulation, and massage most effectively reduces stress and anxiety, as well as fear. Be aware of general contraindications that include open sores, rashes, fever, inflammation, and tumorous growths. It is recommended to stay away from concentrated areas of lymph nodes such as the armpits. Proceed with general Swedish massage, gentle acupressure techniques, and relaxing stretching or range-of-motion exercises. Be sensitive to the child's level of tolerance and encourage open communication and feedback.

Working with Elderly Clients	Along with massage for pregnant mothers, infants, and children, many therapists enjoy working with seniors. Making a connection with elders places the massage therapist in a giving and receiving position (figure 11.6). Therapists find fulfillment working with elders as well as garner insights and perspectives from those who have known other times. Devoting one or two days a week to geriatric clients in a residence home or other setting is an excellent way to reach this population and create a change in your ordinary work routine.

Many people in their middle-aged years find themselves to be part of the "sandwich" generation that is taking care of both children and aging parents. Offering massage to both groups, either for profit or as a volunteer, can help relieve the stresses these groups experience and bring harmony to the home.

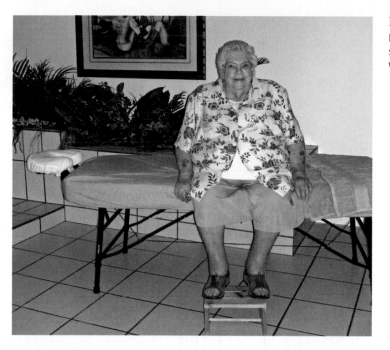

Figure 11.6
Regular massage helps seniors maintain a sense of well-being.

Geriatric Massage

By Linda Rowlands, LMT, NCTMB

The main ingredient in geriatric massage is a loving heart. Many seniors receive their first massage to alleviate muscular aches and pains, then continue treatment after feeling the benefits of massage. Such benefits include becoming more active, feeling more positive, sleeping better, and having a bigger appetite. Seniors also appreciate the benefits of human touch and conversation, both of which improve their quality of life.

As a therapist, listen with your ears, your heart, and your hands to best assess their needs. Many seniors are on medications; be sure you learn the client's specific medications as the massage may interact with them. Ask if their symptoms are under control and if the medications are causing any unwanted side effects. If you have a large geriatric clientele, you will begin to recognize some of the more common prescriptions (see chapter 19).

Common complaints of seniors include frozen shoulder, trouble getting up from a chair, anxiety, stress, sore knees, swollen ankles, insomnia, back pain, and bruising. Use particular caution with skin conditions. Seniors' skin is generally thin from decreased collagen; black and blue spotting often occurs as a reaction to pharmaceuticals.

TECHNIQUE EMPHASIS Identify primary complaints and address those first.

Methodology

The flow of the massage dance for the geriatric client is slow, soothing, and nurturing. Pay particular attention to specific needs and take necessary precautions. The following procedure is a good way to meet the needs of geriatric clients:

1. Call the client a day before to confirm the appointment. As we age, memory lapses are common, and some seniors experience forms of Alzheimer's or **dementia,** an irreversible neurological disorder in which there is a loss of reasoning power. They also like a friendly reminder call if you haven't seen them in a while to book an appointment.

2. Be a good listener and speak up if the client has any hearing loss.

Applications of Theory and Practice for Geriatric Massage

3. Ask them why they want a massage.

4. Take a client intake or history each time you see them; with seniors, as with all clients, each day may bring a change in medical status.

5. Discuss how they feel now and how they expect to feel after the massage.

6. Assess their ability to position themselves on the massage table or chair.

   a. Can they lie down?

   b. Can they lie both prone and supine without straining themselves?

   c. Do they need a pillow or two under their head?

   d. Would side-lying or a sitting position be the best choice?

7. Explain how to get ready for the massage (i.e., disrobing and how to position themselves on the table).

8. Ask them if they need any assistance getting undressed or getting on the table before leaving the room. If not, leave the room but remain close by.

9. With music playing, center yourself and then ask the client to take a deep breath and release. Many seniors breathe quite shallowly and will need to be coached in proper breathing.

10. Massage lighter and more slowly than you do for younger clients.

11. A good length for the massage is 30 to 40 minutes. (The time may be increased after the first few treatments, depending on the physical response of the client.) It is important not to overload the client's body with a lengthy treatment.

12. Be very gentle and slow when checking or performing range of motion.

13. Some clients will chat while others will not talk at all. Remember to keep the massage about them and not you. Do not discuss other clients with them.

14. Use your toolbox (see Procedure 11.1) of modalities and adjust where necessary.

A Special Note

Keep in mind that most seniors are on a fixed income, so it is helpful if you can offer them a reduced price. Geriatric clients can be a wonderful addition to your business; they often are loyal customers, interested in new ways to achieve or maintain good health, and tend to tell their friends about how wonderful they feel with massage.

A "perk" for you, the therapist, is this type of massage is gentler on your body. Therefore, devoting one or two days to working in a senior center or residence not only gives your body a break from the rigors of deeper massage but also strengthens your connection to this special segment of our population.

P R O C E D U R E 11.1 Toolbox of Modalities for Senior Clients

- Swedish—touch and manipulation for stimulation of body, mind, and spirit
- Lymphatic drainage—Activate fluid movement for releasing fluid retention and strengthening the immune system
- Energy work—Balance chakras to assist in destressing the body

- Trager®—A calming, gentle way to free stiffness and release anxiety
- Acutonics—A calming, gentle treatment that uses the vibrations from tuning forks for many ailments
- Aromatherapy—Refreshing fragrances and potent plant health alternatives

Working with the terminally ill in hospice is another opportunity for specializing. Comforting the dying by helping to improve their quality of life is a rewarding, albeit emotionally draining, process for the massage therapist. You are part of a caring team (including nurses and other trained hospice caregivers) whose goal is ultimately to support an individual while treating the prospect of that person's death with dignity.

"Dying can be considered a journey one takes alone with a crowd." These words were spoken by Dr. Roger C. Bone, a physician who was dying of cancer at the same time he was offering suggestions to assist the terminally ill in planning the rest of their lives. "Family and friends," he said, "are the first to gather around you, and they offer the most comfort...but in the end, you must die your own death." The dying process can be an isolating, lonely, painful experience for both the individuals and their family members and friends. Hospice services can provide comfort, care, and pain relief during this stressful time. Part of that care includes the benefits of massage therapy and comforting human touch. Figure 11.7 shows the use of healing touch to comfort a patient.

The terminally ill can benefit from recognizing that dying can be a time of growth, offering opportunities for individuals to reconcile with themselves and loved ones. With guidance from compassionate caregivers, those nearing death can learn to accept their own mortality. Oftentimes, the psychosocial benefits of a gentle, compassionate massage will be more significant than any of the physiological benefits.

Hospice is a comprehensive health care program dedicated to the needs of the terminally ill and their families. Hospice generally encompasses palliative care and support services that address the physical, spiritual, social, and economic needs of the terminally ill and their families. **Palliative care** does not attempt to bring about major physical changes in the condition of the person. It simply aims to achieve comfort and a greater feeling of well-being. Hospice care is not directed toward healing but to making life more comfortable or even bearable to improve the quality of life for the patient and the family.

Although 90% of hospice patient time is spent in a personal residence, some patients live in nursing homes or hospice centers. Hospitals also provide hospice, and a patient requesting these services may be transferred to a special area within the hospital. Hospice patients are cared for by a team of physicians, nurses, social workers, counselors, hospice-certified nursing assistants, clergy, therapists, and volunteers, each of whom provides assistance based on their own area of expertise.

Massage for Hospice and Palliative Care

By Carla DiMauro, BBA, LMT

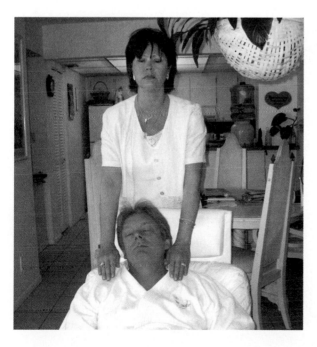

Figure 11.7
Healing Touch is an energy-based approach to provide comforting touch.

Massage therapy is increasingly becoming a part of the care plan for many hospice patients to enhance the more traditional forms of managing symptoms. It has long been recognized that complementary therapies are beneficial where used appropriately. The aim of complementary therapy is to alleviate physical and emotional discomfort in a holistic and safe environment. As a complementary therapy, massage provides a cost-effective therapeutic tool with low risk, if appropriately administered.

Attachment to individuals with a terminal illness is at times fragile for family members, friends, and caregivers. Often they are concerned that medications will prevent the patient from being able to talk or know what is happening. The goal of hospice and palliative care is to have the patient as pain-free and alert as possible (figure 11.8). Much research has lent support to massage therapy's ability to reduce pain and anxiety, and increase alertness. Patients' demands for drugs are often reduced when massage is an integral part of the treatment protocol. Emotional and spiritual pain are just as real and in need of attention as physical pain, and each can be addressed through massage therapy.

Many of the physical and emotional benefits of massage for the hospice patient are similar to those experienced by any other client. These include softening and releasing tight muscles, improving circulation, reducing localized aches and pains, nurturing, and calming.

Indications for Hospice Massage

Indications for massage in the hospice setting include but are not limited to:

- Multidimensional pain, muscle spasms, and contractures
- Anxiety and terminal restlessness
- Depression
- Edema
- Insomnia
- Constipation
- Nausea
- Stress (mental, emotional, and physical)

A 1993 study by the Department of Nursing at the College of St. Scholastica, Duluth, Minnesota, revealed the effects of slow-stroke back massage on relaxation in hospice clients. The study was conducted to investigate a nonpharmacological means of relaxation with 30 hospice clients. It showed that slow-stroke back massage was associ-

Figure 11.8
Enveloping the body requires little or no pressure and is effective in palliative care.

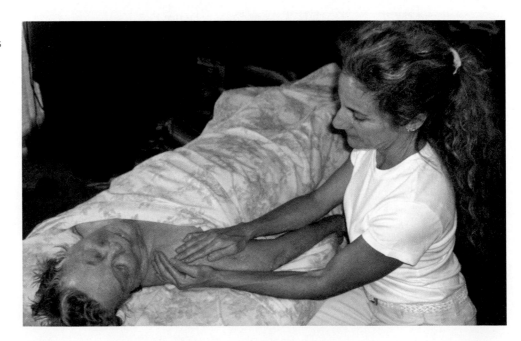

ated with decreases in systolic and diastolic blood pressure and heart rate, and increases in skin temperature. This massage approach also produced changes in vital signs that indicated relaxation. The study concluded that slow-stroke back massage "is a cost-effective treatment which adds to the comfort of hospice clients."

At the Hospice of the Florida Suncoast, a study was made of whether massage could truly be an effective treatment modality for pain and symptom management in hospice. Traditional therapeutic pain-relieving techniques such as neuromuscular and deep tissue massage are not considered appropriate for hospice clients because of their stimulating effects. For hospice patients, techniques that are slow and gentle are most appropriate for their comforting value. In addition, some patients may have conditions that are contraindicated for massage, and strokes may be applied only to unaffected areas. The study involved 151 massage therapy sessions with 32 patients. The positive effects of massage therapy were significant and consistent with those reported for nonhospice patients diagnosed with cancer. Patients reported a 52% reduction in pain scores and experienced similar improvements in anxiety and peacefulness.

Massage therapy is the type of complementary care requested most often by hospice patients. Human touch is one of the most ancient and helpful means for alleviating bodily discomfort and is especially applicable in a hospice setting. Massage can:

- Reduce feelings of isolation, loneliness, and fear
- Restore feelings of self-acceptance and self-esteem
- Provide nurturing and loving touch
- Facilitate emotional release
- Affirm the sense of wholeness, continuity, and completion
- Help to induce a state of peacefulness
- Assist in providing stress relief to family members and caregivers

Precautions for Hospice Massage

Loving, compassionate touch is as basic a human need as shelter, food, and water. Except for certain specific conditions, a little bit of touch is better than no touch at all, particularly when it involves helping to improve the quality of life. With doctors' permission, the only real contraindication would be when the person does not want to be touched. A therapist working with compassion and proper intent can provide a form of touch that may be as simple as holding a hand or foot. Traditional Swedish massage is not always necessary with its effleurage and petrissage strokes that may be damaging to the tissues of an elderly client or patient whose body is compromised by a terminal or life-limiting illness. Touch is not recommended in the following specific areas:

- The site of recent surgery
- The site of tumors or lumps
- Phlebitis (inflammation of a vein)
- Fractures
- Undiagnosed or contagious skin conditions or areas of skin irritation
- Open sores or acute injuries
- Areas of infection or inflammation
- Areas of high acute pain or pain of unknown origin

Training for Hospice

Because working with hospice patients can be very intense, it is essential that massage therapists receive some basic training. Most hospice centers will provide the education and emotional support therapists need in working with patients who are dying or have life-limiting illnesses. This training may include the philosophy and ethics of hospice work, along with the process for receiving referrals, clinical indications and contraindications for interventions with hospice patients, and documentation. The treating physician is always in charge of the whole treatment protocol, and therapists must work under the guidance and authority of hospice staff and family members. Before administering the massage, the massage therapist should review the patient's request, assess the patient's needs, and establish therapeutic goals consistent with the interdisciplinary plan of care. Complementary therapy coordinators at hospice agencies may be available to discuss issues and symptoms of the dying process to facilitate massage therapists in their work. Therapists responding to the physiological needs of the client must also respect the emotional and psychological processes that people experience as they deal with the end of life or a life-limiting illness.

It is important that massage therapists examine their beliefs about death and why they hold them. They need to recognize that each person's beliefs differ and refrain from imposing their own value systems on patients or other therapists. Validation and a listening heart are the best complements to comforting touch during a massage session. "The therapist's own beliefs about death and dying can be a source of strength. However, if they don't know what they believe, they'll find the experience of working with hospice patients much harder," says Heather Lantry, complementary therapies coordinator at Hospice Partners in Lombard, Illinois.

Many people fear dying in pain, of becoming helpless and dependent on others, and losing their dignity. In a society that focuses on freedom and independence, losing control at the end may seem unbearable. Depression may interfere with the patient's ability to embrace self-awareness and is often overlooked by health care professionals. While most dying people are not depressed, those who are can be helped. Massage reduces stress hormones, leaving the terminally ill in a much better place to share their feelings and benefit from just being with another human being. It is a powerful way to be healed, not from their terminal illness but emotionally and mentally along the path of acceptance. Soothing and compassionate touch—the comforting care—can lead to the respect, honor, and dignity that the terminally ill need so desperately.

Applications of Theory and Practice for Hospice and Palliative Care Massage	## Technique When the massage therapist responds to the needs of the hospice client, significant modifications must be made in technique to ensure that massage is safe and appropriate. Adjustments in body mechanics will be necessary where it is not possible to use a massage table, and awareness of these adjustments will prevent injury or stress to the therapist's body. Therapists will work with noncommunicative patients and those suffering from dementia, populations that are unable to request a massage themselves or give valuable feedback. Knowledgeable therapists will work with their eyes wide open and be skilled in nonverbal communication, responding to the physiological as well as psychological needs of the client. The setting for hospice and palliative care massage may vary. Clients may be bedridden, in a recliner, or in a wheelchair. They may be fully or partially clothed. Asian bodywork techniques such as gentle shiatsu or acupressure would be indicated. Geriatric strokes such as "fluffing" and "butterfly techniques" developed by Dietrich W. Miesler, founder of Daybreak Geriatric Massage, may also be effective. All strokes and techniques should be soothing and comforting—never stimulating. Shortness of breath is a common symptom for people who are dying. After careful assessment of why the client is short of breath, the therapist may offer relief using pillows and bolsters to change their position or prop them up. The intention of the therapist is always to provide comfort. Begin the session with long deep breaths to center yourself as you place your hands on the client's shoulders or arms. Relax and be present. All movements should be slow and mindful, creating a peaceful environment that will be safe and appropriate for both the client and the therapist. Centering oneself develops a source of personal inner strength to draw upon and share with the one who needs it.

Respecting the vulnerability of a hospice client to touch at this time ensures that the session will always be within boundaries. Pay close attention to feedback, and be confident in your ability to provide nurturing, compassionate touch. Be informed in dealing with emotional release as it is natural that a client at the end of life who receives touch may experience this.

It is essential that you remain aware of your own vulnerabilities and stay clear within your own boundaries. Without putting aside professional standards, as a therapist who works with hospice clients, you have the right to care throughout the process and to grieve when death comes. You should make every effort to care for your own emotional well-being. Receiving regular massage, writing about your feelings, or sharing them with others may help you maintain your balance.

Massage for the Caregiver

"Grief is one of the most universal human emotions—and one of the most isolating. All the world may love a lover, but few of us know how to honor grief—how to be with a grieving person, or how to handle our own grief."

Sometimes the hardest part of dying or dealing with the terminally ill is seeing the effects it has on the family and primary caregivers. Massage professionals can have a significantly positive impact on stress reduction and provide an additional means of support for family members and hospice caregivers.

A project in Portland, Oregon, used massage therapy to reduce the stress and fatigue of people who were caring for dying loved ones. "Caregiver burnout" is a major reason for the institutionalization of individuals who are in the final phases of a terminal illness. Low-income people, the elderly, and those without extended families may find the caregiver role especially difficult. In this project, postmassage surveys revealed significant improvement in the emotional stress of caregivers and identified massage as an effective intervention that should be considered by hospice agencies.

Instructing families and caregivers in the basic art of comforting touch can also greatly enhance their contact with the terminally ill. Massage is another way they can connect and communicate something positive and useful for their loved one. It can also be very empowering when they receive a positive response in return.

Massage for Children in Hospice

Children are not supposed to die, but they do. Death and dying are confusing and frightening for terminally ill children, and their parents struggle deeply with the realization that they will outlive their child.

Parents of dying children who are treated with massage therapy have reported improved relaxation in the children. They are less irritable and show improved sleep patterns. They radiate an inner sense of self-worth and smile more often.

Again, the aim of massage as complementary therapy is to alleviate physical and emotional discomfort in a holistic and safe environment. Before any complementary therapy is given to children, written consent must be obtained from their parent or primary caregiver.

The environment should be prepared with appropriate warmth and dim lighting. The room should be private with parents or caregiving staff present. Soothing music will enhance the atmosphere of relaxation. A notice should be placed on doors to discourage entry while the massage is in progress. The massage professional should begin with breathing exercises and administer slow, rhythmic massage to the child's legs, feet, arms, and hands. Supine position is recommended at all times to encourage direct eye contact and read facial expressions. Before starting the massage, the child must be assessed for contraindications. Do not massage if the child:

- Has high or low temperature
- Is vomiting or has diarrhea
- Is in seizure or showing sign of seizure

- Is exhibiting abnormal signs of behavior
- Has broken skin, bruises, or recent scar tissue
- Has had a recent injury or surgery
- Shows any concerns
- Does not want to be touched

The massage professional should always ask the child's permission first. Talk with the child during the massage and always look for nonverbal communication, as the child may not be able to tell you whether or not he or she is enjoying the massage. It is essential for the therapist to always remain calm and in control.

It is also helpful for the massage professional to teach some basic massage techniques to parents, lessening their own feelings of helplessness and giving them a way to have positive, nurturing, and caring interaction with their child.

Chapter Summary

Nurturing and compassionate touch is paramount in the provision of comfort care for the terminally ill. Consideration of what the client does or doesn't want lays the foundation for safe and appropriate interaction through massage. Sometimes, simply encompassing a hand or arm between the fullness of the therapist's hands can bring a sense of warmth and peace, permitting the client to just be. A terminally ill client will be facing fears of dying, of losing independence and dignity, of pain, suffering, and loneliness. All of these concerns may be appropriately addressed with nurturing and compassionate touch. The aim of the therapy session is never to heal but always to comfort, allowing acceptance and dignity to pervade as the individual is sheltered on their travel into the great unknown.

Performing massage on the most vulnerable members of our population is quite rewarding. Special needs children's tactile experiences blossom through the power of touch offered by massage therapists, parents, siblings, and extended family members. The power of touch also is extremely important for seniors and patients in a hospice setting. If you choose to work with special populations, you will be rewarded many times over.

Applying Your Knowledge

Self-Testing

1. Effleurage and _____ strokes in a "sawing" motion will help an asthmatic child during an attack.
   a) tapotement
   b) petrissage
   c) vibration
   d) friction

2. Colic in babies may be due to what disorder?
   a) Nervous system
   b) Gastrointestinal
   c) Cardiac
   d) None of the above is correct.

3. How much more weight did preterm infants who were massaged gain compared to the nonmassaged control group in the Touch Research Institute study?
   a) 10%
   b) 20%
   c) 47%
   d) 50%

4. Cerebral palsy is a developmental disability that originates when the parts of the brain that control movement are damaged during gestational development, birth, or early infancy.
   a) True
   b) False

5. Autism includes developmental disorders such as
   a) Asperger's syndrome.
   b) Rett's disorder.

c) pervasive developmental delay

d) All of the above are correct.

6. Children with ADHD can be helped by which modalities?

   a) Craniosacral therapy

   b) Myofascial release

   c) Acupressure

   d) All of the above are correct.

7. Early intervention with educational and other services (including massage therapy) greatly improves the functioning of young children with Down's syndrome.

   a) True

   b) False

8. For blind children, what does massage help to improve?

   a) Posture

   b) Increase body awareness

   c) Ability to see gray areas

   d) a and b

9. What percentage of improvement in language skills did deaf children who were massaged for three months experience?

   a) 13%

   b) 33%

   c) 69%

   d) 73%

10. In what ways can massage benefit the child with AIDS?

    a) Boosting the immune system

    b) Improving circulation

    c) Relieving muscle aches and cramps

    d) All of the above are correct.

11. When working with seniors it is important to listen with your ears, hands, and _____ .

    a) heart

    b) conscience

    c) wallet

    d) All of the above are correct.

12. It is extremely important to obtain client history on seniors, especially knowledge of

    a) any medications being taken

    b) age

    c) weight

    d) height

13. Massage in the hospice setting offers which of the following benefits?

    a) Relief from pain

    b) Relief from insomnia

    c) Relief from nausea and constipation

    d) All of the above are correct.

14. Swedish massage, with its effleurage and petrissage strokes, is always the best modality to use with hospice patients.

    a) True

    b) False

Case Studies/Critical Thinking

A. One of your regular massage clients asks you if she can bring in her 10-year-old son who has been diagnosed with ADHD. He is on ritalin but still having problems in school with focusing and social activities. She would like to know if, in your professional opinion, massage will help. How do you answer?

B. You learned in massage school that the tapotement stroke "cupping" is good for breaking up congestion in the lungs and wonder if it is appropriate for a client's child who has asthma. What type of massage will you perform on this child?

C. A mother of a 4-year-old with cerebral palsy asks you if you can massage her child. Is massage indicated or contraindicated for this condition?

D. You are a newly licensed massage therapist who has decided to devote one day a week to working in a local senior assisted-living center. This center happens to be one with predominantly government-subsidized seniors. Recognizing that massage can be a benefit to seniors but also that they are on a tight budget, how will you proceed?

References for information in this chapter can be found in Quick Guide C at the end of this book.

CHAPTER 12

Massage for Survivors of Abuse

LEARNING OUTCOMES

After completing this chapter, you will be able to:

- Discuss the special considerations in working with victims of sexual abuse.

- Recognize the three phases of sexual abuse effects.

- Identify common indicators of sexual abuse.

- Recognize ways to establish trust with a client.

- Discuss the importance of being a member of a health care team.

- Adapt a protocol for working with survivors of abuse in the massage setting.

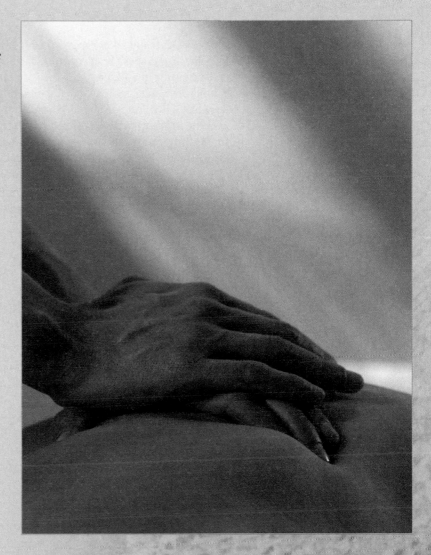

KEY TERMS

client authority *(p. 312)*

disconnection *(p. 312)*

intervention *(p. 311)*

negative behavioral patterns *(p. 308)*

posttraumatic stress disorder
(PTSD) *(p. 311)*

retraumatization *(p. 316)*

sexual abuse *(p. 308)*

three phases of effects *(p. 309)*

touch *(p. 311)*

INTRODUCTION

Abuse is an often overlooked topic not only in massage schools but also in society in general. Sadly, there are too many victims of sexual, verbal, emotional, and physical abuse. Massage therapy can play an important role in an abuse victim's recovery and continued integration with society. As with other special populations, working with abuse survivors requires a particular approach.

This chapter includes sections called "Applications of Theory and Practice." These sections offer additional content for those who want to study these massage specialties in greater depth.

Working with Survivors of Sexual Abuse

By Donna Cerio, MT

As bodywork therapy takes its rightful place as a viable form of health care in the world today, practitioners will reach a wider variety of client populations then ever before.

This chapter introduces the basics of delivering therapeutic bodywork to survivors of sexual abuse. The protocols detailed can be applied to other forms of abuse as well, whether verbal, emotional, or physical.

The belief that "time heals all" definitely does not apply to the wounds of sexual abuse. Healing can be and often is a lifelong process. Years after abuse, abuse survivors may find themselves with chronic body pain, **negative behavioral patterns** such as a pervasive underlying anxiety, a severely damaged self-concept, a fear of intimacy, and many other debilitating results; often these patterns are impossible to change. One of the daunting consequences can be an aversion to being touched, even when the touch is therapeutic, recommended to restore and maintain optimal health, and feels good to most people (figure 12.1).

People can and do make a complete recovery from the trauma of sexual abuse. Massage and bodywork can help clients heal their wounds, reclaim their health and wholeness, and move on to create productive, happy lives free from the obstacles that sexual abuse presents.

Prevalence of Sexual Abuse

The prevalence of sexual abuse is astounding. Writer Patricia Weaver Francisco captures its pervasiveness: "If the occurrence of sexual abuse were audible with its decibel level equal to its frequency, it would overpower us day and night, interrupting every one of our moments, an insistent jackhammer of distress. We would demand an end to it. And if we failed to locate the source, we would condemn the whole structure. We would refuse to live under such conditions."

Sexual abuse includes but is not limited to incest, rape, sexual assault, child molestation, and inappropriate sexual contact by an authority figure. The statistics are staggering and demonstrate that many people suffer from sexual abuse. Even if you do not specialize in clients with a history of sexual abuse, you are quite likely to encounter this client population in your practice. Consider the following:

- "Around the world, at least one woman in every three has been beaten, coerced into sex or otherwise abused in her lifetime" (*Population Reports* published by the Johns Hopkins School of Public Health).

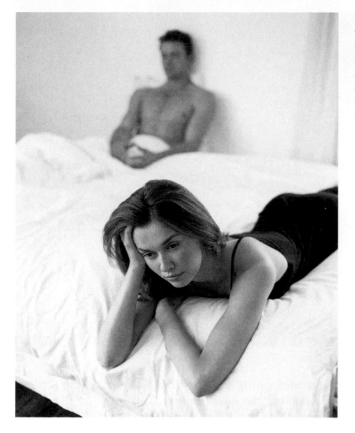

Figure 12.1
Touch experiences that others take for granted are so very difficult for survivors of abuse. They may even have an aversion to the pleasurable touch that others relish.

- "An estimated 302,100 women and 92,700 men are forcibly raped each year in the United States" (U.S. Department of Justice, National Institute of Justice, and Centers for Disease Control and Prevention).
- Only 39% of rapes and sexual assaults were reported to law enforcement (2003 National Crime Victimization Survey).

This last statistic is the most disturbing because it indicates that a significant number of people are suffering in isolation and silence.

Effects of Sexual Abuse

Nearly all victims of sexual abuse will experience **three phases of effects**. These may be indicators that your client has experienced trauma. It is wise for the massage and bodywork practitioner to notice if these effects are present in a client. However, do not conclude that because you see one or more of these effects that your client has suffered sexual abuse. These effects can be indicators of other kinds of trauma. Be aware that they are signs that *may* indicate sexual trauma in the client's history.

Phase I occurs during and immediately following the incident and includes:

- Disorganization
- Disorientation and confusion
- Profound emotional responses such as fear, shame, guilt, humiliation, self-blame, self-degradation, anger, embarrassment, and a desire for revenge
- Avoidance reaction. The person may be quiet, smiling, and dispassionate. In this case, the trauma has been separated from the experience but is still profoundly affecting the abused.

Intervention in phase I can minimize, if not prevent, phase II effects. For intervention to be effective, any law enforcement personnel, medical professionals, psychologists, or other caregivers need to acknowledge the victim's experience. All contact, verbal and

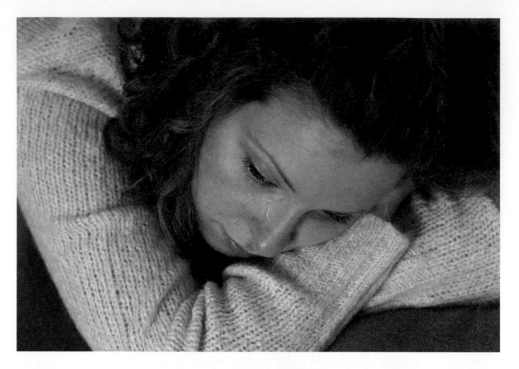

or physical, needs to be made in a calm, caring and respectful way, taking into account any specific personal needs the individual may have (figure 12.2).

Phase II effects appear during the first year after the incident and include:

- Rapid or extreme reorganization of established patterns in their life
- Development of a variety of phobias
- Sleep disturbances
- Gastrointestinal irritability with no known physiological etiology
- Genitourinary discomforts with no known physiological etiology
- Chronic suspicion
- Inability to trust others or self
- Altered interpersonal relationships
- Underlying pervasive anxiety
- Avoidance of sex or unsafe promiscuity
- Depression

Intervention in phase II can minimize, if not prevent, phase III effects.

Phase III effects arise during the ensuing years. These long-term effects of sexual abuse are extensive and can be devastating. Some of the possible serious effects are:

- A greater likelihood of revictimization if the female victim receives no intervention. Repeated incidences of abuse are common.
- Problems with impulse control or being overcontrolling (e.g., compulsive shopping, wanting to control the environment to an excessive degree, making snap decisions).
- Overly concerned with pleasing others. These clients will not tell you something is wrong if they feel upset or distressed by something that happens during a session.
- Difficulties forming relationships beyond the superficial level. This is something the client may tell you indirectly.
- Irritable, distrustful, fearful personalities with unrealistic expectations of others and severe reactions to mistakes, their own or others'. These clients often put themselves down or complain about the ineptitude of others.
- Disturbed pattern of personal interaction (e.g., isolation, foolhardy behavior, failure to protect themselves). A common example is clients who are in abusive relationships and blame themselves for the abuse they endure.

- **post-traumatic stress disorder (PTSD)**—the development of symptoms following an extreme traumatic stressor that involves actual, perceived, or threatened death, serious injury, or other threat to the integrity of a person.
- Inappropriate boundaries, leading to giving too much information about themselves at inappropriate times or being too open about personal matters in situations that may not be safe.
- Inability to identify and maintain boundaries in relationships of all kinds.

Do not assume that a single incident of abuse has less impact than repeated abuse. The effects may vary, but the impact is just as forceful and devastating. **Intervention** can greatly decrease the impact of these effects and increase the quality of life.

Special Needs of Abuse Victims

Sexual abuse, especially of young children, sets the stage for living life as a victim or living in the victim body, which is a state of being in which the person continually expects to be victimized, often consciously but more often unconsciously. The mind tends to interpret events and interactions as abusive, whether or not they merit that interpretation. The emotions easily slip into those of a victim. The physical body automatically responds to stimulus as if it were being threatened.

Sexual abuse undermines a person's trust in her own instinct. For children between the ages of 0 and 7, the connection between the mind and the instinct is not yet developed; therefore, its development is interrupted. Between the ages of 8 to 13, the mind is developing and learning how to relate to the instinct. Sexual abuse at this time interrupts the development of this relationship between the mind and the instinct. Between 14 and the mid-20s, the development of the natural connection to the environment and others in it is distorted. When sexual abuse happens to adults in their mid-20s or later, trust is undermined in all areas of their life. In all these cases, sexual abuse leaves the survivors with a basic ambivalence about touch and a tendency to interpret touch in ways that are not typical.

Survivors of sexual abuse have common characteristics that can complicate touch for them and for those who touch them. The techniques and approaches that usually succeed with the majority of clients can have unintended and unpredictable effects on this client population.

Several factors influence how survivors of sexual abuse perceive **touch**. Two important ones are childhood experience and the context in which the abuse occurred.

Childhood experience plays a significant role in the perception of touch. The first seven years of life are formative in terms of what kind of touch will be expected throughout life. If children experience abusive touch during this time, their expectations and perceptions of touch are radically altered.

The context in which the abuse took place also is a strong determinant of the perception of touch. A therapeutic environment that resembles the context of the original abuse has the potential to trigger a devastating feeling of loss of control. This distorts the perception of the touch so that any touch can feel abusive. The integrity of the environment in which the touch occurs has a profound influence on perception. *Integrity* refers to the values on which the condition of the environment is based. The environment includes the physical, mental, and emotional setting. The Intentional Touch™ principles apply here: "An environment of safety and comfort is necessary for promoting healing in clients," and "We have a moral obligation to deliver our services with responsibility and respect."

Other factors that might affect the perception of touch are alterations in the way the survivor's brain functions as a result of the abuse, social and cultural factors, and the practitioner's approach, training, and experience working with survivors. While some of these factors are out of the practitioner's control, many can be addressed through the practitioner's approach to touch and the therapeutic relationship (figure 12.3).

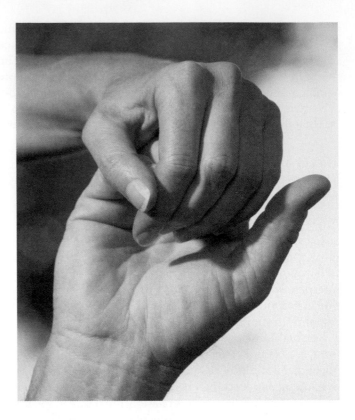

The Therapeutic Relationship and Client Authority

Two of the core experiences of sexual abuse are disempowerment and disconnection from the self and others. Disempowerment is the divestment of one's authority over one's own life. Sexual abuse is like a robber who takes away the victim's authority to have a say over what happens to her body, mind, and emotions. **Disconnection** refers to the disruption in the usually integrated functioning of consciousness, memory, identity, and perception. A person may experience one or more of the following: become unaware of her own feelings; not be able to recall significant events in her past; perceive a situation in a way that is not based on the facts; or sever intimate relationships with people who had been in her life for a long time.

Recovery, therefore, is based on empowering the survivor and creating new connections. Healing takes place in the context of the therapeutic relationship. The basis for all healing lies in two principles: "We, as health care practitioners, do not heal another person," and "Each individual has the authority over his or her own health." The survivor of sexual abuse especially needs to be empowered and given authority while receiving hands-on therapies. When the sexual abuse took place, the power to control how she was touched was taken away. To restore the right to choose, massage therapists must not approach their work as if they know what is best for the client.

In reality, you cannot heal another person, but your techniques can influence the body's own healing mechanisms. Bodywork offers the body the opportunity to heal itself. The actual healing is done by the client's own system. For example, when a person breaks a bone, she sees a doctor to have it x-rayed and set so that it is in the correct position to heal. The actual cellular repair of the break, however, depends on the client's bone cells. The osteoclasts and osteoblasts do the work.

This approach shifts your relationship with your clients, allowing you to view your client's progress as an interactive process. You become your client's ally, her partner in the healing process. Your client is empowered by your recognition of her authority over her own health care, termed **"client authority."** While you are expected to accurately and carefully administrer your treatment, you are relieved of the unrealistic expectation that you are totally responsible for the health of your client.

Bodywork therapy presents the opportunity to help rebuild the shattered relationship structure that is so common in the aftermath of sexual abuse. It is essential to model a healthy, appropriate environment and approach to the therapeutic relationship, as well as a healthy, appropriate touch. Without this, the relationship runs the risk of mimicking the abusive environment. Attention to the relationship structure and environment clears the inherent confusion and distortion that accompanies sexual abuse.

The therapeutic relationship between the massage therapist and the client is an appropriate ground for recovery. Bodywork can promote a healthy, positive relationship with another person. A practitioner who has clear boundaries, no agenda other than to support the client in her path, and is caring and safe is a true treasure for abuse survivors. The clients gain increased stability based on self-trust. They have chosen this therapeutic relationship because it works for them. The result is a stronger base on which to build positive relationships with others.

Applications of Theory and Practice for Massage of Survivors of Abuse: Organized by Category of Clients

The Three Categories of Clients with a History of Sexual Abuse

You may encounter three categories of clients with a history of sexual abuse. Working with each category has unique challenges.

Category One

Category one clients are open and direct with you regarding their history. They seek to work directly on healing from the abuse and see bodywork as a part of their healing strategy. When working with a category one client, the practitioner and client use a team approach with at least one other licensed professional involved. Licensed professionals who are often part of the team include marriage and family therapists, physicians, psychiatrists, and acupuncturists. Often the client has such a team in place already (figure 12.4).

There are three reasons for including another licensed professional:

- Issues may arise that are outside of the practitioner's scope of practice, and a licensed professional can often prevent legal and ethical problems for the practitioner. For example, if a practitioner observes signs that indicate depression, it would be prudent to suggest that the client see a professional who is able to diagnose and treat depression if it is present. Depression may lead to suicide, especially in survivors. If the client does commit suicide and the practitioner had not referred the client, it could be construed as professional negligence.

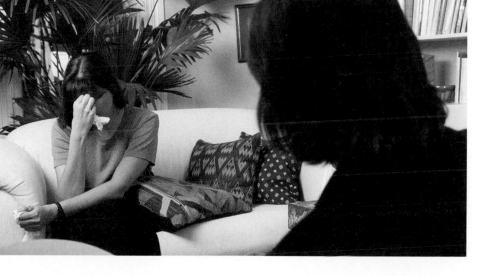

Figure 12.4
A client will often have a health care team that will involve several professionals such as a marriage and family therapist, physicians, psychiatrists, and massage therapists.

Category One

M ay (not her real name) is an example of a category one client. May was referred by a licensed health care professional who knew that the massage therapist specialized in working with sexual abuse survivors. During their phone contact before her first session, May told the therapist of her history. She described exactly what her healing strategy was, at what stage she was in the healing process, and how she saw her potential work with the therapist assisting her further.

- Having a licensed professional involved gives the client the safety net of someone who can intervene to help, if necessary.
- Including licensed professionals gives the client and the bodywork practitioner access to knowledge from the different disciplines of the team members, leading to more effective healing strategies. The team approach contributes to the partnership of alternative and conventional medicine. The opportunity to confer with another professional who is involved in the case is invaluable.

Category Two

Category two clients are aware that they were sexually abused but do not tell you. They may feel shame or fear being judged or rejected. Or, as a survival mechanism, they may have minimized the impact abuse has had on them and not be aware that the abuse is related to their health complaints (figure 12.5).

It is important to address the information about your client's history of sexual abuse appropriately:

- Acknowledge the information verbally by saying something like "I am glad that you told me this." Show appreciation and enthusiasm about receiving the information. Remember, this is a very important step your client is taking toward wholeness and health.

Figure 12.5
Survivors of abuse may feel shame or fear of being judged or rejected.

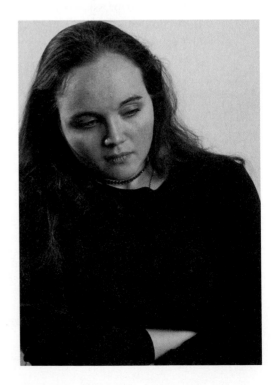

Category Two

Rita (not her real name) is an example of a category two client. She sought bodywork therapy because of a long-term pattern of poor health that had not been responding to conventional medical treatment. She would catch whatever malady was going around, no matter how she tried to protect herself. It would affect her more severely than others, and it would take her longer than average to recover. She was fatigued to the point that it interrupted her daily functioning. She and her massage therapist worked together for a number of years, accomplishing a steady consistent and sustainable improvement in her health. One day, as she was getting onto the table, she said in a casual tone of voice: "Oh, by the way, I was sexually abused as a child and I thought you might like to know."

During the session in which Rita disclosed her history, her muscles were much tenser and less responsive to touch. The therapist was careful not to override the guarding. Future sessions changed in many ways. She became more comfortable with energy work. At the same time, the usual massage she loved became uncomfortable for her. When a client exposes a part of herself to the therapist, she is exposing that part to herself also. It changes her personal relationship with herself, and that changes her relationship with her massage therapist.

Rita needed to build physical and emotional strength to face her past. While her health problems were rooted in her past abuse, her weakness made it impossible for her to deal with it. As Rita grew strong enough to cope, she dealt directly with her past and became even stronger. She is now a marathon runner and top-level executive for a company she helped found. She is seldom ill, and when she is, she recovers faster than most people.

- Thank the client for being forthcoming.
- Create an immediate frame emphasizing the healing process by saying something like "This is important for your healing process."
- Speak with complete acceptance and respect for the information. Make sure your tone of voice reflects acceptance.
- Do not show surprise, anger, disgust, or sadness. Make mental notes of your responses. Work with your responses in your own personal therapy.
- To prevent retraumatizing your clients, do not talk about the details of what they just disclosed to you while you are working on them.
- Create an appropriate time to discuss the implications of the new information on your work together.

Create a list of questions to use when this situation arises. Keep in mind that you want to ask these questions in a way that promotes client authority. Ask at a designated time decided upon by you and the client. The following are useful questions:

- What made this the right time for you to tell me?
- Are there any specific requests you have of me?
- How do you feel this information is going to influence our work?

Address the issue of having a licensed health care professional as part of the team. Inform your client of the benefits of involving others who specialize in treating abuse victims.

As a practitioner, you will ask yourself how knowing about the abuse changes things for your work with this client. Do not assume that because you have seen positive change up until now, everything will continue to progress in the same way. Now that the disclosure has been made, a great deal of significant hidden material likely will surface. You may even find that what has worked with this client before may no longer work and may even have an opposite effect.

Category Three

Category three clients have been sexually abused and have no recollection of it. Therefore, the information never comes out. When people experience serious trauma, they sometimes separate the traumatic event from the conscious mind in order to tolerate what has happened or is happening.

Category Three

Kay (not her real name) is an example of a category three client. Kay, who was 58, sought bodywork therapy for help with several unresolved, long-term chronic ailments, including migraine headaches, depression, fibromyalgia, and chronic fatigue syndrome. She was also dealing with an eating disorder and mental health issues. She had worked with conventional medicine for years without success.

It is not in the massage and bodywork therapist's scope of practice to diagnose. Nor is it ethical to assume that you know from what your client's health problems stem. Even though Kay's symptoms resembled those of a survivor of sexual abuse, her bodywork therapist knew it was best to approach a client like Kay as if she were a category one client.

Two years after starting massage therapy, Kay disclosed to her health care team that she was beginning to have partial memories of sexual abuse in childhood by her grandfather. None of the team members was surprised that there had been severe trauma in her life, but none knew the details of her trauma until she disclosed them.

There is no really "pure" case study of a category three client. Any client could be in this category. It is safest to treat all clients as potentially being in category three, particularly if you notice any of the common indicators listed on page 317.

Each category of client has its own challenges and requirements. Dealing with these calls for flexibility and imagination on the part of the bodywork therapist, along with a willingness to customize the work to the client.

What Bodywork Therapists Need to Know and Why

Sexual trauma has effects on survivors that change the way they respond to health care in general and bodywork in particular. It is important for bodywork practitioners to understand how this client population differs from other client populations. Some consequences of sexual abuse are:

- An aversion to being touched, even if the touch is therapeutic and recommended to restore and maintain optimal health. Because of this aversion, many survivors avoid health care at all costs. For example, a 55-year-old female client had never had a gynecological examination.
- Even well-intended touch can trigger reactions rooted in past traumatic events.
- Sexual abuse leaves deep imprints. Physically and energetically, they are stored at the most basic level of structure, encoded in the cellular levels of the human body. Any touch can activate these imprints, which are sometimes called "landmines," triggering cell memory and retraumatizing the client. **Retraumatization** can have dire consequences for the practitioner as well as the client. In one case, a practitioner lost her license because a client with a history of sexual trauma interpreted a technique that she used as a sexual assault. Sorting out what really happened is difficult since usually only the practitioner and the client are in the treatment room. While they cannot always avoid encountering a landmine, they want to do all they can to avoid triggering its effect.
- The environment in which the bodywork therapy takes place can innocently mimic that of the original abuse. One client reported an experience that occurred when visiting a new physician. Although nothing inappropriate occurred during the appointment, she left the doctor's office feeling traumatized. In her therapy, she discovered the reason: The doctor's office resembled the room in which she had been sexually abused as a child. She and her therapist were able to work through this so that she could continue to receive her health care with this physician. Having a licensed therapist prevents unintended, unwanted consequences.

- Health care practitioners must maintain well-defined boundaries and clarity regarding the client's participation in the decisions regarding treatment. Touch of any kind that is not consented to, or perceived as not consented to, can, and often does, mimic the abuse. A survivor was once seeing a physical therapist for a neck injury. She reacted strongly to being touched on the neck because her neck had been gripped when she was sexually assaulted. The physical therapist, whose training included the idea that body tension was something that intrinsically needed to be released, was not willing to adjust her approach, and the treatment failed.
- Self-care has to be a priority with clients who have been sexually abused. The energy field of abused persons often has an amplified sensory receiving system, making them ultrasensitive to the obvious as well as the subtler elements in the environment. If you have not taken care of and centered yourself before a session, the client may sense this and find it difficult to let go and receive from the session. At those times, the client will almost always ask you how you are doing and be overly concerned about your well-being. Those who do not ask will experience an anxiety for you that will distract from their therapeutic experience. Sexual abuse survivors are often accomplished caregivers but also have trouble accepting care from others.

Common Indicators of Sexual Abuse

A number of signs may indicate that a client has a history of sexual trauma (figure 12.6):

- Micromanaging the session
- Longer recovery time for injuries or illnesses
- Long-term chronic health conditions that do not respond to the usual treatments
- Apprehension about being touched

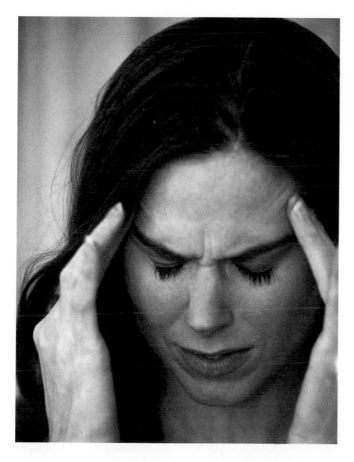

Figure 12.6
Chronic health conditions, such as severe migraines or tension headaches that do not respond to usual treatments, may be indicators of abuse.

- Intensified reactions to common health care procedures
- Undeveloped or unhealthy boundary system
- Self-destructive behavior
- Problems setting limits
- Problems expressing needs and wants
- Black-and-white thinking
- Heightened sensitivity to the environment
- Rigidity: more difficulty handling change than is the norm
- Landmines

If you notice one or more of these signs, do not assume that your client has been sexually abused. Remember the example of the category three client, Kay. If her team of professionals had proceeded on the assumption that they knew what the root of her health problems was, they would have run the risk of sabotaging her healing process by imposing their agenda, thereby undermining the trust between client and professional. As hard as it is to hold back when you think you see what the causes of symptoms are, the results can be disastrous if you do not. Respecting the healing process and its pace is paramount to providing a client-centered service.

Chapter Summary

For survivors of abuse, touch can be a totally different experience than that experienced by other segments of the population. The well-trained massage therapist can be an integral part of an abuse victim's recovery and daily coping. Whether you choose, or are "called," to work with a specific segment of the population, you will be rewarded many times over. We hope you will continue work in one of these specialized fields mentioned in this chapter and the two preceding chapters and that you will have an impact on massage for the human family.

Applying Your Knowledge

Self-Testing

1. How many phases of abuse may be exhibited by a client?
   a) 1
   b) 2
   c) 3
   d) Multiple

2. According to *Population Reports* published by the Johns Hopkins School of Public Health, what is the ratio of women in the world who have been beaten, coerced into sex, or otherwise abused in their lifetime?
   a) 1 in 3
   b) 3 in 10
   c) 5 in 10
   d) 7 in 10

3. Sexual abuse victims have problems with impulse control or being overcontrolling that can manifest as:
   a) Compulsive shopping
   b) Wanting to control the environment to an excessive degree

   c) Making snap decisions
   d) All of the above are correct.

4. Between the ages 8 to 13, the mind is developing and learning how to relate to the instinct. Sexual abuse at this time interrupts the development of this relationship between the mind and the instinct.
   a) True
   b) False

5. Survivors of sexual abuse have a set of common characteristics that can complicate touch for them and for those who touch them.
   a) True
   b) False

6. Two of the core experiences of sexual abuse are disempowerment and disconnection from the self and others.
   a) True
   b) False

7. Bodywork can promote a healthy, positive relationship with another person.
   a) True
   b) False

8. Sexual trauma can create an aversion to being touched in the survivor, even if the touch is therapeutic and recommended, but the practitioner should push forward with the bodywork.

   a) True

   b) False

9. To prevent retraumatizing a client, do not talk about the details of what she just disclosed to you during a massage.

   a) True

   b) False

10. Which of these signs indicate there may be a history of sexual trauma?

    a) Micromanaging the session

    b) Long-term chronic health conditions that do not respond to the usual treatments

    c) Undeveloped or unhealthy boundary system

    d) All of the above are correct.

11. A Category three client has been sexually abused and has no recollection of it.

    a) True

    b) False

Case Studies/Critical Thinking

A. A client has referred a friend for massage. You learn that this friend has been physically abused by a former spouse. How will you approach the first massage?

B. You are working in a chiropractor's office handling mostly insurance clients who have injuries from auto accidents. After performing massage twice on a woman who had been in a car that was rear-ended at 20 miles per hour, you notice that she has bruises all over her body that are not consistent with the accident. How do you handle this?

References for information in this chapter can be found in Quick Guide C at the end of the book.

CHAPTER 13

Sports Massage for Amateur and Professional Athletes

LEARNING OUTCOMES

After completing this chapter, you will be able to:

- Define sports massage and differentiate it from other modalities.

- Explain the physiological effects of sports massage.

- Recognize the indications and contraindications for sports massage.

- List the basic techniques of sports massage and timing parameters for use of each technique.

- Implement sports massage techniques.

- Perform basic muscle testing procedures.

- Explain injury pathology and implementation of cryotherapy and moist heat therapy.

- Develop a working knowledge of massage routines for specific injuries.

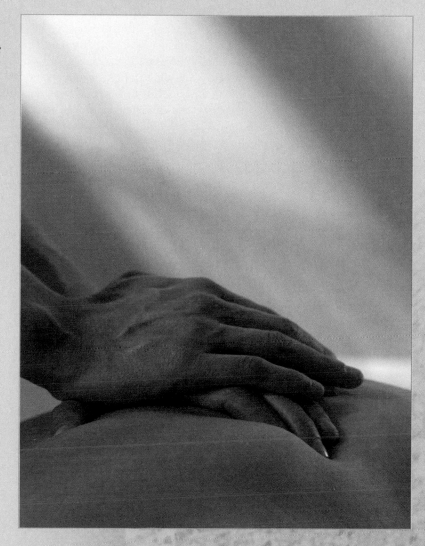

KEY TERMS

bursa *(p. 341)*
cramp *(p. 341)*
cryokinetic therapy *(p. 342)*
cryotherapy *(p. 342)*
ecchymosis *(p. 339)*
Golgi tendon organs *(p. 334)*
Golgi tendon reflex *(p. 334)*
hydrotherapy *(p. 342)*
hyperthermia *(p. 345)*
hypothermia *(p. 346)*

ischemia *(p. 341)*
lactic acid *(p. 323)*
laxity *(p. 340)*
"pain-spasm-pain" cycle *(p. 339)*
positional release or strain-
    counterstrain *(p. 336)*
PRICE *(p. 342)*
proprioceptive neuromuscular
    facilitation (PNF) *(p. 331)*

reciprocal inhibition method
    (p. 335)
RICE *(p. 342)*
spasms *(p. 341)*
"splinting" *(p. 339)*
sprains *(p. 339)*
strain *(p. 340)*
tendinitis *(p. 341)*
tense-relax method *(p. 331)*

INTRODUCTION

Ever since President John F. Kennedy placed an emphasis on health and athletics in the 1960s, the number of professional, semiprofessional, and amateur athletes has swelled. In the early 1980s, the New York City transit strike single-handedly increased the sales of running shoes as millions of people found themselves walking to the office. This boost in sales led to many new designs in athletic footware. Aerobics or "working out" was popularized by personalities such as Jane Fonda, while others, from Bruce Lee (martial arts) to Nadia Comenici (gymnastics) to Magic Johnson (basketball), prompted average people to participate in sports of some sort. Current sports icons such as Lance Armstrong (cycling), Andy Roddick (tennis), and Shaquille O'Neal (basketball) continue to encourage all ages to participate in sports. Decades later, barely a day or evening goes by when the local tennis courts, pools, fitness centers, and ball fields are not filled to capacity with people of all ages. It is not surprising, then, that sports-related injuries and common muscle sorenesses abound. Sports massage helps restore the body's natural balance of strength and elasticity by reducing physiological fatigue and aiding recovery from exercise through dispersion of accumulated by-products (lactic acids).

Sports Massage

Massage is the manipulation of the soft tissues of the body using strokes that are applied with the hand, foot, arm, or elbow. Sports massage takes this definition one step further by using focused strokes within a specific time frame as well as adding hydrotherapy and stretching or range of motion.

A sports massage therapist should possess basic orthopedic skills in order to distinguish between musculoskeletal problems that warrant massage therapy and those that require referral to a physician.

 TECHNIQUE EMPHASIS The sports massage therapist should also have a working knowledge of the application of ice and heat, stretching techniques, strength training, conditioning principles, and all aspects—including the language—of each sport addressed.

For example, repetitive motions such as those performed by a golfer, tennis player, or pitcher can cause medial epicondylitis, lateral epicondylitis, and rotator cuff injuries, respectively. Runners commonly experience "runner's knee," which is trauma to the sleeve of the knee joint; this condition is also referred to as IT band syndrome. Chapter 19 explains stretching and strength training, while chapter 6 examines how the body functions mechanically. Finally, sports massage therapists should embrace both Eastern and Western philosophies so that they view the athlete as a whole and not just as an "injury."

Sports Massage Applications

As chapter 6 showed, muscles cross over joints, acting as levers to decrease or increase the angle between two bones and produce movement. Muscles that are in spasm adversely affect the joints' ability to function optimally. All joints are further complicated by ligaments, connective tissue, and bursae, all of which become stiff when injured and not used during the recovery phase (in the case of an athlete) or when a previously sedentary person begins an exercise routine. Discomfort or stiffness in soft tissues and joints discourages further movement or exercise. This results in a cycle of increasing debility, hampering recovery or discouraging continued involvement in exercise.

A sports massage therapist counteracts this "binding" feeling or restriction by using massage strokes, gentle stretching, range of motion, and applications of ice or heat to release muscle and connective tissue tension, and free joints. Therefore, sports massage can play a part in all phases of an athlete's training, whether professional or amateur. The main applications are preevent, interevent, postevent, recovery, and maintenance massage.

Physiological Effects of Sports Massage

Massage can relax and lengthen shortened or contracted muscles, and it can stimulate weak or stiff muscles. **Lactic acids** build up in muscle tissue shortly after exercise begins. These acids are waste products that contribute to a feeling of pain or "fullness" and "heaviness" with accompanying cramping that exercisers, athletes, dancers, and walkers suffer from during or after workouts or performances. Lactic acids are formed when the glycogen stored in the liver and muscles is burned to produce the energy expended during exercise. These acids must eventually be reconverted to glycogen and stored again or drained out via the lymph and circulatory systems. Pain and fatigue persists until this process of reconverting or excreting is completed. Although some new research suggests the body does an adequate job of removing lactic acids on its own, sports massage can help eliminate the irritation caused by these wastes, thus increasing muscle recovery rates.

This muscle "balancing" can help posture and promote more efficient movement. Although sports massage does not directly increase muscle strength, it can speed recovery from the fatigue that occurs after exercise. In this way, it is possible to do more exercise or training, which in the long run strengthens muscles and improves conditioning. Sports massage also provides a gentle stretching action to both the muscles and the surrounding connective tissues, keeping these tissues elastic.

Indications

The benefits of sports massage are as varied as the numbers of athletic events encountered today. Generally speaking, sports massage will:

- Improve circulation
- Reduce muscle tension and fatigue
- Remove toxins or lactic acids
- Facilitate lymphatic drainage
- Aid in preventing muscle spasms
- Accelerate recovery time

- Lengthen contracted or shortened muscle
- Breakdown scar tissue and adhesions
- Deactivate trigger points
- Aid in the rehabilitation of injury

Contraindications

As with any other massage modality, there are general guidelines that dictate when sports massage would not be advisable. These include:

- Acute stage of an injury or injury with severe pain
- Traumatic joint injuries such as joint instability
- Injuries that do not heal after three weeks
- Broken skin, wounds, or infection

Keep in mind that there are always situations that fall into a gray area regarding whether massage is contraindicated or not. Under normal circumstances, for example, you would refrain from working on an area in which swelling or edema are present. Education in basic orthopedic assessment will help you determine if the situation warrants sports massage (i.e., the muscles need to be flushed due to overexertion or competition). As always, if your common sense, education, or experience tell you to refer the client to the appropriate medical professional, such as a sports medicine doctor or orthopedist, then do so. Many books on orthopedic assessment are available. See appendix A for more information.

Sports Massage Strokes

In addition to the five basic Swedish strokes used in therapeutic massage—effleurage, petrissage, friction, tapotement, and vibration (see chapter 4)—sports massage strokes include compression, direct or sustained pressure, skin rolling, rocking and shaking, compression-broadening, and compression with active movement.

> **EXAM POINT** Generally, preevent strokes are used to "wake up" tissue by increasing circulation and preparing the muscles for a particular sport, while postevent strokes flush the muscle.

Preevent sports massage strokes usually include gliding effleurage, compression, kneading (petrissage), brisk broadening, *superficial* circular friction, percussion, and vibration. Postevent strokes include gliding effleurage, compression, kneading (petrissage), compression-broadening, circular friction, and vibration. On average, both preevent and postevent massage lasts approximately 12 to 15 minutes, although either may be longer depending on the conditions and the athlete. Preevent massage is performed with a quick rhythm and pace with the focus being preparation, while postevent massage is performed slowly with the intent being to flush the muscle. Typically, no lubricant is used. If necessary, a "sports massage cream" (specially formulated to provide enough "glide" so as to not produce unwanted drag on the skin) can be used.

Effleurage

During preevent, recovery, and maintenance sports massage, effleurage (a gliding stroke) is used briskly to warm tissue and assess muscles. Postevent effleurage is done more slowly for a more relaxing effect and to start recovery. Effleurage uses the full palmar surface of the hand to follow the contours of the body (figure 13.1).

Petrissage

Petrissage (kneading, wringing) is not a stimulating stroke and therefore is not usually used in preevent massage.

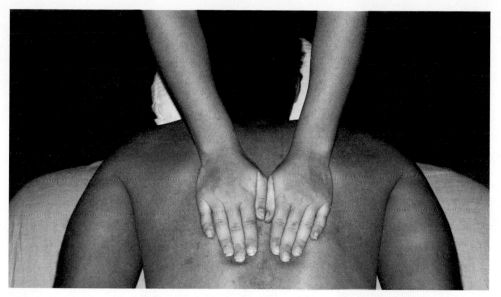

Figure 13.1 Effleurage down back

One- or two-handed petrissage can be used to sink into the muscle, grasp it, pull it up "off" the bone, and release it (figure 13.2).

Friction

Friction is a point-specific stroke that is best used for maintenance massage but can be used, depending on the depth, with other classifications of sports massage. Friction is the best stroke to break up adhesions, thereby increasing muscle elasticity, pliability, and range of motion. Either the thumb, fingers, heel of the hand, elbow, or a T-Bar (see

 EXAM POINT As a postevent, recovery, or maintenance stroke, petrissage "milks," "squeezes," or "wrings out" the muscle.

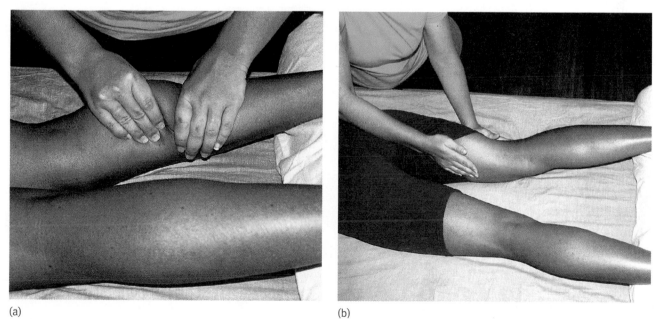

(a)   (b)

Figure 13.2
(*a*) Petrissage on calf. (*b*) Wringing, a form of petrissage, used in sports massage.

chapter 2) can be used with varying depth of pressure (figure 13.3). It is applied in a parallel, circular, or cross-fiber direction. Cross-fiber friction, also known as transverse friction, was developed by Dr. James Cyriax (see chapter 4) and functions best to realign muscle fibers. Friction activates blood flow, increasing oxygenation, and provides for extensive movement (figure 13.4).

Tapotement

Tapotement is a percussive movement in which the hand is immediately pulled off the muscle as soon as the hand strikes it. Hacking/quacking, beating, cupping, slapping, tapping, and pincement are all percussive strokes. Tapotement stimulates and invigor-

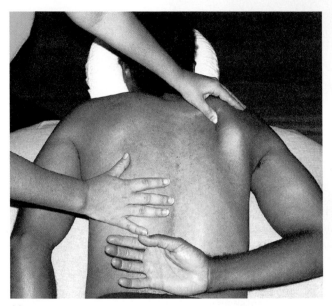

(a)

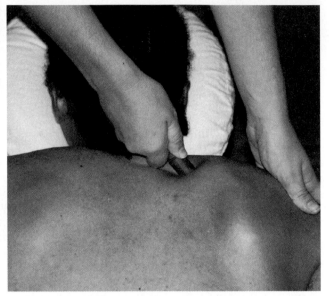

(b)

Figure 13.3
(*a*) Friction with thumb. (*b*) Friction with a T-Bar.

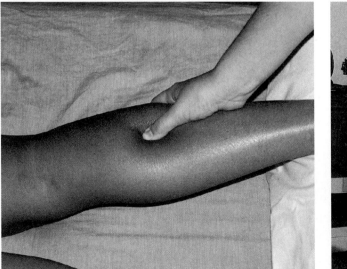

(a)

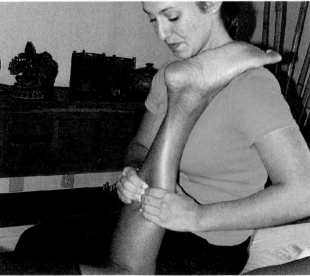

(b)

Figure 13.4
(*a*) Deep cross-fiber friction on gastrocnemius. (*b*) Parallel friction on a relaxed gastrocnemius.

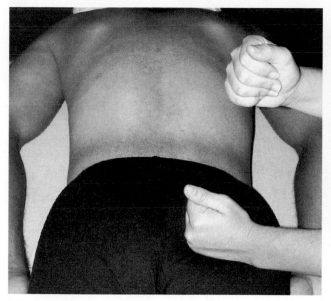

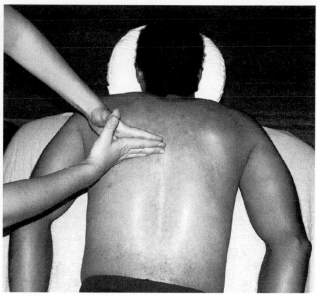

(a)   (b)

Figure 13.5
(*a*) Beating (a tapotement) on gluteals. (*b*) Quacking (a tapotement) on back.

ates the skin, connective tissue, muscles and tendons, and nerve endings, and is, therefore, best used for preevent massage. Tapotement is usually performed using the ulnar side or palmar surface of the hand (figure 13.5).

Vibration

A stroke that can range from quick shaking to slow rocking, vibration can be used in all classifications of sports massage. It can have a stimulating or calming effect on muscles. Used along with deeper work, such as friction, vibration can distract the muscle from guarding. Vibration is performed with the hands or fingers and is most often used on the extremities.

Compression

Compression is applied with direct downward pressure and may be accompanied by a slight twist. The intent is to spread muscle fibers, thus increasing pliability. Note that the more pliable the tissue is, the more depth of pressure is used but with less frequency of thrust; the more resistant the tissue is, the less depth of pressure is used but with greater frequency of thrust. Compression increases the amount of freshly oxygenated blood to the muscle and stimulates the release of histamines and acetylcholine. It is most often used in preevent or interevent massage and is performed with the palmar surface or heel of the hand or a loose fist (figure 13.6).

Direct or Sustained Pressure

Direct or sustained pressure is a technique that is often used for maintenance massage to deactivate trigger points or address specific problems. Direct pressure is performed by placing one thumb near the musculotendinous junction of the muscle origin and the other thumb near the musculotendinous junction of the insertion. Pressure is held for 10 to 15 seconds, or until you feel the muscle respond ("give"). Move the thumb near the insertion and the thumb near the origin 1 inch closer toward the belly of the muscle and repeat sustained pressure. Direct or sustained pressure techniques can be used preevent or interevent if you have worked with this particular athlete before since there will be physiological changes in the body, specifically an interruption in the referred pain. The thumb is usually used to administer direct or sustained pressure (figure 13.7).

Figure 13.6 Compression on hamstrings

Figure 13.7 Direct or sustained pressure on paraspinals

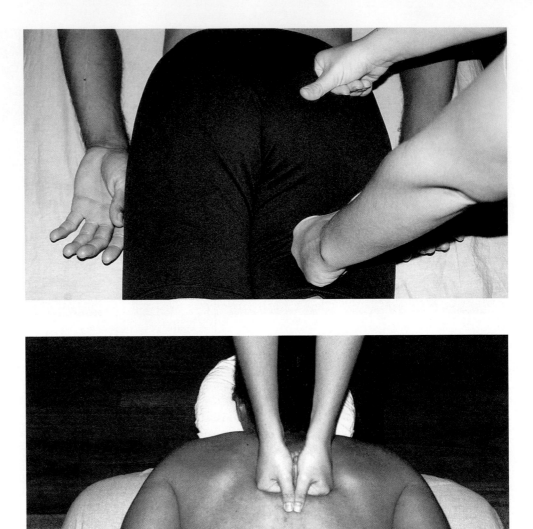

Skin Rolling

Skin rolling is the most effective technique to release spasms in connective tissue. Only the superficial tissue is grasped between fingers and thumb and rolled over your thumbs. Skin rolling is most often used in maintenance/rehabilitation massage and is performed without lubricant (figure 13.8).

Rocking and Shaking

Rocking and shaking can be considered types of vibration strokes. Slow rocking can be used to soothe a tired body after competition, while shaking can help "wake up" muscles during a preevent massage or to halt guarding.

Compression-Broadening

With compression-broadening, the tissue is compressed using a downward and lateral movement (which spreads or broadens the tissue), squeezed, lifted, and then released. This stroke is best used in postevent, recovery, or maintenance/rehabilitation massage. Compression-broadening decreases muscle cramping due to overexertion and aids in flushing out metabolic wastes. Compression-broadening is used on the extremities (figure 13.9).

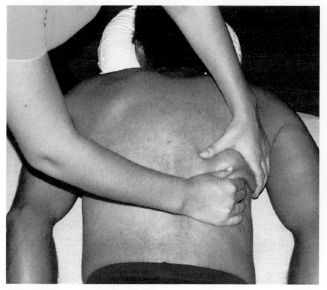

(a)

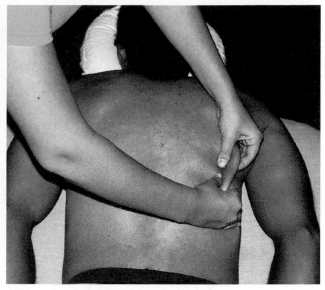

(b)

Figure 13.8

(*a*) Skin rolling begins with grasping superficial tissues (skin and connective tissue only). (*b*) Rolling tissue is the best way to release spasms in connective tissue.

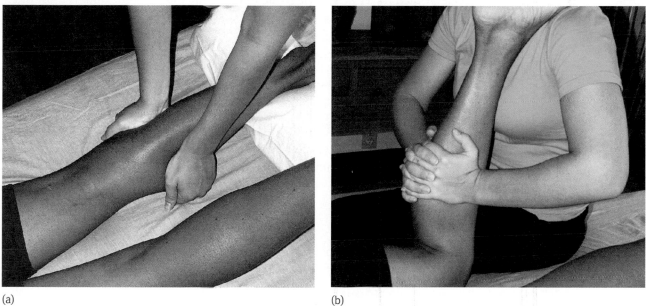

(a)

(b)

Figure 13.9

(*a*) Compression-broadening and lifting. (*b*) A form of compression and lifting is performed by grasping muscle between heels of hands and pulling it away from the bone.

Thumb-Stripping

Thumb-stripping is a deep, gliding stroke on the muscle, usually from insertion to origin, and is used in maintenance/rehabilitation massage.

Pincher Palpation

Pincher palpation ("money sign") is holding the tissue between your thumb and fingers while making the "money sign" or moving your fingers back and forth over the thumb. It is most often used in maintenance/rehabilitation massage.

Figure 13.10 Knuckling

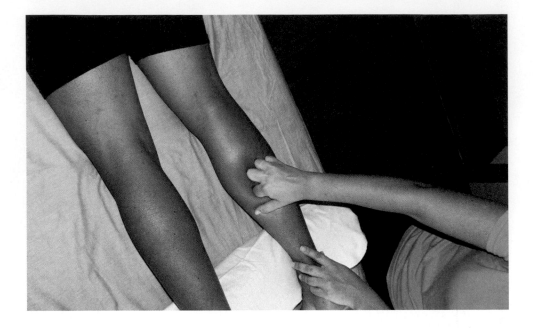

Knuckling

Performed by grasping the muscle between fingers and thumb and alternating the knuckle of each finger across the tissue toward your thumb, knuckling is most often used in maintenance/rehabilitation massage (figure 13.10).

Uncoiling

Uncoiling is performed using the fingertips on one side of the muscle and thumbs on the other side drawing the fingertips toward the thumbs. It is most often used in maintenance/rehabilitation massage.

Compression-torque with Thumbs

Compression-torque with thumbs ("hedge clippers") is usually performed without lubrication by placing the thumbs next to each other, fingers outstretched, elbows out; drop elbows to sides to create a scissor or "hedge clipper" action. It is used in maintenance/rehabilitation massage.

Fanning

Fanning starts with the palmar surface of the hand on the respective body part, and the fingers are separated as the entire hand glides across the muscle.

Prayer

In the prayer stroke, the palms are placed together and heels of the hands positioned on the body part; pressure is applied downward while the hands are separated.

Compressive Active Movement

In the compressive active movement, the therapist compresses the primary mover (agonist) while the athlete contracts the muscle.

Timing Parameters for Sports Massage

The sports massage therapist may customize the length of the treatment session to meet the athlete's wants and needs. Procedure 13.1 outlines suggested strokes or techniques and timing parameters for each of the five classifications of sports massage: preevent, intercompetition, postevent, recovery, and rehabilitation/maintenance.

PROCEDURE 13.1 Sports Massage Techniques and Timing

Pre-event Massage

Timing: one-half to 48 hours before the event, 12 to 15 minutes in duration

Purpose: to assist in warm-up, increase circulation, help maintain flexibility, and help enhance performance

Techniques: effleurage, tapotement, vibration, compression, and brisk rocking or shaking

Interevent Massage

Timing: between events at one competition

Purpose: to assist in warm-up, increase circulation, help maintain flexibility, and help enhance performance

Techniques: effleurage, compression, and direct or sustained pressure

Postevent Massage

Timing: one-half to two hours after the event, 12 to 15 minutes in duration

Purpose: to relieve cramping, decrease soreness, aid in venous return, and promote lymph drainage

Techniques: effleurage, petrissage, slow rocking, and compression-broadening

Recovery Massage

Timing: four to 36 hours after the event

Purpose: to reduce soreness, aid in venous return, promote lymph drainage, and encourage homeostasis

Techniques: effleurage, petrissage, vibration, rocking and shaking, and compression-broadening

Maintenance/Rehabilitation Massage

Timing: between competitions and off-season

Purpose: to address chronic injuries, relieve dysfunctional patterns, increase flexibility, and increase strength

Techniques: effleurage, petrissage, friction, vibration, direct or sustained pressure, skin rolling, compression-broadening, thumb-stripping, pincher palpation, knuckling, uncoiling, and compression torque

Stretching Techniques and Joint Movements

Movement, whether it is gentle stretching or joint movement through a range of motion, is a valuable addition to the basic sports massage strokes. Movement is both an assessment tool, measuring the effectiveness of your strokes, and a "distraction" enabling you to perform deeper work. Positional release is an example of a distraction technique. Figure 13.11 demonstrates various stretches that you can use in working with athletes.

Stretching

There are many valid approaches to stretching, and you should find one that suits your personal tastes. One of the most widely used techniques by sports massage therapists is **proprioceptive neuromuscular facilitation (PNF).** See chapter 19 for an in-depth discussion of stretching and PNF. Figure 13.12 shows a massage therapist using PNF on an athlete.

PNF allows for muscular relaxation through an isometric (static or no movement) contraction of the agonist (prime or involved muscle) or isometric contraction of the antagonist (opposing muscle to the prime or involved muscle). These are referred to as the tense-relax and reciprocal inhibition methods, respectively.

Tense-Relax Method

The **tense-relax method** is the most effective way to increase range of motion. It utilizes the body's own stretch reflex via the Golgi tendon reflex so as to not overstretch any muscle. An understanding of the Golgi tendon organs is important before undertaking any

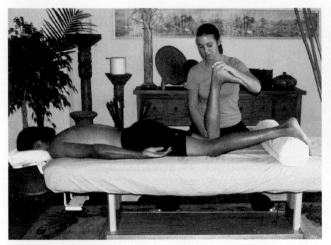

(a)

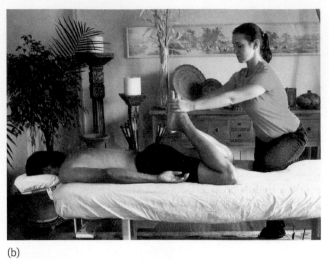

(b)

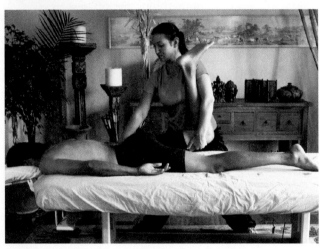

(c)

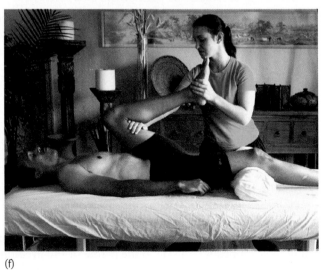

(d)

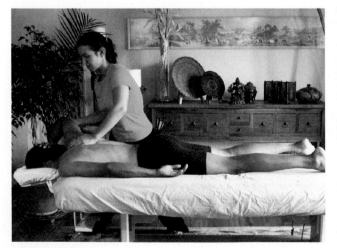

(e)

(f)

Figure 13.11

(*a*) Dorsiflexion of foot sretches gastrocnemius and Achilles tendon. (*b*) Heels-to-buttocks stretch (contraindicated for anyone with knee problems). (*c*) Hip flexor stretch. Right hand is placed on QLs (or gluteus muscles) while left hand raises knee. (*d*) Adduction (followed by abduction) of lower leg addresses rotators. A knuckle is placed at site of rotators' attachment during this movement.
(*e*) Pectoralis stretch. Client's hand is placed on back of head. Therapist's left hand stablizes scapula while right hand raises elbow.
(*f*) Knee-to-chest stretch for lower back. Therapist supports heel/foot while pressing forward on back of thigh.

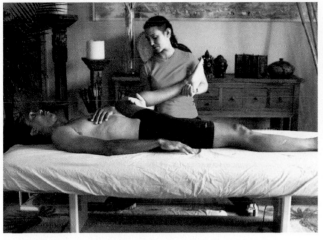

(g)

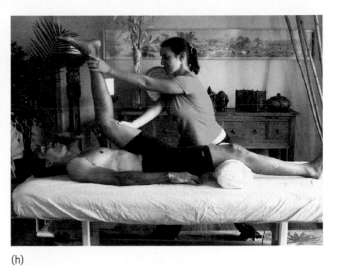

(h)

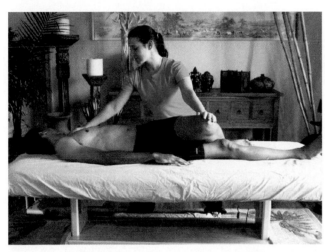

(i)

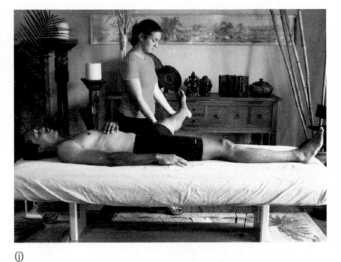

(j)

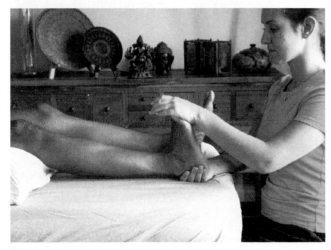

(k)

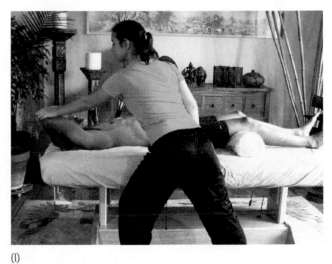

(l)

Figure 13.11 (**Continued**)

(*g*) Abduction of leg to open hip. Therapist supports heel while pressing forward on back of thigh. (*h*) Hamstring stretch. Client's knee remains "soft." Therapist's left hand supports leg while right hand presses back of thigh forward. (*i*) Lying spinal twist. Therapist's left hand adducts client's knee while right hand stablizes left pectoralis attachment. Client is instructed to look left. (*j*) Abduction of leg to stretch adductors. Therapist supports knee and lower leg while abducting. (*k*) Stretching toes, arch of foot, and Achilles tendon. (*l*) Triceps stretch. Client's hand is placed flat on table next to his ear with fingers pointing down. Therapist's left hand is placed on tricep and right hand on hip.

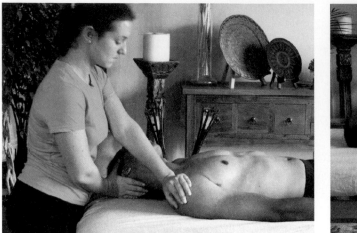
(m)

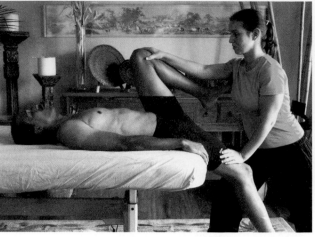
(n)

Figure 13.11 (Continued)

(*m*) Scalenes stretch. Therapist carefully puts client's head in a lateral flexion. Right hand remains on head while left hand stretches shoulder down. (*n*) Iliopsoas stretch. With client at very edge of massage table, therapist allows right leg to stretch down and off table while pushing left knee toward chest.

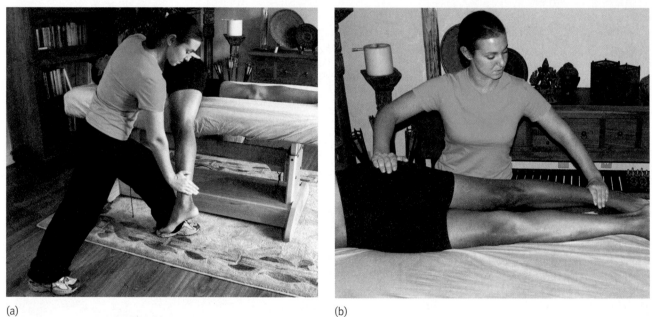
(a)   (b)

Figure 13.12

(*a*) PNF technique for IT Band. With client in a side-lying position, therapist drops client's leg off front of table. Therapist's left hand stablizes hip while right hand provides resistance. (*b*) PNF technique for IT Band. With client in a side-lying position, therapist drops client's leg off back of table. Therapist's left hand stabilizes hip while right hand provides resistance.

stretching movements. **Golgi tendon organs** are proprioceptors (special receptors) in the musculotendinous junction that "register" the muscle contraction and gauge the degree of muscle tension. The response to this tension, known as the **Golgi tendon reflex**, serves to moderate the contraction. This response helps to prevent a tear within the muscle or in the muscle from the bone. Both the sports massage therapist and the athlete need to be mindful of the work being done and the results desired. Tense-relax method is an excellent technique to use before competition and may be used as postevent and maintenance massage. To perform tense-relax:

1. Move the body part through a full range of motion until the stretch reflex is engaged (at the soft-end feel stage).

2. While bracing the body part, have the athlete contract (tense) for five to 10 seconds and then relax.

3. Increase the angle of the same body part, hold for five seconds, and repeat.

4. Repeat the entire process until the desired range of motion is achieved.

Reciprocal Inhibition

EXAM POINT   **Reciprocal inhibition method** is the most effective way to alleviate muscle cramping.

It relaxes a muscle using an isometric contraction of the antagonist or opposing muscle (figure 13.13). To perform reciprocal inhibition:

1. Place one hand on an adjacent body part to "anchor" it.

2. Place your other hand on the antagonist muscle (the one that is the opposing muscle to the cramping muscle) and have the athlete contract the muscle against your resistance.

3. Have the athlete relax, take the body part (muscle) through a range of motion, and repeat if cramping is still present.

4. When cramping has ceased, have the athlete engage the agonist muscle to neurologically reinforce the treatment.

Range of Motion

Normal range of motion (ROM) is determined by comparing both sides of the body as well as questioning the athlete. It is important to restore normal range of motion so muscle imbalances are not created. Both active and passive range of motion are used for

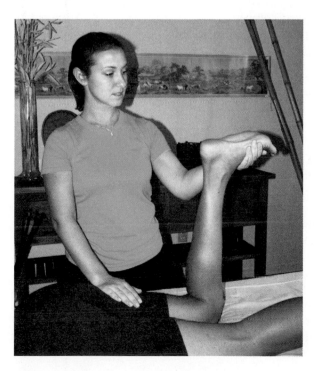

Figure 13.13
Reciprocal inhibition to relieve a cramp in gastrocnemius. Client puts tibialis anterior into flexion while therapist resists.

Table 13.1	Guidelines for Implementing Range of Motion		
Injury Indicated	**Active ROM**	**Passive ROM**	**Active-Resisted ROM**
Joint Injury	Pain exhibited	Pain exhibited	No pain exhibited
Muscle/Tendon	Pain exhibited	No pain exhibited	Pain exhibited
Joint and Muscle/Tendon	Pain exhibited	Pain exhibited	Pain exhibited

Figure 13.14 Range of motion for ankle

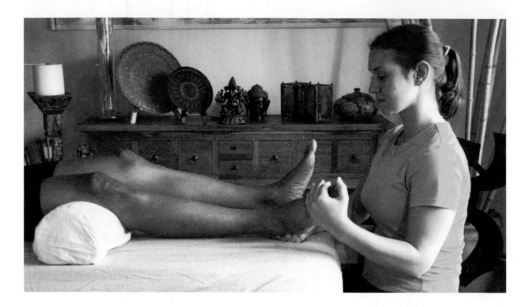

evaluation and treatment (table 13.1). Passive range of motion (PROM) is performed by the therapist, while active range of motion (AROM) requires the athlete to move the joint. ROM exercises performed at the end of a massage session are an effective way to encourage movement of an injured body part, neurologically reeducate muscles, reestablish kinetic (movement) patterns, and reduce compensation patterns (figure 13.14). Note that for any passive ROM to be truly passive, the therapist must instruct the athlete to not "help" with the movement.

General rules to follow using ROM are:

- Acute or subacute injuries should not be stretched, only chronic injuries.
- Pain on active ROM but no pain on passive ROM denotes a musculotendinous problem.
- Pain on both active and passive ROM indicates something other than a muscle problem. Anytime something other than a muscle problem is indicated, it should be checked by the athlete's physician before progressing with massage.

Positional Release

Dr. Lawrence Jones, D.C., developed the technique called **positional release or strain-counterstrain.** It is an effective way to relieve cramping and the pain associated with it, as well as "distract" the area from focusing on the spasm and pain. Simply put, when a tender point is found, move the joint that is closest to this area to a different position, lessening the perception of pain. For example, in the supine position, while holding a tender point with your right thumb on the client's right upper trapezius, slightly shift the athlete's head (which is cradled in your left hand) toward the right shoulder. This maneuver allows you to maintain static pressure on the trapezius while giving the appearance of lessening the discomfort for the athlete.

Muscle Testing

A useful orthopedic skill for a sports massage therapist is muscle testing. Muscle testing will help the therapist to evaluate the muscles that are likely in need of attention to either rehabilitate the athlete or simply ensure that the individual is functioning optimally.

To perform a clinically accurate muscle test, the therapist must have knowledge of each muscle's location and attachments (origins and insertions), actions, and direction of fibers; role of supporting or opposing muscles; proper positioning and stabilizing procedures; and deviations in range of motion. Following are basic muscle testing procedures for muscles listed in the specific sports massage routines given in the "Rehabilitative/Maintenance Massage" section of this chapter. In all cases, the therapist is evaluating if stretching and range of motion are within normal limits or if issues such as spasms and adhesions are adversely affecting the athlete's ability to perform.

Supraspinatus

Position of athlete: Sitting on the treatment table

Position of therapist: Standing in front and slightly to the side of the athlete, hand providing resistance positioned slightly above the athlete's elbow

Procedure: Have the athlete initiate movement to abduct the arm and provide resistance.

Middle Deltoid

Position of athlete: Sitting on the treatment table

Position of therapist: Standing behind the athlete, hand slightly above the athlete's elbow

Procedure: Have the athlete abduct the arm to 90 degrees (shoulder height) and provide resistance.

Infraspinatus and Teres Minor

Position of athlete: Prone on table, head turned toward the testing side, arm abducted 90 degrees with forearm hanging off the table

Position of therapist: Standing at the side of the table, one hand supporting the athlete's elbow, the other hand positioned at the wrist to provide resistance

Procedure: Have the athlete move the forearm forward and upward to the level of the table and provide resistance.

Subscapularis

Position of athlete: Prone on the table, head turned toward the testing side, arm abducted 90 degrees with forearm hanging off the table

Position of therapist: Standing at the side of the table, one hand supporting the athlete's elbow, the other hand positioned at the wrist to provide resistance

Procedure: Have the athlete move the forearm backward and upward to the level of the table and provide resistance.

Biceps Brachii

Position of athlete: Sitting on the treatment table with the forearm supinated

Position of therapist: Standing in front of and to the side of the athlete, one hand positioned at the athlete's wrist and the other hand cupping the shoulder.

Procedure: Have the athlete flex the elbow through a full range of motion and provide resistance.

Flexor Carpi Radialis and Flexor Carpi Ulnaris

Position of athlete: Sitting with elbow flexed and forearm supinated, wrist neutral or slightly extended, fingers relaxed

Position of therapist: Hand under athlete's wrist

Procedure: Have the athlete flex the wrist while you provide resistance over second metacarpal for radialis and fifth metacarpal for ulnaris.

Extensor Carpi Radialis (Longus and Brevis) and Extensor Carpi Ulnaris

Position of athlete: Sitting with elbow flexed and forearm pronated

Position of therapist: Standing in front of the athlete with one hand supporting the athlete's forearm and the other positioned over the metacarpals

Procedure: Have the athlete extend the wrist with resistance over the second and third metacarpals for radialis longus and brevis, and the fifth metacarpal for ulnaris.

Supinator and Pronator

Position of athlete: Sitting with elbow flexed and forearm in pronation for supinator and supination for pronator

Position of therapist: Standing at the side of the athlete, one hand supporting the elbow and the other hand positioned over the wrist for resistance

Procedure: Have the athlete supinate (or pronate) forearm and provide resistance.

Quadriceps Group

Position of athlete: Sitting on the treatment table with hands at sides on the table for stability

Position of therapist: Standing at the side of the athlete with one hand positioned under the knee and the other just above the ankle to provide resistance

Procedure: Have the athlete extend the knee through a full range of motion and provide resistance.

Tibialis Anterior and Posterior

Position of athlete: Sitting on the treatment table

Position of therapist: Sitting in front of the athlete with the athlete's heel resting on the therapist's thigh, one hand placed on top of the foot (dorsal surface) for tibialis anterior or under the foot (plantar surface) for tibialis posterior

Procedure: Have the athlete dorsiflex (or plantar flex) and provide resistance.

Gastrocnemius and Soleus

Position of athlete: Lying prone on the treatment table with feet hanging off the table

Position of therapist: Standing at the end of the table with one hand under and just above the athlete's ankle and the other hand on the bottom (plantar surface)

Procedure: Have the athlete plantar flex the foot and provide resistance.

Hamstring Group

Position of athlete: Lying prone on the treatment table

Position of therapist: Standing at the side of the table with one hand on the back of the athlete's thigh just above the knee and the other on the lower leg just above the ankle

Procedure: Have the athlete flex the leg and provide resistance.

Muscles of Trunk Extension (Quadratus Lumborum and Erector Spinae)

Position of athlete: Lying prone on the treatment table with hands clasped behind the head

Position of therapist: Standing at the side of the table with one forearm placed on the pelvis and the other forearm on the lower legs

Procedure: Have the athlete raise the trunk (extend) off the table.

Muscles of External and Internal Hip Rotation (Lateral Rotators and Gluteals)

Position of athlete: Sitting on the treatment table

Position of therapist: Sitting at the side of the table with one hand positioned on the thigh just above the athlete's knee and the other hand just above the ankle

Procedure: Have the athlete externally (internally) rotate the hip and provide resistance.

Tensor Fasciae Latae and Iliotibial Tract Band

Position of athlete: Side-lying with the uppermost leg forward and on top of the lower leg while the foot rests on table

Position of therapist: Standing behind the athlete with one hand placed on hip (ilium) and the other over the lateral surface of the thigh

Procedure: Have the athlete abduct the leg and provide resistance.

Injury Pathology

Muscles, tendons, ligaments, and connective tissues may all be involved in sports-related injuries. Often the injury occurs due to a blow, tearing, overuse, or insufficient training. The body's first response to injury is inflammation and pain, resulting in formation of a hematoma. This is the body's way of recognizing the injury and is an attempt to guard against further or additional injury. These conditions of response to injury are commonly known as **"splinting."**

The soft tissue first experiences internal bleeding followed by clotting. As blood pools at the injury site, further damage occurs to the surrounding cells and tissues, causing additional tissue death and decreased circulation. This process is termed the peripheral inflammatory response. This process is repeated, applying more pressure to the area and exacerbating already traumatized nerves. Cells called macrophages move to the site to perform a "cleanup" by ingesting debris of the hematoma. This debris is carried away by the lymphatic system. With decreased circulation comes a lack of oxygen and nutrients that are essential for cellular survival, thereby aggravating the pain. As the muscle goes into spasm and the body attempts to "splint" the injured area, more spasm and pain result. This process is known as the **"pain-spasm-pain" cycle.**

Sprains

Sprains are injuries to ligaments that are caused by the ligaments being stretched or compressed beyond their strength and capacity.

★ **EXAM POINT** There are three grades of sprains ranging from mild to severe.

Grade I: A mild stretch with no tear or a tear up to 20%. There is mild tenderness with some swelling. Grade I sprains often heal in five to 14 days.

Grade II: A moderate tear of 20 to 75%. There is visible swelling, **ecchymosis** (bruising), and some loss of use. Grade II tears heal in 14 to 30 days.

Grade III: A 75% to complete tear (rupture). There is obvious swelling, hemorrhaging, **laxity** (instability), and complete loss of use. Grade III tears often take months to heal.

Common Sprains

Ankle sprains usually are caused by twisting or "rolling over" the ankle by stepping on an uneven surface. The most common is inversion (sole of the foot in). The lateral ligaments are weaker and longer, and therefore susceptible to this movement.

Knee sprains usually occur when the foot is planted and a blow is taken from the side, causing an injury to ligaments on the opposite side.

Wrist sprains usually are the result of falling on an outstretched arm.

All sprains are treated with protection, rest, ice, compression, and elevation (PRICE; see section on "Acute Versus Chronic Phase"). Grade II and III sprains may require surgery.

Strains

A **strain** is most often a microscopic tear, usually in the musculotendinous junction, resulting from a violent contraction, overuse, or overstretching of a muscle or muscle group. Often, a "popping" sound can be heard when the injury occurs. A strain differs from a sprain in that the pain associated with the strain is away from the joint.

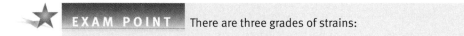

EXAM POINT There are three grades of strains:

- ***Grade I:*** Mild with no loss of use
- ***Grade II:*** Moderate with an incomplete tear accompanied by bleeding into the muscle and some loss of use
- ***Grade III:*** Severe with a complete tear usually resulting from the separation of the musculotendinous or tendinoskeletal junction; usually a result of a sudden or violent blow

Strains usually worsen with activity or continued use. Stiffness, ecchymosis, or edema may be present. Strains are treated with PRICE.

Four-Step Healing Process

Sprains and strains undergo a four-step healing process:

1. Blood flows into the tear, causing swelling.

2. A blood clot forms, which is the beginning of scar tissue.

3. The scar tissue progresses into a stronger scar (in the case of a ligament), or the muscle fibers begin to "knit" together in the case of muscles or tendons.

4. Damaged nerve endings regenerate.

EXAM POINT Ligaments are slower to heal than muscles or tendons because they are avascular (they have a limited number of blood vessels, resulting in a poor blood supply).

Once healing has occurred strengthening the musculature around the area will help rehabilitate the injured site.

Four-Step Treatment Process

1. Reduce inflammation.
2. Decrease muscle spasms.
3. Increase flexibility.
4. Increase strength and endurance.

Spasms and Cramps

Although technically not injuries in the same class as sprains and strains, spasms and cramps cause discomfort or pain and may lead to an injury. Muscle **spasms** are involuntary (convulsive) muscle contractions caused by overexertion or inadequate preparation. Such spasms usually develop gradually. **Cramps** (a tonic contraction) come on rather suddenly and are often a result of dehydration, electrolyte imbalance, or **ischemia** (lack of oxygenated blood).

In both cases, the muscle fibers become entangled, causing fatigue and rendering the muscle incapable of responding when called on to perform. These factors set up the "pain-spasm-pain" cycle. The initial pain impulse moves through the spinal cord and back to cause a reflex contraction. Contractions cause more pain and more contractions, resulting in a cramp. Weakened, overstressed, and improperly prepared muscles are all vulnerable to spasms and cramping. Sports massage breaks up the fibers, allowing the muscle to be useful and resilient.

Bursa

A **bursa** is a small sac that is lined with synovial fluid and located at sites where friction occurs (i.e., joints). Since bursae assist movement in the joints by allowing the tendons to slip over sharp edges, they perform the important function of reducing wear and tear on moving parts. Without the protection of bursae, tendons would eventually fray as they continually slip over bony prominences. The body is capable of growing new bursae where needed or to replace damaged bursae; however, even these new bursae can become inflamed. As bursae become inflamed, they create excess fluid, resulting in a painful condition called bursitis. The cause of bursitis is unknown, but it is thought to be a result of trauma, chronic overuse, or inflammatory arthritis; bursitis often accompanies other inflammatory conditions such as **tendinitis.**

Common sites of bursae that become inflamed are the shoulder, elbow, and knee. There are four bursae in the shoulder joint that may cause the athlete problems: subdeltoid, subacromial, subcoracoid, and subscapular. Subacromial bursitis leads to a condition that is often referred to as "jack hammer's shoulder." The olecranon bursa is located on the posterior side of the elbow and functions to allow the tendons to move over the elbow. Inflammation of the olecranon bursa leads to a condition referred to as "student's elbow." There are 13 bursae in the knee, four of which are anterior: superficial infrapatellar, suprapatellar, prepatellar, and deep infrapatellar. The popliteal bursa and semimembranosus bursa are located in the popliteal region (back of the knee); the remaining bursae are found on the lateral and medial aspects of the knee. Inflammation of the anterior bursae leads to a condition referred to as "housemaid's knee."

Acute Versus Chronic Phase

Determining where the athlete is in the injury phase is essential to being a good sports massage therapist.

Although the first method of treatment for sprains, strains, and localized spasms has always been **R**est, **I**ce, **C**ompression, and **E**levation **(RICE),** today many professionals follow National Safety Council guidelines and recommend **P**revention/**P**rotection, **R**est, **I**ce, **C**ompression, and **E**levation **(PRICE).** Prevention takes the form of a supportive wrap or taping; protection, a removable cast, splint, wrap, or sling prevents movement that may exacerbate the injury. Rest prohibits further use and therefore injury. Ice decreases the pooling of blood and lowers the tissue temperature, decreasing metabolic needs. Compression limits swelling. Elevation keeps the injury above the heart and aids in draining fluid off the injured area.

Timing parameters vary depending on factors such as the athlete's age, fitness level, type of injury, and so forth. Below are guidelines for appropriately addressing sports injuries:

Acute phase—from onset up to 72 hours; a result of sudden trauma (new injury), accompanied by swelling, redness, heat, inflammation, and moderate amount of pain

Subacute phase—72 hours to two weeks after onset; slight inflammation may still be present

Chronic phase—beyond two weeks with the incidence of reoccurrence for three months and beyond

Hydrotherapy in Treatment of Athletic Injury

Hydrotherapy is the use of water, via thermal, mechanical, or chemical application, in the treatment of a sports-related injury. Thermal application examples are hot packs or cold packs and have the most important physiological effect.

A mechanical application example for the athlete is a whirlpool bath. Use of hydrotherapy in other settings such as a spa can be found in chapter 14. **Cryotherapy** involves the use of ice. **Cryokinetic therapy** combines ice therapy with movement (stretching or range of motion).

Physiological Effects of Hydrotherapy

It is important to understand that the human body constantly makes adjustments to maintain physiological stability. These adjustments occur in response to environmental factors, social conditions (stress), and internal considerations (food, water, disease). Hydrotherapy produces an effect in the body through application of water at varying temperatures (also see chapter 5).

Temperature Ranges

Normal body temperature is 98.6° Fahrenheit (37° Celsius). Table 13.2 shows the temperature ranges for hydrotherapy.

Note that there is no thermal effect for the client when the water temperature is in neutral range of 94 degrees to 97 degrees.

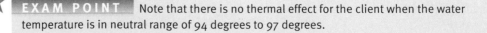

Table 13.2	Hydrotherapy Temperature Ranges
Very hot	104° and higher
Hot	100° to 104°
Warm	92° to 100°
	Neutral: 94° to 97°*
Tepid	80° to 92°
Cool	70° to 80°
Cold	55° to 70°
Very cold	32° to 55°

*No thermal effect

Three C's of Transfer of Heat

⭐ **EXAM POINT** Transfer of heat occurs in one of three ways:

1. Conduction: from one solid to another (e.g., hot pack)
2. Convection: movement of currents through a liquid or gas (e.g., steam bath, paraffin bath)
3. Conversion: conversion of energy into heat (e.g., UV lamps).

Effects of Heat

⭐ **EXAM POINT** Generally, heat increases all physiological functions such as vasodilation, diaphoresis (sweating), hyperemia (increased blood flow), oxygen content in blood, and respiration.

Local effects of heat are vasodilation, erythemia (redness of skin due to histamine release), analgesia (decrease in pain), and decreased muscle spasms.

Effects of Cold

⭐ **EXAM POINT** Generally, cold penetrates deeper than heat and decreases all physiological functions such as vasoconstriction, blood flow, respiration, and metabolism.

Local effects of cold are vasoconstriction, analgesia, decreased blood flow, and decreased muscle spasms.

⭐ **EXAM POINT** Contralateral effect occurs when the application of a therapy to one extremity causes an identical response in the opposite extremity.

Cryotherapy

Cryotherapy is the most effective manner of treating a soft tissue injury during the actue phase. It is also the most accepted method of treating localized spasms. Ideally, ice should be applied within five minutes of an acute injury with repeated applications after the tissue has returned to a more normal temperature (figure 13.15).

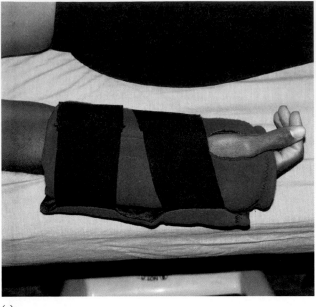
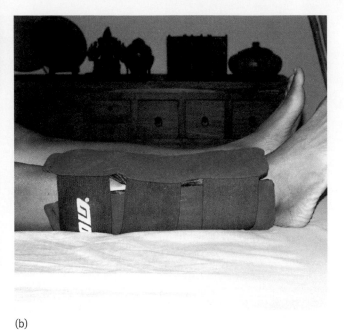

(a)   (b)

Figure 13.15

(*a*) Cryotherapy applied to wrist and hand. (*b*) Cryotherapy applied to lower leg.

The success comes not so much from the ice itself but rather from the effects afterward. Ice reduces the tissue temperature, which in turn reduces nerve conduction, muscle excitability, and the need for oxygen in the tissues. Blood vessels constrict, which allows for reduced swelling and inflammation, thus decreasing spasms and cramps. When the ice is removed, the tissue warms up to a more normal body temperature, blood vessels dilate, and blood flows into the injury site. This fresh, oxygenated blood flushes the wastes and debris from the area (especially when combined with stretching and range of motion techniques), promoting healing.

Application of Ice

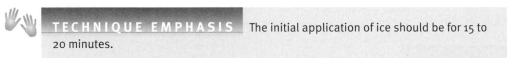

TECHNIQUE EMPHASIS   The initial application of ice should be for 15 to 20 minutes.

Remove the ice and allow the tissue to warm before reapplying. A cycle of 20 minutes on and 40 minutes off during the acute phase is the most widely accepted method for achieving the best results. After the acute phase, ice may be alternated with moist heat for contrasting effects to further promote healing. Ice should not be used on anyone who has a hypersensitivity to cold.

Four Sensations of Ice Application

1. Feeling of cold and pain
2. Warming sensation
3. Aching or throbbing
4. Tissue numbness

Ice used in conjunction with stretching and range of motion—cryokinetic therapy (or cryostretch)—not only promotes healing but also encourages correct neuromuscular facilitation and realignment of injured tissue. Application can be in the form of gel ice packs (see chapter 2), ice bath, or ice in a Styrofoam or paper cup (with the edge peeled away). In a pinch, a frozen bag of peas can be used. Applications of ice (with the exception of the ice cup, where movement prevents "burn") should not be made directly to the skin; use a towel or other cloth between the ice pack and skin. (At an event, where supplies might be limited, the athlete's T-shirt can be used instead of a towel.)

Six Steps of Cryokinetic Therapy

1. Application of ice for 10 to 15 minutes

2. Passive stretch for 20 seconds and relax

3. Active contraction for 5 seconds and relax (tense-relax)

4. Passive stretch for 20 seconds and relax

5. Repeat stretch sequence two more times

6. Repeat complete treatment two more times with ice being applied for only 3 to 5 minutes each time

Remember, perform gentle stretching or range of motion *only* when the injured area is numb (ice, movement, ice, movement, etc.). To reiterate, it is the *movement* (stretching or range of motion) that rehabilitates the area, not the ice.

Moist Heat Therapy

Moist heat therapy is an effective method of treating *chronic* injuries by warming the superficial tissues before massage. Moist heat can also be used after massage in conjunction with stretching techniques to further increase range of motion. Application of moist heat can be in the form of Hydrocollator packs, hot baths, or Thermaphores and Fomenteks (see chapter 3).

Core Body Temperature Issues

Sports massage therapists need to be mindful of the physiological changes that take place in the athlete's body during competition. You may observe one of the following indications that an athlete is having a problem with core body temperature: hyperthermia (including severe muscle cramps), heat exhaustion, and heat stroke, or hypothermia.

Hyperthermia

Hyperthermia is having a body temperature higher than normal. It is a result of the body's rate of heat production exceeding its ability to dissipate (or give off) heat. Contributory factors to hyperthermia are high air temperature, humidity or altitude, and dehydration. A loss of fluids is a primary reason for developing hyperthermia. Be sure your athlete replaces lost fluids *before* the postevent massage.

Signs of hyperthermia are clumsiness, stumbling or dizziness, cramping, nausea and headache, and excessive or lack of sweating.

Heat Exhaustion

Signs of heat exhaustion are nausea and headache, hair on back of neck and arms or chest standing up, chills and cool skin, fatigue, and sweating. While waiting for the attending medical professionals, place ice on the back of the neck and offer cool liquids to drink; help the person into shade if possible.

Heat Stroke

Signs of heat stroke are incoherent speech, confusion, aggressive behavior, and lack of sweating. Wait for attention from medical professionals and do not offer cool liquids to drink.

Hypothermia

Hypothermia is having a core body temperature lower than normal. It is a result of the body's rate of heat loss exceeding the rate of heat production (body heat is lost too quickly). Contributory factors to hypothermia are cool, wet, or rainy weather, and high altitude.

Signs of hypothermia are shivering, appearance of intoxication, blue lips or nails, and combative behavior. While waiting for attention from medical professionals, wrap the athlete in a warm blanket and offer warm liquids to drink. *Remember: In all cases, the athlete should be immediately referred to the medical professionals in attendance at the sporting event.*

Sports Massage at Events

Depending on the type of sporting event, it is advisable to have either massage chairs or tables (or both) on hand. Work can begin at the chair and finish with stretches on the table (figure 13.16). Your background knowledge of injury pathology and any previous experiences using hydrotherapy, principles for stretching and range of motion, and recognition of core body temperatures will serve you well when you work with athletes during competitions.

Preevent Massage

Preevent massage is most often performed within a half hour of competition. Many athletes are quite superstitious and have their own specific routines before competing. It is a good idea to ask the athlete what type of warm-up he or she would like. Of course, you will be focusing on the main muscle groups used in competition, but the athlete may not want stretching, for example.

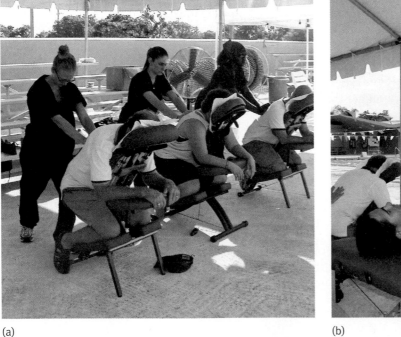
(a)

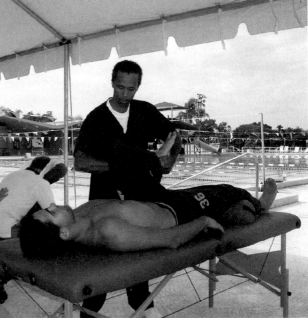
(b)

Figure 13.16
(*a*) Chair massage works at any sporting event for both competitors and spectators. Work can begin on chair and finish with stretches on table. (*b*) Table work is valuable for stretching out athletes before or after competition. Begin supine with knee to chest.

Preevent Warm-up Massage

Begin prone. Moving quickly, palm press up the leg as a form of compressive effleurage; with heels of hands or fingertips, press and rock each muscle group from both the insertion and origin toward the belly of the muscle; finish with a tapotement such as hacking/quacking or beating. Apply leg stretches. Repeat on other leg.

Move to the back and begin with a diagonal cross-stretch (scapula to pelvis); with heels of the hands, press and rock up the paraspinals; drop arms off the table to use vibration down the arms; use a tapotement such as tapping on the trapeziuses; finish with presses to the shoulders.

Position the athlete supine. Moving quickly, palm press up the legs; rock insertion and origin toward the muscle belly; use tapotements such as pincement on lower legs and beating on quadriceps stretch and repeat on other leg. Palm press arms; press and rock insertion and origin; use vibration all down the arm. Repeat on other arm. Alternate presses on shoulders.

Postevent Massage

All strokes are slow and even with the idea of flushing the muscles. Athletes usually appreciate some gentle stretching in postevent massage. Keep in mind the information presented earlier in this chapter regarding body temperatures and act accordingly. Make sure any possible injury is also brought to the attention of medical professionals.

Postevent Massage

Begin supine. Slowly palm press or effleurage leg followed by petrissage. Use compression-broadening and gentle rocking. Apply stretch and traction. Repeat on the other leg. Use effleurage, petrissage, and compression-broadening on the arms, and finish with gentle rocking. Slowly press shoulders toward feet. Use fingers to glide up the back of the neck holding traction at the occipital ridge.

Position the athlete prone. Use effleurage, petrissage, compression-broadening, and gentle rocking on the leg. Apply stretch and traction. Repeat on the other leg. Perform cross-stretch on the back. Palm press down the back and hold traction over the sacrum. Use palmar circles as effleurage over paraspinals and gently rock. Use petrissage on the trapezius and down the arms; follow with a stretch and traction. Use one-handed petrissage and finger glides up the neck. Press shoulders down to finish. Figure 13.17 features massage being performed before and after an event.

Following are common sports injuries and suggested routines for treating these injuries. Keep in mind that the routines are recommendations and should be modified to fit the athlete. If there is an injury, such rehabilitative/maintenance sports massage routines should be performed only after the athlete has been seen by the appropriate medical professional.

Rehabilitative/ Maintenance Massage

★ **EXAM POINT** The routines that follow are for off season or massage between separate competitions; deep work, such as that suggested in the following routines, is never performed pre- or postevent.

Common causes for musculotendinous injuries are improper warm-up, insufficient conditioning, and poor technique. Remember, in all cases of acute injury, the first treatment is RICE. Any massage and stretching or ROM is introduced when appropriate.

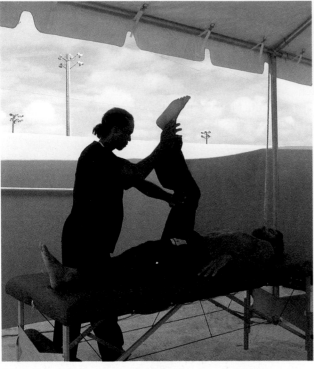

(a)

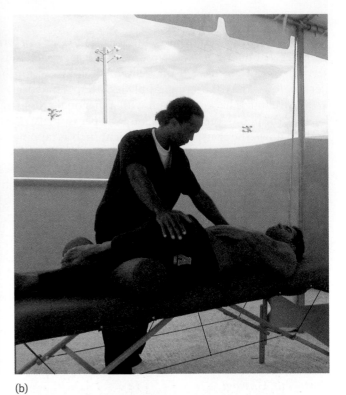

(b)

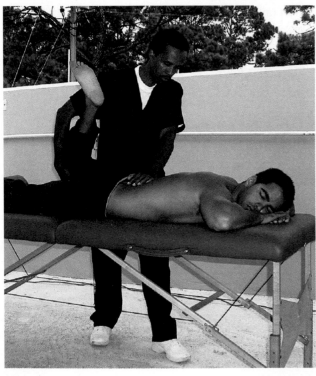

(c)

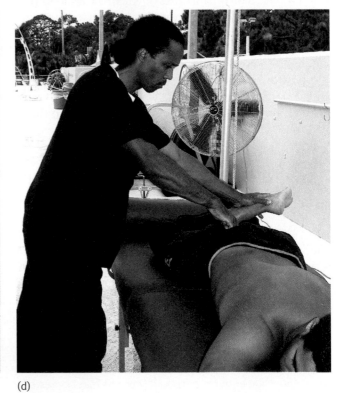

(d)

Figure 13.17

(*a*) Straighten leg to provide hamstrings with a good stretch. (*b*) Bend knee, drop foot down to table, extend opposite arm out to side, and perform lying spinal twist stretch. (*c*) Position client prone, bend knee to 90 degrees, stabilize low back, and lift up on knee. This stretch is for hip flexors. (*d*) Release knee to table, stabilize hip rotators, and adduct lower leg.

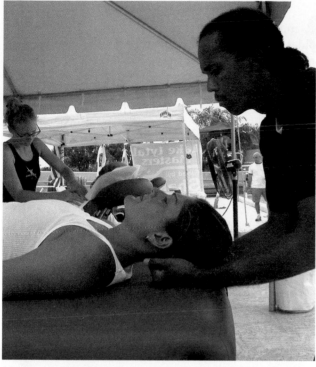

(e)

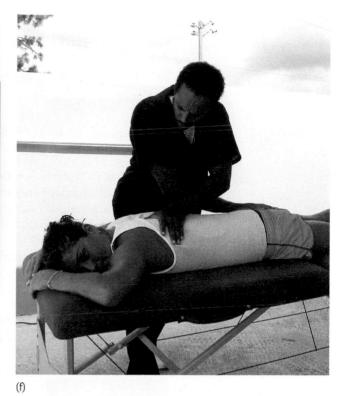

(f)

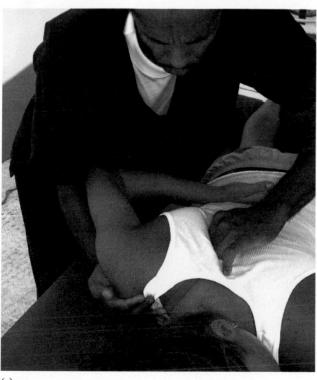

(g)

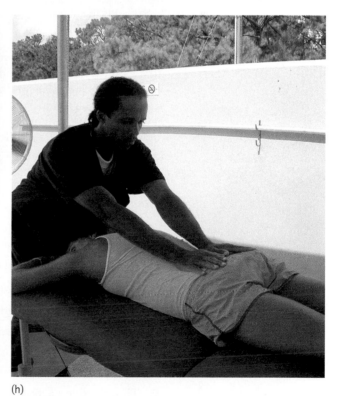

(h)

Figure 13.17 (Continued)

(*e*) Begin work on upper body by depressing shoulders for a mild stretch followed by traction of neck. (*f*) In prone position, perform a myofascial release cross-stretch. (*g*) Warm up shoulders with a stretch by stabilizing scapula and lifting shoulder. (*h*) Palm press down paraspinals and conclude with a lumbosacral stretch.

Shoulder Injuries

Shoulder pain can be a result of a multitude of causes. Wear and tear on the biceps tendon is a common cause of shoulder pain. Clicking or popping sounds are indicative of the tendon slipping out of the groove, and frayed tendons or a tear may be the result.

> ⭐ **EXAM POINT** Rotator cuff tendinitis (impingement syndrome) is the supraspinatus tendon being squeezed at the acromioclavicular (ac) joint.

Each time the arm is held out to the side, the rotator cuff tendons (especially the supraspinatus tendon) are squeezed, resulting in inflammation and impingement. The arm may be nonfunctional above shoulder level, and there may be difficulty finding a comfortable sleeping position.

Rotator muscle cuff strain involves all of the SITS (supraspinatus, infraspinatus, teres minor, and subscapularis) muscles as well as the teres major. Besides improper warm-up, falling on an outstretched arm or a violent pull to the arm can be the cause. Often there is no initial pain, but pain develops over six to 12 hours.

Shoulder bursitis occurs when the bursa lubricating the rotator cuff tendons becomes inflamed. This is common in racquet and throwing sports. The pain may start slowly and intensify over six to 12 hours, with excruciating pain being felt when the arm is abducted.

> ⭐ **EXAM POINT** Adhesive capsulitis (frozen shoulder) is a tightening of the sleeve that holds the humerus in place.

This is most often caused by a lack of use or immobilization from a previous injury. Pain may be jabbing and range of motion restricted.

Acromioclavicular sprain (separation) occurs when the clavicle separates from the scapula at the acromioclavicular joint and the ligaments are stretched. The athlete may have a problem horizontally adducting or abducting the arm. Pain may be worse at night, leading to difficulty sleeping, or when the arm is raised over the head. (A dislocated shoulder occurs when the humerus pops out of the glenoid fossa and the ligaments are stretched.)

Shoulder Routine

Muscles involved: rotator cuff (SITS), deltoids, bicep brachii (figure 13.18)

Position of athlete: Prone

Position of therapist: Standing at the side of the table facing the athlete's head

1. Compare affected side to the unaffected side.
2. Evaluate rotator cuff with muscle testing techniques.
3. Use compression effleurage and loose-fist compression on infraspinatus muscle.
4. Apply finger petrissage on infraspinatus muscle.
5. Drop arm off the table and use compression-broadening.
6. Thumb glide starting inferior to spine of the scapula and from vertebral border of scapula out to the humerus.
7. Use cross-fiber friction on the infraspinatus, teres major, and teres minor muscles and their tendinous attachments.
8. Place the arm back on the table to apply effleurage and cross-fiber friction to the supraspinatus muscle and tendon.
9. Use compressive effleurage over the entire area with a loose fist.

Figure 13.18
(*a*) Anterior view of shoulder
muscles. (*b*) Posterior view
of shoulder muscles.

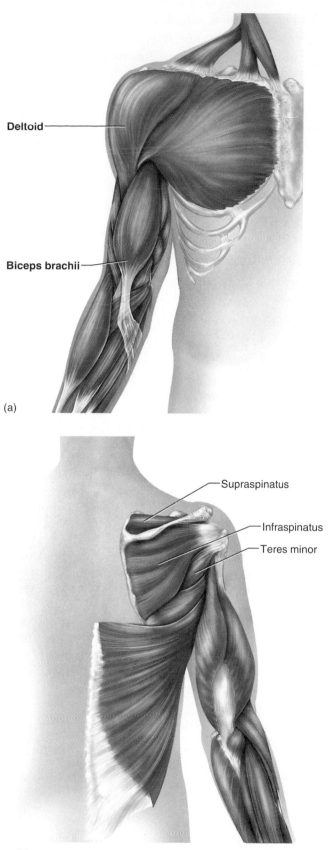

Deltoid

Biceps brachii

(a)

Supraspinatus

Infraspinatus

Teres minor

(b)

10. Perform petrissage and thumb strip the surrounding muscles (rhomboids, trapeziuses, etc).

11. Compress the posterior and middle deltoids. Apply pincher palpation (money sign) to the middle deltoid. Use cross-fiber friction on the deltoid tuberosity.

Position of athlete: Supine

1. Use compressive effleurage on the bicep brachii.

2. Apply compressive petrissage to the biceps.

3. Perform loose-fist glide and thumb glide on the biceps.

4. Use finger glide to the tendon of the long head of bicep and apply cross-fiber friction.

5. Apply cross-fiber friction from above the elbow to the tendon of the long head of the bicep.

6. Use compression effleurage on the biceps.

7. Perform compression active movement technique (apply palm pressure while the client flexes the bicep).

8. Use compressive effleurage over the entire area.

Tennis and Golfer's Elbow

Common elbow injuries are tennis elbow and golfer's elbow. Tennis elbow is a result of stressing the supinator and pronator muscles, specifically the tendinous attachments at the lateral and medial epicondyle. Ninety percent of tennis elbow injuries are due to the backhand stroke, which stresses extensor and supinator attachments at the lateral epicondyle. The remaining 10% are a result of the forehand stroke, which stresses flexor and pronator muscles attaching to the medial epicondyle. Both golfer's elbow and pitcher's elbow involve the attachments at the medial epicondyle. Symptoms come on gradually and progressively get worse. There is often stiffness upon awakening.

Elbow bursitis (olecranon elbow bursitis) is an irritation of the bursa sac and is usually caused by direct fall on the tip of the elbow. Excess fluid distends off the tip of the elbow.

An elbow sprain is a partial tearing of the sleeve or stretching of the ligaments and is commonly caused by an arm that is forced out straight (hyperextended). There is pain on straightening. (Dislocation of the elbow is displacement of the radius or ulna on the humerus.)

Ulnar neuritis is a stretching of the ulnar nerve with pain that may develop and then go away, only to return a few weeks later. It is common in throwing and racquet sports. Symptoms include the sensation of "pins and needles" and numbness in the little finger and half of the ring finger (mimicking Thoracic Outlet Syndrome, TOS).

Elbow Routine

Muscles involved: Extensor and flexor carpi radialis and ulnaris, supinator, pronator teres (figure 13.19)

Position of athlete: Supine (with arm pronated)

Position of therapist: Standing at the side of the treatment table facing the athlete's head

1. Compare the affected side with the unaffected side.

2. Evaluate extensor carpi group with muscle testing techniques.

3. Apply compressive effleurage.

4. Perform compression-broadening.

5. Use effleurage (draining effleurage) with the forearm held at a 90 degree angle.

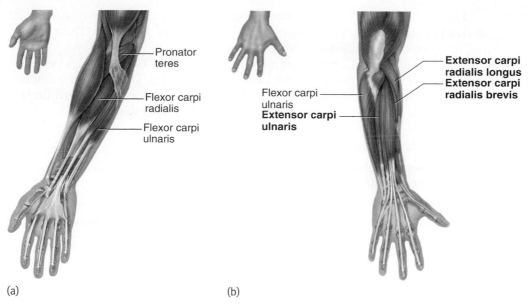

Figure 13.19

(*a*) Anterior view of forearm. (*b*) Posterior view of forearm.

6. With arm pronated, apply thumb glide along the extensor muscle group (holding the arm extended) from wrist to elbow, lateral to medial. Supinate the arm and do the same.

7. Place the arm in a medially rotated position with the upper arm abducted 45 degrees. Stand between the athlete and the abducted arm. While one hand flexes the wrist within the flexibility range of the athlete, the other hand supports the elbow and applies deep cross-fiber friction on and around the extensor muscle attachments at the lateral epicondyle.

8. Supinate and do the same on and around the medial epicondyle.

9. Use direct/sustained pressure for 10 to 15 seconds.

10. Apply deep tissue knuckling on the forearm.

11. Perform compression active movement technique (compress extensors and flexors while the athlete extends and flexes elbow).

12. Use compressive effleurage on the entire arm.

Quadriceps Injuries

Quadricep muscle strains (or pain in the upper anterior leg) are caused by overstretching or a quick contraction resulting in a rupture of the musculotendinous unit. This strain is most often in the rectus femoris or vastus intermedius muscles. Besides improper warm-up, common causes are a mistimed kick (in football or soccer) or one leg being shorter than the other. Symptoms are a tearing sensation, limited knee flexion, and pain down the rectus femoris.

A contusion of the quadriceps is caused by a sudden blow rupturing blood vessel, fatty tissue, muscles, and bone. The most serious is when the periosteum is ruptured, causing osteoblasts to leak into the area and lead to new bone formation, or myositis ossificans. Decreased range of motion and apparent ecchymosis are signs of contusion.

Patella tendon rupture is a tear of the tendon from the tibial tuberosity. It is often caused by landing on a leg off balance. The knee usually gives or buckles. Surgical intervention is likely.

Patella tendinitis, or "jumper's knee," is inflammation of the tendon at the tibial tuberosity caused by repetitive jumping or misalignment of the patella. There may be pain on awakening and resisted knee extension.

"Runner's knee," or IT band syndrome, is an overuse (3,000 foot strikes per mile) causing microtrauma or tearing of the sleeve of the knee joint. There is pain on the lateral aspect of the knee. Footware should be checked to confirm, as the sole over the ball of the foot will still appear new even in a worn pair of running shoes.

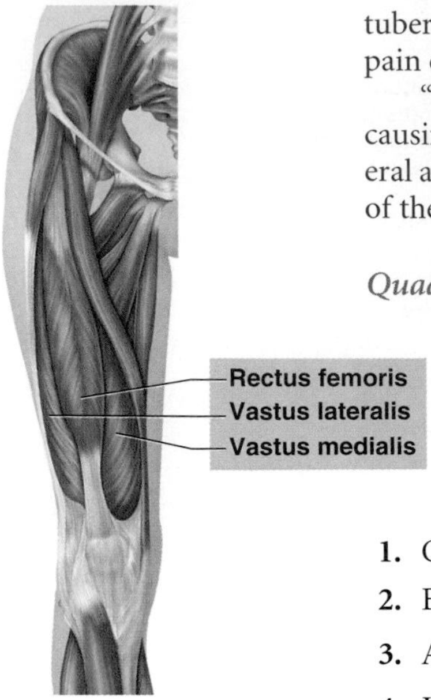

Quadriceps Routine

Muscles involved: Quadriceps group (rectus femoris, vastus intermedius, vastus lateralis, vastus medialis) (figure 13.20)

Position of athlete: Supine

Position of therapist: Standing at the side of the table facing the athlete's head

1. Compare the affected side to the unaffected side.

2. Evaluate quadriceps with muscle testing techniques.

3. Apply compressive effleurage and petrissage to the quadriceps.

4. Use compression-broadening and lifting on quadriceps.

5. Glide with loose fist and thumb strip.

6. Perform wringing and knuckling strokes.

7. Bend the knee and place the foot on table; sit next to foot. Using fingertips, pull muscle back and forth (also a Thai massage technique).

8. Interlock fingers and perform compressive effleurage. Place thumbs on medial and lateral aspect of thigh; drop elbows to "press" medial and laterally knee to hip (also a Thai massage technique).

9. Palm circle the area pressed by thumbs knee to hip (also a Thai massage technique).

10. Use cross-fiber friction on the patellar tendon.

11. Place leg back down on the table and move hands in figure eights up and down thigh (fists placed together with thumbs interlocked).

12. Apply compressive effleurage.

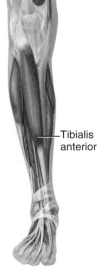

Figure 13.20 Anterior view of quadriceps

Rectus femoris
Vastus lateralis
Vastus medialis

Anterior Lower Leg Injuries

Shin splints, a lay term referring to lower leg pain, is a result of playing many sports such as running; dancers may suffer from this condition as well.

Posterior tibial shin splints (medial tibial stress syndrome) is an inflammation or strain to the tibialis posterior musculotendinous unit. In fact, 75% of shin splints are due to strain of the posterior tibialis muscle with causes being training on poor surface such as concrete or asphalt and excessive foot pronation or flat feet. Initially, pain occurs after two to three hours of exercise and later pain begins immediately upon exercise; lumps may be palpable. Additionally, injury to the tibialis anterior muscle may appear after a sudden increase in activity or running downhill.

Tibial paeriostitis is an irritation to the covering of the tibia bone and is caused by running on a very hard surface. Many runners and dancers are prone to this.

Anterior Lower Leg/Shin Splints Routine

Muscles involved: tibialis anterior and posterior (figure 13.21)

Position of athlete: Supine

Position of therapist: Standing at the side of the table facing the athlete's head

Tibialis anterior

Figure 13.21 Anterior view of lower leg

1. Compare the affected side to the unaffected side.

2. Evaluate tibialis anterior and tibialis posterior with muscle testing techniques.

3. Use compressive effleurage and petrissage on foot and lower leg by moving hand over hand up shin. Apply palmar circles medial and lateral from ankle to knee.

4. Use compression-broadening with more pressure on the lateral side.

5. Stabilize the medial malleous and compress from the lateral malleous to the head of the fibula with heel of the hand.

6. Slightly lift the lower leg and apply effleurage with alternating hands from ankle to knee.

7. Perform cross-fiber friction with thumb to the lateral side of the tibialis anterior.

8. Facing the table, lightly apply longitudinal cross-fiber friction to the tibialis posterior.

9. Apply digital gliding with the thumb moving in strips laterally from the tibia to the fibula.

10. Using the pads of the thumbs, apply effleurage to the plantar surface of the foot while plantar flexing the foot. At the tender areas, apply static pressure with thumbs for eight to 12 seconds.

11. Use direct pressure at insertion and origin of the tibialis anterior.

12. Perform compression active movement technique.

13. Use compressive effleurage on foot and entire lower leg.

Posterior Lower Leg (Gastrocnemius and Soleus) Injuries

Gastrocnemius muscle strain is pain in the back of the lower leg that results from over-stretching and causes a rupture, most often of the medial head of the musculotendinous unit, because of quick acceleration, quick stops, or side-to-side movements. Along with apparent ecchymosis, the athlete is unable to stand on his or her toes.

Achilles tendinitis is inflammation of the Achilles tendon caused by a sudden burst of speed, landing with the heel pointing inward or outward, or improper footware. Pain may be intense upon awakening or on resisted plantar flexion or forceful passive dorsiflexion.

Achilles tendon rupture is a complete tear of the Achilles tendon. Likely causes are sudden acceleration, landing from a jump, or a direct blow to the Achilles. The athlete may hear a popping sound, be unable to walk, and test positive for the Thompson test (the athlete kneels on the table while the therapist squeezes the gastrocnemius. If there is no movement, it is a positive test).

Lower Leg Routine

Muscles involved: gastrocnemius and soleus (figure 13.22)

Position of athlete: Prone

Position of therapist: Standing at the side of the table facing the athlete's head

1. Compare the affected side to the unaffected side.

2. Evaluate gastrocnemius and soleus with muscle testing techniques.

3. Apply compressive effleurage and petrissage.

4. Use compression-broadening, followed by knuckling (medial and lateral) lower leg.

5. Perform thumb strip on the gastrocnemius medial and lateral and up the center for soleus.

6. Bend the knee, sit on the table, and place the foot on your shoulder. Glide with fingertips together ankle toward knee (medial and lateral) and center.

7. Dorsiflex the foot with one hand while treating the Achilles tendon with thumb and index finger gliding down.

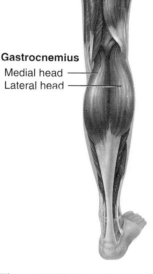

Gastrocnemius
Medial head
Lateral head

Figure 13.22 Posterior view of lower leg

8. Apply one-hand petrissage to the entire calf.

9. Dorsiflex the foot and place it on your chest. Push thumbs into the Achilles, alternating to create a "wave."

10. Apply compressive effleurage.

Hamstring Injuries

Hamstring strain is pain in the back of the upper leg that is often due to overstretching or a quick contraction causing a rupture in the musculotendinous unit, most often the bicep femoris. Athletes may hear a popping sound, feel a tearing sensation, experience pain from the ischial tuberosity to the knee, and exhibit ecchymosis.

Hamstring Routine

Muscles involved: hamstring group (bicep femoris, semimembranosus, semitendinosus) (figure 13.23)

Position of athlete: Prone

Position of therapist: Standing at the side of the table facing athlete's head

1. Compare the affected side to the unaffected side.

2. Evaluate hamstrings with muscle testing techniques.

3. Apply compressive effleurage and petrissage to the hamstrings.

4. Perform compression-broadening from insertion to origin (using heels and palms, then switch to thumbs higher up on the thigh).

5. Uncoil (muscle roll) in a medial to lateral direction from insertion to origin.

6. Facing the table, apply "prayer fashion" stroke to hamstrings. Use compression-broadening and pincher palpation (money sign) and/or knuckling.

7. Perform thumb strip medial to lateral with cross-fiber frictioning.

8. Use compression active movement technique.

9. Apply compressive effleurage.

Low Back Problems

Many people suffer from low back pain. Treat not only the low back muscles but also the buttock muscles (gluteals and rotators) and hamstrings for maximum effectiveness.

Figure 13.23 Posterior view of thigh

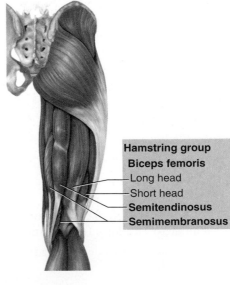

Hamstring group
Biceps femoris
Long head
Short head
Semitendinosus
Semimembranosus

For suspected sciatica, perform straight-leg raised test (athlete is positioned supine; straight leg is raised, producing pain; leg is lowered until pain dissipates; the foot is dorsiflexed, causing the pain to return).

Low Back Routine

Muscles involved: quadratus lumborum, erector spinae, piriformis (all rotators), quadriceps, IT band and tensor fasciae latae (TFL), and hamstrings (figure 13.24)

Position of athlete: Prone

Position of therapist: At the side of the table facing the athlete's head

1. Apply compressive effleurage to the hamstrings and gluteus.
2. Use a loose fist to compress hamstrings and gluteus.
3. Perform thumb strip on hamstrings, especially the attachment at the ischial tuberosity.

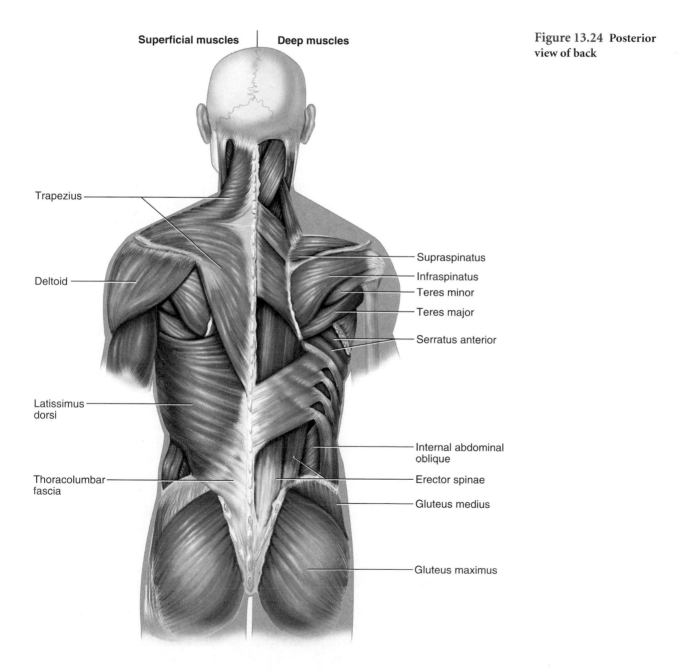

Superficial muscles | **Deep muscles**

Trapezius

Deltoid

Latissimus dorsi

Thoracolumbar fascia

Supraspinatus

Infraspinatus

Teres minor

Teres major

Serratus anterior

Internal abdominal oblique

Erector spinae

Gluteus medius

Gluteus maximus

Figure 13.24 Posterior view of back

4. Perform thumb strip on attachments along the sacrum and gluteus; finish with compression.

5. Standing at the athlete's head, use deep tissue sculpting (with fists, no lubricant) down the paraspinals.

6. Apply compressive effleurage on quadratus lumborum with forearm and elbow and use thumb strip from crest to twelfth rib. Repeat (standing at the head of the table) superior to inferior.

7. Apply compressive effleurage down and back up the paraspinals.

8. Treat the rest of the back as needed.

Position of athlete: Side-lying

1. Use "hedge clippers" up IT band.

2. Apply compressive petrissage and effleurage up the IT band.

3. Perform thumb glide and cross-fiber friction up the IT band.

4. Standing behind the athlete, hold static pressure around hip attachments.

5. Use a forearm roll off the hip.

6. Treat adductors on other leg with loose-fist compression.

Position of athlete: Supine

1. Use compressive effleurage on quadriceps.

2. Perform thumb glide three or four passes up the quadriceps, then strip up the rectus femoris and cross-fiber friction the origin of rectus femoris (2 inches below hip bone).

3. Apply compressive effleurage using the forearm.

4. Bend the knee, placing the foot on the table, and perform movements from quadriceps routine. Also, use cross-fiber friction on the iliopsoas attachments and the attachments at the knee.

5. Stretch.

Knee Injuries

As the largest and most complex joint in the body, the knee is a frequent site of injury—quite often involving one of the many ligaments found in the joint. Another common injury is to the menisci, the fibrocartilagenous pads that cushion the femoral and tibial articular surfaces. Meniscus injuries are often due to rotational stress on the weight-bearing leg. All knee injuries require appropriate medical attention. However, since the surrounding muscles and tendons act to support the knee, massage on these areas is beneficial.

The knee is critical to stopping, bending, squatting, ambulation (walking), and standing. It is mobilized and stabilized by muscle groups, primarily the quadriceps and hamstrings. The most frequently strained hamstring muscles are the bicep femoris due to overstretching.

Knee Routine

Performing the leg routines—especially the quadriceps routine—as well as the low back routine will aid in alleviating knee pain, rehabilitate knee injuries, and prevent knee injuries.

Chapter Summary

Sports massage is a specific discipline within the field of massage therapy. Information on certification in sports massage is available by calling the American Massage Therapy Association (AMTA) or logging on to the AMTA website to request a sports massage packet. See the Online Learning Center and appendix A for AMTA contact information.

You will find sports massage training useful whether or not you specialize in this area. Both professional athletes and "weekend warriors" alike will benefit from and seek out your services for sports massage. In addition, experience with orthopedic assessment techniques will help you identify when an injury (your own or another's) requires medical attention. Being able to distinguish when to use or not use certain strokes is a valuable tool. Sports massage is one of many avenues to explore to increase your possibilities for employment.

Applying Your Knowledge

Self-Testing

1. Which stroke can be used fast (to invigorate) and slow (to relax)?
   a) Effleurage
   b) Petrissage
   c) Tapotement
   d) Percussion

2. What is the duration for both preevent and postevent massage?
   a) 15–30 minutes
   b) 30–60 minutes
   c) 2 hours
   d) 10–15 minutes

3. What is the best stroke to break up adhesions in maintenance massage?
   a) Cross-fiber friction
   b) Effleurage
   c) Hacking
   d) None of the above is correct.

4. Which PNF method neurologically "wakes up" a muscle?
   a) Reciprocal inhibition
   b) Tense-relax
   c) Active
   d) Passive

5. Which stroke involves squeezing or wringing out a muscle?
   a) Compression
   b) Effleurage
   c) Petrissage
   d) Vibration

6. What is the primary goal of postevent massage?
   a) To remove toxins
   b) To decrease circulation
   c) To prepare the athlete
   d) To increase muscle tonicity

7. What is the purpose of preevent massage?
   a) To cool the athlete down
   b) To restore the athlete
   c) To assist in warming up the athlete
   d) To correct muscle imbalances

8. What is the most effective way to increase range of motion?
   a) Tense-relax
   b) Reciprocal inhibition
   c) Strain-counterstrain
   d) Positional release

9. Which stroke works best to flush toxins out of the muscle?
   a) Effleurage
   b) Petrissage
   c) Vibration
   d) Pincement

10. Which method of PNF uses the agonist (prime mover) muscle?
    a) Reciprocal inhibition
    b) Tense-relax
    c) Strain-counterstrain
    d) Positional release

Case Studies/Critical Thinking

A. *You are doing pre- and postevent massage at a local 10K race. It is June with above-record temperatures and humidity for the area. On completion of his race, a runner comes to your table for a massage exhibiting aggressiveness and slurred speech. The runner likewise shows no sign of sweating. How do you proceed?*

B. *A swimmer is manifesting signs of nervousness before her meet. She would like a preevent massage but asks you not to perform any quick strokes as she is "rattled" already. Do you follow her wishes and perform soothing massage to help her relax?*

References for information in this chapter can be found in Quick Guide C at the end of the book.

CHAPTER 14

Spa Therapy: Peace, Beauty, and Massage

LEARNING OUTCOMES

After completing this chapter, you will be able to:

- Describe the growing trend of more people taking advantage of spa treatments.

- Describe the therapeutic effects of heat and ice on the body.

- Identify the types of treatment commonly found in a spa setting.

- Demonstrate various body treatments such as basic facials, friction baths, paraffin treatments, parafango treatments, and herbal wraps.

- List the terminology of the spa setting.

- Explain contraindications of various treatments.

- Explain precautions, hygiene, and safety as practiced in a spa setting.

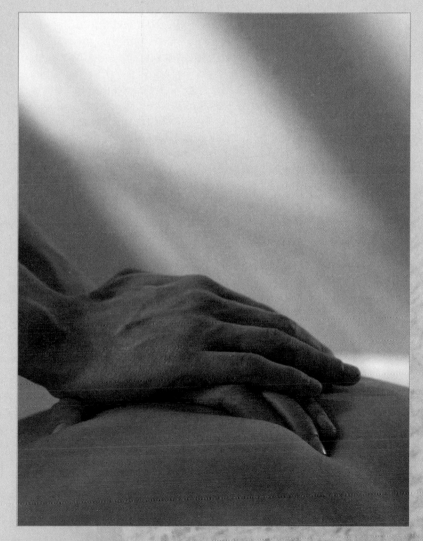

KEY TERMS

aromatherapy *(p. 383)*

cryotherapy *(p. 375)*

Dead Sea mud treatment *(p. 383)*

dry brush exfoliation *(p. 375)*

dulse scrub *(p. 375)*

exfoliate *(p. 375)*

frostbite *(p. 376)*

herbal wrap *(p. 383)*

hydrotherapy *(p. 374)*

immersion bath *(p. 375)*

parafango *(p. 377)*

paraffin *(p. 377)*

salt rub or salt glow *(p. 375)*

sauna *(p. 374)*

Scotch hose *(p. 375)*

steam *(p. 373)*

stone massage therapy *(p. 363)*

Swiss shower *(p. 374)*

Vichy shower *(p. 374)*

INTRODUCTION

With the increase in the number of spas and their expanding services during the last decade has come an increase in opportunities for massage therapists who may want to work in this environment. Perhaps more than ever before, people are starting to focus on maintaining their health and pampering themselves. Bottled water, for example, has become such a mainstay of the modern lifestyle that vending machines offer water alongside sodas. Water is likewise an essential element of the spa experience. The origin of the word *spa*, although somewhat debated, involves water. *Spa* possibly came about as an acronym of the following Latin terms: *sanus per aquam* (meaning "health by (or through) water"), *solus per aqua* (meaning "enter by means of water"), *salut per aqua* (meaning "health (or relaxation) through water"), or *espa* (meaning "fountain").

Centuries ago, humans enjoyed the Roman baths or Japanese bathhouses as a social environment that also relaxed the body and soul, and contributed to the relief and often the healing of chronic illness. Today, that same communal bathing center has been refined to include numerous types of spa facilities. Now persons of even modest incomes can enjoy the benefits of being guided toward relaxation and wellness. Massage therapists are likewise able to take advantage of the largest industry to employ them.

This chapter contains information the massage therapist needs to successfully practice within a spa environment. Procedures for typical spa treatments are described. Many of the types of spa facilities are explained. Whatever your interest as a massage therapist, there is a place in this vast and fast-growing market for your particular skills and level of education. Most spas also employ cosmetologists, estheticians, and nail technicians. Depending on the type of spa, a dermatologist, nutritionist, orthopedist, and fitness trainer may be part of the staff as well as a naturopath and holistic or spiritual counselor.

In many states, a facial cannot be legally given by someone who has not obtained the certification of an esthetician. However, a general facial procedure is included in this chapter to give you information about the facial process because a number of states allow persons to perform facials if they are trained by the product line the spa uses. This training is limited to using the specific products the company sells for this service and does not grant certification as an esthetician and the ability to legally perform procedures within the scope of practice for an esthetician. A massage therapist should always be aware of what the law allows within their scope of practice in the city and state in which they are working.

Types of Spas

Destination spas are hotel-type properties that function only to support guests' spa activities. Usually, there are no outside clients. Depending on the theme of the spa, guests may receive fitness training, weight loss and dietary education, horseback riding or sports training, and dancing or lessons in the performing arts. Some destination spas may also provide a serenity-enhancing setting and stress-reduction activities. All of these, however, include massage to some degree.

Medical wellness spas incorporate the services of physicians and emphasize lifestyle changes by encouraging optimal health and well-being. Programs usually include back care, neuromuscular and deep tissue massage, manual lymph drainage (see chapter 16), and smoking cessation. Medical spas are becoming very popular as places to recover from plastic and gastric bypass surgery.

Fitness and beauty spas cater to clients who want to maintain a high level of fitness with an emphasis on beauty goals. Counselors and usually dermatologists are on staff to guide the client's approach to becoming physically fit and to educate the client in various beauty maintenance regimes. Facials, manual lymph drainage, body wraps, and other services such as hair care, nail care, and body waxing are staples here. A personal trainer is available to put together an exercise and nutrition program that fits a client's specific profile. These spas range in price from business-class affordable to expensive for the ultimate in luxury and extras.

Weight-loss spas concentrate on modifying the behaviors that may have contributed to the client's eating problems. Such spas also focus on diet and nutrition counseling, exercise, detoxification, and stress-maintenance strategies.

Day spas focus on clients who require same-day service. The clients spend the day—or part of a day—receiving treatment. This type of facility is popular with the general public and especially businesswomen, club groups, and wedding parties. There is a growing trend of day spa gift certificates being given to young women as a coming-of-age activity.

Cruise ship and resort spas employ a large number of massage therapists as part of their relaxation and adventure packages.

Today, you will find a broad range of spa facilities to fit every pocketbook and lifestyle. The benefits and opportunities are enormous for a competent and experienced therapist. The American Massage Therapy Association (AMTA) Foundation reports that currently 22% of licensed therapists are working in a spa setting. Some therapists work in more than one facility during a week to achieve a greater opportunity for income. With so many opportunities for employment in a spa facility, it is important to know what is required and how to perform as a spa massage therapist.

What Makes a Spa a Spa?

Client service to the point of pampering and the focus on the specific needs of the client at all times are what makes a spa. Creating a special place of peace and well-being by using color, fragrances, air temperature, relaxing music, and special lighting can provide the ultimate experience for you and your client. With the stress of family and jobs creating chaotic days, an escape to a quiet, sensual setting, where a confident and professional therapist takes charge of your well-being, can bring about amazing lifestyle and health changes.

If you apply the following rules for treatment of your clients, you will have the joy of seeing customer satisfaction, health and lifestyle redirection, changes in client self-esteem, and repeat business (box 14.1.). Repeat business means that your clients are so satisfied with their service that they return again and again. They will also tell their friends and family members, which will lead to new clients.

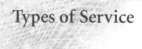

Types of Service

Swedish massage (see chapter 4), a full-body massage technique used to provide deep relaxation, is the type of massage most often offered in a spa facility. Swedish massage works with the soft tissue of the body as well as the muscles, ligaments, and tendons. This type of massage increases the circulation of blood and lymph.

Stone massage therapy is used for both facial and full-body massage. The use of marine or river stones is extremely effective in delivering cold or heat. The use of cold stones can increase microcirculation and compression, effecting a change on the cellular level. Stones may be placed on the meridian, trigger points, or chakra points, depending on the type of treatment given. Deep tissue and neuromuscular massage may also be added in sports or fitness settings. In most spas, an esthetician will provide face massage when doing a facial with products to clean, exfoliate, tone, and stimulate the skin. However, a face, scalp, and neck massage may be part of the full-body program and would be performed by a massage therapist.

1. Schedule your clients so that they will not feel rushed, and arrive at least 15 minutes before their appointment to ready your room.

2. Greet the client by name, warmly shake hands, and offer the client refreshment or an opportunity to relax in a steam room, sauna, or quiet room with aromatherapy and music before the massage begins.

3. Make sure you are totally focused on the client, not answering phone calls or handling personal business during his or her visit.

4. Make sure the client is warm and comfortable during the massage and in a private area with soft music and soothing light.

5. Use warm towels, eye packs, and bolsters or pillows during treatments.

6. When the client is finished, have a robe and slippers within reach. Offer water, fruit, juice, or tea. If the client is to have further service, walk the client to the area and introduce him or her to the next technician. If not, allow the client an unhurried time to shower and redress, and walk the client toward the exit.

Box 14.2	Facial Changes Brought About by Aging and Benefits of Facial Massage

- Skin grows paler, sometimes gray or yellow.
- Lips grow thinner.
- Eyebrows and eyelids droop and worry lines appear.
- Jawline and mouth corners sag.
- Skin on the neck grows loose or double chin develops.

Regular facials or facial massage can provide the following benefits:

- Fresher-looking and rosier skin tone
- Less undereye puffiness
- Raised eyebrows and fewer worry lines and furrows around the mouth
- Fuller lips
- Toned jawline
- Diminished double chin

Face Massage

As we go about our lives, gravity acts upon the body to pull and stretch our muscles. When we add toxic elements, makeup, and nutrient-poor diets to the equation, it is easy to see why so many women (and men) seek facial treatments on a regular basis. As we age, many changes occur to our facial structure. Facials or facial massage can provide benefits by countering some of these changes (box 14.2).

To understand how massage can bring about facial changes, let's look briefly at the facial muscles. Without the facial muscles, we would not be able to laugh, smile, yawn, or kiss. These muscles also give your face its shape. Firm muscles—devoid of toxins and plump with increased circulation—will give you the appearance of a young and toned person. Refer to figure 14.1 to locate the muscles as we study the muscles of the neck, face, and scalp.

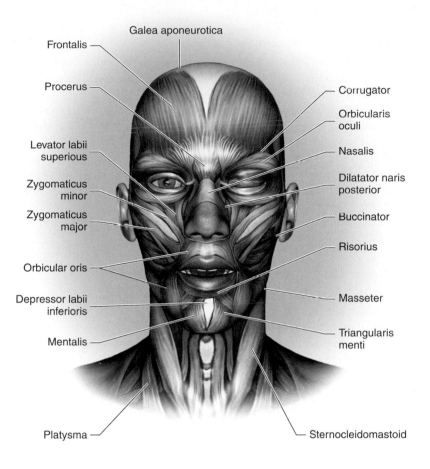

Muscles of the Neck

The muscle that works to move the lower jaw is the platysma. It is the broad group of fibers that lies beneath the skin on each side of the neck. The sternocleidomastoid is responsible for the rotation of the head and pulls the head toward the shoulder on either side. The trapezius is found at the back of the head and shoulders, and pulls the head back and from side to side.

Muscles of the Mouth

The triangularis menti is the pyramid-shaped muscle that connects from the lower jaw up to the mouth. It draws down the corners of the mouth. The risorius is a narrow bundle of muscle fibers that retracts the corners of the mouth toward the back teeth.

The zygomaticus major and the zygomaticus minor are two muscles comprised of slender cords of muscle fibers that raise the corners of the mouth and extend into the cheek. They are also known as the "laughing muscles" for the role they play when you smile or laugh.

The fibers of the thin levator labii superioris muscle converge in the upper lip. The quadratus menti is a small, four-sided muscle. It draws down the lower lip. Containing body fat intermingled with its fibers, this muscle contributes to the fullness of the lips when it is properly toned. The mentalis is a very small muscle in the front of the chin. The quadratus labii superioris is a large muscle that lies beneath the upper lip and connects to muscles in the cheek.

The buccinator is a wide, thin muscle beneath the cheek. It works to compress the cheek, as when you blow up a balloon, purse your lips, or whistle. The orbicular oris completely encircles the mouth. It consists of numerous strands of muscle fibers that go in different directions and connect with fibers in the upper and lower lips, cheeks, nose, and surrounding areas.

Muscles for Chewing (Mastication)

When clients hold tension in their jaws, these are the muscles involved. If they do not relax properly, the clients will lose muscle tone in their face, and these muscles may even contribute to temporomandibular joint syndrome (TMJ).

The pterygoid internus helps to close the mouth and move the jaw.

The external pterygoid also works to close the mouth and rotate the jaw. This muscle is short, thick, and cone-shaped.

The temporal is a large muscle on the side of the head that closes the jaws with force. It goes diagonally back from the cheekbone to the outer jaw hinge. The masseter works in conjunction with the temporal to clench the jaws. Working with this muscle can firm the jawline and tighten the skin of the neck.

The digastricus runs down from the chin into the top of the neck. Toning this muscle can aid in reducing the double chin effect.

Muscles of the Nose

The pyrimadalis nasi spans the bridge of the nose. It draws down the middle of the eyebrows and wrinkles the nose.

The dilatator naris posterior is a small muscle situated above and behind the nostril. This muscle is responsible for the contour and length of your nose.

The dilatator naris anterior lies directly above the middle of each nostril and is very thin and delicate. This is the muscle responsible for the flaring of your nostrils.

The depressor alae nasi extends across the base of the nose and closes the nasal opening by pulling down the septum.

The compressor nasi begins at the bridge of the nose and extends up over the bridge, compressing the nostrils.

Muscles of the Eye

The levator palpebra superioris in the upper eyelid is extremely thin but vital to maintaining firm, toned upper eyelids.

The orbicularis oculi is a strong muscle that surrounds the orbit of the eye. It acts to open and close the eye. When you squint, the orbicularis oculi raises the lower eyelid. Often these muscles are affected by a stroke, and their inactivity will lead to drooping eyelids.

The corrugator muscle juts out from the top of the forehead and runs into the muscle within the upper eyelid. Strengthening and toning this muscle can erase brow or worry lines on the forehead.

The epicranius raises the eyebrows. Massage applied to this area helps increase oxygen and blood circulation throughout the forehead and eyes. Regular treatment to the epicranius can soften tension in the face and give the client a relaxed appearance.

Muscles of the Ear

The following muscles lie around the ear. They have little effect on the appearance of the face. However, learning to flex the three muscles that lie just under the skin around the ears can help the jaw and scalp muscles to strengthen and tone. This action can give a natural face-lift appearance by interacting with the muscles supporting the eyebrows and eye sockets, and can relieve the "crow's feet" or frown lines at the corners of the eye.

The anterior auricular is the smallest of the ear muscles. It is very thin and fan-shaped. Its action is to draw the ear forward.

The largest ear muscle, the superior auricular, raises the ears.

The posterior auricular draws the ear backward.

Muscles of the Scalp

The skin on your scalp is the thickest layer of skin on your entire body. Two types of scalp muscles lie under the skin.

The frontalis is a very thin muscle located over the forehead. It draws the scalp forward and produces horizontal wrinkles in the forehead.

The occipitalis is about an inch and a half long and lies at the back of the head. Its action is to pull the scalp backward.

The galea aponeurotica is a wide, flat tendon joining the frontalis and the occipitalis muscles.

Now that you know the structure and function of the muscles of the face, you can understand how important a correctly done facial massage or treatment can be to the health and appearance of your client.

Facial Treatment Procedures

Every client procedure must begin with a consultation. This is where you establish what service the client has scheduled and what the client expects as the outcome of the service, and gain information about the client's condition. Contraindications to a facial include a rash or other visible skin condition, recent burns that have not completely healed, or sutures or open wounds on the face and scalp. Always check to make sure the client is not allergic to the product you are using. The management of the spa or clinic may set the guidelines for the treatment you are performing. Most product lines also have representatives who visit the spas that use their products and train the therapists in the way they want their products applied. Procedure 14.1 outlines a basic facial treatment procedure, and Figures 14.2 and 14.3 illustrate it.

Facial Massage

Before beginning the client's facial massage, make sure that the client is in a comfortable and relaxing position. Soft music, muted lighting or candles, and aromatherapy fragrances enhance the massage. The manipulations used on the facial area are of the same type as in a body massage. They include effleurage or gliding strokes, used to skim the surface; petrissage, or a kneading movement that uses grasping of the skin between the thumb and the forefinger; tapotement, which consists of light digital tapping; and vibration, fine or tremulous movements that cause a reflex response.

It is extremely important that massage movements are directed toward the origin of the muscles to avoid damaging delicate muscular tissues. Correct hand position allows for slightly curved fingers with only the fingertips touching the skin. After much practice, the massage therapist should be able to give a facial massage in a series of rhythmic movements, as if completing a dance program.

Figure 14.4 shows the correct steps in performing a facial massage.

P R O C E D U R E   14.1   Performing a Basic Facial Treatment

Objective: To perform a basic facial treatment for your client

Items to be used:

- Small towel or cape for the client's shoulders
- Cap or small towel to cover the client's hair
- Mild cleansing cream or lotion
- Mild astringent or skin-toning lotion
- Cotton pads or sponges to apply and remove cosmetics
- Cotton-tipped swabs and facial tissues to remove makeup from eye and lip areas
- Cool or warm aromatherapy towels

Continued next page—

Cleansing Procedure—Applying Cleanser

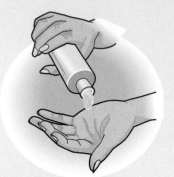

(a)

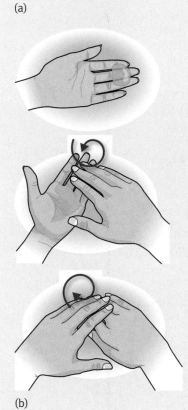

(b)

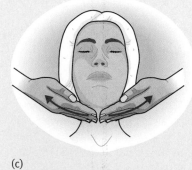

(c)

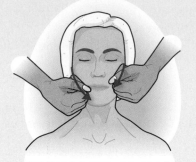

(d)

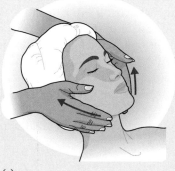

(e)

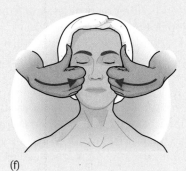

(f)

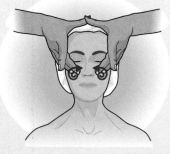

(g)

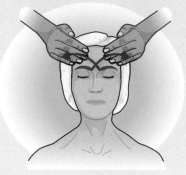

(h)

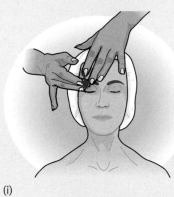

(i)

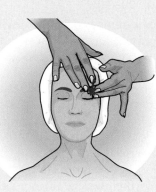

(j)

Figure 14.2 Cleansing procedure

(*a*) Check your nail length. Wash hands thoroughly using soap and warm water. Wipe hands with alcohol or antibacterial gel. (*b*) Apply facial cleanser on finger tips of one hand. Spread evenly to back and front of the fingers on both hands. (*c*) Begin on client's neck, palms down. Work hand back toward the client's ears. (*d*) Slide the back of the fingers along the jawline toward the chin. (*e*) Slide the front of the fingers up and over the cheeks. (*f*) Slide the back of the fingers over the cheeks toward the nose. (*g*) Using light pressure make small circular motions on the flare of the nostrils. Use the pad of the fingers. (*h*) Move the finger pads toward the forehead then out toward the temples. Stop at the temples and apply slight pressure. (*i*) Using the left hand, lift the right eyebrow with the middle and fourth fingers. With the middle and fourth finger of the right hand, very gently apply the cleansing product to the eyelid with downward strokes. (*j*) Repeat the previous procedure using the right hand and lifting the left eyebrow.

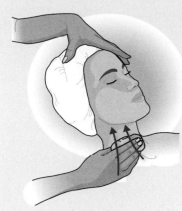

(a)

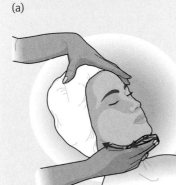

(b)

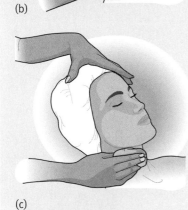

(c)

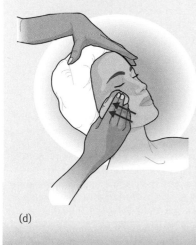

(d)

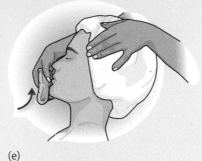

(e)

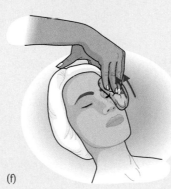

(f)

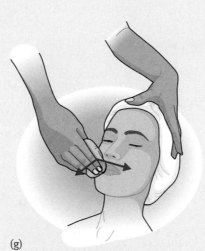

(g)

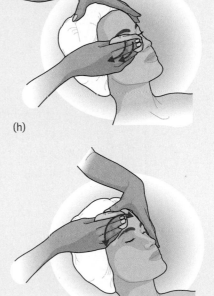

(h)

(i)

(j)

Figure 14.3 Cleanser removal procedure

(*a*) Begin by stroking upward. Remember to remove cleanser in the direction of the beard growth with male clients. (*b*) With the pad directly under the chin, slide the pad upward along the jawline toward the ear. (*c*) Repeat on the other side of the client's neck. (*d*) Use upward movements begining at jawline, to cleanse the cheek. (*e*) With continous upward movement, cross over the chin area. (*f*) Repeat the procedure to cleanse the other cheek. (*g*) Begin at the center and work outward toward the corners of the mouth to cleanse above the lips. (*h*) Cleanse the sides of the nose by moving the pad up and down the cheeks. (*i*) Cleanse the forehead by placing the pad in the center and moving toward the temple. Apply slight pressure on the temple, then cleanse the other side. (*j*) Cleanse the lid area by using the middle and ring finger of the left hand to lift the eyebrow. Use the right hand to cleanse gently with downward strokes toward the lashes. Repeat on the other eyelid. Pat dry with a tissue to remove all residue, and you are ready to begin a facial massage.

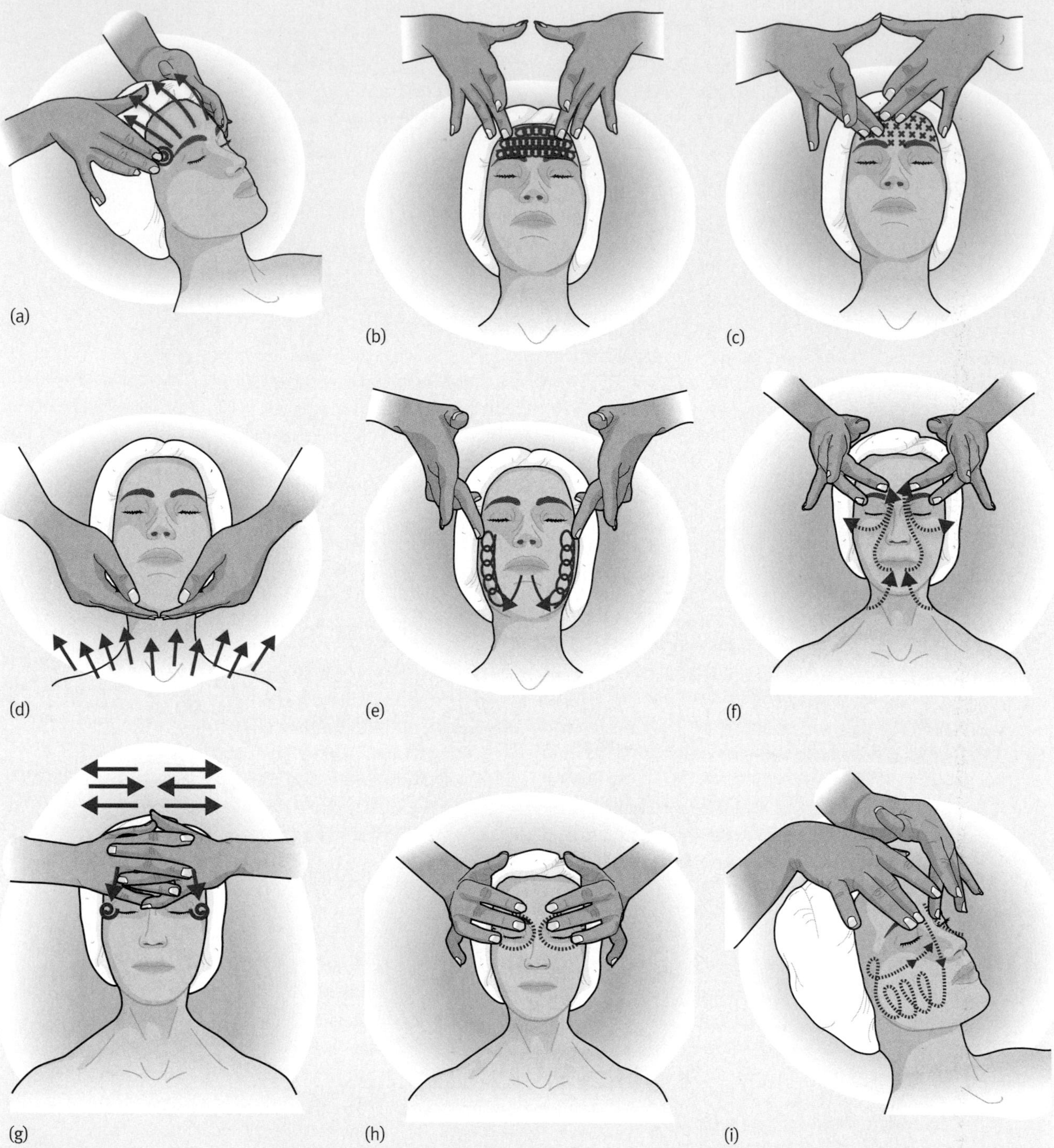

Figure 14.4 Facial massage

(*a*) Apply massage oil or lotion over the face and neck using the same movement that was used in applying the cleanser. Begin with linear movement over the forehead. Use circular motion over the temples. (*b*) Using the middle finger pad, continue circular movement over the entire forehead. Work from the brow line and move toward the hairline. (*c*) With the middle and the fourth finger pad, begin crisscross movements at one side of the forehead, move across, and then work back. (*d*) Use gentle pressure to lift the chin. (*e*) Use the middle finger pad to move in a circular motion from the jawline to the ear. (*f*) Make gentle circular movements from the chin, around the mouth, on the sides of the nose, and out on the cheeks. (*g*) Interlace the fingers at the middle of the forehead and slide them apart using light pressure. Do this motion three times, and then use slight pressure and a circular motion at the temples. (*h*) Place the index finger over the brow line. Place the middle finger at the inner corner of the eyes and slide the fingers to the outer corners of the eyes. Circle under the eyes and back. (*i*) Begin circular motions at the bridge of the nose and between the corners of the eyes, and with your middle finger, move across the cheeks, apply pressure at the temple, and slide across the cheek toward the nose.

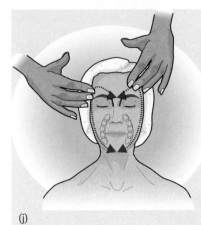
(j)

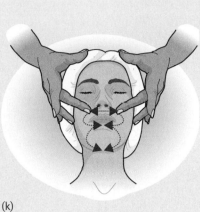
(k)

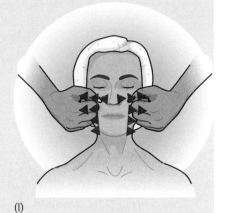
(l)

(m)

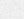
(n)

(o)

(p)

Figure 14.4 Facial massage (Continued)
(*j*) Begin circular movements from the corners of the mouth to the sides of the nose and slide fingers over the brow line and back down to the corners of the mouth. (*k*) Use the middle finger pad to slide above the upper lip, around the mouth, and under the lower lip and chin. (*l*) Use the knuckles to lift lightly from the mouth toward the ears. (*m*) Use a circular movement of the middle fingers to massage the cheeks from the chin upward toward zygomatic arch (*n*) Light tapping movements can be used from the chin to the ear on both sides of the face. (*o*) Upward strokes are applied over the front of the neck. More pressure can be used along the sides with downward strokes. (*p*) Apply circular movement along the sides of the neck and across the chest.

Scalp Massage

Scalp and hair manipulation is very beneficial. Manipulation increases circulation of blood to the scalp and hair follicles, and empties clogged oil ducts. It can also increase lymph flow and stimulate hair growth, and is wonderful for releasing tension. A massage therapist should never treat the scalp if any condition or disease process is present. Remember to never pull the hair away from the scalp or put undue pressure on the client's neck. Figure 14.5 shows the correct technique for scalp massage.

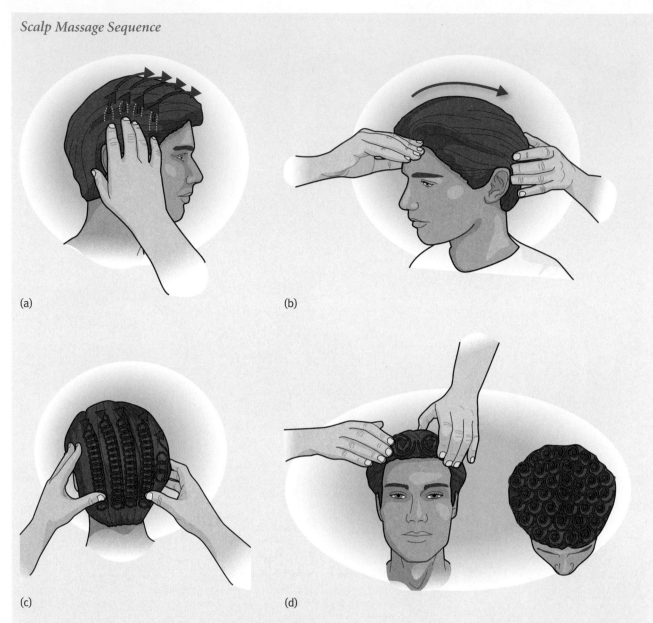

Figure 14.5 Scalp massage

(*a*) Place the fingertips on each side of the client's head at the hairline. Slide the fingers upward, while spreading them apart. Stop at the center of the scalp when the fingers meet. Repeat three times. (*b*) Stand at the side of the client. Place your left hand at the back of the head and your right hand on the forehead. Use the thumb and fingers to massage upward on the forehead toward the crown. The strokes should be slow and firm. (*c*) Stand behind the client and place your hands on the sides of the head. Hold the head with the fingers and drop your thumbs to the back hairline. Use your thumbs to massage the scalp with small circular movements toward the crown. Repeat three to five times. (*d*) While standing behind the client, use the fingertips to make circular movements at the front hairline. Use a quick, upward, twisting movement, firm enough to move the scalp. Continue over the entire scalp. Repeat once.

Therapeutic Modalities Commonly Used in a Spa Facility

One of the oldest therapeutic modalities is the use of heat and cold. Prehistoric humans probably discovered that standing in a cold stream would soothe tired feet and that sitting with their backs toward a warm fire would relax muscles that were tense from the hunt. The accepted normal body temperature for human beings is 98.6°F. Our body reacts physiologically to keep itself at the normal temperature. When heat or cold is applied, many bodily changes occur. With the application of heat, the body temperature rises: blood vessels dilate, profuse sweating occurs, and the white blood cell count elevates. Applying heat

Box 14.3   Heat Types, Sources, and Applications

- Dry heat
    - Heating pad
    - Infrared radiation
    - Sauna
    - Hot stones
- Moist heat
    - Spray baths
    - Immersion tub baths
    - Moist heat packs
    - Steam and moist sauna treatments
- Diathermy (heat using an electric current)
    - Microwave and shortwave

to a specific area will cause vasodilation—a widening of the lumen of blood vessels, reddening of the skin due to vasodilation, and increased metabolic activity. Leukocytes are sent to the area, and the white blood cell components reduce inflammation, destroying viruses and bacteria.

A controlled heat application of short duration has a precise therapeutic value, but the therapist must avoid extreme levels of heat for long periods of time. Prolonged treatment with high temperatures can cause irreversible tissue damage. The choice of how the heat is administered is based on the sources available as well as the objective of the treatment. Box 14.3 lists the types of heat and their sources.

Heating Pads and Moist Heat Packs

Heating pads containing an electrical element and moist heat packs that have been filled with clay and placed in a Hydrocollator for heating, as well as heating pads that are heated in a microwave oven, are used to treat a localized area. You must carefully follow the operating instructions so that the client is not injured. Heated pads or packs are of tremendous value in bringing about therapeutic benefits.

Infrared Radiation

Heat lamps and other forms of infrared radiation simulate the sun's rays by allowing radiation to penetrate the skin. Infrared heat can alleviate pain, reduce soreness or stiffness in muscles, and increase superficial circulation.

Steam Baths, Showers, and Sauna

Steam is the vapor state of water. It is a mist that is created as heated water begins to cool. The small particles of water emitted into the air as steam penetrate body tissues very easily. The steam bath can be taken in a cabinet that encompasses the whole body except for the head or in a steam room. In the steam room, the steam is generated mechanically and pumped through a duct system, as with a home furnace or air conditioner, to fill the room where the client is seated. The temperature for most steam baths is 120° to 130°F. The client's body will become saturated with steam and will be unable to perspire to cool down, so extra caution is needed when steam is used. A tent with a steam pump attached can also be placed over clients while they lie supine on a covered massage table. The tent covers the entire body with the client's head extended through an opening. Aromatherapy can be used with either treatment to enhance the elimination of toxins and create a more relaxing environment.

A **Vichy shower,** which is a unit composed of many pulsating showerheads with an adjustable force, is one of the types of shower equipment used to deliver warm water and mild compression to the client. The client is placed on a table (prone position, face to the side) that is topped with a waterproof mat, and water is showered onto the client through several showerheads mounted on a track of pipes hung just below the ceiling. The water drains through special holes around the edges of the table and falls to the floor to enter a larger drain (figure 14.6). The gentle force of the warm shower (95° to 100°F) is a very relaxing form of hydromassage. The use of water in any form for therapeutic purposes is known as **hydrotherapy.**

A Vichy shower is an easy way to cleanse the client after using muds, herbal products, or salts, especially if the client has limited mobility. The client may find the procedure very stimulating when a faster tempo or slightly stronger force of water is used.

A **Swiss shower** is a shower stall with usually four showerheads that can be aimed where water is needed on the client. The water temperature is adjusted to be the same for all of the showerheads, or to be very warm in some and cold in others for use in contrast hydromassage therapy.

A **sauna** is always in a room that fills with dry heat that is mechanically produced. The sauna's dry heat creates profuse sweating, which aids the body in the release of toxins and relieves pain and stiffness. The sauna's temperature may be between 180° to 190°F, so make sure the client does not overheat and replaces body fluids by drinking plenty of water. Clients who are pregnant or have diabetes, heart or blood pressure conditions, or other health concerns should be referred to their physicians before using extreme heat as a modality. The general length of treatment is 10 to 15 minutes. You should never leave a client unattended while using a sauna or steam treatments. If the client complains of discomfort, headache, throbbing at pulse points, weakness, or nausea, discontinue the treatment.

Figure 14.6

The Vichy shower consists of a series of multiple shower heads mounted horizontally over a special purpose "wet" table.

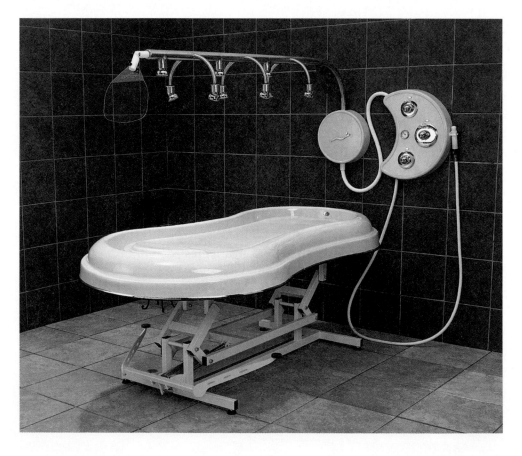

Before a steam or sauna treatment, a dulse scrub or dry brush **exfoliation** may be given. A **dulse scrub** is a treatment whereby the body is scrubbed with a blend of seaweed and oil to remove the top layer of skin and supply nutrients. A **dry brush exfoliation** uses a brush with special bristles to remove layers of dead skin and improve surface circulation.

A **salt rub**—a body rub using coarse salt for exfoliation—may be given to refresh the client. The salt rub is often called a **salt glow** because of the radiant appearance of the skin after treatment.

> ⭐ **EXAM POINT** A salt glow or salt rub should not be done after a steam bath or sauna treatment as the pores of the skin will be open and susceptible to a salt burn. Remember: Special consideration is always necessary when treating the feet of diabetics and persons who may have phlebitis.

To stimulate the client's immune system, increase circulation, and enrich the skin, a salt glow or rub can be used. It usually lasts about 30 to 45 minutes and exfoliates and energizes the skin. The client is placed in a wet room area, such as on a Vichy shower table, and a gentle spray of warm water (some spas use mineral waters) is applied to the skin. The therapist wears a special mitt and applies sea salt or mineral salts to the skin. After one area is finished, a rinsing spray is applied before moving on. After the treatment, the client should receive a final cleansing rinse, and safety precautions for a wet floor or area should be followed. The area should be cleaned with disinfectant after the treatment.

For removing salt or sugar after a rub, the therapist may use a Scotch hose on clients who can stand. The **Scotch hose** consists of two high-pressure hoses that alternately spray very warm and cold water. The alternating temperature of the water will force the muscles to contract and relax continually.

An **immersion bath** in which the body part is submerged in water is used when a medium is needed to surround the body and conduct heat or cold. The objectives of all baths are external cleansing and stimulation of bodily physiology. Table 14.1 indicates water temperature standards.

Application of Cold

Using cold or ice for therapeutic purposes is called **cryotherapy.** You would use cold whenever there is a need to control a client's tissue temperature. When cold is applied to an area of the body, heat is pulled away from the tissues. This procedure is very beneficial in relieving pain, swelling, and inflammation to an area or injury. The cold constricts the small blood vessels close to the surface and stops the body's inflammatory

Table 14.1	Water Temperatures for Spa Treatments	
Temperature		
Fahrenheit	**Celsius**	**Type of Bath**
40° to 65°	4.4° to 18.3°	Cold
67° to 75°	18.3° to 23.8°	Cool
85° to 95°	29.4° to 35°	Tepid
90° to 94°	32.2° to 35.5°	Salt and mineral baths
95° to 100°	35° to 37.7°	Warm
100° to 115°	37.7° to 43.3°	Hot

PROCEDURE 14.2   Performing a Friction Bath

Objective: **To learn how to give your client a friction bath**

Items to be used:

- Cotton bath towels
- Loofah, friction mitts, or natural sponge
- Cotton bath blanket
- Water temperature between 40° and 75°F
- Sink, basin, or small tub

Procedure steps:

1. Prepare your room before the client arrives. Make sure the air temperature is comfortable and items to be used are placed within reach. Cover your massage table with waterproof padding and a bath blanket.

2. Explain the procedure to the client and have the client lie prone with the face to one side.

3. Drape the client so that only the part of the body you are bathing is exposed.

4. Apply friction massage movements to the part of the body being treated.

5. Dip the loofah, sponge, or mitt into the water and rub the body part for 10 seconds.

6. Apply light friction as you dry the body part with a towel.

7. Cover the treated area and move to another body part, or let the client rest for a few minutes.

---

response. As with heat applications, a client must be observed when using cold. If a bath treatment is used, make sure the client is not overly chilled. A cold bath of short duration—three to five minutes—may be better tolerated if rubbing is used. Procedure 14.2 gives instructions for performing a friction bath.

Additional application methods for cold are listed in box 14.4.

Benefits of Cold

Since the normal temperature of the skin surface is 92°F, a change of temperature of only a very few degrees will begin vasoconstriction. This will slow the swelling and inflammation of an injured area; that is why ice is the first type of application for trauma or injuries to muscle and tissue. Cold can also greatly reduce the neural response that signals the brain that pain is present. This response is called analgesic, meaning that the ice or cold acts to deaden the pain sensation and bring relief to the injured party.

Alternating heat and cold can restore circulation to the area as well as reduce swelling and pain. However, cold for a long duration can lead to **frostbite**—a condition brought about by the freezing of tissue. More information concerning the therapeutic use of heat and cold for injury can be found in chapter 13, along with more in-depth guidelines on the indications and contraindications for heat and cold use. Working in a cosmetically oriented spa, you would seldom be asked to treat injuries.

Box 14.4	Other Applications for Cold

- Ice packs, bags, or ice cups
- Massage using ice
- Vasoconstricting coolant sprays and gels
- Iced or cold towels

Mud, Clay, and Paraffin Treatments

Masks

Contrary to popular belief, masking with clay as well as gel and other products can benefit dry skin. Dry skin has as many toxins, impurities, and dead cells as oily or normal skin may have.

The mask used for "pulling out" of the skin is made with a natural clay.

Most clays that are beneficial to skin come from the ocean. These clays contain minerals and vitamins that will enrich the skin and can come in a wide range of colors. Although clay can work to provide treatment alone, adding essential oils and other ingredients can contribute to a specific treatment goal. In the past, many practitioners mixed their own blends, but today, it is possible to select from a large array of quality products that are tested and guaranteed to produce a desired effect. Make sure that your client does not have an allergy to seafood as the clay may contain seaweed and marine animals.

Clay masks can also be used along with essential oils to treat skin trauma, such as sunburn, rash, acne, or lines on a mature face. A mask for sunburn or a rash can be done as a soothing treatment. Acne facials have a medicinal and oil treatment factor, while a mask for mature and lined skin may be applied specifically to cleanse, tone, and rehydrate the skin.

Fine vellum hair follicles that cover the surface of the face act as sensors to send the brain a message and register the amount of moisture available. If these sensors register with the brain that there is little hydration present on the skin, then the brain will send the message to pores to release the oil that may be needed to protect the skin later. That is why drinking the proper amount of water can increase skin beauty. With a facial and steam or a shower mist to enhance the moisture levels, a mature face with fine lines can improve with only one treatment.

Paraffin is a waxy substance used in treatments to hold in heat, trap moisture, and return it to the skin, allowing nutrients to be absorbed. A paraffin wrap treatment can be used to tone and firm, detoxify, and smooth the skin. The paraffin is heated and nutrients or oils are added. In the basic treatment, the paraffin is applied to the skin and the body or body part is then wrapped. Many types of equipment are specifically designed to heat the paraffin. It is wise to follow the directions given by the manufacturer of the equipment for safety purposes and use only the products specified for that particular appliance. Procedure 14.3 provides instructions for a basic paraffin treatment. The treatment should last 20 to 30 minutes after application. Although immediate results are often present, weekly treatment for three to seven weeks provides maximum detoxification and toning.

Parafango

Parafango is the ultimate mud wrap experience for the day spa patron as well as the out-call client. Sea mud from off the coast of Italy or France is combined with paraffin to create a mixture that is easily applied to and removed from the skin. This sea mud,

PROCEDURE 14.3   Performing a Basic Paraffin Treatment

Objective: To give your client a paraffin treatment

Items to be used:

- Detoxifying gel
- Paraffin
- Wraps (disposable)
- Thermal blankets
- Body brush
- Paraffin heating unit
- Disposable drape sheets
- Gloves
- Protective table covering
- Timer

Procedure Steps:

1. To protect your table, cover it with a cotton thermal blanket, drape sheet, and disposable wrap sheet.

2. Have the client lie face down and apply the detoxifying gel to the treatment area.

3. Brush paraffin onto the skin, covering the entire treatment area.

4. Cover the client with a wrap sheet and place a drape sheet and thermal blanket over him or her.

5. Allow the treatment to process for 20 to 30 minutes.

6. Unwrap the client and remove the paraffin. Discard the wrap sheets. Apply body toner or herbal lotion to the treated area. Usually a shower is not needed.

packaged as a small brick, is rich in minerals such as selenium, calcium, magnesium, and potassium. Parafango provides benefits similar to other wrap treatments, including moisturizing or rehydrating the skin, promoting relaxation, and acting as an anti-inflammatory. Additionally, the high temperature of the sea mud, approximately 110 degrees, boosts the immune and lymphatic systems to release metabolic wastes or toxins. The total effect is to normalize all body functions and create homeostasis. Procedure 14.4 explains the guidelines for parafango spa treatments.

Although the mud can be somewhat messy to apply, it does not require an elaborate shower facility—found only in full-service spas—to remove. It peels off quite easily, usually as a whole unit (figure 14.11). Therefore, parafango is a treatment that therapists can take on out-calls to clients' homes or conveniently use in a small office. Some proponents of aminocel serum cream believe that in addition to increasing circulation and eliminating toxins, the cream can remove cellulite and decrease stretch marks.

 EXAM POINT   Contraindications for a parafango treatment include pregnancy, heart problems, tumors, and fever, to name a few. Further, an allergy to seafood and shellfish is considered a contraindication as the sea mud may contain kelp or other seafood-based allergens.

Stone Therapy

Many spas offer stone therapy, a massage treatment using hot basalt stones in combination with energy. This modality includes balancing and aromatherapy for release and renewal of the physical, emotional, and spiritual body (figure 14.12).

The main premise of stone therapy is to balance and ground the recipient to the earth with the use of stones. With their natural low frequency, stones assist people in being grounded and more able to handle everyday stresses. The second premise of stone therapy is the use of cold as well as hot stones (thermotherapy) in the massage. By honoring the elements of fire, water, earth, and air, stone therapy helps unify the human mind, body, and spirit with the universal life force. Hot water bathes the black basalt

PROCEDURE 14.4 Performing a Parafango Treatment

Objective: **To give your client a parafango treatment**

Items needed:

- Four-inch-wide natural bristle paintbrush
- Parafango bricks
- Aminocel ampoules
- Parafango heating unit
- Film cutter (similar to a tongue depressor)
- Plastic wrap
- Reflective blanket and flannel sheets (figure 14.7)

Procedure steps:

1. Brush the skin with a soft brush.

2. Apply aminocel serum cream.

3. Paint or brush melted parafango on one body part at a time (start applying to the legs in prone position) (figure 14.8).

4. Wrap the client's skin in plastic and a thermal blanket, and allow the client to rest.

5. Use the film cutter to make one cut in the parafango and peel it off (e.g., "slicing" up the leg once, followed by peeling the mud off the entire leg as a whole) (figures 14.9 and 14.10).

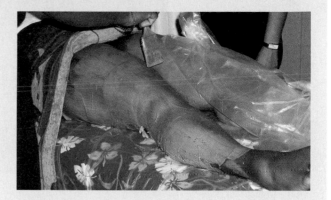

Figure 14.8
Parafango is brushed on the body using a 4-inch-wide natural bristle paint bursh.

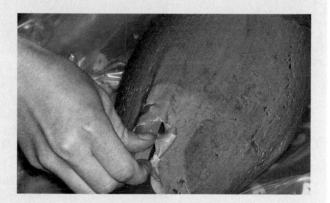

Figure 14.9
Parafango is loosened with a wooden tongue depressor.

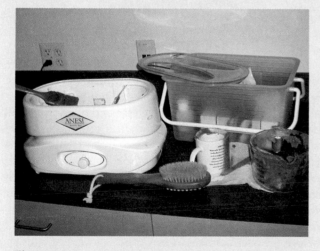

Figure 14.7
Parafango equipment.

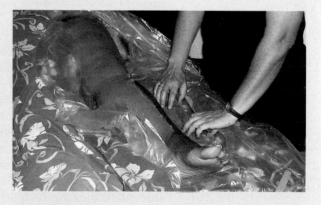

Figure 14.10
Dried parafango is peeled off the body.

Figure 14.11
Parafango removes easily, leaving skin soft and moisturized.

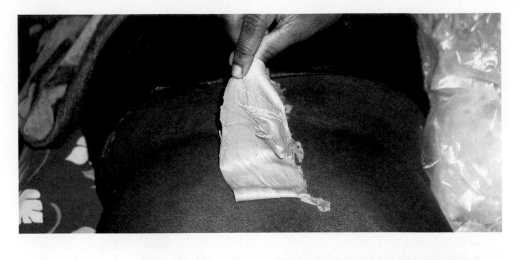

Figure 14.12
Stones are placed on the spine corresponding to the chakras.

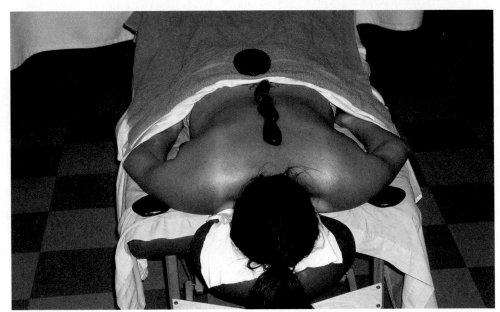

stones that are then used to cradle and massage the body. The use of cold marble pieces along with hot basalt stones creates a thermodynamic effect on the individual's physical (blood, lymph, digestive fluids, and muscle tissue), mental (release and memories), and spiritual (sense of connection) aspects. The thermodynamic effect accelerates movement, which in turn promotes healing. With the additional use of essential oils and energy balancing in the stone treatment, the higher frequencies are incorporated to assist in balancing the spiritual and emotional aspects of the individual with the physical body.

The stone treatment is a dance with nature and spirit; this dance begins with clearing the room and making a sacred space. One way to do this is by burning sage and fanning the smoke through the room with feathers while calling in the energies of the four directions. This can be done before the client arrives. If this is not allowed in your spa or healing center, a chime bar, Tibetan tone bowl, or music chosen with the intention of clearing the space will be more than adequate.

There are a variety of stone treatments and all are personalized by the therapist doing the work. Figure 14.13 illustrates an example of stone therapy performed by a therapist. As with any massage, the therapist can add techniques of other modalities to the stone treatment (e.g., lymph drainage, deep tissue, shiatsu, etc.). Some treatments are mainly for energy balance and the client is fully clothed. Other treatments are a balance of bodywork and energy balancing. In this type of treatment, the client is instructed to

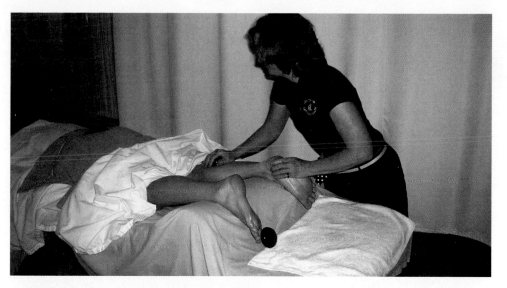

Figure 14.13
Therapist massaging with a hot stone.

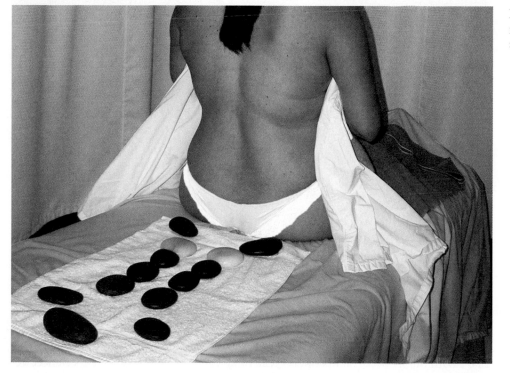

Figure 14.14
Stones are laid out in a specific pattern.

lic on a row of hot and cold stones (covered with a sheet or a towel) that cradle the spine (figure 14.14). Hot stones are placed in the client's hands, between the toes, under the neck, and on the abdomen, chest, and forehead (figures 14.15 and 14.16). Essential oils are chosen with the individual client in mind. The chakras are opened as the essential oils are dropped on the hot belly stones, and spirit energy is invited to assist the treatment. The therapist touches each of the belly stones, mixing the essential oils with the fingertips and feathering them on the client's shoulders. The therapist then begins to massage the client with the hot and cold stones while maintaining a clockwise movement around the massage table. Stones are selected from the roaster and ice chest as needed and replaced to recycle for later use during the treatment. The clicking of the stones and the mixture of the water and oil, hot and cold, music, and a variety of aromas all add to the stone massage experience.

Figure 14.15
The smallest stones are placed between the toes.

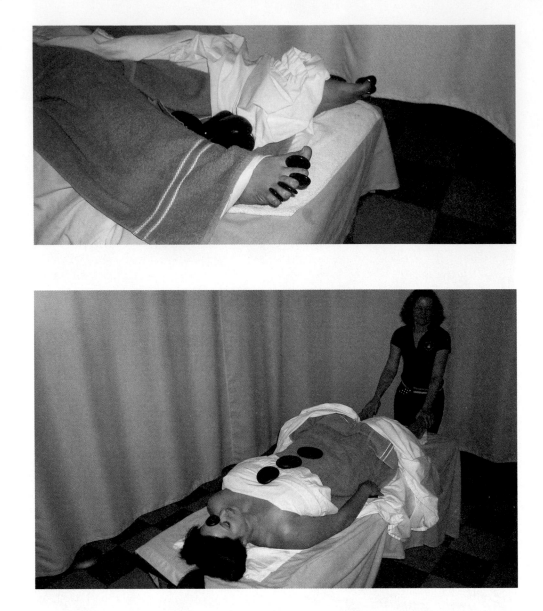

Figure 14.16
Stones are placed on each chakra.

A session lasts approximately 90 minutes, concluding with a gratitude prayer for the energy present and tapping of the stones as the therapist circles the table to seal the treatment. Clients are offered bath salts infused with essential oil and encouraged to take a bath before bed. Clients often speak of an intense, never-before-experienced relaxation after the massage as well as vivid dreams after a night of deep sleep.

Aromatherapy and Herbal Treatments

Aromatherapy and herbal treatment are widely used in spas. Aromatherapy, in its most basic form, is present in virtually every spa as spas generally burn scented candles to promote relaxation and client well-being, and essential oils are usually found in spa products such as facial treatments. Herbal wraps are extremely beneficial and are likewise used in many full-service spas.

History of Aromatherapy

Aromatherapy is one of humankind's oldest methods of treatment. The Greeks, Romans, Egyptians, and Native Americans all used aromatherapy and essential oils in the treatment of disease as well as to enhance daily life. When used properly, aromatherapy can be a powerful aid to healing. As early as 8000 BCE, the people of India used aromatherapy as part of ayurvedic medicine and still practice it today using the same ancient methods. The Egyptian physician Imhotep prescribed aromatic oils for bathing, massage, and embalming of the dead nearly 6000 years ago. Native Americans used aromatherapy in their healing rituals and especially in their sweat lodges where often magnolia bark, cedar, and dried lobelia were used to cure rheumatism, tuberculosis, and asthma. Nostradamus used rose petal infusions and myrrh to purify the air during the plagues in Europe. The list goes on and on. Every culture has used aromatherapy for centuries and most continue to do so.

What Is Aromatherapy?

Aromatherapy is the use of essential oils in treatments such as massage, facials, body wraps, and baths for both physical and emotional well-being. Aromatherapy can also be as simple as lighting a fragrant candle. Essential oils are made from compounds that occur naturally in plant materials, such as leaves, stems, flowers, and resin. They are a strong concentration of the compounds and should be used with caution and never taken internally or used directly on mucous membranes, such as the eyes or genitals.

Essential oils can be purchased alone or in a combination that has been mixed to obtain specific therapeutic properties. When mixed with lotions, massage oils, clay, or other treatment mediums, they can be applied to the skin or used in herbal wraps. These oils have many soothing and healing properties, and can be absorbed into the skin. On the skin surface, they can stimulate nerve endings and blood circulation. They can tone and strengthen skin texture, and are used extensively in facials, to massage burn scars, or in massages for cellulite and stretch marks. When the fragrance of the essential oils is inhaled, minute droplets of the oils enter the body through the lining of the nose. Herbal steam treatments are very beneficial for relaxation, depression, or anxiety.

The most amazing property of essential oils is how quickly and easily they reduce stress and bring relaxation. When the body is stressed, the brain is sending signals to increase heart rate, breathe less deeply, and send more oil to the skin surface. Blood vessels constrict and muscles become tense. Aromatherapy stops these signals and sends the brain the information that all is well, that you are a healthy, happy being. Many studies by research scientists are being done today to see how this happens. We all know that when we smell grandma's apple pie or roses or the ocean, we can experience a change in our attitudes and feelings. Marketers use this process to their advantage. Used car dealers spray the interior of older cars with "new car smell" so that people feel thrilled to purchase them. Real estate agents scent houses that they are trying to sell with cinnamon and vanilla to make the houses feel homey. So too can you use aromatherapy to direct the emotional and spiritual experience of the client during treatment.

Herbal Wraps

One of the most relaxing treatments found in spas is an herbal wrap. During an **herbal wrap,** a warm herbal solution is spread over the body, which is then wrapped to trap perspiration. The trapping of the body's moisture can help the skin absorb essential nutrients while herbs or essential oils in the mixture may tone the skin or pull toxins from the body. Procedure 14.5 details the steps for a basic herbal wrap.

This type of treatment, applying a product and wrapping, can benefit the lymphatic system and will stimulate the elimination of toxins, if using the detoxifying herbs, or soothe, relax, and restore calm to the body. Some of the other popular treatments are **Dead Sea mud treatment,** which uses mud from the Dead Sea that is excellent for detoxification and skin disorders, and an herbal wrap using kelp or other seaweed. All of the herbal wraps can be used to put vitamins, minerals, and other nutrients into the skin for beautification.

Herbal, essential oil, and salt solutions can be used to treat the hands and feet as well as the rest of the body. Using the essential oils of lavender, geranium, sage, or green tea along with coarse sea salt can soften calluses, and cool and heal tired feet and hands.

PROCEDURE 14.5 Performing a Basic Herbal Wrap

Objective: To give your client an herbal wrap treatment

Items needed:

- Unit for heating herbal solution
- Detoxifying herbs
- Two herbal linen wrap sheets
- Disposable wraps
- Thermal cotton blankets

Procedure steps:

1. To protect your table, cover it with a cotton thermal blanket, sheet, and disposable wrap sheet.

2. Place an herbal linen wrap soaked in detoxifying or soothing herbs on the bed and have client lie on the linen, then wrap the entire body. You can wrap the lower body alone if this is a cellulite treatment.

3. Place a second, soaked linen over the client.

4. Wrap the treated area with disposable wraps.

5. Cover the client with a thermal blanket.

6. Allow the client to lie quietly while the product works for about 20 to 30 minutes.

7. Apply toner and begin Swedish massage, or have the client take a tepid shower and then apply the toner.

Quick Guide F explains the categories of herbal and essential oil preparations and the properties present in the oils that can be used for the client. Pay close attention to the contraindications, as essential oil and herbal blends can be harmful if not properly used.

Treating Clients with Allergies

Massage therapists will often encounter clients who have allergies to products that they may wish to use. In these cases, you will need to determine what the client can have put on his or her skin. The rule of thumb is that if the client can ingest a substance, then it will probably not cause a reaction on his or her skin. If the client can eat foods containing or cooked with canola, corn, or coconut oil, those oils can be used as a base. You can add cinnamon (very small amounts), coconut milk, vanilla flavoring, peppermint flavoring, ginger, and orange, lemon, or peach extracts. Citrus extracts work well to remove toxins from the skin of tobacco smokers. Oatmeal, almond oil, honey, and crushed strawberries can make an excellent detoxifying, softening, and toning mask. With a little research and preparation, even the most allergy-prone client can be given treatment.

Sanitation of Equipment

Safety and sanitation are discussed in depth in chapter 2. The most important point to remember is that cleanliness is crucial. A dirty, unkempt environment will lead to the possibility of transmission of disease and ineffective treatments. Always be aware of the surrounding to which you submit your clients, and be sure to follow the directions of the supplier of the products you use. Make sure any and all equipment you use is working properly and that you have followed the manufacturer's guidelines.

Chapter Summary

Spa facilities are continually changing and growing as the industry moves forward. The future of massage therapy is firmly established in this type of practice and offers unlimited possibilities for employment. Colleges are offering programs in spa management, and major hotel and resort chains are hiring and training a large number of professional therapists. This avenue of the profession can lead you toward a very lucrative and enjoyable future as a massage therapist.

Applying Your Knowledge

Self-Testing

1. What is the normal temperature of the skin?
   a) 110°F
   b) 85°F
   c) 96°F
   d) 92°F

2. What is the main purpose of paraffin?
   a) To soften the skin
   b) To hold in heat and trap moisture
   c) To add a glow to the skin
   d) To chill sore muscles

3. What makes the day spa different from other types of spa facilities?
   a) Clients go there to lose weight.
   b) Clients receive same-day service.
   c) It provides smoking cessation treatments.
   d) Clients go there for medication management.

4. Which of the following Latin terms may be the origin of the acronym from which we derive the word *spa?*
   a) *Sanus per aquam*
   b) *Servo par ora*
   c) *Santus alumni*
   d) *Salut per aquarius*

5. What are the stones used in stone massage effective for the delivery of?
   a) Cold, moisture, and lotion
   b) Cold, heat, and mild compression
   c) Lotion, oil, and herbs
   d) Cold, ice, and pressure

6. What are five facial changes that can occur with aging?
   1. _____
   2. _____
   3. _____
   4. _____
   5. _____

7. In what area is the sternocleidomastoid muscle located?
   a) Scalp
   b) Tongue
   c) Shoulder
   d) Neck

8. List five steps you can take to ensure that your client is satisfied.
   1. _____
   2. _____
   3. _____
   4. _____
   5. _____

9. Which muscle is responsible for the flaring of the nostrils?
   a) Dilatator naris anterior
   b) Levator palpebra
   c) Pyrimadalis nasi
   d) Digastricus

10. Which water temperature is considered tepid?
    a) 45°F
    b) 85°F
    c) 100°F
    d) 115° F

Case Studies/Critical Thiinking

A. *Judy, a 45-year-old female, comes into your spa for a facial that includes neck and shoulder massage. This is her first appointment at your facility. You realize that Judy has a raised red rash covering most of her face and neck. Do you continue with the appointment?*

B. *Jamala, a 36-year-old female, was referred to you by her fitness trainer for immersion therapy using hot water. While asking questions during the consultation, you find that Jamala is elated because she just found out that she is pregnant. Should you continue treatments as requested?*

References for information in this chapter can be found in Quick Guide C at the end of the book.

PART IV

Complementary Massage and Bodywork Modalities

CHAPTER 15   Eastern Practices and Energy Work

CHAPTER 16   Introduction to Other Modalities

CHAPTER 15

Eastern Practices and Energy Work

LEARNING OUTCOMES

After completing this chapter, you will be able to:

- Recognize the basic philosophy of Eastern healing practices.
- Recognize the concepts of Qi, yin and yang, and the five element theory.
- Locate and identify the Chinese meridians and the organs associated with them.
- Identify other Eastern massage modalities such as *Tui Na*, Acupressure, Shiatsu, Jin Shin Do®, *Amma, Ayurveda*, Thai massage, Reflexology, Moxibustion, and Cupping.
- Explain how energy work, such as Reiki and Polarity therapy, function.
- Recognize the similarities and differences among all Eastern healing practices.

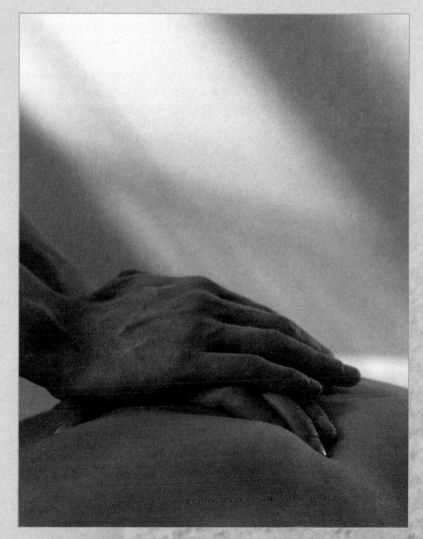

acupressure *(p. 405)*

Amma or *Anma*(p. 411)

Ayurveda (p. 411)

cun (p. 409)

cupping *(p. 411)*

dosha (p. 412)

five element theory *(p. 401)*

hsueh (p. 397)

lomi lomi (p. 418)

meridians *(p. 391)*

moxibustion *(p. 391)*

polarity therapy *(p. 423)*

Qi or *Prana (p. 390)*

reflexology *(p. 421)*

Reiki *(p. 418)*

sen (p. 416)

shiatsu *(p. 410)*

Thai massage *(p. 414)*

yang *(p. 391)*

yin *(p. 391)*

INTRODUCTION

Historically, many Westerners do not embrace the wellness philosophies and approaches that the Asian countries accept as part of daily life. In the West, we are conditioned to follow the modern Western medical model or "reductionist" theory. That is, we treat disease and illness after the fact, rather than prophylactically. Emphasizing prevention requires addressing the entire person—mind, body, and spirit—by focusing on every aspect that touches his or her life. Today, as more and more people search for therapies that are outside the Western medical model, they turn to Eastern practices such as Chinese medicine, acupressure (and acupuncture), energy work, and bodywork (discussed in this chapter), as well as herbs (see chapter 22) and traditional stretching and strengthening exercises (see chapter 19). In fact, many Western-trained physicians are also acquiring instruction in various Eastern therapies to meet the needs of their patients. For this same reason, it behooves the well-rounded massage therapist to be conversant in Eastern practices and therapies.

The various sections on the modalites discussed in this chapter have been contributed by noted practitioners in each respective field. Quick Guides B and C list books and websites as valuable references to use in furthering your studies in those areas that are of particular interest.

Chinese Medicine, Meridians, and Acupressure

By Marc H. Kalmanson, BSN, MSN, ARNP, LMT, RYT

The study of Traditional Chinese Medicine (TCM), *Tui Na*, the corresponding meridians, and all massage modalities that are based on an acupressure-style delivery remains quite avant-garde for most students in the Americas and Europe. As your clients' knowledge and desires grows, you may find it necessary to, at the very least, acquaint yourself with Eastern practices.

Philosophical Concepts in Chinese Medicine

One cannot have a discussion of Chinese medicine without, at first, laying a brief foundation of the philosophical concepts upon which almost all Asian traditions are based.

EXAM POINT   At the core of those traditions are the concepts of yin and yang, (pronounced "yong" as in gong), meridians, and **Qi**, (pronounced "chee") or *prana*, translated as "life force" or "universal life force energy."

These terms describe the presence and movement of subtle energies within all living things as well as the life-sustaining, life-enhancing, and life-giving of Qi.

The earliest known documentation of Chinese medicine is in the book *Nei Jing*, believed to have been written by the Yellow Emperor, Huang Ti (2697-2596 BCE). The concepts of yin and yang may be attributed to the *Book of Changes* (*Yi Jing*), written about 700 BCE, but some writers suggest that the concepts of yin and yang date back to the beginnings of Chinese medicine. Others suggest the use of the words *yin* and *yang* began at about 400 years BCE.

Based on these simple, intuitive descriptions, Chinese scholars extrapolated states of human existence and nature.

Yin and yang are used to contrast and compare all things. These contrasts and comparisons are applied to factors such as time of day, year, season, gender, individual constitution, organ systems, types of food or activities, as well as many other characteristics.

While **yin** is associated with stillness, settling down, slow movement, coolness, moisture, night, or darkness, **yang** is related to fire, heat, sun, day, dryness, rising up, fast movement, and speed.

While the concepts of yin and yang are fundamental to Chinese medicine, they are general and nonspecific in and of themselves and do not explain the full range of physiological phenomena that are identified by the various methods of diagnosis and identification of signs and symptoms.

Diagnostics

Most schools of Eastern medicine teach Traditional Chinese Medicine (TCM) and the five element theory, which deals with the theory of the system of correspondences as they relate to life and health.

⭐ **EXAM POINT** Within those programs, the diagnostic procedures taught and used include an extensive asking diagnosis as well as a tongue, facial, and pulse diagnosis.

There is a difference between the academic programs taught with respect to pulse diagnosis. During the era of Mao Tse Tung and other Chinese Communist Party leaders, some of the wisdom of the ancient practitioners was lost. Pulse diagnosis relied on methods that were based on limited information. However, a few schools of Eastern medicine teach "Contemporary Pulse Diagnosis," developed by Shen and Hammer.

Meridians explain the movement of specific energetic pathways in the body. These meridians are not based on the Western understanding of their function but on their Eastern designation and understanding of function and relationship.

⭐ **EXAM POINT** There are 12 principle meridians as well as extra channels and "special points."

Within these channels are located hundreds of points that, when stimulated by acupuncture, acupressure, or **moxibustion** (the burning of a special herb called artemisia), effect changes to the energetic flow of the human system. These changes can result in decreased pain, increased range of motion, lowered blood pressure and heart rate, and improvement in both acute and chronic conditions, including diabetes mellitus, high blood pressure, drug and alcohol addiction, and orthopedic injuries, to name but a few. It is a practice that truly provides real hope and optimism for the ill and

Think About It

A good analogy to keep in mind as you study this material is that the TCM practitioner corresponds to the doctor or physician in Western medicine, while the modalities, such as shiatsu, correspond to the medicine or pharmaceuticals that the doctor would prescribe.

injured without the complications of drug reactions or medical mistakes so common in Western medicine.

To begin a discussion, we must first look at the concepts that form the foundation of the practice.

The Concept of Qi

The concept of Qi (or Chi) does not translate well into English or Western thought but may be illustrated by a few examples. When one speaks about Qi, a distinction must be made between universal Qi (in our environment) and the human Qi that inhabits the human body. Universal Qi is a fluidly dynamic entity that can neither be created nor destroyed. However, human Qi can be deficient or abundant. Human Qi responds to both internal and external influences, while universal Qi embodies both form and spirit, and persists even after the death of the tangible form; universal Qi is therefore never-ending. Qi exists in the space around us, within us, and in all things. It is quantified and qualified by the nature and character of that which encompasses it.

Qi is the foundation of all that exists. It is the driving force of all things, and yet it is subtle. It is the rabbit and the tortoise; it is both ends of the spectrum and everything in between. It is both the light and the dark, the up and the down; it is both that which is and that which is not; it is constantly expressing itself in myriad and unlimited form. Admittedly, these concepts are difficult to comprehend for those who have not been exposed to Eastern thought.

Yin and Yang

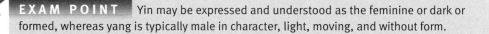

EXAM POINT Yin may be expressed and understood as the feminine or dark or formed, whereas yang is typically male in character, light, moving, and without form.

One cannot exist without the other, and, in fact, each gives rise to the other. The well-known symbol for yin and yang expresses this interdependent relationship (figure 15.1). Ideally yin and yang exist in harmony and balance with each other. But they may both be in excess or deficient. A deficiency or excess of one does not necessarily mean that the other is deficient or excessive. Yin can be deficient without yang being in excess; however, deficient Qi can cause yang to appear in excess and vice versa. When one is abundant, the other is not always deficient or excessive.

Try to understand that it is not a dualistic concept but rather a universal one. All aspects of the one are expressed in myriad forms. Yin and yang can be expressed and contrasted in table 15.1.

People who have a predominance of yin energy tend to be more cold-natured, slower in their movements and deliberations, and less outgoing, while yang-predominant individuals are more outgoing, gregarious, and restless, and may have fiery tempers or react quickly. People with a "type A" personality are usually those with more than adequate yang. They may also be more prone to agitation and excitement.

Table 15.2 examines the differences in how disease is expressed with respect to signs and symptoms that are typically yin or yang.

Think About It

Yin is from the earth up, and yang is down from the heavens to the earth.
Yin covers the "yinnards," and these meridians run anteriorly; yang is like a strong "yawn" and runs posteriorly.

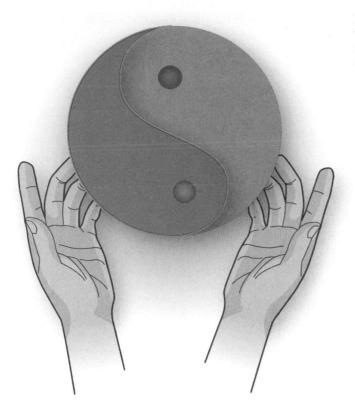

Table 15.1	*Contrasting Aspects of Yin and Yang*
Yin	**Yang**
Water	Fire
Quiet	Restless
Cold	Hot
Soft	Hard
Slow	Rapid
Wet	Dry
Inhibition	Agitation or excitement
Substantive/solid	Unsubstantial/formless
Conserving	Transforming
Storing	Changing
Interior	Exterior
Front	Back
Structure	Function

For individuals with yang deficiency, for example, illnesses tend to come on gradually, linger, and become chronic. When these persons become ill with even an acute process, it tends to manifest more slowly and stay a longer time. Pathogens and injuries tend to be driven deeper into the body, whereas those with sufficient yang tend to heal more quickly, have more superficial types of injuries with less complications, and recover faster. Because of the yang energy, they have more reserve energy, but there is a

Table 15.2	Yin and Yang Expressed as Signs and Symptoms	
Yin	**Yang**
Chronic	Acute
Gradual or insidious	Rapid
Lingering	Rapid and frequent changes
Lethargic	Restlessness and hyperactivity
Cold or cool extremities	Hot extremities
Pale	Reddened
Prefers warm beverages	Prefers cold or cool
Weak voice/dislikes talking	Talkative/loud
Symptoms usually more interior	Symptoms usually more exterior

Table 15.3	Yin and Yang Organs	
Yin Organs	**Yang Organs**
Heart	Small intestine
Liver	gallbladder
Lungs	Large intestine
Spleen	Stomach
Kidneys	Bladder
Pericardium	"Triple Burner" or triple warmer "Triple heater"

downside. Yang-predominant persons can also burnout more quickly. (Recall the story of the race between the tortoise and the hare.) Another aspect of yin and yang is their relationship to the blood. Qi is yang in the blood, but as blood is dense, fluid, and thick, it is also yin. Yang is defensive Qi manifest in all of yang qualities. It is skin and the inherent qualities of skin as a protection, and it is in the muscles due to their strength to initiate movement and create heat. But yin is nutritive as it is more internal, circulating in the blood and body fluids. Yang transforms food into energy, but yin stores it. The interaction of yin and yang is as a finely tuned and practiced symphony orchestra. They function in concert with each other for the fullest expression of Qi. Table 15.3 lists the designations of yin and yang organs.

As these designations show, yin organs have a commonality of storing, preserving, and maintaining, contrasted with the yang organs, which digest, metabolize, transform, and eliminate.

The Meridian System

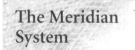

EXAM POINT There are 12 regular meridians and 2 extra meridians, resulting in 14 total meridians.

The extra meridians are the Conception Vessel (Ren) and the Governing Vessel (Du). Most of the yang channels begin in the upper body and descend, while one-half of the yin channels begin in the lower body and ascend. The Conception Vessel regulates all yin meridians and is the reserve for yin energy. The Governing Vessel regulates all yang meridians and is the reserve for yang energy.

All of the meridian channels have a two-hour period of maximum energy flow when treatment is optimal for each particular channel. These energy flows occur as three parts of a continuing cycle within a 24-hour period composed of four channels in each cycle. The first begins at 3 a.m. In traditional care, these times are followed, but in the West, this would be impractical to follow due to the major disruption to peoples' schedules and the necessity of often treating several meridians.

In Chinese Medicine, the anatomical position is similar to the Western one with the following exception. In the Chinese system, the upper arms are at a 90 degrees angle to the body and the elbow is also flexed at 90 degrees with the palmar aspect of the hands facing in the same direction as the anterior aspect of the body (figure 15.2).

The Lung meridian is represented by *L* or *Lu* (yin). Its time of maximum energy is between 3 a.m. and 5 a.m., followed by the Large Intestine (LI) (yang) from 5 a.m. to 7 a.m. The Stomach (ST) (yang) is at its maximum from 7 a.m. to 9 a.m. Ending this first cycle is the Spleen (SP) (yin) from 9 a.m. to 11 a.m.

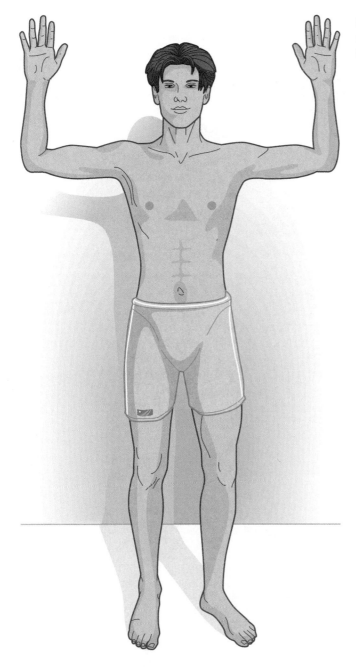

Figure 15.2
Anatomical position used in traditional Chinese medicine.

The second daily cycle begins with the Heart (H) (yin) at 11 a.m. to 1 p.m., followed by the Small Intestine (SI) (yang) at 1 p.m. to 3 p.m., proceeding to the Urinary Bladder (UB/BL) (yang) channel from 3 p.m. to 5 p.m., and ending with the Kidney (K) (yin) at 5 p.m. to 7 p.m.

The third daily cycle begins at 7 p.m. with the Pericardium (P/PC) channel (yin). It ends at 9 p.m. and is followed by the "triple warmer" (TW) (yang), which is predominant until 11 p.m. From 11 p.m. until 1 a.m. the Gallbladder channel (GB) (yang) is at its maximum. Completing the 24-hour cycle is the Liver (Liv) (yin) from 1 a.m. to 3 a.m.

TECHNIQUE EMPHASIS As stated previously, most of the yang meridians or channels begin in the upper parts of the body and for the most part descend inferiorly, while the yin channels mostly ascend.

Figure 15.3 Lung meridian The lung channel begins on the lateral aspect of chest, at the 1st inter-coastal space (ICS) and runs to the radial aspect of the thumb at the posterior corner of the nail.

LU 1
Treats coughs, asthma and emphysema, tight and congested/phlegmy lungs/chest, shoulder and back pain.

LU 5
Treats coughs with mucus, sore throat, stiff and painful arm.

LU 7
Treats cough and cold symptoms, headaches, elbow, wrist, and hand pain.

LU 9
Treats weakness and chronic lung problems, cough, asthma and sore throat, shoulder and back pain.

LU 10
Treats acute or painful sore throat, carpal tunnel.

The 24-hour flow of energy begins in the lungs, as already noted, and ends with the liver channel, but because the liver channel, flows to the lung channel, this cycle never ends. What comprises this flow? It is both the flow of Qi and the flow of blood and lymph fluids known as **hsueh.** Note in the following descriptions of the locations of the channels' beginning and ending points how this occurs.

The *Lung* channel begins on the lateral aspect of the chest, at the first intercostal space, and runs to the radial aspect of the thumb, at the posterior corner of the nail (figure 15.3).

The *Large Intestine* channel begins at the radial margin of the index finger, at the posterior corner of the nail, and ends between the nasolabial groove and the midpoint of the outer margin of the nasal ala on the contralateral side of the body (figure 15.4).

The *Stomach* channel begins between the globe of the eye and the midpoint of the infraorbital ridge and ends at the lateral aspect of the tip of the second toe posterior to the corner of the toenail (figure 15.5).

The *Spleen* channel begins at the medial aspect of the great toe at a point just posterior to the corner of the toenail and ends at the midaxillary line, in the sixth intercostal space (figure 15.6).

The *Heart* channel begins at the center of the axilla, on the medial side of the axillary artery, and completes its path at the radial aspect of the tip of the fifth finger, just posterior to the corner of the fingernail (figure 15.7).

The larger intestine channel begins at the radial margin of the index finger, at the posterier corner of the nail and ends between the naso-labial groove and the midpoint of the outer margin of the nasal ala on the contralateral side of the body.

LI 4
Treats colds, fever, headache, toothache, nasal discharge. **Caution**: do not use during pregnancy (induces labor).

LI 10
Treats pain in elbow (tennis elbow), abdominal pain and diarrhea.

LI 11
Treats fever, high blood pressure, digestive problems. Cooling and tonifying.

LI 15
Treats stiff and painful shoulder.

LI 20
Treats cold, hayfever, stuffy nose, facial paralysis.

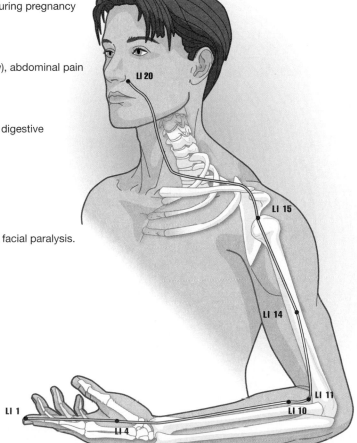

Figure 15.4 Large intestine meridian

The stomach channel begins between the globe of the eye and the mid point of the infra orbital ridge and ends at the lateral aspect of the tip of the 2nd toe posterior to the corner of the toenail.

ST 6

Treats ringing in the ear, toothache, dizziness.

ST 21

Treats indigestion, nausea, vomiting, colitis.

ST 25

Treats constipation, diarrhea, vomiting, colitis.

ST 36

Treats all stomach and intestinal disorders. Assists in digestion of food.

ST 40

Treats phlegm in chest, dizziness.

ST 41

Treats headache, knee and ankle pain.

ST 44

Treats headache, knee and ankle pain.

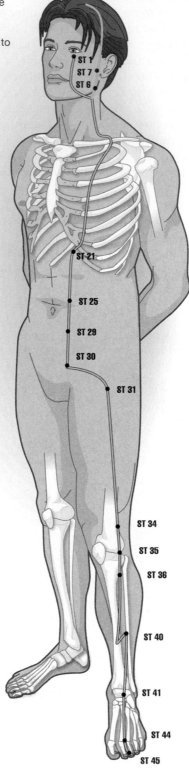

Figure 15.5 Stomach meridian

The spleen channel begins at the medial aspect of the great toe at a point just posterior to the corner of toenail and ends at the mid-axillary line, in the 6th intercostal space.

SP 6
Treats impotence, infertility, menstrual disorders. **Caution**: Do not use during pregnancy.

SP 9
Treats pain and swelling in the knee, abdominal pain.

SP 10
Treats itching and rashes, menstrual disorders.

Figure 15.6 Spleen meridian

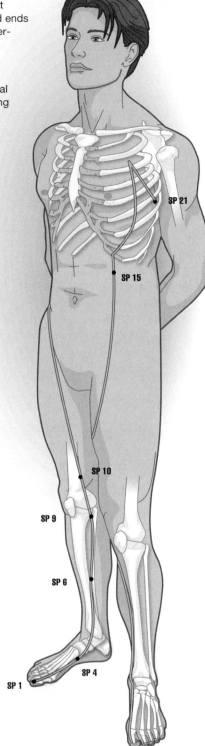

Chapter 15 Eastern Practices and Energy Work

Figure 15.7 Heart meridian

The heart channel begins at the center of the axilla, on the medial side of the axillary artery and completes its path at the radial of the tip of the 5th finger, just posterior to the corner of the fingernail.

H 3
Treats pain in chest, numbness of hand and arm.

H 7
Treats insomnia, palpitations.

H 9
Treats palpitations, pain in chest, heart attack.

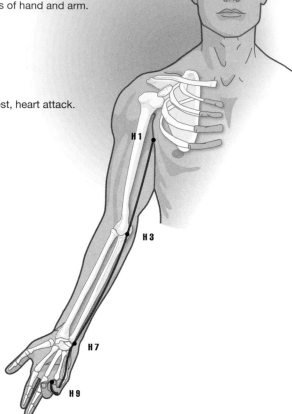

The *Small Intestine* meridian begins at the posterior corner of the lateral edge of the fifth finger and ends in the depression between the tragus of the ear lobe and the temporomandibular joint when the mouth is minimally opened (figure 15.8).

The *Urinary Bladder* channel starts at the laterosuperior aspect of the inner canthus, near the medial orbital border, and ends at the lateral edge of the fifth toe, at the posterior corner of the nail (figure 15.9).

The *Kidney* meridian begins in the shallow space at the junction of anterior and middle third of the palmar aspect of the foot in the depression between the second and third MP (metaphalangeal) joint when the toes are flexed. This point is called the "Bubbling Well" or "Bubbling Spring," because the kidneys receive energy bubbling up from the earth into the soles of the feet. Actually, the first point of each meridian is called the Jing or "well" point because of the energy bubbling up into the channels. The Kidney channel ends in a shallow between the first rib and the inferior aspect of the clavicle (figure 15.10).

In the last of the cycles, the *Pericardium* meridian begins just lateral to the nipple in the fourth intercostal space and approximately in line with the coracoid process. It ends at the midpoint of the tip of the middle finger (figure 15.11).

The "*Triple Heater*," also called *San Jiao* (S), begins at the ulnar aspect of the fourth finger, just posterior to the corner of the nail and ends at the lateral border of the orbit at the lateral aspect of the eyebrow (figure 15.12).

The small intestine meridian begins at the posterior corner of the lateral edge of the 5th finger and ends in the depression between the tragus of the ear lobe and temporo-mandibular joint when the mouth is minimally opened.

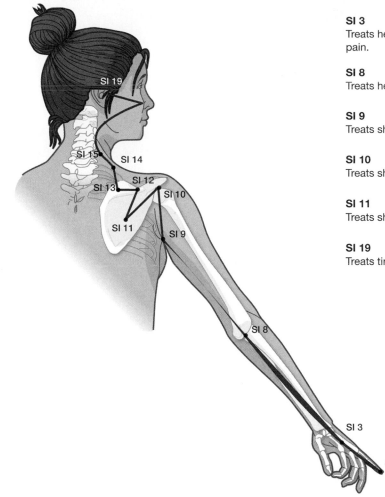

SI 3
Treats headaches, neck stiffness, back and neck pain.

SI 8
Treats head, neck, shoulder, back, elbow, arm pain.

SI 9
Treats shoulder pain.

SI 10
Treats shoulder pain.

SI 11
Treats shoulder pain.

SI 19
Treats tinnitus and deafness.

Figure 15.8 Small Intestine meridian

The *Gallbladder* meridian begins at a point just lateral to the outer canthus of the eye and ends at the lateral aspect of the distal fourth toe, just posterior to the corner of the toenail (figure 15.13).

The final meridian, the *Liver*, begins at the dorsolateral aspect of the distal phalanx of the great toe. It ends at the midclavicular line, directly below the nipple, in the sixth intercostal space (figure 15.14).

The Conception Vessel begins at the perineum and runs anteriorly up the mid-sagittal line to the end at the lower lip. The Governing Vessel begins at the perineum and runs posteriorly and runs up the mid-sagittal line, over the top of the head, anteriorly on the face to end at the upper lip.

The Five Element Theory

Somewhere between 476 and 221 BCE in the "warring states" period of Chinese history, the **five element theory** or "seats of government theory" began, according to Macioccia.

Chapter 15 Eastern Practices and Energy Work

The urinary bladder channel starts at the latero-superior aspect of the inner canthus, near the medial orbital border and ends at the lateral edge of the 5th toe at the posterior corner of the nail. Urinary bladder (UB) aka bladder (BL).

BL 10
Treats headache, neck, shoulder and back pain, cervical vertebral disorders.

BL 11
Treats osteoporosis and bone problems, shoulder pain, cough and fever.

BL 17
Treats blood problems and difficiencies, diaphragm tension, chest pain.

BL 40
Treats low back pain, lumbago, sciatica, knee pain and swelling, hip pain and leg cramps.

BL 60
Treats low back pain, sciatica, ankle and heel pain.

BL 57
Treats lower leg pain, hemorrhoids.

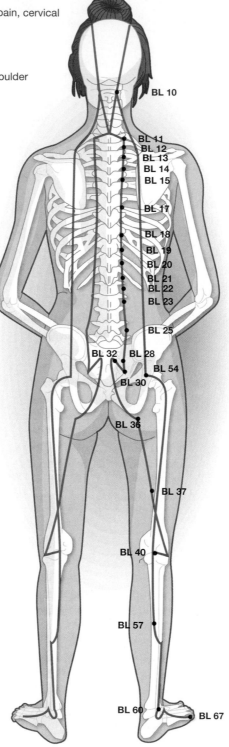

Figure 15.9 Urinary Bladder meridian

The kidney meridian begins in the shallow space at the junction of anterior and middle third of the palmar aspect of the foot in the depression between the 2nd and 3rd M-P joint when the toes are flexed and ends in a shallow between the first rib and the inferior aspect of the clavicle.

K 1

Treats headaches, shock, fainting, infantile convulsions.

K 3

Treats long-term chronic weakness or exhaustion, impotence or infertility.

K 6

Treats insomnia and irregular menstruation.

K 10

Treats knee pain and impotence.

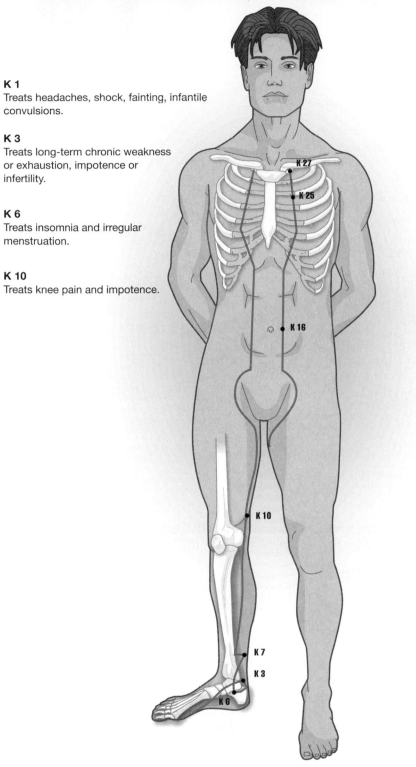

Figure 15.10 Kidney meridian

Figure 15.11 Pericardium meridian

Pericardium meridian begins just lateral to the nipple in the 4th inter-costal space and approximately in line with the coracoid process. It ends at the midpoint of the tip of the middle finger.

P 6
Treats chest pain, insomnia, nausea and vomiting, morning sickness.

P 7
Treats palpitations and gastric disorders.

P 8
Treats anxiety and emotional distress.

P 9
Treats coma, sun stroke.

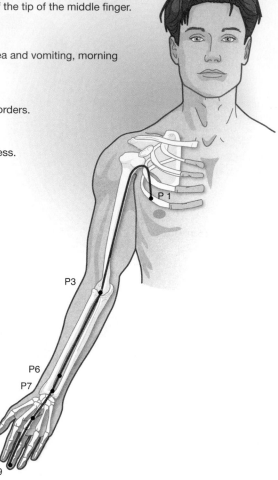

This theory was developed by the same school of thought that devised the theory of yin and yang and was led by Zou Yan, who lived from 350 to 270 BCE.

 EXAM POINT These elements, or "abilities" as they were also called, were recognized as powers, forces, or entities in nature that had the ability to effect changes in or create states of nature. The elements are water, fire, metal, wood, and earth.

Each one has an effect upon and is affected by the others. Moreover, there are also intervening factors that cause each of the five elements to influence, impact, and modify each other in varying ways.

The Five Elements are seen to embody differences in taste, direction, consistency, and type of movement or flow. They have several other characteristics as well.

EXAM POINT Seasonal variations are acknowledged with Wood representing spring and being related to birth. Metal is assigned to fall as it is associated with the harvest, while Water is believed to relate to winter and the "storing" activities that occur at that time of year. Earth, however, does not correspond to any season as it is thought that the other elements circle around Earth as the center or core of the five.

The triple heater also called San Jiao (S) begins at the ulnar aspect of the 4th finger just posterior to corner of nail and ends at the lateral border of the orbit at the lateral aspect of the eyebrow.

SJ 3
Treats headache, earache, sore throat, hand pain.

SJ 5
Treats ear disorders, fever, shoulder pain.

SJ 17
Treats facial paralysis, deafness, ear disorders.

SJ 23
Treats headache, eye disorders.

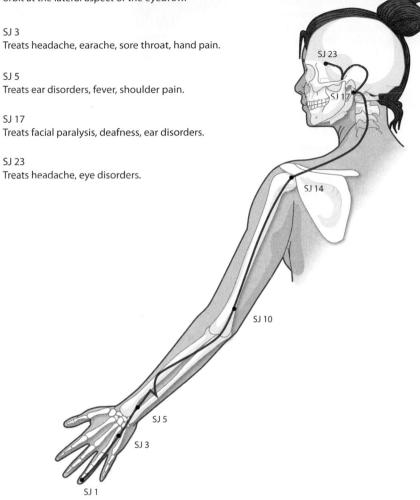

Figure 15.12 Triple heater or *San jiao* meridian

In looking at how each element arises, we see direct relationships between the elements. These relationships are called The "Generating Sequence," and in this sequence, we see that each element is generated by another (figure 15.15). Wood generates Fire, Fire generates Earth, Earth generates Metal, Metal generates Water, and Water generates Wood. Table 15.4 details the correspondences of the Five Elements from Macioccia.

Acupressure

Acupressure stimulates the same points as does acupuncture. It does not use needles, however, so it is better tolerated by those who are averse to needles. The techniques are usually done with the distal tip or pad of the finger or thumb.

There are acupressure points that massage therapists can safely use for some common complaints. Below is a description of these acupressure points for such nonemergent complaints. Three criteria are followed in applying acupressure:

1. Which point(s) to use for the specific complaint or problem

2. How to locate the point

3. How to apply the appropriate pressure

Figure 15.13 Gallbladder meridian

The gallbladder meridian begins at a point just lateral to the outer canthus of the eye and ends at the lateral aspect of the distal 4th toe, just posterior to the corner of the toenail.

GB 1
Treats eye problems, headaches.

GB 14
Treats pain in forehead, eye disorders.

GB 20
Treats flu and cold symptoms, headaches, hypertension, cervical vertebral disorders.

GB 21
Treats shoulder and neck pain.

GB 30
Treats hip pain, sciatica, weakness or paralysis of lower extremities.

GB 34
Treats sciatica, hip pain.

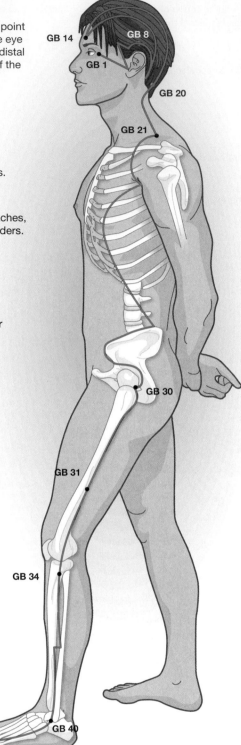

The liver begins at the dorso-lateral aspect of the distal phalanx of the great toe. It ends at the mid-clavicular line, directly below the nipple, in the 6th inter-costal space.

LV 1
Treats hernia, enuresis, dysmenorrhea.

LV 3
Treats irregular menstruation, headaches.

LV 8
Treats knee pain.

LV 14
Treats chest pain, abdominal distention.

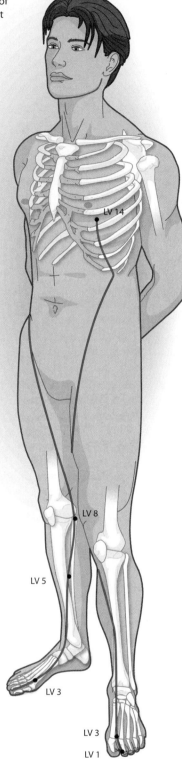

Figure 15.14 Liver meridian

Figure 15.15 **The Generating Sequence**

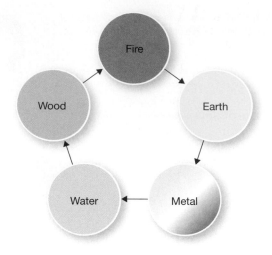

Table 15.4	*Correspondences of the Five Elements*				
	Wood	**Fire**	**Earth**	**Metal**	**Water**
Seasons	Spring	Summer	None	Fall	Winter
Directions	East	South	Center	West	North
Colors	Green	Red	Yellow	White	Black
Climates	Wind	Heat	Dampness	Dryness	Cold
Stages of development	Birth	Growth	Transformation	Harvest	Storage
Yin organs	Liver	Heart	Spleen	Lungs	Kidneys
Yang organs	Gallbladder	Small Intestine	Stomach	Large Intestine	Bladder
Sense Organs	Eyes	Tongue	Mouth	Nose	Ears
Tissues	Sinews	Vessels	Muscles	Skin	Bones
Emotions	Anger	Joy	Pensiveness	Grief	Fear
Sounds	Shouting	Laughing	Singing	Weeping	Groaning

Taking the criteria in reverse order:

3. Pressure should be applied gently and gradually increasing to a level that is tolerated by the client.

TECHNIQUE EMPHASIS Increases in pressure should be mediated by increased movement of weight of the body, extension of the arm, or whichever is most appropriate.

The pressure is usually maintained for 30 seconds to one or two minutes. The length of time depends on the client's tolerance. If a point is tender, it is usually held for a longer time (but with less pressure), while a nontender point may be held for a shorter time but at a deeper pressure. Applications to points may also be repeated one or two times and only one or two times a day so as not to overstimulate a point or its channel.

2. They are located through the use of bony prominences and other corporeal landmarks. The term **cun** (pronounced "soon") is also used. It equals the width of the client's thumb at the middle joint. Another method that is used is the distance of the space between the creases formed on the middle finger when a circle is formed by the middle finger touching the end of the thumb. The *cun* is used as a measure from a known point on the body and is designated as 1 *cun*, 2 *cun*, and so on. For example, a point for treating nausea is located 3 *cun* proximal to the wrist crease between the two tendons on the anterior aspect of the forearm.

1. The appropriate points are listed in a number of texts on acupressure and acupuncture. The correct point is one that describes signs and symptoms that best coincide with those offered by the client.

Many excellent texts offer more detailed information and explanations; several of these are noted in the reference list in Quick Guide C. But now, we will look at how acupressure is used for specific complaints.

A common complaint is headache; many people experience daily- or weekly-occurring headaches of a nonserious nature that are nonetheless quite disruptive. Several acupressure points are used for headaches:

- Gallbladder 20 is located at the depression between the sternocleidomastoid muscle and the splenius capitis at the base of the posterior skull. Pressure is applied in a direction toward the nose.
- *Yin Tang* is located just above the bridge of the nose and between the eyebrows.
- Large Intestine 4 is found at the end of the crease formed when the thumb is adducted and pressed against the second MP (meta phalangeal) joint. It is treated with the hand in a relaxed position. LI 4 is also helpful for toothache, temporomandibular joint (TMJ) pain, coughing due to the common cold, and pharyngitis.

🖐 **TECHNIQUE EMPHASIS** This point is never used during pregnancy!

- Gallbladder 41 is found on the dorsal aspect of the foot approximately 2 *cun* distal to the joint between the fifth and fourth toes in the natural hollow.
- Small Intestine 3 is located at the apex of the crease on the ulnar side of the hand formed by a fist.

Another very disturbing and potentially debilitating problem is nausea. It can be treated using Pericardium 6, found between the tendons on the anterior aspect of the forearm 3 *cun* proximal to the wrist crease when the wrist is flexed.

Pain in the wrists, hands, and fingers may be relieved with pressure on the Triple Heater or Triple Warmer point located in line with the fourth finger when the wrist is flexed minimally.

Pain in the upper back, neck, and shoulders can be remedied by pressure at Gallbladder 21, found on the superior aspect of the shoulder midway between the C7-T1 interspace and the acromion.

Low back and hip pain can be treated with pressure at:

- Urinary Bladder 40, located at the center of the popliteal fossa. It is also useful for knee joint pain, disorders of the hip joint, and leg cramps.
- Urinary Bladder 60. It may also be helpful in treating sciatica and injury to the ankle joint.

- Gallbladder 30, found one-third of the distance from the greater trochanter to the base of the coccyx.
- Gallbladder 34, found anterior to the neck of the fibula. It is also useful for treating lower extremity and knee pain.

For pain in the shoulder joint, use Large Intestine 15, found in the depression in the deltoid muscle when the arm is abducted at 90 degrees laterally.

In keeping with the Chinese meridians, shiatsu and other forms of acupressure-style massage evolved to treat the whole person.

Shiatsu

Shiatsu is a massage technique developed in Japan and based upon the *Nei Jing*, a book of healing written by the Yellow Emperor.

EXAM POINT Shiatsu uses the theories of acupuncture and the meridian system and its channels of energy to affect healing through the application of direct pressure with the therapist's fingers.

TECHNIQUE EMPHASIS Deep and firm pressure is applied at a 90 degrees angle to the *tsubo* point to stimulate healing to the specific channel affected by the illness, injury, or disease.

Work on the point may also involve stretching. While the pressure is deep, it is applied with a slow progression and rhythm to allow the client to tolerate the depth and intensity while remaining relaxed, open, and accepting of the treatment. The experienced and sensitive therapist will also match the rhythm of the technique to the client's inherent rhythm so as to be in a synchronous mode with the client.

The depth and maintenance of the pressure applied allow both the therapist and the receiver to communicate verbally and through nonverbal cues. The therapist should remain open, aware, and sensitive to client responses to provide the most successful therapy. While the majority of treatments are administered slowly with deep pressure, when there is an excess of Qi at a point or points, a faster and shorter-duration technique is used.

Jin Shin Do

Jin Shin Do was developed by Iona Marsaa Teeguarden.

EXAM POINT This modality is a synthesis of Teeguarden's studies of acupuncture technique blended with information gathered from studying Asian breathing techniques, Taoist philosophy, and contemporary psychology.

EXAM POINT Jin Shin Do, which translates as "the way of the compassionate spirit," uses acupressure to increase the flow of energy through the meridians or channels to relieve pain and reduce stress and tension.

Relieving pain and reducing stress and tension are essential to prevent a vicious circle of causation from forming.

Through a proper assessment of imbalances in the meridians, the therapist can determine which channels are out of balance and make corrections with direct application of acupressure to the appropriate point or points. Jin Shin Do uses the same system of meridians and five elements that is used in Chinese medicine.

EXAM POINT *Amma*, also spelled *anma*, is another Asian bodywork technique based on the *Nei Jing*; it literally means "push-pull."

Amma

Amma also uses the 14 energy channels, cutaneous regions, and tendinomuscle and connecting channels to both gather information and treat.

TECHNIQUE EMPHASIS In *amma* therapy, the therapist must be intuitive and sensitive to the client's needs.

The therapist also must have a thorough knowledge of human anatomy and physiology. Through direct application of the fingers and hands, the therapist observes subtle changes in skin and muscle tension and energy flow. The therapist then effects changes in the client's tissues by remaining sensitive to the client's energy channels based on those assessments.

The technique is applied with both the thumbs and the palmar surface of the hands and fingers. The movements are slow and deliberate, yet gentle. They may be circular or linear. A main difference in technique when compared to Western massage technique is that *anma* (*amma*) and all Asian techniques are administered with respect to the lines of energy (the channels) as well as the tissues themselves.

Moxibustion

Moxibustion is a traditional Chinese treatment using the burning of an herb, *moxa* (or artemisia), over an acupuncture point. The intent is to stimulate the flow of Qi by increasing the flow of blood. There are two types of moxibustion, direct and indirect, with direct moxibustion being further divided into scarring and nonscarring. Scarring moxibustion involves burning the *moxa* completely down to the skin, hence the name. With nonscarring moxibustion, the herb is not allowed to burn all the way down to the skin.

Cupping

Another traditional Chinese treatment is Cupping. The intent of **Cupping** also is to stimulate Qi or blood flow. Traditionally, the cups are made of either bamboo or glass and remain stationary on the dry skin or are moved around. The first method uses a burning taper held inside the cup briefly to consume the oxygen, thus forming a vacuum when placed on the skin. The second method is to use a small amount of oil under the cup and move it around. With both methods, the vacuum draws the skin up and encourages localized blood flow. Some ancient evidence suggests that cupping may also have been used for bloodletting and pulling toxins from the skin.

Cupping is still practiced today, although most modern-day methods employ plastic cups rather than bamboo. A vacuum pump instead of a flame is used with plastic cups to create the suction.

Ayurveda

By Donald J. Glassey, MSW, DC, LMT, NCTMB

From the Far East to the Near East, we see a similar yet different approach to healing. *Ayurveda* focuses on the whole being, as does traditional Chinese medicine, but this system is based on traditions found in the Indian culture.

The Sanskrit term *Ayurveda* means the science (*veda*) of life (*ayus*) and longevity. This East Indian system of wellness is several thousand years old. It is similar to Chinese medicine in that both procedures use a total examination of the client (including pulse, temperature, skin condition, eyes, psychological characteristics, and other factors) when making a diagnosis.

> **EXAM POINT** *Ayurveda* uses diet, herbs, water therapy, massage, attitude training and behavior modification, detoxification regimens, and meditation along with other procedures to encourage restoration of the body to a condition of balance.

The goal of the procedures is to balance the three subtle element influences of air and space, fire and water, and earth and water. These subtle elements govern physiological functions and influence psychological states. These element influences are also described as the body's three fundamental energies, called **doshas,** the mind-body constitution called *prakruti* in Sanskrit. Table 15.5 provides information on charting *prakruti*. The names of the *doshas* are *Vata* (air), *Pitta* (fire), and *Kapha* (earth). Table 15.6 describes the *doshas*. Health is a perfect balance of the three *doshas* and an equal balance of body, mind, and soul or consciousness. Most individuals, however, have one or two *doshas* predominant and characteristics in all three categories.

Ayurveda is the art of living in harmony with the laws of nature and encompasses the entire life of the individual. The aims of this science are to maintain the health of a healthy person and to heal the disease of an unhealthy person. Both maintenance and healing are carried out by entirely natural means.

Doshas

Vata: The force in the body that represents all kinetic activity, all movement of any sort in the organism.

Pitta: The force in the body that is responsible for all forms of digestion in the organism and balances kinetic and potential energies.

Kapha: The force in the body that represents stability and structure of all sorts in the organism. Figure 15.16 illustrates the placement of the *doshas* within the human body. See box 15.1.

Ayurvedic Massage

Massage is an essential part of the Ayurvedic approach to health and well-being.

> **EXAM POINT** *Ayurveda* suggests massage with specific oils and procedures to be of greatest benefit according to an individual's *dosha*.

In general, *Vata* people require oil massage more frequently than *Pitta* and *Kapha* types. Sesame oil is recommended for the *Vata* constitution, with sunflower or sandalwood oil for *Pitta* and corn or calamus root oil for *Kapha* types. *Vata* and *Pitta doshas* need a lighter massage, while *Kaphas* require a heavier massage.

> **EXAM POINT** A classic ayurvedic massage is given with the oil heated slightly above the body temperature for *Vata* and *Kapha* constitutions and slightly below body temperature for *Pitta* types.

The oil must be heated to the correct temperature and up to a gallon of oil may be used for the procedure.

Aspect of Constitution	Vata	Pitta	Kapha
○ Frame	Thin	Moderate	Thick
○ Body weight	Low	Moderate	Overweight
○ Skin	Dry, rough Cool, brown Black	Soft, oily Warm, fair Red yellowish	Thick, oily Cool, pale White
○ Hair	Black, dry Kinky	Soft, oily Yellow, early gray, red	Thick, oily, wavy Dark or light
○ Teeth	Protruded, big and crooked; gums emaciated	Moderate in size; soft gums, yellowish	Strong, white
○ Eyes	Small, dull, dry, brown, black	Sharp, penetrating, green, gray, yellow	Big, attractive, blue; thick eyelashes
○ Appetite	Variable	Good, excessive, unbearable	Slow but steady
○ Taste	Sweet, sour, saline	Sweet, bitter, astringent	Pungent, bitter, astringent
○ Thirst	Variable	Excessive	Scanty
○ Elimination	Dry, hard, constipated	Soft, oily, loose	Thick, oily, heavy, slow
○ Physical activity	Very active	Moderate	Lethargic
○ Mind	Restless, active	Aggressive, intelligent	Calm, slow
○ Emotional	Fearful, insecure	Aggressive, irritable	Calm, greedy
○ Temperament	Unpredictable	Jealous	Attached
○ Faith	Changeable	Fanatical	Steady
○ Memory	Recent memory good, remote memory poor	Sharp	Slow but prolonged
○ Dreams	Fearful, flying, jumping, running	Fiery, anger, violence, war	Watery, river, ocean, lake, swimming, romantic
○ Sleep	Scanty, interrupted	Little but sound	Heavy, prolonged
○ Speech	Fast	Sharp and cutting	Slow
○ Financial status	Poor; spends money quickly on trifles	Moderate; spends on luxuries	Rich, money saver; spends on food
○ Pulse	Thready, feeble; moves like a snake	Moderate, jumping like a frog	Broad, slow; moves like a swan
○ Climate	Likes hot	Likes cool	Likes dry

Table 15.5 Charting the Human Constitution (Prakruti)

Note: Circles have been provided next to the aspects for those who wish to determine a general idea of individual constitutional makeup. Mark V for *vata*, P for *pitta*, or K for *kapha* in each circle according to the description best filling each aspect.

TECHNIQUE EMPHASIS   The massage begins by "drizzling" the appropriate heated oil onto the supine client's forehead. The oil continues to be "slowly dripped" over the rest of the face and then onto the neck and shoulders, arms and hands, torso, legs, and feet.

The next step is to massage the oil into the skin with the appropriate pressure for the individual's *dosha* on the front of the body in the same sequence that the oil is applied.

The massage continues prone in the same sequence of slowly dripping the heated oil on the back of the head, neck, and shoulders, arms and hands, torso, legs, and feet.

Table 15.6 *The Three Doshas*

Dosha	Effect of Balanced *Dosha*	Effect of Imbalanced *Dosha*	Factors Aggravating *Dosha*
Vata	Exhilaration Mind clear and alert Perfect functioning of bowels and urinary tract Proper formation of all bodily tissues Sound sleep Excellent vitality and immunity	Roughness of skin Weight loss or gain Dark complexion Anxiety Restlessness Worry Constipation Decreased strength Arthritis Hypertension	Excessive exercise Wakefulness Falling Bone fractures Tuberculosis Supression of natural urges Cold Fear or grief Agitation or anger Fasting Pungent, astringent, and bitter foods Late autumn and winter (November–February)
Pitta	Lustrous complexion Contentment Perfect digestion Softness of body Heat and thirst mechanisms perfectly balanced Balanced intellect	Yellowish complexion Excessive body heat Insufficient sleep Weak digestion Inflammation Skin diseases Heartburn Peptic ulcer	Anger Strong sunshine Burning sensations Fasting Sesame products Linseed Yogurt Wine, vinegar Pungent, sour, or salty foods Late summer and autumn (July–October)
Kapha	Strength Normal joints Stability of mind Dignity Affectionate and forgiving nature Strong and properly proportioned body Courage Vitality	Pale complexion Coldness Laziness Excessive sleep Dullness Asthma Excessive weight gain Looseness of joints Depression	Sleeping during daytime Excessive acid intake Heavy food Sweet, sour, or salty food Milk products Sugar Spring and early summer (March–June)

Again, the next step is to massage the oil into the skin with the appropriate pressure for the client's constitution on the back of the body in the same sequence that the oil is applied.

The final step in the massage is to rub the client's skin with graham flour to absorb the oil. The entire posterior of the body is done first, starting with the head and working down to the feet, and then the anterior of the body, starting with the face and working down to the feet. The individual is then given the opportunity to rest and relax on the massage table for five to 10 minutes or longer. The massage is concluded with the client taking a shower to wash off the graham flour.

Thai Massage

Geographically positioned between China and India is Thailand, the "Land of Smiles." As with the other Eastern modalities, **Thai massage** focuses on the whole person.

Thai massage, or *Nuad Bo-Rarn*, is the ancient massage of Thailand that "manipulates" the body's muscular and connective tissue structures using acupressure-style

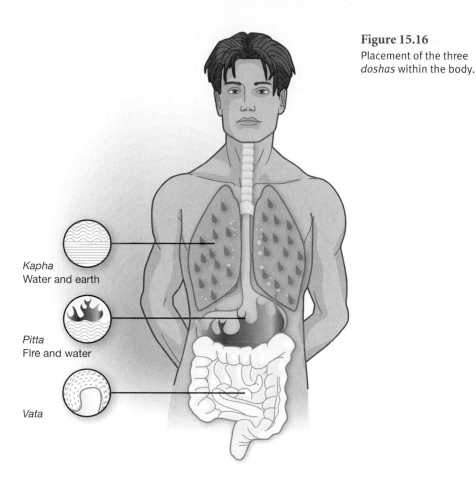

Figure 15.16
Placement of the three *doshas* within the body.

Kapha
Water and earth

Pitta
Fire and water

Vata

Think About It | The Three Doshas

Structures in the Body that Represent the Three Doshas
    Vata: Nervous system, bones, and tubular organs, especially the colon
    Pitta: Eyes, skin, liver, spleen, small intestine, and stomach
    Kapha: Joints and synovial membranes

Mind-Body Characteristics of the Three *Doshas*
    Vata: Light, thin frame and build
        Tendency to dry skin and hair
        Aversion to cold weather
        Irregular hunger and digestion with tendency to constipation
        Tendency to have worry, anxiety, and fear
        Usually quick to learn new things and quick to forget
    Pitta: Moderate build
        Tendency to light skin and hair, moles, and freckles
        Aversion to hot weather
        Sharp hunger and strong digestion
        Tendency to irritability and anger
        Usually quick to learn new things, and remember what seems necessary
    Kapha: Solid, stocky build
        Oily, smooth skin with plentiful head of hair
        Can endure climatic extremes easily
        Slow digestion, including hunger
        Tending to complacency and possessiveness
        Slow to grasp new information and slow to forget

massage combined with passive yoga stretches. Chongkol ("John") Setthakorn, founding physician of the Institute of Thai Massage, Chiang Mai, Thailand, refers to Thai massage as "lazy man's yoga"; it is a therapy in which you get a massage and have yoga done to you! Often, with this method of massage, the skeletal structure is affected, allowing for correction of postural imbalances. Indeed, there are not many chiropractors in Thailand; those who do practice are often serving Western visitors. In traditional Thai massage, the massage is only one aspect of healing and is often used in concert with medicinal herbs and spiritual focus.

Thai massage actually began in India, having its roots in *ayurveda*. Shivago Komarpaj, a contemporary of Buddha and some say Buddha's doctor, was thought to be the "father of Thai medicine." Thai massage has similarities to Chinese medicine. Traditional Chinese medicine works with energy channels called meridians.

★ **EXAM POINT**   Thai massage works with energy pathways referred to as *sen lines*.

Although Thai massage is similar to other Eastern bodywork, it has the unique ability to blend all facets of healing within one session. In other words, besides the physical aspect of Thai massage, most recipients also report experiencing spiritual or nirvanalike sensations during treatment; such sensations leave them feeling fully integrated and possessing equanimity (*upeksa*). Additionally, physicians in Thai hospitals employ the use of herbs to provide a well-rounded or thorough treatment.

The teachings of Thai massage were closely guarded in the *Wats*, or temples and monasteries. Historically, only the monks were versed in and allowed to practice Thai massage. Today, Thai massage is taught and practiced outside of the *Wats* throughout the country.

Even though Thai massage has moved out of the temples, Buddhist doctrine remains crucial to the work. For Buddhists, it is necessary to adhere to the "four divine states of consciousness," which assure complete happiness. These state are:

Metta—the desire to make others happy and the ability to show loving kindness

Karuna—compassion for all who suffer and the desire to ease their sufferings

Mudita—rejoicing with those who have good fortune and never feeling envy

Upekkha—regarding one's fellows without prejudice or preference

Practicing and Receiving Thai Massage

There are two styles of Thai massage, one found in the northern part of the country around Chiang Mai and the other found in the southern regions around Bangkok. The northern style is considered the "gentle" approach, while southern-style Thai massage is more "aggressive" and some recipients say is analogous to sumo wrestling!

To perform Thai massage correctly and efficiently requires the practitioner to possess strength, balance, focus, and intention. Practicing yoga, Tai Chi, or Qi Gong maintains the aforementioned qualities, while breathing exercises and meditation help you focus. Hands, feet, and elbows are all used to deliver the acupressure point techniques; thumbs "walk" the 10 main energy lines, or *sen,* in the body. Walking the energy lines intrinsically opens up the energy channels, allowing for an unrestricted flow of energy through the body. Unrestricted flow of energy is paramount to a properly balanced physical, emotional, and mental being. According to Buddhist philosophy, the intent of the giver should be one of altruisim, or bestowing kindness and being totally concerned with the receiver's well-being while expecting no personal gains.

To receive Thai massage, wear loose, comfortable clothes to allow for a wide range of stretching movements without restriction. Ideally, warm clothes such as sweats should be worn even in warm climates to prevent body heat loss over the two hours you will be receiving massage. Whether you are flexible or not, everyone can receive Thai massage. Many clients report an increased level of flexibility and range of motion after only a few treatments.

The benefits of Thai massage are numerous. It promotes deep relaxation and quiets the mind, releases tension, increases flexibility, improves circulation and neurological functioning, relieves pain, and assists in relieving degenerative conditions associated with the normal aging process.

Thai massage has several rules to be followed:

- Never practice in a public place or boast about your knowledge (outwardly exhibiting your skills for recognition)
- Do not hope for any gains (allow the Universe and the "Father," Doctor Shivago Komarpaj, to decide what works)
- Do not take patients from another (convincing clients to leave a practitioner and come to you is unethical)
- Ask for advice and listen to people who know more than you (learn from mentors)
- Bring a good reputation to the work (do your best work and work within ethical standards)
- Always give thanks to the Father Doctor.

As with other massage modalities, obtain a thorough client history. Many contraindications such as high blood pressure and herniated discs hold true for certain positions in Thai massage. For example, do not perform certain stretches, such as the Cobra, if the client has a herniated disc in the low back. However, Thai massage is often an excellent alternative to Swedish or circulatory massage for clients who are experiencing conditions that are considered contraindications for massage such as breast cancer (after recovering from surgery or chemotherapy).

Thai Methodology

TECHNIQUE EMPHASIS Always work with a relatively straight back and arms. Use your body weight and position to perform each movement or stretch. Pressure is often applied by rocking the body back and forth while palm pressing. Know your center of gravity and learn to move your client's body from your balanced position.

In palm pressing, use the full palm of the hand, not the heel of the hand, and never press directly on bone. Thumb walking is accomplished using the pads of the thumbs, rather than the joint or thumbnail. A foot press is performed using the arch of the foot rather than the heel or ball of the foot. Be mindful of the condition of your hands and feet. Have nails short and clean on both hands and feet before each massage.

Whether working in supine, side-lying, or prone position, begin work on a woman on her left side and on a man on his right side. The Thai people believe that energy runs through women's and men's bodies differently.

Thai Techniques

Palm pressing prepares the body for work, is used as a transition, and relaxes or "finishes" the work much the same as effleurage does in Swedish massage.

To *thumb walk* the energy lines, thumbs face each other and alternately move up the body part with "thumb chasing thumb."

Circular strokes are done with thumbs, fingers, and palms.

Quacking (or hacking in Swedish massage) is performed by pressing palms together, fingers held apart from each other and heels of palms held apart. Wrists and fingers remain loose, while the ulnar sides of the hands strike the body. Immediately pull the hands off upon striking. The "quacking" sound can be heard each time the hands strike the body.

Forearm rolls begin with the arms placed over the body palms down. Simply roll the forearms over once, lift the arms off, turn the arms palms down, place the forearms back on the body, and repeat.

The *elbow press* is a unique method of applying pressure to a specific spot.

TECHNIQUE EMPHASIS Increased pressure is the result of the elbow being opened, not pushing harder into the tissue.

A *knee press* is used when both hands are already being used elsewhere on the body (as in knee on the quadratus lumborum muscles of the low back while both hands are used to raise the leg for a stretch).

As mentioned earlier, Thai massage is performed fully clothed on a dense floor mat. The session usually lasts approximately two hours and is begun supine at the feet, working toward the crown of the head. Side-lying, prone, and sitting may follow in any order. Palm pressing is done first, followed by energy line walking, followed by several stretches all based on yoga asanas.

A tutorial would be too lengthy to include in this text, but seminars for continuing education credits are offered in many places; these short courses are fun ways to be introduced to this marvelous ancient massage. Training in Thailand can be done at the Old Traditional Medicine Hospital or the International Training Massage Institute in Chiang Mai, Thailand. Figure 15.17 features Thai massage techniques.

Lomi Lomi

Lomi lomi is a traditional Hawaiian form of health care that emphasizes spirituality and healing through prayer, ceremonies, massage, stretching, and joint mobilization. Adjunctive modalities are herbal medicine (*la'au lapa'au*), exercise (*ha'i ha'i*), nutrition (*mea 'ai pono*), and relationship-centered care (*ho'oponopono*). Lomi lomi represents a holistic approach (*lokahi*) to health and wellness.

A renaissance of Hawaiian cultural medicine occurred three decades ago as the legacy of native ways of healing began to surface following two centuries of political suppression. Islanders began to look toward the traditional treasures of wellness that were safeguarded by elder masters (*kahuna*) of the healing arts and culture. Of these life-saving gifts, *lomi lomi* has emerged as a premier source of relief and respite from the constant stress and strain of contemporary lifestyles.

Lomi lomi uses long, gliding strokes with the forearms and hands along with movement. As with Thai massage, a *lomi lomi* massage session often begins and concludes with a prayer or ritualistic practice.

Energy Work

Three modalities—Reiki, Reflexology, and Polarity—are energy or energy-based methods of treatment. The information provided in this section is intended to familiarize you with these methods. It is not intended to teach you the method, as all three modalities require certifications beyond massage therapy basic certification or licensure. Should you choose to incorporate energy work into your massage routine, you will find it greatly enhances your work. Please be advised that anytime you are working with energy, the transference of energy between client and therapist or from therapist to client is a possibility. For a discussion on this phenomena, see chapter 17.

Reiki

In Japan, **Reiki** is a generic word used to describe any type of healing work based on life force energy. It includes many systems of energy healing. The Reiki system of healing known to most Westerners was founded by Dr. Mikao Usui, who was born in Japan in

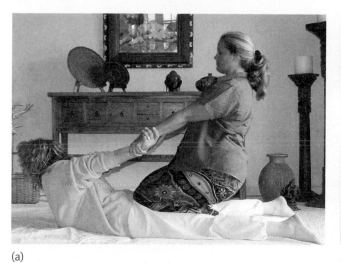

(a)

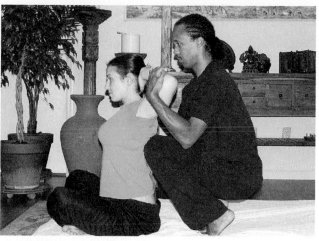

(b)

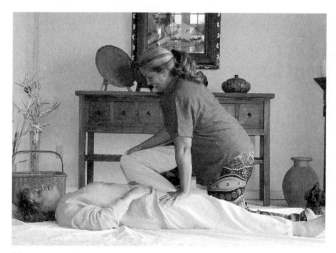

(c)

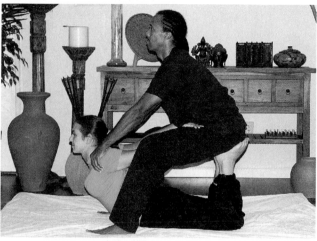

(d)

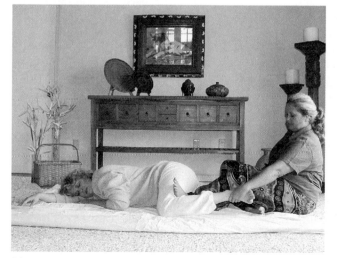

(e)

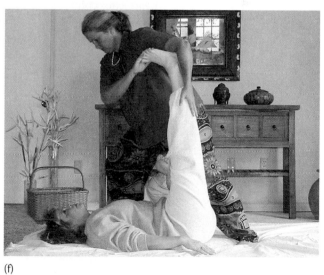

(f)

Figure 15.17

(*a*) Thai stretch using knee presses based on the Cobra yoga asana. (*b*) Thai stretch using knee presses under scapula stretches chest muscles. (*c*) Thai stretch using palm presses (knee to chest). (*d*) A more advanced Thai technique. (*e*) Pressure points on hamstrings using foot presses. (*f*) Thai stretch for hamstrings.

the mid-nineteenth century. Usui was impressed with the Buddha's quest for knowledge and enlightenment. He had an extreme desire to help others and noted in his study of the Buddha that the Buddha and his many disciples could heal by using the energy of life force surrounding an individual.

Usui believed that we are alive because life force is flowing through us.

★ **EXAM POINT** Life force flows within the physical body through pathways called chakras, meridians, and *nadis*.

It also flows around us in a field of energy called the aura. This life force nourishes the organs and cells of the body with energy and supports them in their vital functions. When this flow of life force is disrupted, it causes diminished function in one or more of the organs and tissues of the physical body.

Usui also discovered that the life force is responsive to thoughts and feelings. It becomes disrupted when we accept, either consciously or unconsciously, negative thoughts or feelings about ourselves and others. These negative thoughts and feelings attach themselves to the energy field and disrupt the flow of energy. This diminishes the ability to be at peace and to make decisions.

Reiki heals by allowing universal energy to flow through the affected parts of the energy field and charge them with positive energy. It raises the vibratory level of the energy field in and around the physical body where the negative thoughts and feelings are attached. This causes the negative energy to break apart and fall away. In so doing, Reiki clears, straightens, and heals the energy pathways, thus allowing the life force to flow in a healthy and natural way.

★ **EXAM POINT** Reiki focuses on strengthening the Qi and clearing the chakras of negative energy.

Reiki is both powerful and gentle. In its long history, it has been used in healing a vast array of illnesses and injuries, including serious problems such as multiple sclerosis, heart disease, and cancer, as well as skin problems, cuts, bruises, broken bones, headache, colds, flu, insomnia, and fatigue. Reiki is likewise used to treat emotional problems such as a lack of confidence, indecisiveness, depression, and hyperactivity. It is used on animals, plants, and negative energy within structures, as well as humans.

Although Reiki is spiritual in nature, it is not a religion. It has no dogma or specific doctrine you must believe to learn or practice it within the United States. Reiki training, however, is governed by a lineage system. Usui's method, which legend states he was given while fasting and meditating on Mount Kori-yama, is called the Usui System of Natural Healing, or *Usui Shiki Ryoho*. Usui trained Dr. Chujiro Hayashi to succeed him, and Hayashi in turn trained Hawayo Takata. Mrs. Hawayo Takata trained 22 disciples, and the lineage of most Western practitioners comes from one of these 22.

Reiki Levels

Reiki training is divided into three levels. In First Degree Reiki, an attunement is given to open the chakras of the student. Hand positions are also taught at this level. In Second Degree Reiki (Reiki II), the student is taught the symbols given to Usui on the mountain and how to use them. There are five Reiki symbols that represent the five levels of mind (table 15.7). The symbols were originally used not for healing but rather to enlighten others in the five levels of Buddhist wisdom used to attain enlightenment (Buddhist nirvana). Reiki II is used to heal specific conditions and unwanted habits. A procedure known as scanning and long-distance healing are also taught in Reiki II.

In Third Degree Reiki (Reiki III), the student is taught the use of meditation, expanded consciousness, techniques used to solve problems and heal emotional illnesses, and the use

Table 15.7	Reiki Symbols and Meanings
Symbols	**Meaning**
Cho-Ku-Rei	The light switch, nonattachment to earth
Sei-He-Ki	Emotional healing, cleansing, and purification
Hon-Sha-Ze-Sho-Nen	Past/present/future, healing karma, distance healing
Dai-Ko-Myo	A healing of the soul
Raku	Lightning bolt, completion, and grounding

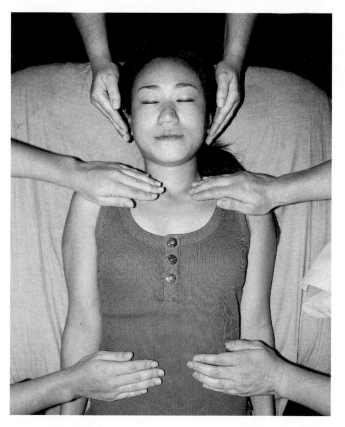

Figure 15.18
Person receiving Reiki from three Reiki practitioners.

of crystals and stones to empower healing. Only a Reiki III/Master Teacher can train others in the Usui method of Reiki and use all three levels of healing (figure 15.18). A number of Reiki associations and training centers are located across the United States.

Reflexology

★ **EXAM POINT**   For many centuries, **reflexology**—a system of stimulating the body to heal by applying pressure to points on the body (hands and feet) that affect organs or their functions—was practiced in Asia.

Carvings and drawings show health care practitioners in India, Egypt, and Greece using reflexology for the treatment of disease as far back as 2300 BCE. Reflexology as a system of treatment moved into the modern world in the 1920s, when Dr. William

Fitzgerald and Dr. Joe Shelby Riley converted the knowledge from their research into reflexology into a usable form. Eunice D. Ingham further developed and taught their findings to the public, beginning in the 1930s.

The scientific basis for reflexology began when Sir Charles Sherrington proved that the nervous system as a whole unit adjusts to a stimulus when it is applied to any part of the body. Sir Sherrington won a Nobel Prize in the 1890s for this work. Today, research studies are being conducted throughout the world that are validating reflexology as a treatment. Several countries have incorporated reflexology into the general health care community.

Reflexology is a form of compression massage that uses certain points on the hands, feet, and ears to bring about changes in corresponding organs and tissues. (See figure 15.19 for a sample foot reflexology chart.) Activation of these points can contribute to normalizing body functions by increasing circulation, lymph drainage, and stress reduction.

In reflexology practice, the body is divided into 10 zones, all vertical and on the left and right sides. Using the spine as a center point, each side has five zones. The right side of the zone represents the right side of the body, and the left side represents the left side of the body. Compression is applied to all of the zones during a treatment session. Figure 15.20 illustrates reflexology techniques.

The treatment session is divided into two parts: the exploratory phase and the implementation phase.

TECHNIQUE EMPHASIS In the exploratory phase, a practitioner uses slight pressure on meridian points to determine soreness or tenderness.

You would do this to find "crystals" that collect and slow down the blood and lymph flow. These crystals are deposits of calcium, uric acid, and other toxins. There are a number of contraindications for performing reflexology, especially on the feet, and you should only do so after extensive training from a certified reflexologist.

Figure 15.19 Sample foot reflexology chart

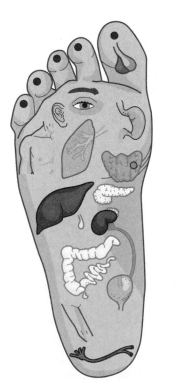
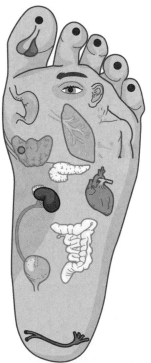

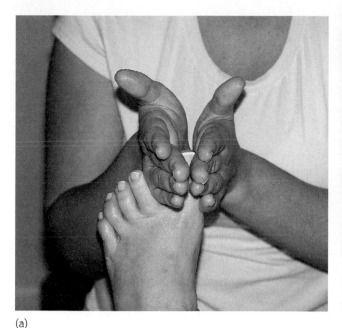
(a)

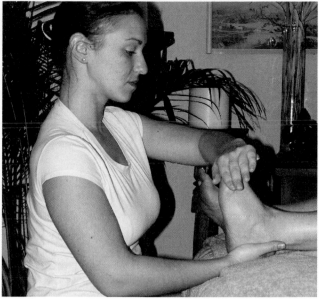
(b)

Figure 15.20
(*a*) Toe boogie. (*b*) Ankle rotation.

After the completion of the exploratory phase comes the implementation phase. It is at this stage that detailed manipulations are performed to offer release of the recipient's problems.

TECHNIQUE EMPHASIS To perform reflexology, you must have a deep understanding of the meridian points and the direct links to the parts of the body.

On the foot, the left foot corresponds to the left side of the body, and vice versa; the big toe is the corresponding area for the head. At the base of each toe is the area representing the eyes and sinuses. The spinal column runs the length of the foot from the big toe toward the heel along the inside edge of the foot. On the ear, the head is represented by the top of the outer edge, and the spinal points run the edge of the ear toward the lobe. Most Western practitioners use only the foot for treatment sessions. See the Online Learning Center and the References and Resources section of this book for resources on reflexology and contact information for reflexology training and certification.

Polarity Therapy

Polarity therapy is a method of energy-based bodywork that includes diet, exercise, and self-awareness. This system was developed by Dr. Randolph Stone (1890–1981) and focuses on life energy, charkas, and the elements (earth, water, fire, air, and ether.)

EXAM POINT Throughout Stone's long years of research and practice, he wrote seven volumes on polarity healing. His theory is that the body's energy field is affected by both emotional and physiological factors.

He believed that the basis of the energy field is a pulsation of expansion/contraction or repulsion/attraction that is known as yang and yin in Eastern therapy.

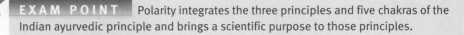

Stone used hermetic philosophy by showing how the caduceus—a staff with two entwined snakes and two wings at the top—corresponded with the energy field of flow within the body. In this example, the wings of the caduceus represent the two hemispheres of the brain. The knob in the center is the pineal body, and the upper right staff is the flow of the energy that produces the center of the brain. He felt that the two serpents represented the mind principle with the fiery breath of the sun as the positive pole of vital energy, called yang by Chinese practitioners. The left side of the body was said to flow with the cooling energy of the moon or the yin.

In the study of Polarity, it is believed that these two currents cross over the body in a grid that alternates positive and negative energy. The imbalance of the flow of energy is believed to contribute to disharmony and lead to disease in the individual. Stone's Polarity Therapy is used by natural health care practitioners, chiropractors, and osteopaths today. The practice of polarity therapy requires extensive knowledge and training. More information on training and certification requirements is available from the American Polarity Association; its contact information is listed in the Quick Guide A.

Chapter Summary

The common denominator among all of the Eastern practices is their approach to healing by viewing the person as a whole. Body, mind, and spirit are all important and equal aspects in contributing to health and balance. We recognize this approach is different from our Western practices, which view the parts of each person as separate entities apart from the whole. Further, Western medicine tends to treat conditions after they have developed, whereas Eastern practices strive to prevent disease. All Eastern practices—whether massage, energy line work, or diet—seek to establish balance and optimal health.

Applying Your Knowledge

Self-Testing

1. In what modality do you work 10 vertical zones?
   a) Thai massage
   b) Reflexology
   c) Shiatsu
   d) Trigger point

2. What is energy known as in different languages?
   a) Qi, *ki*, chi
   b) *Prana*
   c) a and b

3. Yang is associated with which organs?
   a) Hollow organs
   b) Solid organs

4. The liver is what kind of organ?
   a) Hollow
   b) Solid

5. What season is associated with the wood element?
   a) Spring
   b) Summer
   c) Fall
   d) Winter

6. Fear is the emotion of which element?
   a) Wood
   b) Water
   c) Fire
   d) Metal

7. What are the energy lines in Thai massage called?
   a) Meridians
   b) *Sen*
   c) *Nadis*
   d) Qi

8. What are the acupressure points used in shiatsu called?
   a) *Sen*
   b) Meridians
   c) *Tsubos*
   d) Elements

9. In *Ayurveda*, what are the body's three fundamental energies?
   a) Five elements
   b) *Doshas*
   c) a combined with b
   d) None of the above is correct.

10. In Reflexology, where is the spine located on the foot?
    a) Along the big toe side
    b) Along the little toe side
    c) In the middle of the foot
    d) On the heel

Case Studies/Critical Thinking

A. One of your regular clients comes in for her appointment and asks you about two types of energy work called Reiki and Polarity Therapy. How would you describe or explain these modalities to her?

B. A new client has informed you of an illness that is normally considered a contraindication, at least for circulatory massage. He still would like you to work on him. Is there a massage modality you can safely use on this client? If so, what modality would you use and why?

References for information in this chapter can be found in Quick Guide C at the end of the book.

CHAPTER 16

Introduction to Other Modalities

LEARNING OUTCOMES

After completing this chapter, you will be able to:

- Recognize and be familiar with various types or modalities of massage.

- Be acquainted with the history behind the development of these massage modalities.

- Identify the basic steps for performing the different modalities.

- Recognize the indications and contraindications for these modalities.

- Be aware of specialized training required to perform specific modalities.

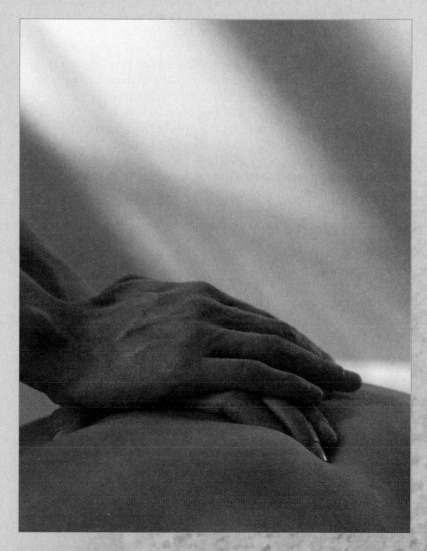

KEY TERMS

Alexander Technique *(p. 449)*

Cerebrospinal Fluid Technique
   Massage (CSFTM) *(p. 453)*

CranioSacral Therapy
   (CST) *(p. 457)*

fascia *(p. 439)*

Hellerwork *(p. 438)*

Lymphatic Drainage
   Therapy (LDT) *(p. 449)*

meninges *(p. 454)*

myofascial release *(p. 440)*

neuromuscular massage *(p. 429)*

neuropeptides (nerve
   proteins) *(p. 456)*

referred or radiating pain *(p. 428)*

Rolfing *(p. 434)*

somatoemotional release *(p. 457)*

Trager® *(p. 445)*

trigger point *(p. 428)*

INTRODUCTION

This chapter contains submissions from noted people in the field. Upon completing your basic massage school training, you will most likely find yourself drawn to a particular modality or type of massage. Here, we give you an insight to well-known and established modalities as well as innovative ones; there are many more modalities that you will discover in your journey as a massage therapist. In addition to his tutorial on myofascial release, John Barnes offers an interesting discussion of the whole body approach from Eastern practices versus the reductionist approach of Western medicine by emphasizing the importance for massage therapists to blend Eastern and Western philosophies of healing.

Career opportunities in such modalities could include working with chiropractic physicians by performing trigger point or neuromuscular massage, or working with structural integration such as Rolfing and Hellerwork. You may choose the more subtle approaches of Trager®, Lymphatic Drainage Technique, Cerebrospinal Fluid Technique Massage, or CranioSacral Therapy. Any of the various movement therapies such as Alexander Technique and Fledenkrais may appeal to you as well. Or perhaps you will choose to include one or more of these modalities to complement your Swedish massage. Notice that many of these modalities overlap in their approach and treatment goal. Often, it is a matter of finding which modality works best for your clients and the therapy or therapies with which you work best.

Of particular note, we include a piece on intuitive neuromuscular massage with a somewhat different approach to this long-standing work and a piece on Cerebrospinal Fluid Technique Massage (CSFTM), which is a cutting-edge procedure based on the latest science. It is a completely different analysis and protocol than CranioSacral Therapy(CST) or any other type of body work. Unlike in CST, in which practitioners analyze for a craniosacral rhythm, CSFTM practitioners palpate for impedence to cerebrospinal fluid circulation from the coccyx to the top of the cranium—at every single vertebral level. Therefore, the clinical effect is totally distinct from that of any other body-energy work.

Trigger Point Therapy

Trigger Point Therapy is a technique that many practitioners find to be an extremely useful tool to learn and use throughout their professional careers. Developed by Janet Travell, MD (John F. Kennedy's personal physician during his presidency), and David G. Simons, MD, Trigger Point Therapy can be practiced alone or in combination with general massage, bodywork, chiropractic work, and many other therapies.

> ★ **EXAM POINT** Dr. Travell defines a **Trigger Point** as a hyperirritable spot in the muscle or the fascia that is painful when compressed. She further classifies these points, or spots, as either latent or active.

Active trigger points are areas of pain at rest or in motion, are always tender, and prevent the muscle from lengthening. Active points refer or radiate pain on direct compression. (**Referred or radiating pain** is pain that is experienced or occurs at a distance

PROCEDURE 16.1 Performing Trigger Point Therapy

Cryotherapy (use of ice or other cooling agents) may be used in conjunction with Trigger Point Therapy. The point is usually held with fingers, thumbs, or elbows; a knobble or T-bar may also be used. It is extremely important to have client feedback when performing this modality, especially if using an implement such as a T-bar.

Procedure steps:

1. Identify the hyperirritable spot.

2. Ask your client to rate the pain on a scale from 1 to 10 (with 10 being most painful).

3. Hold static pressure at a level of 7 to 8.

4. Have your client inform you when the pain level starts diminishing.

5. Release the spot when the pain level has been reduced to approximately 2.

6. Gently stretch the muscle afterward.

---

from the trigger point.) Latent trigger points exhibit pain only when palpated. Both active and latent trigger points result in dysfunction.

The trigger point may reflexively relate to contracture in a muscle, hypersensitivity in the skin, increased pressure in the joints, decreased visceral activity in the visceral organs, or vasoconstriction in local circulation. More often than not, trigger points are found in areas of the body that receive the most postural stress and palpate as "knotted" tissue.

Normal muscle and fascia do not contain trigger points. The trigger point can be found in the belly of the muscle, the musculotendinous junction, or the tendinoperiosteal junction. Deactivation of the trigger point is performed with ischemic (static) compression or digital pressure directly into the point. Pressure must be enough to affect a response but not so much that the result is counterproductive.

Methodology

Trigger Point Therapy is relatively easy to perform and may be performed in a variety of situations: during a Swedish (circulatory) massage, during a chair massage, or during an athletic event. The intent is to interrupt the nerve impulses to the muscle through some sort of manual static pressure. See procedure 16.1.

Trigger Point work stands alone as a therapy but is also considered an important component of neuromuscular massage.

Neuromuscular massage, developed by Dr. Stanley Leif, is the manipulation of the soft tissue, which normalizes its function. This is accomplished by assessing the patient's condition through observation and palpation, and manipulating the affected musculature.

Neuromuscular Massage Therapy

⭐ **EXAM POINT** The purpose of **Neuromuscular massage** is to correct the shortening of the tendon, muscle, and tendon (T-M-T) unit, thereby rendering the tension of the T-M-T unit equal.

To achieve this, it is most appropriate to work the muscle segment to achieve the proper length of the T-M-T unit. In other words, the practitioner is able to achieve the greatest differential in length by working the muscle. The specific neuromuscular therapy approach that is described below is a bit different from commonly practiced neuromuscular therapy in that it works origin to insertion rather than the standard insertion to origin.

Intuitive Neuromuscular Massage

By Lewis Rudolph,
BS, AAS, LMT

Being intuitive is being perceptive and insightful. Intuitive Neuromuscular Massage (INM) involves taking your skills and training in observation and palpation, and applying them to assessing and correcting muscular and physiological abnormalities. I began doing massage with minimal training and just did what made sense. I looked at what was "wrong" and "intuitively" pushed until it was "right." I was able to picture the area and try to correct it. Intuitive Neuromuscular Massage evolved from my work (figure 16.1).

History of INM

Intuitive Neuromuscular Massage started when I noticed some trends in muscular reaction in massage school in 1991. There were differing results from what I was doing in a massage session. The difference was the direction of the massage strokes that I used. I thought very little about this, leaving it behind in the classroom when venturing out to make my fortune in the practice of massage therapy.

My first job as a massage therapist was working with chiropractic physicians. I was asked to work on many injured people with both acute and chronic pain. During this time, I became very interested in Trigger Point Therapy and pain patterns. I worked at learning the trigger points and their associated pain patterns to help people through the recuperative process. The results were very good—both the clients and the doctors were happy with the outcomes of the therapy. Most important, I was able to help many patients by doing trigger point work.

Subsequently, I noticed that the doctors were doing a lot of stretching of the patients that I had just worked on. I thought that I was not accomplishing all that was possible if the doctors had to stretch a patient after I had just massaged them. Over several months, I experimented with using different pressure, direction, and speed. There were some very interesting results that I did not expect, yet I should have, given what I had noticed in massage school.

The change that made the most difference was in the direction of the massage strokes. I changed the direction of the massage stroke from the usual insertion-to-origin to origin-to-insertion. As this direction was used, the results from the treatment were much better. In addition, I experimented with the pressure and speed of the massage stroke. I noticed that when the pressure was too great, the patient's muscle contracted even farther. I began to work with less depth of pressure (see chapter 4) and

Figure 16.1
INM developer Lewis Rudolph demonstrates the technique.

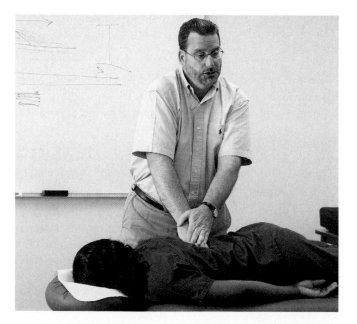

found that the appropriate level of pressure was just the amount required to move the muscle. The pressure needed to be within the tolerance level of the patient, however. If the pressure was beyond the patient's tolerance or not deep enough, the stroke was not as effective in reducing the spasm or increasing the range of motion.

After working on those two elements of the technique that I was developing, I started to adjust the speed with which I worked with the muscle. As with the depth, if the speed was wrong, the effectiveness decreased. If the muscle was worked too quickly, the muscle contracted, and it became almost impossible to reduce the spasm or increase the range of motion. If I went too slowly, patient feedback was negative because there was not enough movement and I was unable to finish the massage completely due to lack of time. Additionally, there were times that the patient didn't feel as if anything was going on—or rather, as if enough was going on.

Since I put these first three elements together and made slight adjustments, the technique has evolved and has been proven through the test of time. Adjustments are made at the "contact point," or the body part that you, the practitioner, use to work on a certain body part of the patient, and in the amount you work on an area. Lastly, the phrase "less is more" is apropos in the use of this method (figure 16.2). Overworking, as well as underworking, any area can cause the results to be less than optimal.

The Approach

Five very specific elements are important in intuitive neuromuscular massage. It is crucial to understand the proper usage of each of these elements, or the treatment results will be less than optimal. With patience and practice, the practitioner can become very successful using this method.

Five Elements of INM

The first element is the direction of the stroke. The word *stroke* is actually a misnomer, because the stroke is not in reality a stroke. As you read in the history of INM, this work is based on Trigger Point Therapy. The movement of the practitioner is not gliding at all; rather, it is contacting a spasm, or trigger point, at its proximal edge and stretching the muscle from the origin to the insertion. To accomplish this, the massage therapist must know the muscle that he is working on and the origin and insertion of the muscle. If the practitioner does not know these things, then he should at least be able to feel the muscle from the origin to the insertion. If the muscle does not move, the practitioner

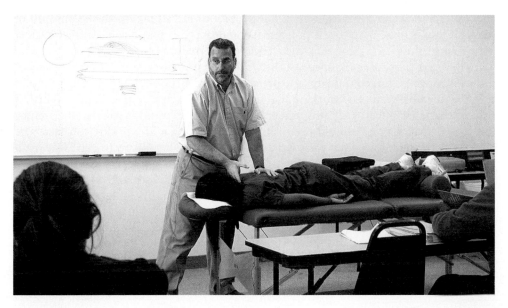

Figure 16.2
In performing INM, the adage "less is more" in terms of pressure often applies.

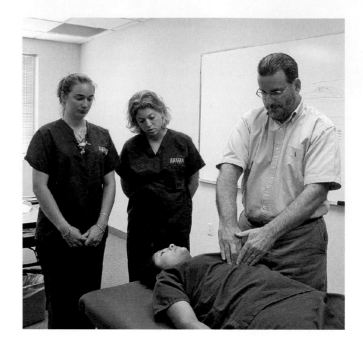

Figure 16.3
A spasm is contacted at the muscle's proximal edge.

should adjust the direction of the stretch. This should be done slowly and deliberately to allow the muscle to react properly (figure 16.3).

What does it feel like? It first feels like the skin is moving; when the skin has reached its maximum elasticity, the stretch will stop or at least slow down. After this happens, the muscle and or fascia will start to stretch, depending on the contact point (the larger the point, the more fascia is going to move) and the depth of the pressure (the deeper the pressure, the more likely you will be moving muscle instead of fascia). If the muscle or the fascia does not move after the skin has "stretched," you need to change direction slowly and deliberately, paying close attention to the change in movement and resistance against your pressure. If you are changing from the wrong direction to the right direction, you will know the difference because the resistance will decrease and the movement of the muscle will increase.

The second element is the amount of the pressure the practitioner uses. This varies according to the patient and the type of muscle as well as the size of the muscle. The amount of the pressure that should be used is just enough to move the muscle, without causing much pain to the client. This is, however, a difficult balance to achieve. The client's tolerance and her condition and expectations are all factors in the amount of pressure that is to be used. If the pressure is too deep, the muscle will contract against the pressure, thus decreasing the effectiveness of the treatment.

The third element is the speed of the work. The practitioner must work slowly. A muscle cannot be forced quickly to expand. Think of a rubber band to help you picture the negative results of working too fast. If you stretch a rubber band too fast, it will contract just as fast. Keep this rubber band analogy in mind as you carefully gauge the speed at which you should be working, and try to avoid working too fast. The client will let you know when you work too fast because she will try to run away from your "stroke."

The fourth element is the contact point used by the practitioner. The contact point is the body part that the practitioner uses on the body part of the patient that is being worked on. Generally speaking, the larger the area being worked, the larger the contact point used by the practitioner. Another factor is the size of the practitioner and the size of the patient. If the practitioner uses a smaller contact point, the sensation will feel deeper than if the practitioner uses a larger contact point. For example, if a practitioner uses his thumb in a rhomboid muscle, it will feel much more severe than if the practitioner uses the palm of his hand, given the same amount of pressure. This is due to a dispersion of the weight over a larger area.

Now that we have four of the elements, it is time to put them all together and try to make more sense of it. Remember that the four elements we have discussed so far are direction, pressure, speed, and contact point. Each of these elements is difficult enough to do properly, yet, for a treatment to be optimal, all four elements must be done correctly. The fifth element, which we will add later, is the amount of time that should be spent on a muscle or an area.

When palpating, the practitioner will feel a muscle in spasm. This may present itself in a "banding" or a "clustering" when the practitioner comes into contact with the muscle in spasm. Once the muscle is identified and the corresponding origin and insertion are identified, the practitioner will put pressure directly perpendicular to the plane of the body. The contact point of the pressure is on the proximal edge of the muscle in spasm. This should be done very slowly, keeping in mind the patient's tolerance. If the practitioner goes beyond the patient's tolerance, the muscle will contract against the practitioner's pressure. If the practitioner goes into the muscle too fast, the muscle will contract against the practitioner's pressure. Once contact is made with the muscle in spasm and the patient is comfortable with the pressure, the direction of the pressure should slowly be changed toward the insertion of the muscle. It should feel like the practitioner is "hooking in" to the muscle and then pushing (or pulling) the muscle toward the insertion of the muscle. The direction should be deep and move laterally slowly and with consistent pressure. See procedure 16.2.

P R O C E D U R E 16.2 Performing an Intuitive Neuromuscular Massage

Objective: **To learn how to give your client an Intuitive Neuromuscular Massage**

Procedure steps:

1. Start working at one of these three points:
   - The proximal edge of the belly of the muscle
   - The proximal edge of the trigger point
   - The proximal edge of a muscle in spasm

2. When working on a muscle, keep it in the most neutral position possible.

3. The action of the movement of the stroke is like the Nike™ "swoosh." The muscle is contacted at one of the points stated in step 1, then pushed (or pulled) toward the insertion.

4. Remember that the pressure that is to be used is just enough to move the muscle tissue.

5. The contact point used will depend on the size of the area being worked. The smaller the area, the smaller the contact point used.

6. It is very important not to overwork the muscle. The muscle will follow a pattern when it is worked:

   - As pressure is applied to the area, the skin will stretch slightly and then stop.
   - As pressure continues, fascia will stretch, and then, sometimes simultaneously, the muscle will stretch.
   - The muscle then stops stretching. Leave the area.

7. It is imperative that the pressure at the osseous attachments is lessened to reduce the risk of increased pain at the attachment.

8. Once the stretch has been completed, application of cross fiber friction of the attachments (both proximal and distal) is recommended.

9. This process can be repeated with increasing pressure after the muscle has been allowed to relax in its elongated state. The effects of the treatment will continue even after the treatment is completed, so don't try to do too much at once. Overstretching the muscle will cause the muscle to contract posttreatment.

Overview

1. Before any palpation is done, survey the body both standing and lying down.

2. Ask questions during this time:
   - Is this a result of a trauma?
   - What physical activities are you involved in (include work, home, exercise programs)?
   - Is this pain chronic or acute?
   - When does it hurt more, and is it after a specific activity?

3. Palpate the body while continuing to ask questions. Palpation and answers to your questions are the primary sources of information. Use this time to familiarize yourself with the client's body, especially tight areas and possible areas of dysfunction. Develop a plan of action for treating the client based on this information.

4. Note whether the muscle is in spasm or hard. Also note the muscle texture.

5. Warm up the body further by applying either compressions or effleurage, depending on the use of lubricants. The purpose is to warm up the muscles through increased blood flow.

6. The primary difference between this treatment and others is that the direction of the movement is from the origin toward the insertion. That is, the direction of the movement is from the most stable toward the least stable attachment.

7. Use your own personal strength to accomplish the goal of stretching the musculature to the proper length. It is appropriate to use your fingers, fists, hands, elbows, forearms, or whatever works best for you with this technique.

8. You can work with or without lubrication. The lesser the amount of lubrication, the more effective the work. This does not mean that you should necessarily work with or without lubrication; just do as you are used to and be open to trying a different approach.

9. The most important aspect of the work is achieving the proper pressure and speed. It is imperative that the tissue be worked slowly. If the tissue is worked too fast, the muscle will "fight" against the work and contract. Do not work too deeply for the same reason. Use pressure that is just enough to move the muscle and no more than that.

10. The contraindications for Intuitive Neuromuscular Massage are the same as for any other bodywork. There are no additional contraindications for doing this work.

11. Patient variables to consider in this treatment include:
    - Age
    - Physical condition
    - Emotional condition
    - Diseases
    - Tolerance to treatment

Rolfing

By Don Curry, LMT, Certified Advanced Rolfer

Rolfing as a bodywork modality emerged from the work and research of Ida Pauline Rolf.

A biological chemist, Rolf went to Europe in the late 1920s to pursue studies in mathematics and atomic physics at the Swiss Technical Institute in Zurich and homeopathic medicine in Geneva. On her return to the United States, Rolf began to seek answers to fundamental questions about health for which the mainstream therapies of the day had no answer. Her insights that formed the groundwork for what became Structural Integration emerged through her work in New York during the 1940s treating chronically disabled people who turned to her after traditional medicine was of little or no help to them.

The application of Rolf's work as a holistic technique for enhancing human potential began to emerge in the 1950s, when she spent time in England working with John Bennett, a student of G. I. Gurdjieff. In the mid-1960s, she worked at Esalen Institute. Fritz Perls, the developer of Gestalt psychology, saw our posture as an emotional hieroglyph, expressing how we feel about ourselves and the world around us, and viewed a technique such as Structural Integration, which sought to balance the body, as a valuable adjunct to psychological work.

It was at Esalen that Rolf began training the first practitioners and instructors in what would later become the Rolf Institute. The institute eventually settled in Boulder, Colorado, where it remains today, training and certifying Rolf practitioners.

Until her death in 1979, Ida Rolf continued writing, teaching, and promoting Structural Integration. Her book *Rolfing: The Integration of Human Structures* (see Quick Guide C) presents the principles and theories of her work.

The Goal of Structural Integration

> ★ **EXAM POINT** The goal of Structural Integration is to take the body from a structurally imbalanced and stressed position, or "randomness" (as Rolf characterized it), to a place of alignment and balance based on the inherent design of the body.

To reach this goal, Rolf proposed three main insights or principles:

1. *The body is segmented:* Though the body is a single structured organism, it is made up of discrete segments. For the body as a whole to become balanced, each segment must be restored to its natural function. Once restored, each segment becomes balanced within itself and in relation to each of the other segments.

2. *The body is plastic:* Rolf proposed that the primary tissue that shaped our posture was fascia. Fascia, in traditional anatomy, was often considered to be a web that is found everywhere in the body but as a passive container of the more important structures (muscle, bone, viscera, etc.) that were named and studied by the anatomist.

   Fascia is the tissue that really "connects" the whole body. This connective tissue lies beneath the skin and follows the general shape of the body, surrounding and investing the musculature and forming the periosteum over the matrix of the bones. The third layer (subscious fascia) surrounds and supports the visceral organs. Called "the organ of form" by Rolf, fascia flows throughout the body from head to toe and from the skin to the dura of the central nervous system.

   Subscious fascia is comprised of collagen, which has the ability to respond to the manner in which energy travels through it by changing its structure and form. Our bodies bear the history of our traumas. Our habitual movements and the postures we assume—to avoid pain, earn a living, play a character, and control or express emotion—have the cumulative effect of taking us out of balance in the gravitational field. The resulting stress begins to accumulate in the structure. When the fascia is stressed, it thickens, shortens, and forms adhesions until the stress is relieved. The effect is that the area is braced and splinted but at the expense of resilience, elasticity, and vitality. In continuing to move and attempt to balance ourselves, the compensations we make for those areas of diminished vitality are expressed in the structure as tipping, rotation, and strain throughout the joint system.

   That responsiveness of fascia to energy is used in Structural Integration to organize the body. Just as the energy of injury, emotional trauma, and stress disorganizes the structure, Rolf's work uses deep fascial manipulation to lengthen chronically shortened areas, free adhesions, and move the body back to a position where the fascial planes are clearly delineated and the web is open and resilient.

3. *Gravity is the therapist:* Rolf set the goal of the manipulation as restoring the body to balance. She stated that if the body could achieve balance in the gravitational field—stand without effort—then gravity would no longer be a disorganizing force that it struggled against but would be an energy that reinforced its inherent structure and encouraged its organization. Rolf called this position of balance and connection in the body "the line" and stated that from this position, the body would lengthen along its vertical axis, the fascial planes would delineate, and the body would relax, unwind, and open.

The 10 Sessions of Rolfing

To achieve this goal of balancing and aligning the body, Rolf divided the work into 10 sessions that she called the "recipe." Drawing on her vision of a segmented body, each of the first seven sessions focuses on a different structural element of the body with a goal of restoring it to design position and function. The last three sessions seek to align the segments and render the body in balance with each block positioned properly.

The first three sessions focus on the superficial fascia, de-stressing and shaping the body generally in preparation for the deeper work of the later sessions.

The first session's goal is increased vital capacity. It works on the rib cage, thoracic outlet, and those areas synergistic with the opening of the breath. The second session opens the arches, aligns the feet, ankles, and knees, and begins the process of providing the necessary support for the integration and balance for the structures above. The third session defines a lateral line connecting the segments from trochanter to shoulder and alignment of the ribs. The twelfth rib, in particular, was considered by Rolf to be a primary transfer point connecting movement and support; its proper positioning was an essential preparation for the rest of the sessions (figure 16.4).

The next four sessions accomplish the transformational work of structural integration. Session four differentiates the function of adductors from the pelvic floor, freeing the pelvis from underneath. Depending on the rotation of the legs, the adductors sometimes—inappropriately—work as synergists to flexors or extensors. In the fourth session, the adductor compartment is centered correctly on the medial aspect of the thigh.

The fifth session releases tension from the anterior lumbar spine and restores the ilio-psoas to more proper position and function. For most people, the ilio-psoas is not controlled consciously, but the patterns of tension it holds determine the relation of lumbar spine, pelvis, and legs. Postural patterns such as scoliosis and lordosis involve an

Figure 16.4

Don Curry, Certified Advanced Rolfer, demonstrates the third session of organizing lateral midline and alignment of the twelfth rib.

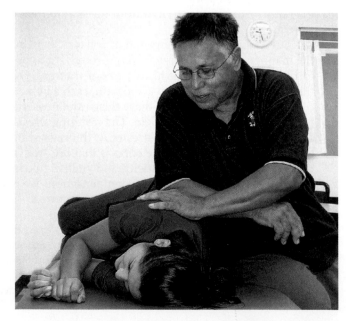

imbalance of tension in the psoas. When the psoas is functioning properly, movement in the lower body is initiated from the axial skeleton rather than solely from the appendicular skeleton (legs).

Freeing the sacrum and restoring the pelvis' ability to "breathe" in the sixth session completes the three-session series that balances the pelvis on horizontal joint surfaces. The role of the pelvis shifts from acting as a solid block under compression to functioning as a spacer that transmits the energy of support and balance through it.

Completing the work of the middle four sessions, the seventh session balances the head on top of the spine. Deep work on the cervical fascia seeks to bring a horizontality to its support and movement, which reflect and reinforce the new stability and order in the pelvis. Additional opening of the connective tissue of the skull and face, decompresses the facial bones and improves breathing by opening constricted nasal passages.

The last three sessions are where integration occurs. The work of the first seven sessions was to differentiate, organize, and balance the segments individually. To bring the segments into relationship and have them support and balance each other—as a whole—is the goal of sessions eight and nine.

The tenth session finishes the work of giving the body the ability to access the "line." This session looks mainly at the joint surfaces. To Rolf, the hallmark of a balanced body was one in which the structure was supported on functionally horizontal joints and was erect and balanced when at rest.

So, what exactly are the effects and benefits of becoming more upright and balanced? Rolf presented ideas and concepts that explained changes observed when a person went through her process, which seemed to transcend being a more balanced and efficient machine (see chapter 6). Rolf talked often in her classes about "core" and "sleeve." This is an additional perspective that sees an organization in the body that relates the way its inner core is supported by the peripheral musculature.

Through the years of her teaching, Rolf described the core at times as the intrinsic musculature (which, to her, was the braid of the deep spinal muscles and the diaphragms that spanned the body horizontally) and at other times as the fluid inner volume of the abdominal/thoracic space. In any case, the idea is that in the process of the body becoming more erect, balanced, and relaxed, the energetic core of the body is free from the impingement caused by the body's struggle with gravity and bracing against collapse. Depending on how it is defined, the core is the seat of imagination, emotion, metabolism, and other such processes. It would follow that a body that is balanced and open would exhibit more balance in all its vital processes.

Training

Practitioners trained by the Rolf Institute have the sole right to use *Rolfer, Rolfing*, and other derived terms in their practice. While the Rolf Institute is the best known, other schools have opened since Rolf's death that also teach her work and methods. Notably, the Guild for Structural Integration split off from the Rolf Institute in the 1990s and its faculty includes teachers who were trained by Rolf.

The depth and quality of training in structural integration vary with the different curriculums of the schools that teach it. They range from a bachelor's degree in massage (with a 10-session structural integration training as a specialty track) to brief survey courses that are taught in a series of weekends or personal presentations by individual practitioners of the work. These brief survey courses generally cover some aspect of structural work or treatment strategies based on experiences of the individual practitioners.

In general, to be trained as a practitioner of Structural Integration, you must first be trained as a massage therapist with grounding in anatomy and physiology and some mastery of massage. The technique of structural integration is then taught as an advanced modality. The requirements and cost of the training vary with the variety of curricula and intentions of the different schools.

In 2001, the International Association of Structural Integrators (IASI) was formed as an umbrella organization for practitioners who are heirs to the Rolf technique. This organization also serves as a forum for exchanging ideas and perspectives. The IASI is a good point of contact for information about schools, training, and developments in the field.

Hellerwork

Developed by Joseph Heller in 1978, **Hellerwork** evolved from his experience with Rolfing and is also a structural integrative approach to balancing the body. It consists of 11 one and one-half hour sessions that use deep tissue bodywork techniques to restore proper posture. Creating awareness of one's movement is also a component of Hellerwork.

Myofascial Release
By John F. Barnes, PT

The health professions have generally ignored the importance of an entire physiological system—the fascial system that profoundly influences all other structures and systems of the body. This glaring omission has severely affected our effectiveness and the lasting quality of our efforts. Including myofascial release in our evaluatory and treatment regimes allows us to provide a more comprehensive approach to our clients that is safe, cost-efficient, and consistently effective.

Fascial restrictions can exert tremendous tensile forces on the neuromuscular-skeletal and other pain-sensitive structures. This enormous pressure (approximately 2000 pounds per square inch) can create the very symptoms that we have so long been trying to eliminate. This knowledge frees us from only trying to relieve symptoms and gives us the tools we need to find and eradicate the cause-and-effect (symptoms) relationship for a permanent resolution of our client's complex problems.

Myofascial release techniques are utilized in a wide range of settings and diagnoses: pain; movement restriction; spasm; spasticity; neurological dysfunction (i.e., cerebral palsy, and head and birth injury); cerebrovascular accident; scoliosis; menstrual and pelvic pain and dysfunction; headaches; temporomandibular pain and dysfunction; geriatrics; sports injuries; pediatrics; chronic fatigue syndrome; fibromyalgia; traumatic and surgical scarring; and acute and chronic pain.

Development of the John F. Barnes Myofascial Release Approach

What has come to be known as the John F. Barnes **Myofascial Release Approach** represents a journey that began in my teens with a devastating weightlifting accident. Over four decades of exploration and refinement have led to a widely practiced and highly effective approach to the evaluation and treatment of pain and postural anomalies based on restrictions in the fascial system (figure 16.5).

My initial back injury at age 17 led to over a decade of debilitating chronic pain. Surgery to remove a crushed vertebral disc provided improved function and lessened pain. However, my back continued to be problematic. Throughout this experience, I began to experiment with self-treatment techniques to relieve my pain symptoms. These techniques centered on the very prolonged holding of specific stretch positions. I began to successfully apply these techniques with my patients without an understanding of the mechanism by which they worked. Upon attending an osteopathic course dealing with connective tissue and soft tissue mobilization, I realized that the techniques I had developed were very similar but had several important differences. I found that I was holding the positions for much longer periods of time—at least 90 to 120 seconds. The time factor proved to be pivotal for releasing the entire elastocollagenous complex, leading to permanent elongation of the tissues and relief of pain-producing pressure on other structures. Older forms of myofascial release used forces that were applied too ag-

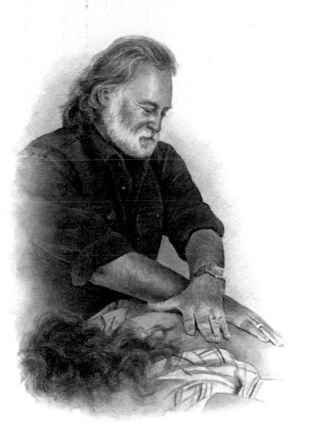

Figure 16.5
John F. Barnes, PT, using Myofascial Release for back pain.

gressively and for too short a time; my approach used prolonged application of gentle but firm pressure, permitting the practitioner to feel the release of progressive myofascial barriers and "follow" the tissues as they release. Older approaches yielded only temporary results, while my experience taught me that the fascial system could not be forced but permanent changes could be achieved by "finessing" the tissues. Building upon my knowledge of the fascial system, I began to visualize the body as an integrated whole through the complex interrelationships of the fascial network. The result is a body of refined concepts and treatment principles that can allow clients and therapists to accomplish true, authentic healing.

My personal history with pain that "trapped" me in my body provided deep experimental lessons, enabling an enhanced appreciation of my clients' physical and emotional suffering. I have had the opportunity of training over 50,000 therapists in my Myofascial Release Approach, and the demand for information on Myofascial Release is growing exponentially.

Anatomy and Physiology of Fascia

Fascia is a tough connective tissue that spreads throughout the body in a three-dimensional web from head to foot without interruption. The fascia surrounds every muscle, bone, nerve, blood vessel, and organ of the body, all the way down to the cellular level. Therefore, malfunction of the fascial system due to trauma, posture, or inflammation can create a binding down of the fascia, resulting in abnormal pressure on nerves, muscles, bones, or organs. This can create pain or malfunction throughout the body, sometimes with bizarre side effects and seemingly unrelated symptoms, not always following dermatomal zones. It is thought that an extremely high percentage of people suffering with pain or lack of motion may be having fascial problems, but most go undiagnosed, as the importance of fascia is just now being recognized. All of the standard tests, such as x-rays, myelograms, CAT scans, electromyography, and so on, do not show the fascial restrictions!

The fascia can be broken down into three divisions: superficial fascia lies directly below the dermis; deep fascia surrounds and infuses with muscle, bone, nerves, blood vessels, and organs of the body all the way down to the cellular level; and the deepest fascia lies within the dura of the cranial-sacral system.

Fascia at the cellular level creates the interstitial spaces and has extremely important functions of support, protection, separation, cellular respiration, nutrition, elimination, metabolism, and fluid and lymphatic flow. In other words, it is the immediate environment of every cell of the body. This means that any trauma or malfunction of the fascia can set up the environment for poor cellular efficiency, necrosis, disease, pain, and dysfunction throughout the body.

Other important aspects of fascia are:

- It supports and stabilizes, thus enhancing, the postural balance of the body.
- It is vitally involved in all aspects of motion and acts as a shock absorber.
- It aids in circulatory economy, especially in venous and lymphatic fluids.
- Fascial change will often precede chronic tissue congestion.
- Such chronic passive congestion creates the formation of fibrous tissue, which then proceeds to increase hydrogen ion concentration of articular and periarticular structures.
- It is a major area of inflammatory processes.
- Fluid and infectious processes often travel along fascial planes.

The central nervous system is surrounded by fascial tissue (dura mater) that attaches to the inside of the cranium, the foramen magnum, and at the second sacral segment. Dysfunction in these tissues can have profound and widespread neurological effects. *Myofascial Pain and Dysfunction* by Dr. Janet Travell, beautifully illustrates the myofascial element: every muscle of the body is surrounded by a smooth fascial sheath, every muscular fascicule is surrounded by fascia, every fibril is surrounded by fascia, and every microfibril down to the cellular level is surrounded by fascia that can exert pressures of over 2000 pounds per square inch. Therefore, it is the fascia that can ultimately determine the length and function of its muscular component.

We must be clear that medicine, modalities, muscle energy techniques, mobilization and manipulation, massage, and flexibility and exercise programs do not alter the powerful fascial restrictions that occur in a high percentage of our patients. These restrictions are only altered via Myofascial Release.

Myofascial Release is a whole-body hands-on approach to the evaluation and treatment of the human structure. The therapist is taught to evaluate the fascial system through visual analysis of the human frame three-dimensionally in space, by palpating the tissue texture and various fascial layers, and by observing the symmetry, rate, quality, and intensity of strength of the craniosacral rhythm. Proper Myofascial Release requires ongoing reevaluation, including the above procedures and observance of vasomotor responses and their location as they occur after a particular fascial restriction has been released. This provides instantaneous and very accurate information that enables the therapist to proceed intelligently and logically from one treatment session to the next, to the ultimate resolution of the patient's dysfunction (figure 16.6).

When the therapist has determined where the fascial restrictions lie, he will apply gentle pressure into the direction of the restriction. At first, the elastic component of the fascia will release, and at some point, the collagenous barrier will be engaged. This barrier cannot be forced (it is too strong). The therapist waits with gentle but firm pressure, and as the collagenous aspect releases, he then follows the motion of the tissue, barrier upon barrier, until freedom is felt.

The development of the practitioner's tactile and proprioceptive senses enhances the "feel" necessary for the successful completion of these techniques. We were all born with this ability to feel the releases and the direction in which the tissue seems to move from barrier to barrier. When we first learn Myofascial Release, we can perform these

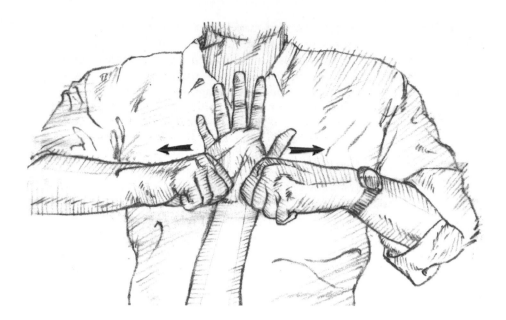

Figure 16.6
Therapist performing
Myofascial Release.

effective techniques mechanically, and with a little practice, we can discover the "feel" and move to a higher level of achievement.

Each time we experience a trauma, undergo an inflammatory process, or suffer from poor postures over time, the fascial system becomes restricted. These restrictions act like the concentric layers of an onion. These adaptive layers slowly tighten until we begin to lose our physiological adaptive capacity (our margin of error). We slowly tighten, losing our flexibility and spontaneity of motion, which sets us up for trauma, pain, or restriction of motion. These powerful restrictions begin to pull us out of our three-dimensional orientation with gravity. The goal of Myofascial Release is to help return the individual's physiological adaptive capacity by increasing space and mobility, restoring three-dimensional balance, and returning the structure to as close as potentially possible to its vertical orientation with gravity. This equilibrium allows the individual's self-correcting mechanisms to come into play and alleviate symptoms and restore proper function.

The Myofascial Release Approach, when combined with the valuable skills we now possess, acts as a facilitator and intensifier of treatment for more consistent effectiveness and lasting results for our clients. This is a total approach incorporating a physiological system that, when included with traditional massage therapy or bodywork, acts as a catalyst, yielding impressive, clinically reproducible results.

The Function of Fascia

The fascia serves a major purpose in that it permits the body to retain its normal shape and thus maintain the vital organs in their correct positions. It also allows the body to resist mechanical stresses, both internally and externally. Fascia has maintained its general structures and purposes over the millennia. These functions are evident in the earliest stages of multicelled organisms, in which two or more cells were able to stay in contact, communicate, and resist the forces of the environment through the connective tissue.

Fascia covers the muscles, bones, nerves, organs, and vessels down to the cellular level (figure 16.7). Therefore, malfunction of the system due to trauma, poor posture, or inflammation can bind down the fascia, resulting in abnormal pressure on any or all of these body components. It is through that process that this binding down, or restriction, may result in many of the poor or temporary results achieved by conventional medical, dental, and therapeutic treatments.

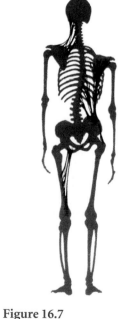

Figure 16.7
The fascial skelton

As Travell has explained, restrictions of the fascia can create pain or malfunction throughout the body, sometimes with bizarre side effects and seemingly unrelated symptoms that do not always follow dermatome zones. It is thought that an extremely high percentage of people suffering with pain, loss of motion, or both, may have fascial restriction problems. Most of these conditions go undiagnosed, however, as many of the standard tests, such as radiographs, myelograms, computerized tomographic scans, and electromyograms, do not show the fascia. If we can't see it, we can't look for restriction with our eyes.

The therapist or physician is taught to find the cause of symptoms by evaluation of the fascial system by visually analyzing the human frame, palpating the tissue texture of the various fascial layers, and observing the symmetry, rate, quality, and intensity of the craniosacral rhythm. The technique requires continuous reevaluation, including observance of vasomotor responses and their location as they occur after a particular restriction has been released. This provides instantaneous and accurate information, enabling the therapist or physician to proceed intelligently and logically from one treatment session to the next, to the ultimate resolution of the patient's pain and dysfunction.

When the location of the fascial restriction is determined, gentle pressure is applied in its direction. This has the effect of pulling the elastocollagenous fibers straight. When pressure is first applied to the elastocollagenous complex, the elastic component is engaged. This has a springy feel. The elastic component is slowly stretched until the hands stop at a firm barrier. This is the collagenous component. This barrier cannot be forced; it is too strong. Instead, gentle sustained pressure will release it.

This fact has to do with viscous flow phenomenon, that is, a low load (gentle pressure) applied slowly will allow a viscous medium to flow to a greater extent than a high load (quickly applied pressure). The viscosity of the ground substance has an effect on the collagen, since it is believed that the viscous medium that makes up the ground substance controls the ease with which collagen fibers rearrange themselves. Viscoelasticity "causes it to resist a suddenly applied force but results in gradual elongation to a constantly applied force over time. Creep is the progressive deformation of soft tissue due to constant low loading over time. Hysteresis is the property whereby the work done in deforming a material causes heat and hence energy loss." The therapist or physician follows the motion of the tissue, barrier to barrier, until freedom from restriction is felt.

The Arndt-Schultz law also explains how the gentle, sustained pressures of Myofascial Release can produce such consistent changes and improvement. The law states that "weak stimuli increases physiologic activity and very strong stimuli inhibit or abolish activity."

The biomechanical, bioelectrical and neurophysiological effects of Myofascial Release represent an evolutionary leap for our professions and our patients. This is a total approach incorporating a physiologic system that, when included with traditional therapy, medicine, or dentistry, acts as a catalyst and yields impressive, clinically reproducible results.

Touching patients with skilled hands, however, can be one of the most potent ways of locating fascial restrictions and effecting positive change. Touching patients through mobilization, massage, and various forms of exercise and movement therapy, coupled with the gentle, refined touch of Myofascial Release and the sophisticated movement therapy called myofascial unwinding, creates a sensorimotor interplay. This experience of contact and movement is the very experience we need to reprogram our biocomputer, the mind-body, the basis for learning any new skill. Those practicing Myofascial Release use the skin and fascia as a handle or lever to created new options for enhanced function and movement of every structure of the body. Myofascial Release helps remove the straightjacket of pressure caused by restricted fascia, eliminating symptoms such as stiffness, pain, and spasm. Then, through its influence of the neuromuscular and skeletal systems, it creates the opportunity for patients to "learn" new enhanced movement patterns.

Myofascial Unwinding: Tissue Memory

Mind and body act together, immutably joined, inseparable, connected, influencing, and intercommunicating constantly. Myofascial Release techniques and the sophisticated movement therapy called myofascial unwinding seem to allow for the complete communication of mind with body and body with mind, which is necessary for healing (see chapter 17). I believe that the body remembers everything that ever happened to it. Mind-body awareness and healing are often linked to the concept of "state-dependent" memory, learning, and behavior, also called déjà vu. We have all experienced this, for example, when a certain smell or sound of a particular piece of music creates a flashback phenomenon, producing a visual, sensorimotor replay of a past event or an important episode in our lives with such vividness that it is as if it were happening at that moment.

My experience has shown that during periods of trauma, people form subconscious, indelible imprints of the experience that have high levels of emotional content. The body can hold information below the conscious level, as a protective mechanism, so that memories tend to become dissociated or amnesiac. This is called memory dissociation or reversible amnesia. The memories are state- (or position-) dependent and can therefore be retrieved when the person is in a particular state (or position). This information is not available in the normal conscious state, and the body's protective mechanisms keep us away from the positions that our mind-body awareness construes as painful or traumatic. It has been demonstrated consistently that when a Myofascial Release technique takes the tissue to a significant position or when myofascial unwinding allows a body part to assume a significant position three-dimensionally in space, the tissue not only changes and improves, but memories, associated emotional states, and belief systems also rise to the conscious level. This awareness, through the positional reproduction of a past event or trauma, allows the individual to grasp hidden information that may be creating or maintaining symptoms or behavior that deters improvement. With the repressed and stored information now at conscious level, the individual is in a position to learn which holding or bracing patterns have been impeding progress and why. The release of the tissue with its stored emotions and hidden information creates an environment for change.

Technique Required for Facilitation of a Release

Myofascial Release and myofascial unwinding free the fascial tissue restrictions, thereby altering the habitual muscular response and allowing the positional, reversible amnesia to surface, producing emotions and beliefs that are the cause of the holding patterns and ultimate symptoms. To allow this spontaneous motion to proceed without interference, it is important for the therapist to quiet her mind and feel the subtle inherent motions in the patient. Quietly following the tissue (Myofascial Release) or body part (myofascial unwinding) three-dimensionally along the direction of ease, the therapist guides the patient's movement into the significant restrictions or positions. With myofascial unwinding, the therapist eliminates gravity from the system, unloading the structure to allow the body's gravity-oriented righting reflexes and protective responses to temporarily suspend their influence. The body is then free to move into positions that allow repressed state- or position-dependent physiological or flashback phenomena to recur. As this happens within the safe environment of a treatment session, the patient can facilitate the body's own inherent self-correcting mechanism to obtain improvement.

Myofascial Release and myofascial unwinding bring the tissue or support the body part into a position eliminating gravity as the patient moves spontaneously. This allows the individual to be more fully aware of her divided consciousness. Reactivating the original conditions and the resultant physiological responses by influencing the fascia to release results in a flashback phenomenon, brings the repressed memory to conscious awareness and then allows the patient to have the choice to change. No longer do patients habitually find themselves holding or stiffening to protect themselves from future pain trauma. Genuine release of fear and emotion takes place simultaneously with physical fascial release and physiological release of the associated hormones. As a result of observing the outcomes of many patients who have benefited from Myofascial Release and unwinding, I have concluded that Myofascial Release is more than just an assemblage of techniques. Instead, it helps create a whole-body awareness, allowing the health professional to facilitate more than just structural change but also growth and the possibility for a more total resolution of restrictions, emotions, and cognition. Thus, this treatment is holistic in nature and complements traditional therapy based on reductionism.

Therapists of the near future will function quite differently from those of the past. Building on and respecting the foundation developed by various health professions, they will treat the whole person intellectually, emotionally, and structurally. They will have a wide variety of techniques with which to help others, thanks to continuing advances in scientific technology. With highly developed sensitivity and creativity, they will be able to interact with the patient intelligently and humanely, on an individual level and as part of an interdisciplinary team.

The therapist skilled in Myofascial Release is concerned with releasing and reorganizing the body's fascial restrictions mechanically and reorganizing the neuromuscular system. The reorganization occurs by supplying the central nervous system with new information (awareness) that allows for change and improved potential and consciousness.

It is important for those providing treatment to realize that the body is a repository of information. The body can be used as a biofeedback system for the master therapist's finely trained, sensitive hands. It can then be used as a handle or lever to provide access to emotions and belief systems and allow for structural and biomechanical change.

Mastery means achieving not only a certain level of skill but also an attitude. Masters are fully aware of what they are doing. They understand the importance of touch as an expression of acceptance, nourishment, and a form of biofeedback to glean information from clients' mind-body awareness. Their touch should be applied with focused awareness and conscious purpose. The focus should be fluid, moving from tight, narrow (logical, analytical thought) to open—feeling everything at once without thought or effort (intuition, insight).

Tell your clients not to view the cause of their dysfunction as a defeat but rather to see it as a lesson. By looking for the positive, they can see its value, learn from it, and allow themselves to heal. Help them to understand that one of the best lessons is that they may not be able to change the circumstances of their life, but they can change their reaction to their circumstance; they can move from being passive, helpless recipients to active participants. This important change in perspective creates a partnership between you and your patients where you can help them help themselves.

Thus, mastery is teaching through example. The master therapist is real, calm, nonjudgmental, intelligent, sensitive, strong yet flexible, supportive, compassionate, empathetic, and joyful.

Bindegeweb-massage	Connective Tissue Massage, or *Bindegewebmassage,* was developed by Elizabeth Dicke in Germany. It also functions to relieve myofascial restrictions in the fascia using light pressure or strokes without lubricant. Strokes are long and finished with a "hook" or comma shape.

Trager By Deane Juhan, MA	Trager psychophysical integration was the discovery of Milton Trager, MD. He first encountered its simple principles and surprising effects intuitively, and almost accidentally, at the age of 18. He spent the next 50 years, first as a lay practitioner and later as a

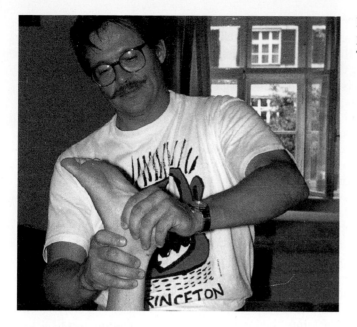

Figure 16.8
Deane Juhan performing
Trager.

medical professional, expanding and refining his discovery. This long, successful career as a therapist was behind him before he tried to teach anyone his innovative form of bodywork, so that in spite of its almost silent incubation and development, Dr. Trager's work reached his first students at a very ripe stage, with a wide variety of demonstrably successful applications.

Dr. Trager's manner of manipulating the body is not a technique or a method, in the sense that there are no rigid procedures that are claimed to produce specific symptomatic results (figure 16.8). There is no formula, no recipe, no standardized practical procedure. Rather, it is an *approach,* a way of learning and of teaching movement reeducation. He stresses that his patients should come to him ready to absorb a lesson, instead of ready to simply receive a treatment. His concern is not with moving particular muscles or joints per se but with using motion in muscles and joints to produce particular sensory feelings—positive, pleasurable feelings that enter the central nervous system and begin to trigger tissue changes by means of the many sensory-motor feedback loops between the mind and the muscles.

Trager practitioners do not change the condition of tissue with their hands but use the hands to communicate a quality of feeling to the nervous system, and this feeling then elicits tissue response within the client. When a body feels lighter, it begins to stand and to move as though it were lighter.

Elements of a Trager Session

A Trager session takes from one to one and a half hours. No oils or lotions are used. The client wears swim trunks, briefs, or bathing suit and lies on a well-padded table in a warm, comfortable environment. During the session, the practitioner makes touch-contact with the body of the client—both as a whole and in its individual parts—in such a gentle and rhythmic way that the person lying passively on the table actually experiences the possibility of being able to move each part of the body freely, effortlessly, and gracefully on her own. The practitioner works in a relaxed, meditative state of consciousness that Dr. Trager calls "Hook-up." The state allows the practitioner to connect deeply with the recipient in an unforced way, to remain continually aware of the slightest responses, and to work efficiently without fatigue.

After getting up from the table, the client is given some instruction in the use of MENTASTICS®, a system of simple, effortless movement sequences developed by Dr. Trager to maintain and even enhance the sense of lightness, freedom, and flexibility that was instilled by the table work. MENTASTICS is Dr. Trager's coinage for "mental gymnastics"—a "mindfulness in motion"—designed to help his clients recreate for themselves the sensory feelings produced by the motion of their tissue in the practitioner's hands. It is a powerful means of teaching the client to recall the pleasurable sensory state that produced positive tissue change, and because it is this feeling state that triggered positive tissue response in the first place, every time the feeling is clearly recalled, the changes deepen and become more permanent and more receptive to further positive change.

It is evident, based on most recipients' experiences, that the effects of a Trager session penetrate below the level of conscious awareness and continue to produce positive results long after the session itself. Changes described have included the disappearance of specific symptoms, discomforts, or pains; heightened levels of energy and vitality; more effortless posture and carriage; greater joint mobility; deeper states of relaxation than were previously possible; and a new ease in daily activities. "When a body feels lighter, it begins to stand and to move as though it were lighter"—Milton Trager.

Unlike many movement reeducation approaches, in Trager, the client has no task to perform but rather becomes increasingly passive to the steady, rhythmic motions imparted by the practitioner's hands. But perhaps what most distinguishes Trager from other disciplines is the particular focus and intent of the practitioner's manipulations. Most other methods direct their attention to one or another of the body's tissues—the skin, the fascia, the muscles, the joints, the lymph and blood circulation, overall structural relationships, and so on—and the various properties of these tissues determine the sort of touch and manipulation required by the practitioner.

Trager seeks to specifically influence the feeling states in the sensory and the unconscious elements of the mind, which most directly control tissue response, metabolism, postural habits, and behavioral patterns. Of course, as with all other kinds of bodywork, the goal of the practitioner determines the manner in which he works: in seeking to produce particular kinds of feeling, the Trager practitioner can contact the tissues only in ways that will actually stimulate those specific sensory and emotional responses. In an hour-long Trager session, there are several thousand light, rhythmic contacts, and each one of them is an opportunity to create and deepen the feelings of lightness, freedom, relaxation, ease, and peace. When the practitioner encounters stiffened limbs or hardened muscles, his response is never to bear down on them, to work harder to soften them, or force them to stretch. On the contrary, his response is immediately to become lighter, more sensitive, more searching. The practitioner never asserts his idea of how soft or free an area should be; he deliberately retreats from such assertions and instead projects through the motions of his hands the questions, "What can be lighter and freer than that? Yes. And lighter than that? Fine. And freer than that?" And so on.

Trager avoids undue pressure and effort so that the manner of working will be wholly consistent with its goal of creating sensations of lightness, freedom, and ease. In the first place heavy pressure on spasmed muscles or forced stretching of stiffened joints normally causes a painful response; the involved area is usually hypersensitive in the first place and is already braced against painful motions. This generation of pain is precisely the opposite sensory effect of the desired response, and it seriously interrupts the repetitive rhythmic flow of pleasurable sensations to the mind. More than that, pain inevitably triggers reflex contractions, and this merely produces another defensive pattern rather than dispersing the ones that are already there. Second, the feelings of lightness and effortlessness simply cannot be imparted by means of heavy pressure and hard work on the part of the practitioner.

Dr. Trager holds that the moment the practitioner *tries* to relax the tissue, he is doomed to failure. Trying is effort, effort is tension, and relaxation is quite the opposite. The practitioner's touch, then, must be as light as the feelings he wishes to instill. The point is not to impose a preconceived structural or functional model on the client's body but to transmit a pleasurable and continual questioning, "What is freer, what is lighter?" The point is not to arrive finally at a specific goal—after all, we don't know what "freest" or "best" might be—but to instill in the mind of the client the constant renewal of the question, "What is better, and what is better?" This is not the imposition of a postural or behavioral model but rather the initiation of an open-ended developmental process, both for the client and the practitioner.

This developmental process is of primary importance to the Trager practitioner. These questionings and these feelings have to be established in his character, have to be part of his mind and body, before he can successfully project them into another person's sensibilities. No one can give what they do not genuinely have. This is why the cultivation by the practitioner of the mental state Dr. Trager calls "Hook-up"—a relaxed, meditative alertness—is crucial to effective Trager. The state of "Hook-up" is not fundamentally different from a state of deep meditation, even though the practitioner in "Hook-up" is physically active. Achieving this state of active meditation is not an incidental addition to Dr. Trager's work: it is of the essence. "Hook-up" is the practitioner's source of the enriched and relaxed feelings that he projects, his own contact with the qualities of gracefulness, effortlessness, and nonintrusive presence. "It is," Dr. Trager says, "like floating in a vast ocean of pleasantness," and it is the gentle rocking of that ocean that is imparted to the client's body. Dr. Trager maintains that the attributes of mind and body are holistically interrelated in the whole energetic force field that composes all matter and life:

> We are surrounded by a force which sustains everything. You don't have to go beyond the surface of your skin to get it. But people are blocked within themselves, so negative, so tense, that this force cannot enter their consciousness. Once this force comes into them, they are changed people and will function differently and much better than they have ever done before.

It is the conscious contact with this force, this ocean of pleasantness, that gives the practitioner the pleasurable feelings they project through their motions into the sensations of the client, and as the client's consciousness is opened to these feelings, it is this force that it becomes the active source of vitality and health.

The principle is elegantly simple: We learn to love by being loved, we learn gentleness by being gentled, we learn to be graceful by experiencing the feeling of grace. The goal of a Trager session is no more complex than this—to bring to the surface of consciousness an awareness of this force and the pleasurable and positive feelings that are inherent in it. These feelings will do the rest. As the Maharishi Mahesh Yogi said to Dr. Trager in 1958, "It is natural for the mind to want to go to the field of greater happiness," toward deeper understanding, toward expansiveness, toward connecting with the sources of our being. Trager was developed as a sensory means of redirecting the footsteps of someone who has lost the way.

Application of the Trager Approach

The appeal of the Trager approach is broad. Many kinds of people have been attracted to the work, all of them searching for more effective ways of producing more immediate and more lasting results in psychophysical and neuromuscular conditions. Classes have drawn students from such disciplines as holistic health care, psychology, counseling, medicine, nursing, physical therapy, massage, sports, and performing arts, among others that regard movement as a primary means of learning and an integral part of exercise.

Ever since his early success with paralysis, Dr. Trager's particular interest has been the application of his approach to severe neuromuscular disturbances that do not respond well to conventional approaches. However, both he and the practitioners he has trained achieve excellent results with a wide range of conditions that are more common and less overwhelmingly debilitating—the aches, pains, depressions, poor postures, limited movements, and aging processes that plague many daily lives to one degree or another. Most of these troublesome and inhibiting conditions do not respond any better to drugs and surgery than do many kinds of paralysis and spasm, but they often prove to be very responsive to the soothing sensory intervention of Trager.

Since birth, we have had in our day-to-day lives many good and bad experiences that have shaped us physically and psychologically. Every individual carries within herself an exceedingly intricate computer system, a recorder that has no erase button. Whatever experiences have been put there will always be there, influencing every function of the mind and body. Since it is not possible to avoid a variety of traumas, and since none may be erased once they have occurred, help should be directed toward bringing appropriate positive feeling experiences to the client. These help directly to influence the mind and body, so that the physical patterns can be alleviated. We are all familiar with the degenerative effects that negative feelings and attitudes can have on the body, but it is possible to turn this potent force of feelings to a constructive purpose as well.

The sensory and emotional feelings associated with healthy response to stimulation may be blocked by social or psychological difficulties as well as by disease or trauma. Because this is true, Trager has produced dramatic instances of success in helping psychological and behavioral pathologies as well as physical pathologies. These kinds of behavioral changes can be elicited in many varieties of psychological and physical conditions.

Dr. Trager contends very firmly that he is not a "healer" or a manipulator of esoteric energies and that his successes have nothing of the miraculous about them. The kinds of reflex responses, tissue changes, and behavioral changes he is able to elicit are possible because of the intimate neurological associations between sensory stimulations, emotional feelings, attitudes and concepts, and the body's motor responses to all of them. At this time, no one can say with certainty just exactly how these sensations, feelings, and actions are materially interrelated, but the fact that they profoundly influence one another is abundantly clear. And it is equally clear that the unconscious forces that control their relationships may be turned back from a vicious circle into a fruitful one.

Dr. Peter Levine, a neurophysiologist, took one of Dr. Trager's early trainings and discussed possible mechanisms of psychophysical integration with him. Dr. Trager told him that he felt it had a sound scientific basis but that it was difficult to explain it and have it accepted. Dr. Levine's response was, "If an accepted scientific theory cannot explain a particular phenomenon, it is not because the phenomenon is unscientific, but because science itself is not appropriately refined." Dr. Trager's is a subtle and intuitive approach to the elusive and complex problem of the physiological manifestation of psychological distress, and all degrees of this distress and its manifestations have the positive potential for improvement as long as the nerve circuits themselves are not destroyed by disease or trauma.

Trager work is not in itself a medical treatment. It is actually a learning experience. You are learning how your body can move. You are learning what it is like to be freer and lighter. It is really a learning approach to using yourself well, to being a whole person—to having all your pieces and parts well integrated and coordinated, to feeling yourself connected to the energies that sustain you.

All of it is directed toward the mind. In the final analysis, people do not respond to a technique or procedure; they respond to the skill with which it is used. Any technique may be applied with little or no connection to the actual awareness of the client and with poor results. What constitutes skill for Dr. Trager is, more than anything else, the ability to be there with the client, to be "Hooked-up," open to the client's needs, intimately aware of responses, intimately responsive to response. It is this connection that Dr. Trager strives above all to impart to his clients and to teach to his students. And it is this feeling of calm, peaceful connectedness that is, indeed, the essence of Trager work.

"Not until we experience it is it more than just words," Dr. Trager tells his students. "After we experience it, there is no need for words. The importance of words is to stimulate the desire to experience. Feeling is experience, and by this experience, we develop."

Named for its creator, F. M. Alexander, the **Alexander Technique** uses gentle touch along with awareness of movement to teach people to recognize habitual movements, such as poor posture, and correct them. Alexander Technique is actually more of an educational process to help people recognize how and why they move or how and why any given activity is performed, rather than a modality that seeks to correct imbalances. The role of the practitioner is more one of a teacher who assesses and then offers guidance based on that assessment.

Alexander Technique

Moshe Feldenkrais broadened his work from martial arts training and an educational background in engineering to develop an approach to the body that he termed "functional integration." Clients are guided through a series of movements that establish a new pattern of movement that the body then recognizes as the correct way to move. Thus, "awareness of movement" replaces formerly learned deterimental habits, with new beneficial ones thereby increasing flexibility and range of motion.

Feldenkrais

The lymphatic system is still a very mysterious system. It wasn't until the 17th century that medical science even recognized the presence of lymphatic vessels in the body. (Aselli, 1627).

The physiology and physiopathology of the lymphatic system slowly unraveled by group of scientists interested in the knowledge of the unusual system. Within the medical communities as well as the field of bodywork, there is unfortunately a significant lack of education about this important component of the body.

The proper functioning of the lymphatic system is critical to our body's ability to drain stagnant fluids, detoxify, regenerate tissues, filter out toxins and foreign substances, and maintain a healthy immune system.

Lymphatic Drainage Therapy (LDT)

By Bruno Chikly, MD, DO (Hon.)

The Importance of Lymph Drainage for Health

The lymphatic system is a complex system comprised primarily of lymph vessels and nodes working in cooperation to accomplish the tasks.

> ⭐ **EXAM POINT** Unlike the circulatory system—which uses the pumping of the heart to circulate its blood flow—lymph vessels rely on hundreds of tiny muscular units (lymphangions) contracting throughout the body to propel lymph flow.

These contractions enable the lymph vessels to transport numerous substances (proteins, toxins, hormones, fatty acids, immune cells) to lymph nodes, which can then process them (figure 16.9). The action of these muscular units can be hindered or stopped, however, due to surgery, trauma, burns, infections, substantial swelling, fatigue, stress, or age. When the lymph circulation stagnates, fluids, proteins, cells, and toxins accumulate, and cellular functioning is significantly compromised. This may open the way to many physical ailments and hasten the aging process.

Lymphatic Drainage Therapy (LDT) is a gentle and non-invasive hands-on technique designed to attain and sustain proper functioning of the human fluid system.

> ⭐ **EXAM POINT** Its origins can be traced to two traditions in particular: the published research of Frederic Millard, a Canadian osteopathic physician (1922), and Emil Vodder, a Danish massage practitioner and doctor of philosophy (1932).

Figure 16.9
Developer Bruno Chikly performing Lymphatic Drainage Therapy.

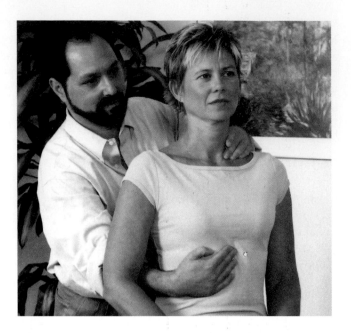

Over the years, methods based on the discoveries of these pioneers have been honed, refined, and expanded. Today, lymphatic drainage therapy are employed as standard scientific practice throughout Europe and continue to gain recognition in the United States—both from healthcare providers and national insurers such as Medicare.

Taking the Techniques to a New Level

Lymph Drainage Therapy (LDT) is a hands-on method of lymphatic drainage developed by Dr. Bruno Chikly, MD, DO (hon.). Created out of his award-winning research on the lymphatic system, LDT takes traditional lymph drainage techniques and adds a new level of precision in keeping with the latest scientific discoveries and exact anatomical science.

LDT is the first technique to teach practitioners how to detect the specific rhythm, direction, depth, and quality of the lymphatic flow. As a result, therapists can achieve profound, more precise outcomes in shorter periods of time. For clients, the process is very pleasurable and induces deep states of relaxation.

How LDT Is Performed

The LDT process involves the use of gentle manual maneuvers to aid in the recirculation of body fluids. While the exact amount of pressure applied depends on the area and pathology involved, it averages an extremely light 5 grams—or the equivalent weight of a nickel.

Using this technique, trained therapists are able to detect the specific rhythm, direction, depth, and quality of the lymph flow anywhere in the body. From there, they can use their hands to perform Manual Lymphatic Mapping (MLM) of the vessels to assess the overall direction of lymphatic circulation, areas of stagnation, and the best alternate pathways for draining lymph and other body fluids.

Benefits of LDT

Due to the nature and role of the lymphatic system, LDT can prove beneficial in the correction of numerous conditions as well as in preventive health maintenance. This is why you'll find a wide range of practitioners using LDT. Among them are medical doctors, osteopathic physicians, doctors of chiropractic, physical therapists, occupational therapists, naturopaths, nurses, lymphedema specialists, dentists, massage therapists, and other bodyworkers. It is reimbursed by numerous insurance companies in North America for its efficiency with edema (Lymphedema) and is increasingly taught in manual therapy schools.

In essence, Lymph Drainage Therapy works to help recirculate body fluids, stimulate functioning of the immune system, and promote a state of relaxation and balance within the autonomic nervous system. It is shown that when these actions are accomplished, the results may be:

- Reduction in edemas (swelling) and lymphedemas of many origins
- Detoxification of the body
- Regeneration of tissues (e.g., from burns and pre- and postsurgical scarring) and antiaging effects
- Relief of chronic inflammation and conditions such as acne, eczema, and allergies
- Immune system stimulation for preventive and therapeutic effects
- Reduction in the symptoms of chronic fatigue syndrome and fibromyalgia
- Relief of chronic pain
- Deep relaxation to aid insomnia, depression, stress, loss of vitality, and loss of memory
- Antispastic actions to relieve conditions such as voluntary or involuntary muscle hypertonus
- Alleviation of adiposis and cellulite tissue

The Difference between LDT and Vodder's Work

Emil Vodder was a very inspired man who made remarkable discoveries. LDT is based on and follows the natural progression of Vodder's work, using scientific discoveries and improvements in bodywork techniques and osteopathy to take his findings a step further. In particular, LDT specifically attunes to areas and or works with applications that other schools usually do not, including:

- The specific rhythm of the lymph flow, consistent with the discoveries of W. Olszewski (see Quick Guide B, page B-1.)
- The specific direction of the lymph and interstitial fluid flow in the superficial and deep tissue layers
- The specific pressure and depth (helps specify the level of treatment: superficial tissue, deep layer, subcutaneous tissue, mucosa, muscles, viscera, periosteum, organ of the senses, etc.)
- The quality of the lymph and interstitial fluid flow ("potency")
- The specific drainage of the muscles, bones, periosteum, and articulations (articulations release)
- The abdominal and thoracic viscera, including the liver, spleen, uterus, large and small intestines, prostate, lungs, pleura, kidneys, adrenal glands, pericardium, etc.
- Manual Lymphatic Mapping to assess the specific direction of the superficial and deep lymph and interstitial fluids in physiological and pathological conditions
- Fibrotic techniques: 15 different techniques to apply on the collagen fibers/fascia before applying the lymphatic strokes (used for lymphedema, postsurgery, postradiation, etc.)
- Applications for fascia restrictions (Lymphofascia Release)/Connective Tissue Fibers Release (CTFR)
- Applications for chronic scars: Scar Release Therapy
- Clinical connection between deep breathing and the lymph flow
- Working with three different lymphatic rhythms
- Working with other fluids, including the interstitial fluid, synovial fluid, cerebrospinal fluid, and blood (veins and arteries)
- Specific maneuvers to access the cisterna chyli
- Drainage of the central nervous system, including drainage of the pia and dura maters
- Drainage of the sciatic nerves and other peripheral nerves
- Applications for trigger points, Chapman reflexes, and acupressure points
- Extensive breast protocol (lymphatic breast care)

- Drainage of the chambers of the eyes
- Drainage of the ears, including the cochlea and the semicircular canals
- Drainage of the nasal cavity
- Drainage of the oral cavity, including tonsils and eustachian tubes, temporomandibular joint (TMJ), gums, and teeth
- Drainage of the synovial fluid; applications for body joints/articulations, including the spine, rib cage, skull, and cranial sutures as well as the upper and lower extremities
- Full-body fluid diagnosis

Manual Lymphatic Mapping (MLM) and Its Clinical Application

Manual Lymphatic Mapping (MLM) represents one of the most recent advances in lymph drainage techniques. A noninvasive process, it enables trained practitioners to manually assess the specific direction of lymphatic circulation, and then use that information to determine the most efficient alternate pathways for draining areas of fluid stagnation.

For example, in a case of postmastectomy lymphedema presenting in the upper extremity, the obstructed lymph flow must reroute to an unaffected lymph territory (lymphotome). There are some 20 anterior and posterior alternate pathways from which it may choose to accomplish this task, including the axilla, inguinals, clavicles, intercostals, Mascagni's pathways, and vasa vasorum. It may be difficult for a practitioner to determine which pathway the lymph flow will take. Making a wrong assumption can cause a significant loss of time and resources. Using Manual Lymphatic Mapping, the therapist can find the specific alternate pathway preferred by the lymph.

Manual assessment of the lymphatic rhythm and direction requires time and dedication to learning this modality. It is recommended that therapists new to the method first develop their skills for assessing the rhythm of the lymphatic flow. With training and practice, most therapists are able to attain the sensitivity required to evaluate the rhythm, and determine the specific direction of lymphatic flow.

While the scientific means for measuring the accuracy of client mapping are not yet available at the time of this book's publication, investigations are currently underway using protocols to help measure and document the efficacy of this technique (lymphangioscintigraphy).

In LDT, we use our hands to aid nature in her work. LDT can be applied to a wide range of ailments. There is almost no limit to the number of indications already discovered. This technique is usually extremely light and non-invasive as well as highly effective.

Bodyworkers enjoy the amazing effects of fluids running unimpaired throughout the body, affecting multiple aspects of the organism, from the circulatory and detoxification mechanisms, the immune system to the autonomic nervous system.

I tell my students that LDT is so gentle that if they respect the few contraindications of this work they can feel assured that they can safely use this techniques for most all of the clinical conditions they encounter. LDT will simultaneously release so many body systems, they will be continually surprised as I am by amazing results.

Cerebrospinal Fluid Technique Massage

By Donald J. Glassey MSW, DC, LMT, NCTMB

The Cerebrospinal Fluid Technique Massage (CSFTM) procedure incorporates cutting-edge science with the philosophical principles underlying massage as a healing art. Historically, it is well-documented that the philosophical foundations of massage are vitalistic (see chapter 1).

Philosophy and Science

The basic principle of vitalism states that there is an inherent or inborn intelligence that animates, motivates, heals, coordinates, and inspires living beings. (Since the body is organized in such a varied and complex manner, it must be "intelligent.") Vitalism assumes that life is self-determining and self-evolving. Healing is seen as a process of personal evolution, growth, self-development, and self-discovery. Growth and development need mutual support, and that support is a feeling state, an emotion.

Feelings are just information (just as touch is information) that needs to be listened to and not "manipulated." When the feeling state is experienced, the body can make a physiological shift. For example, a "gut feeling" is a visceral response to one's external environment. The feeling state then is a response to internal and external life conditions, which are recorded when information is received by the nervous, muscular, and other systems. The memory of the information is related to the feeling at that time, and a biochemical condition correlates to the healing experience.

According to Ida Rolf (Structural Integration, or Rolfing), Dr. Janet Travell (Trigger Point Therapy), John Barnes (Myofascial Release), Dr. John Upledger (CranoSacral Therapy), and others, muscular patterns are formed in psychological arrangements. The chemical of emotion intersects with the muscular patterns, and muscles respond to psychological states. Feelings and motor patterns develop together where the feelings are "fluid"-born chemicals whose emotional chemistry and muscular behavior are linked.

The clinical objective of **Cerebrospinal Fluid Technique Massage (CSFTM)** is to free up the flow of cerebrospinal fluid (CSF) around the cerebrospinal axis comprised of the brain and spinal cord.

What is cerebrospinal fluid, where is it found, and why is it so important? Cerebrospinal fluid comprises a continuous fluid system whose circulation is very important to the functioning of the brain itself. Far more than a "shock absorber" cushion of protection for the brain and spinal cord, CSF is essential to the proper functioning of the central nervous system. Cerebrospinal fluid bathes the neurons (nerve cells) and glial cells (connective tissue) of the brain and spinal cord, carrying nutrients to and removing metabolic wastes and toxic substances from the central nervous system.

CSF also has a major influence on the body's homeostatic pH balance of acidity-alkalinity. Recent research also suggests that CSF may be the primary factor that produces the electromagnetic environment of neurons and other cells of the central nervous system. Further current scientific research indicates that CSF acts as a chelating (binding) agent, removing metallic toxins from the brain and spinal cord, and providing protection against free-radical, cell-damaging oxidation and the accumulation of nonmetallic toxins.

Physiologists currently state that carbon dioxide levels in CSF have a more direct influence on chemoreceptor respiratory mechanisms in the brainstem than do carbon dioxide levels in the blood. Thus, carbon dioxide levels in CSF have a major influence on the critical acid-base balance of body homeostasis, which is partly regulated by carbon dioxide. In addition, electrolytes (sodium and potassium) present in CSF have a great influence on the body's electromagnetic environment, allowing the central nervous system to work by the conduction of electricity. (Electrolytes are substances that when dissolved in water can conduct electricity.)

These two mechanisms involving carbon dioxide levels and electrolyte elements are severely impaired by impeded CSF circulation.

Approximately 500 milliliters (about 1 pint) of CSF are formed per day from cavities in very center of the brain called the lateral ventricles. Spongy masses of specialized cells in the ventricles called the choroid plexus, as well as the ependyma (membranes) that line the ventricles, weep CSF from the blood. According to Dr. Chikly, the leading expert in the lymphatic system, up to 60% of circulating CSF is exchanged from lymph fluid and about 40% from the choroid plexus. This is enough to completely replace the entire volume of CSF three to five times daily.

CSF formed in the lateral ventricles (cavities) within the right and left cerebral hemispheres flows through canals into the third ventricle in the mid-brain area. It then continues through another canal into the fourth ventricle within the region of the middle and lower brainstem. The fourth ventricle narrows to form the central canal of the spinal cord, which extends to the level of the second lumbar vertebrae. From the fourth ventricle, CSF flows down through the central canal of the spinal cord, or it can circulate up through three small canals around the outer surface of the brain.

In either pathway, CSF is now circulating between the three layers of the **meninges** (Saran Wrap-like membranes covering the brain and spinal cord). CSF circulates between two membranes—the pia mater ("soft mother"), which is thin and adheres to the exterior surface of the brain and spinal cord, and the arachnoid mater ("spider mother"), which is the middle layer of the three membranes called meninges. The outer layer of these coverings is the dura mater ("tough mother"), which adheres to the inner surface of the cranium and some of the osseous cervical and sacral spinal segments. Dr. Jon Upledger, founder of CranoSacral Therapy, claims that CSF also circulates between the arachnoid and dura maters. The spinal cord begins at the foramen magnum, a large hole at the base of the skull, and extends to the second lumbar vertebrae, where it terminates.

Although the spinal cord itself ends at the second lumbar vertebrae, it separates into numerous lumbosacral nerve roots that together are called the cauda equine, which means "horses tail," which they resemble. These lumbosacral nerve roots are surrounded by a reservoir of CSF called the lumbar cistern that begins at the second lumbar vertebrae and ends at the second of five sacral segments. Strands of the cauda equina called the filum (threadlike) terminale (terminating point) attach the spinal cord to the coccyx, where it ends.

The circulating CSF is reabsorbed into the blood through the arachnoid villi bodies of the superior sagittal sinus cavity at the top of the cranium. However, Dr. Chikly's scientific literature search has led him to conclude that up to 90% of the circulating CSF may actually be absorbed into the lymphatic system.

CSFTM Procedure

The CSFTM procedure uses variations of the major categories of Swedish massage strokes, including effleurage, petrissage, friction, and tapotement. These Swedish massage stroke variations emphasize certain parameters: a specific amount of pressure, pace of the stroke, and a designated angle when applying the stroke. These guidelines are designed to free up areas of impeded CSF circulation around the cerebrospinal axis. The procedure also addresses massaging particular muscles whose action facilitates the CSF pumping mechanism, as well as certain spinal and cranial muscles (figure 16.10).

The CSFTM protocol is designed primarily to affect the five layers of muscles whose action moves the vertebral column and cranial muscles, as well as other muscles

Figure 16.10
Dr. Don Glassey, LMT, facilitating a posterior cranial sweep as part of the Cerebrospinal Fluid Technique Massage procedure.

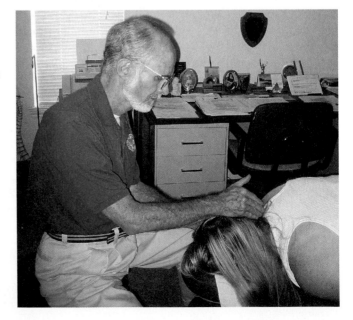

that directly affect the CSF pumps. The contractions of these five layers of spinal muscles affect not only the spinal column as a whole but also other structures that they attach to, such as the arm, scapula, diaphragm, and ribs. Certain layers of these spinal muscles affect movement of large sections of the spine, such as the erector spinae group, while other deeper muscles affect individual or multiple vertebrae, such as the transversospinalis group.

CSF circulates immediately underneath the spinal bones, which together comprise the vertebral column. Consequently, the flow of CSF can be impeded by misalignments of these bones. Since the actions of the five layers of muscles directly affect the position and movement of the spinal bones individually and in sections, it is imperative that these muscles be functioning properly for CSF to circulate freely.

Although the actions of the cranial muscles do not directly affect the movement of cranial bones, according to Upledger and others, the cranial bones may in fact move in response to the primary respiratory mechanism (PRM). It is theorized that the primary respiratory mechanism is a rhythmic motion independent of the heartbeat and breath, although it can be enhanced by deep breathing. The PRM, or cranial-sacral rhythm, has been attributed to the bending of cranial bones and a subtle motion between the bones. Living bone (unlike dry, dead bone) is flexible like plastic and therefore could expand and contract, as the fibrous sutures (joints) between the cranial bones may allow small amounts of movement. Since CSF also circulates directly underneath the cranial bones, potential misalignments of these bones may also impede CSF circulation around the cranium. Misalignments of cranial bones will most certainly affect the functioning of cranial muscles and vice versa. Therefore, it is essential that the cranial muscles be functioning appropriately for CSF to circulate freely.

Cerebrospinal fluid circulation around the brain and spinal cord is affected primarily by the action of two coordinated pumping mechanisms. The cranial pumping mechanism occurs at the spheno-basilar junction, where the sphenoid bone articulates with the basilar portion (anterior, inferior part) of the occiput bone. The sphenoid bone is in the center of the skull and articulates with many other cranial bones.

Upon inspiration, as the nasal conchae fill up with air, pressure is applied on the speno-basilar junction. This pressure causes the junction to move slightly posterior and inferior. On expiration, the spheno-basilar articulation relaxes as the pressure created by the inhaled air is released. This release of pressure causes the junction to move slightly anterior and superior. This to-and-fro movement of the spheno-basilar junction pumps CSF down through the spinal canal on its journey toward the second sacral segment.

A simultaneous movement also occurs between the spheno-basilar junction and the other major pumping mechanism, which is the sacrum. Upon inspiration, the diaphragm contracts down, resulting in a series of muscle contractions in the thoraco-abdominal region that cause the sacrum to "pump." Specifically, the following muscles contract inferiorly to cause the sacrum to extend up upon inspiration where the narrow sacral apex (bottom) goes anterior and the broad sacral base (top) goes posterior. The rectus abdominis, internal oblique, transverse abdominis, quadratus lumborum, and serratus posterior inferior contract inferior synergistically as the diaphragm contracts down upon inspiration. These muscles are assisted in the sacral pumping by the actions of the iliocostalis and longissimus relays of the erector spinae group and the inferiormost portions of the multifidus muscles of the transversospinalis group, which also contract inferiorly.

Upon expiration, the diaphragm relaxes upward, also affecting a series of muscle contractions in the same region that complete the "pumping" (up-and-down movement) of the sacrum. The following muscles contract superiorly to cause the sacrum to flex down upon expiration where the apex goes posterior and the base goes anterior. The ilio-psoas, external oblique, and serratus posterior inferior contract superior synergistically as the diaphragm relaxes.

This extension and flexion (up-and-down movement) of the sacrum causes a synchronistic flexion, and extension of the spheno-basilar junction in the cranium. In flexion, the junction rises, and in extension, the junction falls. The cartilaginous articulation of these two bones (sphenoid and basilar portion of the occiput) allows for the bones moving up and away from each other on flexion and down and toward each other on extension. Therefore, for CSF to circulate freely, the muscles that affect the pumping mechanisms must be functioning appropriately as well.

Neuropeptides

Aside from the significance of unimpeded CSF circulation, another aspect of its importance to health and well-being involves neuropeptides. In the early 1970s, neuroscientist Dr. Candace Pert discovered the "neuropeptide" opiate receptor site on cells, which was to become one of the most important advances in the scientific understanding of the body-mind connection.

Neuropeptides (nerve proteins) are biochemicals that regulate almost all life processes on a cellular level and thereby link all body systems. Dr. Pert uses the analogy that cells (the basic functional unit of life) are the engines that drive the human body, and a specific peptide is the spark that starts the engine.

Neuropeptides are produced primarily in the brain, although almost every tissue in the body produces and exchanges neuropeptides. Scientists such as Dr. Pert have discovered almost 100 different neuropeptides, the first of which to be found were hormones because they are larger molecules. Neuropeptides are one of three types of the most powerful biochemicals in the body, categorized as ligands from the Latin ligare, meaning "that which binds." Neurotransmitters and steroids (sex hormones) are the other types of ligands; however, neuropeptides constitute 95% of all ligands.

Neuropeptides circulate throughout the body in the blood, lymph, and CSF. (It is interesting to note that if the formed elements are removed from these body fluids, blood plasma, lymph, and CSF all have a similar chemical composition—the same as seawater.) Neuropeptides are called messenger molecules because they send chemical messages from the brain to receptor sites on cell membranes throughout the entire body. It is like a "lock-and-key" mechanism where the neuropeptide is the "key" that opens the "lock" on the cell membrane to cause complex and fundamental changes in the cells they lock onto. Dr. Pert, however, feels the standard scientific "key fitting into a lock" analogy is too static an image for this dynamic process. She uses the description of two voices, peptides and receptor site, hitting the same note and resulting in a resonance that rings the doorbell of the cell to open it.

The information message of the neuropeptide enters the cell membrane and readies the nucleus of the cell to communicate with surrounding cells to bring about a physiological change in tissues, glands, organs, and systems of the body. Dr. Pert describes neuropeptides as the sheet music that allows the body to orchestrate the physiological and emotional prosesses.

Another indicator for release of impeded CSF circulation involves carbon dioxide and oxygen. Recall that levels of carbon dioxide and oxygen in CSF are more influential than in the blood in regulating respiration. The mechanism of an increase in hydrostatic pressure in an area of CSF stasis or "pooling" related to impeded circulation has a similar effect on oxygen and carbon dioxide levels in CSF. Since the molecular weight of a carbon dioxide molecule is one and one-half that of an oxygen molecule, more of the heavier carbon dioxide than oxygen molecules filter through the semipermeable meningeal membrane.

This results in a decrease in carbon dioxide molecules circulating in CSF in the area of impedance (stasis). This decrease in carbon dioxide levels in CSF causes an increase in pH (a more alkaline condition) in the acid-base balance in the CSF specifically and the body in general.

This increase in pH affects the homeostatic chemoreceptors that control respiration in the brainstem. Consequently, the body responds to the change in pH, due to a decrease in the carbon dioxide levels in the CSF, by a decrease in the amount of oxygen that needs to be taken in through inspiration. The respiratory control mechanisms in the brain register a decrease in carbon dioxide levels related solely to impeded CSF circulation. However, this is a false reading of the overall carbon dioxide-oxygen concentration in the CSF and subsequent acid-base balance—"false" because the imbalance is created by an "abnormal" condition of impeded CSF circulation rather than by a "normal" change in overall carbon dioxide-oxygen levels (acid-base balance).

Conversely, when the impeded CSF circulation is corrected, the stasis and "pooling" in the area of impedance are eliminated. The condition of increased hydrostatic pressure is no longer present, and carbon dioxide molecules are no longer pushed through the meningeal membrane in the area of impeded CSF circulation. Consequently, carbon dioxide levels in the CSF return to a "normal" level, that is, a level not related to the "abnormal" condition of impeded CSF circulation. At the same time, the respiratory control mechanisms in the brainstem register this change as an overall increase of carbon dioxide levels in the CSF, and the body responds by increasing oxygen intake, which lowers the pH.

This is observed clinically by the immediate response of a spontaneous diaphragmatic breath as the body increases oxygen intake through inhalation. This creates a balance in the carbon dioxide-oxygen concentration of the CSF and a subsequent balance of acid-base levels in the CSF and the body. Thus, the correction of impeded CSF circulation can be observed clinically as an immediate spontaneous diaphragmatic breath each time an area of impeded CSF circulation is corrected. We call this the "ah, that's better breath," which can be observed in other types of bodywork that may also release areas of impeded CSF circulation.

Therefore, the correction of an area of impeded CSF circulation can be palpated by the change in resistance on the skin surface over the area of impedance. Thus, the physiological condition created by impeded CSF circulation, caused by vertebral or cranial subluxations, produces detectable clinical indicators. These clinical indicators allow the trained practitioner to detect the presence and location of areas of impedance to CSF circulation, and provide a method of evaluating or checking for the correction of the area of impedance.

⭐ **EXAM POINT** **CranioSacral Therapy (CST)** is a very gentle, hands-on method developed by osteopath John Upledger for evaluating and enhancing the function of the CranioSacral System.

CranioSacral Therapy
By Don Ash
PT, CST-D

This system provides nutrition to the central nervous system through the production and reabsorption of cerebrospinal fluid. This system is made up of the mid-brain ventricles where CSF is produced, the menningeal membranes that surround the brain and spinal cord where CSF circulates, and the connective tissue and bony structures that support the spinal column and brain. Cerebrospinal fluid is essential to the brain and spinal cord providing nutrition, removing wastes, and creating a soft watery environment in which the organs of the head reside.

The therapist performing CST uses extremely light touch (usually 5 grams) on connective tissue and bony structures to encourage the body to release restrictions that may be inhibiting the flow of CSF to the central nervous system and thereby inhibiting the health of the client (figure 16.11).

Releases are defined in three major ways with this work. First, there can be a change in tone of connective tissue, fascia, muscles, ligaments, organs, or menningeal membranes. This is characterized by muscle fasciculation, softening, or spreading; borborygmus (digestive tract noise); flutter of eyes; or breath change. There may also be the liberation of energy from the body in forms including heat, pulsing, vibration, sense of fluid flow, energy flow, or repelling. And finally, there can be ventilation of feelings or pent-up emotions from the body, characterized by spontaneous tears, laughter, and expressions of feelings, thoughts, or recall of traumatic events. This response is known as **somatoemotional release.**

Figure 16.11
CranioSacral Therapy is all about gentle, well-intentioned touch, listening to the CS rhythm, and encouraging change.

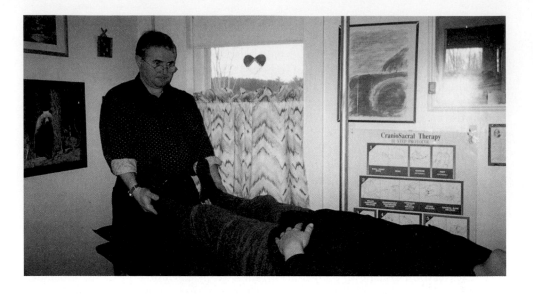

Like the pulse of the heart and breath in the lungs, the craniosacral system has a palpable rhythm that can be felt throughout the body. Once a source of restriction of movement is identified, the therapist can gently assist the natural movement of the fluid and related soft tissue to help the body self-correct. We use the bones as handles to access the system. Holding the sacrum may help release the lower spine, and holding the temporal bones may help with headaches, hearing, and balance. This simple action is often all it takes to help the body heal. The interesting thing about CST is that the system includes the head and spine in a dynamic way. A person who has suffered head and neck pain for years may be relieved of his problem by balancing the craniosacral system from the tailbone (sacrum). Evaluating and treating what you find in a craniosacral way is very interesting for the therapist and rewarding for the client. The client is viewed as a whole person and not just a back client or a headache client. For this reason, CST is a wonderful modality to include with massage and other complementary and integrative therapies.

Benefits of CST

The purpose of CST is to neither heal nor cure. CST enhances the body's ability to heal itself by encouraging release of restrictions to the systems of the body. The therapist takes on the role of the facilitator of change for the client. The client and his body are viewed as the catalyst for healing.

CST promotes health, well-being, and resistance to disease. It can be effective with stress-related problems such as insomnia, fatigue, chronic headaches, anxiety, and temporomandibular joint dysfunction. It is an excellent complement to chemotherapy, surgery, and rehabilitation. Due to its neurologic orientation, CST can effectively assist with sensory disorders, including vision problems, autism, loss of taste or smell, tinnitis, vertigo, and neuralgias. CST encourages release of restrictions that may be the result of trauma, strain, or injury. Examples include head, neck, and back injuries from traumatic events such as motor vehicle accidents, falls, sports, and work-related injuries.

Because of the extremely light touch the CST practitioner uses, CST can safely be done with newborns and children who have suffered birth trauma, cerebral palsy, anoxia, hyperactivity, learning disability, dyslexia, attention deficit, or developmental delay.

CST is contraindicated in conditions where variation or increase in intercranial pressure would be detrimental, such as acute aneurysm, cerebral hemorrhage, or other preexisting severe bleeding disorder.

Responses to CST vary from client to client. Some feel relaxed and desire sleep. Others experience increased energy and alertness. Reduction of pain or increase in function may occur immediately after a session or may become noticeable over a few days. Since CST helps the body resume its natural healing processes, it is common for improvements to continue weeks after a session. Some clients experience a "reorganization phase" as the body adapts to the release of previously held patterns. Minor discomfort can sometimes temporarily occur, much like the release of lactic acid from muscle tissue after a thorough massage.

Working with CST

CST complements massage work in many ways. It can prepare the body for massage, exercise, and other bodywork by softening tissue and reducing tension. The only equipment required is a quiet, private space, a massage table, and a therapist stool. Many therapists add an air mattress to the treatment table as the optimal work surface. Treatment time, much as with massage, is usually 45 to 90 minutes, based largely on the therapists' schedule and the needs of the client.

Frequency of client visits varies with outcome, but one to two times per week are common. Intensive treatment sessions sometimes can be more frequent and with more than one therapist. The therapy can be delivered at two levels with Upledger work. The Upledger Institute has two levels of certification (see Quick Guide C). Strictly manual therapists can use the work to make structural changes in the body with softer tone, improved range of motion, and decreased pain. Others may use the work as a body-mind approach to healing and self-awareness with somatoemotional release. One of the greatest contributions of Dr. Upledger's work to the bodywork field is the idea that the body has a consciousness that can be accessed by monitoring the craniosacral rhythm.

The therapist can manually bring the rhythm to gentle, slow, still point. This encourages the body to try to release restrictions in the craniosacral system that were there before the still point was induced.

And sometimes the nonconscious of the body can express itself in the rhythm. If there is trust and recognition of good intention on the part of the therapist, the craniosacral rhythm will spontaneously and abruptly stop. We have come to know this as a "siginificance detector." The significant awareness for the patient (and the therapist) is that the position the patients's body is in and what the patient is thinking at the time may be very important in the healing process. The patient may move an arm or leg. The rhythm stops abruptly, and suddenly, the patient recalls the traumatic event that occurred when the leg or arm was in that exact position. Release occurs often spontaneously, pain subsides, and the patient recalls and therefore understands and releases the reason for the original restriction. The body becomes softer and better able to return to normal function or respond to massage or other therapies.

Dr. Upledger's most recent work in the somatoemotional release process is using the craniosacral rhythm to respond to yes-no questions posed by the skilled therapist. Through this process, dialogue with the nonconscious of the body can lead to understanding for the consciousness of the patient. The patients can finally come to terms with their disability or dysfunction, and resolve, accept, or forgive the origin; they can move on into the rest of their lives without the baggage that sometimes lingers after therapy, treatment, or surgery, or remains unaffected by medications. Dr. Upledger is now working with creating awareness for the patient about the consciousness of separate organs of the brain and even types of cells in the immune system of the body.

Dr. Upledger has lectured for 30 years that anyone with good intention and a desire to listen to the inner wisdom of the body can use CST to make the world a touch better.

Clinical applications of CST can include hospitals, nursing homes, rehabilitation centers, schools, and private practices. Documentation and referrals are frequently cross-referenced among physicians, physical therapists, occupational therapists, chiropractors, and massage therapists. Standard practice guidelines concerning hygiene, sanitary work space, confidentiality, honor and respect for the client, and the process of growth and healing are of the highest importance in delivering this service. Such topics are referenced extensively in other sections of this book.

Chapter Summary

A good beginning for all students is to achieve familiarity with the various modalities and choose those that appeal to them. Keep in mind that some people are better suited to work with certain modalities, such as the gentle touch of Lymphatic Drainage Therapy and CranioSacral Therapy versus the strength required to perform Rolfing or neuromuscular work. Do your research so you'll know which modalities are in demand in your area (see Chapter 21). Also, focus on the specialized training required for becoming proficient in the different modalities outlined in this chapter: are courses easily available to you in your modality of choice?

Applying Your Knowledge

Self-Testing

1. Rolfing is based on what theory or principle?
   a) Reintegration of the body
   b) Structural changes in the body
   c) Rebalancing of the body
   d) All of the above are correct.

2. What massage modality uses gentle rocking?
   a) Esalen
   b) Trigger Point
   c) Swedish
   d) Trager

3. What massage modality recognizes restrictions in more superficial tissue?
   a) Myofascial Release
   b) Polarity
   c) Trager
   d) Acupuncture

4. What modality seeks to recognize a hyperirritable spot?
   a) Trager
   b) Trigger Point
   c) CranioSacral Therapy
   d) Lymphatic Drainage Therapy

5. Who developed Lymphatic Drainage Therapy?
   a) Lewis Rudolph
   b) Don Glassey
   c) Bruno Chikly
   d) Don Curry

6. In which modality does the practitioner feel for subtle movement of fluids in the body?
   a) CSF
   b) CranioSacral
   c) Intuitive neuromuscular
   d) a and b

7. Which modality builds on 10 sessions?
   a) Rolfing
   b) Trager
   c) Neuromuscular
   d) Chair

8. In which modality is it described that the therapists feel as if they are "hooking in" to the muscle?
   a) Myofascial Release
   b) Neuromuscular
   c) CSF
   d) Lymphatic Drainage Therapy

9. Which modality describes the tissue as "unwinding"?
   a) Myofascial Release
   b) Neuromuscular
   c) Trager
   d) Lymphatic Drainage Therapy

10. Which modality discusses the importance of neuropeptides to the body-mind connection?
    a) Trager
    b) Trigger Point
    c) CranioSacral Therapy
    d) Cerebrospinal Fluid Technique Massage

Case Studies/Critical Thinking

A. A client has recently undergone a mastectomy for breast cancer. What modality would you encourage her to seek out and why?

B. A new client has an unblanced posture (one shoulder is held higher than the other and one hip is leading). What modalities would you suggest to correct such postural imbalances?

References for information in this chapter can be found in Quick Guide C at the end of the book.

PART V

Wellness for Body and Mind

CHAPTER 17   **Body-Mind Connection**

CHAPTER 18   **Nutrition and Wellness**

CHAPTER 19   **Eastern and Western Principles
of Movement**

Body-Mind Connection

LEARNING OUTCOMES

After completing this chapter, you will be able to:

- Understand the balance of mind and body and its connection to our state of health.

- List the steps in the fight-or-flight response path.

- Explain the placebo effect and how it relates to our well-being.

- Describe common methods for reducing stress.

- Discuss how energy work balances and transforms to connect mind to body.

- Discuss the role that Native American spiritualism and indigenous massage practices play in the body-mind connection.

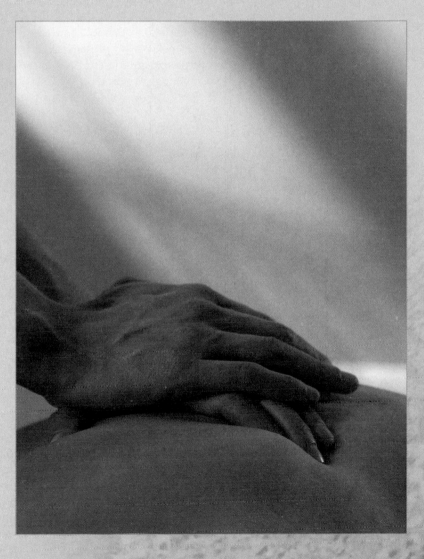

KEY TERMS

cortisol *(p. 466)*

countertransference *(p. 470)*

electroencephalogram
(EEG) *(p. 470)*

fight-or-flight response *(p. 466)*

guided imagery *(p. 472)*

meditation *(p. 469)*

neuropeptides *(p. 466)*

placebo *(p. 467)*

placebo effect *(p. 468)*

psychoneuroimmunology *(p. 466)*

relaxation response *(p. 468)*

seven aural planes *(p. 470)*

transference *(p. 470)*

INTRODUCTION

We are entering an age in which scientific research is shifting its focus from finding a solution to a specific problem to finding out how the brain works to guide the body to health and happiness. Many colleges in the United States have recently increased their program offerings to include classes in mind-body medicine as scientists map the pathways that connect the mind to the body.

The fact that our thoughts and feelings can affect our health has been known since ancient times by most of the people of the world. Many early cultures created rituals and healing techniques that continue to be used today. These techniques linking the body to the mind to bring about balance and the resulting good health are finally making their way into mainstream America.

In the late 1970s, **psychoneuroimmunology** emerged as a valid field of science and a method of treatment that understood the mind-body interaction. After decades of study at such renowned research centers as Duke University, Harvard Medical School, and the Mind/Body Medical Institute in Boston, scientists now realize that although disease is a presence we may have trouble stopping, the survivor rate depends on the behavioral patterns and mind-set of the individual. In this chapter, we will explain the complex system by which our psychological (mind) affects our physiological (body) state of health and the role massage therapy plays in the mind-body connection.

Fight-or-Flight Response

The physiological state known as the **fight-or-flight response** is a complex system our bodies use to respond to changes that may be dangerous or life-threatening. When we are confronted with a stressful situation, either real or imagined, our brain sends out **neuropeptides** (chemical messengers) that allow the mind to communicate with the body. The body responds with a sudden rise in blood pressure, our heart rate escalates, and our muscles tense in preparation for immediate action. If the threat continues, our breathing rate quickens, and the hypothalamus secretes a chemical called CRH that stimulates the pituitary gland. The pituitary then makes ACTH, which travels to the adrenal glands and stimulates the release of cortisol. **Cortisol** keeps the blood sugar at a higher-than-normal level so that extra energy for flight is available. The adrenal glands have already released epinephrine to increase the heart and breathing rates, so the legs and arms fill with blood to increase energy and endurance (figure 17.1).

As all of this happens, digestion stops, sex hormone secretion ceases, basal metabolism slows to conserve energy, and our brains function only in automatic response mode and not in judgment mode. After the event passes, our bodies return to normal and the extra hormones are eliminated from the body. This response saved the lives of our ancestors who had only two choices when faced with danger: fight or run. But when this response is recurring daily due to constant stress, we have stomachaches, weight gain, and malnutrition; women have reproductive problems or "hot flashes," and men may have lower sperm counts and impotence. The elevated blood sugar from stress can lead to diabetes, and the extra cortisol in the bloodstream slows our metabolism, causing weight problems.

Today, our civilization has led to many changes in our lifestyles that make the two choices of fight or flight ridiculous. When we are stressed by our boss, the response

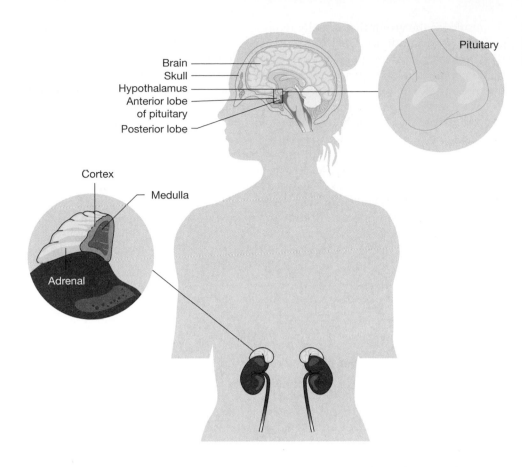

Figure 17.1
Fight or flight hormones prepare the body for action.

Brain
Skull
Hypothalamus
Anterior lobe
of pituitary
Posterior lobe

Pituitary

Cortex
Medulla
Adrenal

kicks in, but we cannot fight, and most times we have to overrule our brain and stay put. We tell ourselves, "I would leave this job in a heartbeat, but I can't live without the money" or some other rationale that keeps the cycle of stress going.

If we could fight or flee, our response network would play out and calm down. A type of euphoria would result, and when the epinephrine left our system, we would re-balance ourselves. When we cannot fight or flee, the cycle continues, unresolved, until we develop ulcers, cancer, or other health disorders. We then may receive medication for the anxiety and fear, but if the stressor is not removed, the cycle continues until our illness makes our choice for us. It has recently been discovered that major events such as divorce, job loss, and death of a spouse (although horrible situations) are not the greatest stressors to the body. It is the chronic agitation of interruption, job site stress, noise, lack of enough money for basic needs, and alienation that leads most quickly to heart attacks and cancer.

Our society's "get more, go more, work more" attitude is destroying the healthful balance we should have. Massage plays a major role in reducing stress, which can in turn contribute to having a healthier body. A number of other techniques are used to "re-train the mind and body" to bypass and control the flight or fight responses and thereby lessen their effects on our body. We will review a few of the more common methods in the following paragraphs.

Placebo Effect

The word **placebo** comes from the Latin for "I shall please" and is known in the research field as "an inactive substance or treatment given to satisfy the patient's/client's need for drug therapy or health care intervention." When research scientists first began test studies on medications, they would give a control group a placebo or "sugar pill" and then give another group the actual medication. As they documented the changes in the groups, they soon came to realize that at least 50% of the placebo group often showed the results of the group that actually received the medication. Sugar pills may still be given to hypochondriacs. Doctors treat imaginary illnesses with placebo medications with remarkable results. Based on this information, scientists came to the conclusion that if people thought they were taking the real pill, their body followed suit and made the appropriate changes as if the medication were used, thus creating the **placebo effect.**

Scientists went on to perform tests that concluded that what you held in your mind, or thought, could cause the body to transform. In other words, the body could be controlled by the mind. This concept was already familiar to indigenous peoples and the Eastern world. This fact has brought about many changes in how illness is approached. The scientists went on to discover that if ill persons were told they would die in six months, they usually did die six months later—almost to the day. They also discovered that if patients who might be too sick for surgery were told that they had indeed received the surgery, they often recovered and lost the evidence of the condition for which the surgery was to be performed.

About 20 years ago, the medical world scoffed at the idea that massage could alleviate the harmful effects of stress. Medical professionals generally attributed the benefits of massage to the placebo effect. Now with current research, we can prove that the physiological benefits of regular massage are not just in the mind.

Methods That Connect Body and Mind

Another phrase that has evolved from recent study is the "relaxation response." The **relaxation response** is the state reached by having a calm mind. During this state, the blood pressure drops, your muscles lose their tension, and the neuropeptides stop transmitting messages. These actions in turn cause the heart and breathing rate to slow down. Numerous methods are used to reach this state of relaxation. Massage, meditation, repetitive motion, chanting, sound, breathing exercises, energy work, and yoga are some of the specific methods we have discussed in this text (figure 17.2). Participants in stress or body-mind balancing techniques report better health, more energy, a more focused approach to work, and less pain. (See chapter 19 for more information on yoga.)

Meditation

Through the centuries, humankind has meditated (figure 17.3). Meditation is a major part of all religions, from Buddhism and Native American spiritual rituals to Christian

Figure 17.2
Yoga is an excellent practice for balancing the body, mind, and spirit.

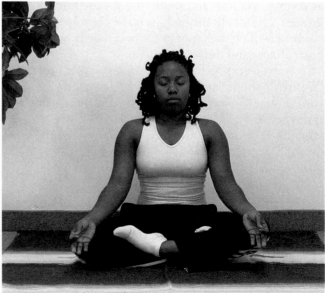

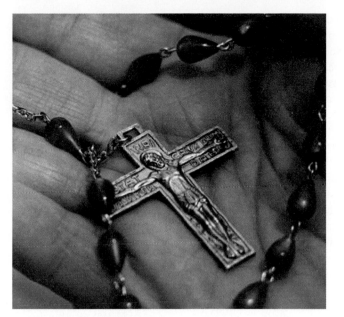
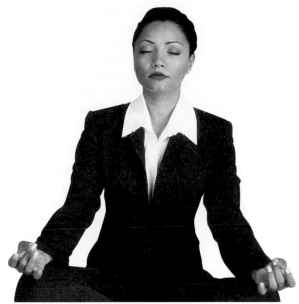

Figure 17.3
Many religions incorporate meditation as part of their prayer or rituals.

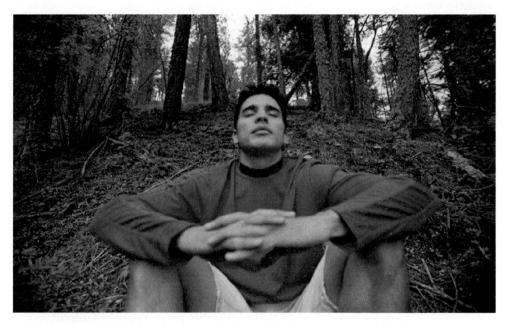

Figure 17.4
Meditation can simply be a part of sitting still and focusing inward.

prayer. At the same time, many methods of meditation have nothing to do with religion, such as affirmations, staring at a candle flame, or simply closing your eyes and centering your thoughts.

When you look for the definition of *meditation,* you will get as many answers as places you look. The accepted scientific definition of **meditation** is any act of mind-body focus that brings about an altering of the psychophysiological state of an individual that in turn brings about the opposite of the usual reactions to stress (figure 17.4). This definition encompasses a broad area of practices that can be considered meditation. In fact, meditation can be as individual as the person who is meditating.

In years past, people who meditated were sometimes considered "out there" or eccentric, but now there is scientific and medical proof that meditation practices can alter the brain waves. When doctors first placed electrodes on the body of meditating individuals, they were astounded to discover that the breath and heart rate slowed, and oxygen consumption decreased, although oxygen saturation seemed more consistent and muscle spasms ceased. Brain waves that were monitored with an **electroencephalogram (EEG)** by recording the electrical currents in the brain showed a different pattern than during sleep. The person was still able to respond to external stimuli as in a waking state. However, none of the stress-associated fight-or-flight mechanisms remained in play. These facts led scientists to believe that meditation can alleviate the ravages of the stress response on the body, and when the body is focused and calm, it can begin to heal itself.

A very real aspect of meditation can be utilized when you, as the massage therapist, meditate before giving a massage. When you are focused and balanced, there can be limited **countertransference,** which is the redirection of your desires and feelings, especially unconscious childhood negativity, to the client. You are also better able to redirect the **transference,** which is transference to you of the client's negative feelings, thought, and desires. Have you ever just felt bad or were sad when you gave a certain individual a massage? It may have been the transference of negativity from something in the client's life of which you are not aware. The same sensation can happen to the client. Your client may have feelings that are not explained when you are having a very bad day, even if your massage is technically perfect.

Balancing the Spirit

We have mentioned the chakra and energy systems in other chapters, so we will only touch on these concepts briefly in reference to stress reduction and transference. The chakras are considered to be the keys to our body-mind-spirit health and well-being. By acting as a conduction system between the glands of our body and our **seven aural planes** (levels of energy), the chakras constantly assess, filter, and balance the body's mental and emotional state to communicate what the physical body needs (figure 17.5).

The basic process of balancing our spirit, which leads to a better mental clarity and physical health, begins with looking deeply into ourselves. Sometimes this balancing is hard because we must learn to love and accept our own individuality and forgive ourselves for the things we feel guilt over or times we feel we have failed. It seems to be easier to forgive others than to forgive ourselves and accept who we really are, but by doing so, we gain the wisdom to transform our thinking about past experiences, we affirm our worth, and we begin to focus on our contributions to family, friends, clients, and the world.

Chakra Balancing

Practice chakra balancing by breathing into each chakra, beginning with the root chakra, *Muladhara.* Work your way up through each chakra, visualizing its corresponding color as a spinning vortex opening out in all directions from your body. Finish with the crown chakra with protective white light falling down around you. Return to the solar plexus chakra, *Manipura,* and create a word or phrase that is particular to you. It might be a quality you admire or a goal you would like to achieve in your life. By centering your breath in the solar plexus and repeating this mantra, you will witness the manifestation of this affirmation. It is in the solar plexus that you plant the seed for growth and the area to which you return to when you need peace.

Begin with the root chakra, *Muladhara.* Envision a swirling vortex of red at the perineum. In women, it spins counterclockwise; in men, clockwise. See it opening down toward your feet and floor. Repeat its mantra, if you wish, *Lam,* representing survival and existence.

Move up to the sacral chakra, *Svadisthana.* Envision a swirling vortex of orange just above the pubic bone. In women, it is spinning clockwise; in men, counterclockwise. See it opening to the front of your body. Repeat its mantra, *Vam,* representing creativity and sensuality.

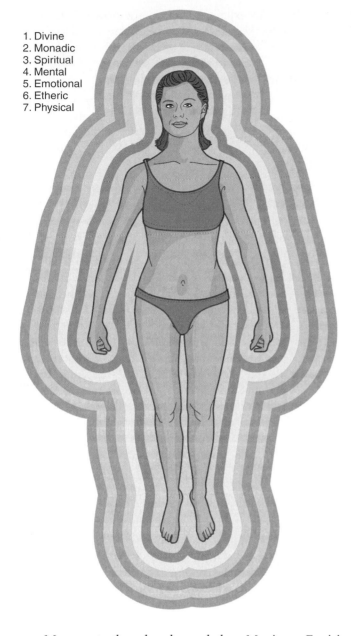

1. Divine
2. Monadic
3. Spiritual
4. Mental
5. Emotional
6. Etheric
7. Physical

Figure 17.5
Seven levels of energy surround our body. These energy layers reflect the body, mind, and spirit as one continuous connection.

Move up to the solar plexus chakra, *Manipura*. Envision a swirling vortex of yellow at the navel. In women, it is spinning counterclockwise; in men, clockwise. See it opening to the front of your body. Repeat its mantra, *Ram,* representing strength and self-empowerment.

Move up to the heart chakra, *Anahata*. Envision a swirling vortex of green at the heart center. In women, it is spinning clockwise; in men, counterclockwise. See it opening to the front of your body. Repeat its mantra, *Yam,* representing unconditional love.

Move up to the throat chakra, *Visshuddha*. Envision a swirling vortex of blue at the base of your throat. In women, it is spinning counterclockwise; in men, clockwise. See it opening to the front of your body. Repeat its mantra, *Ham,* representing speaking truth.

Move up to the third-eye chakra, *Ajna*. Envision a swirling vortex of violet between your brows. In women, it is spinning clockwise; in men, counterclockwise. See it opening to the front of your body. Repeat its mantra, *Om,* representing awareness and intuition.

Finally, move up to the crown chakra, *Sahasrara*. Envision a swirling vortex of white (gold or silver) emanating from the crown of the head and opening out above it in all directions. Some believe this chakra has no mantra for it is beyond sound; others believe the *Om* mantra is used. This chakra represents cosmic consciousness.

Take your breath up through each chakra, exhaling as if from the crown chakra protective white light down around you. Do this several times to fully balance and integrate all of the chakras.

Finish for Meditation or Chakra Balancing

Draw your hands together, rubbing them briskly to create heat. Place your palms over your eyes and repeat, "I am Light." Rub your hands together again, place them over your heart and affirm, "I am Love." Rub your hands together one more time. Place them over the solar plexus and affirm, "I am Strength." You may also finish with placing your hands over any area of your body that needs healing.

Energy Work and Guided Imagery

The practice of Reiki, healing touch, and guided imagery can bring about spiritual as well as physical changes. Many hospitals have begun using these and other energy techniques before and after surgery, chemotherapy, and physical therapy with amazing results. Patients who have energy work before surgery often require a remarkably low amount of anesthesia, have less pain afterward, and heal at twice the rate. Cancer patients often have fewer chemotherapy sessions and less recurrence of disease when regular energy work and guided imagery are involved in the overall treatment. Guided imagery has been used as a method of dispelling fear before a medical procedure. It also works great before a really hard test or performance.

Guided imagery, often called visualization, is a method of taking your brain and body through a preplanned outcome or a release of negativity. It is a state of meditation that uses a technique of active involvement. This relaxation technique is not nearly as mysterious and deep as it sounds. It is simply the holding of images in your mind, almost like daydreaming. While daydreams may ramble and are an excellent way to relax and refresh your mind, guided imagery is more specific in its outcome goals.

A guided imagery session can be done by yourself (as in thinking and visualizing a relaxing image such as the ocean) or with professionals to help carry you and your body responses on a determined course. Many cancer patients visualize a laser or something else going through their bodies and attacking the cancer cells or tumor. This visualization seems to help sluggish phagocytes move with a purpose and destroy diseased cells more efficiently. One woman visualized Pac-Man characters surging through her veins and eating the cancer cells that were metastasizing from her breast cancer. She has been cancer-free for five years and says that every couple of months, she meditates and visualizes Pac-Man on patrol, just in case. An example of a guided imagery visualization is detailed in box 17.1.

Indigenous Massage and Native American Practices

Some of the most dramatic methods of the body-mind connection to wellness come from the traditions of indigenous peoples of the Americas, Africa, Australia, India, and Europe (figure 17.6). Every culture on the planet developed methods for health and well-being long before doctors and formal medicine emerged. If you study some of these fascinating methods, you will find that massage played a large part in the healing rituals and techniques. Learning one of these methods may also help you to strengthen your skills as a massage therapist and bodyworker.

The following paragraphs give a general overview of Cherokee massage practices, but please understand that many books, documentaries, travel experiences, and seminars on other indigenous massage techniques can add insights to greatly enhance your abilities and understanding of how the body-mind connection works.

To practice the art of Cherokee massage, you must first understand the Cherokee belief that energy comes from the heart and soul of the therapist and flows through the hands and into the energy field of the client. It is also a belief that all and everything is connected and what the therapist does and thinks affects the clients, their families, and

NOTE: This guided imagery can be recorded and played back, or performed as a group with one person with a soothing voice reading it.

Lie down or sit on the floor, leaning against a wall. Close your eyes. Breathe deeply and slowly. Imagine the room becoming warmer and the air softer. Breathe in the soft, warm air; breathe out the poisons in your body. Breathe in, breathe out, breathe in, breathe out. Continue to breathe slowly and deeply. Imagine a gold light forming in the ceiling of the room. The light slowly flows down and forms a golden ball of misty light above your head. Imagine the golden mist leaving the ball and flowing in with your breath and then out, taking the poisons and anything causing worry and negativity into the ball. When all of the negativity is gone, imagine the ball slowly rising to the ceiling and out into the sky until it disappears. Continue to breathe slowly. Become aware of the room around you as you slowly open your eyes. When the room feels solid, clap your hands three times to break the connection. Rise slowly and record any images or feelings in a journal.

This is a basic scenario. You can change colors or let your mind make the colors for you. You can pretend you rise and go through the wall to enter a garden or seascape. Focus on whatever scenes or images help you to feel relaxed and in control. If you are at a desk or waiting in a line, you can close your eyes and imagine colors surrounding you for only a few minutes. This guided imagery strategy will help you to alleviate stress. Do not use guided imagery while driving.

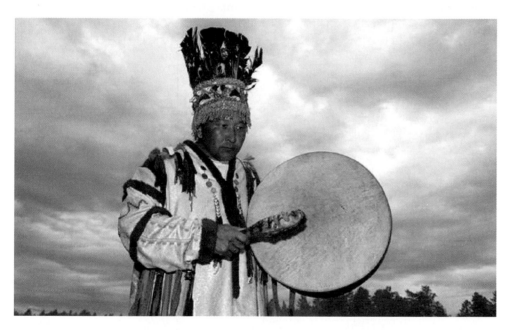

Figure 17.6
Present-day shaman performing ancient Siberian ritual for healing.

their community. This belief is part of the difference between the traditional indigenous massage and today's core massage techniques. It is more than a knowledge and ability to massage tissue. A Cherokee massage therapist of the traditional ways will not touch someone if they are not of right spirit and calm mind.

Cherokee massage therapists, however, used and are still using some of the same techniques that you are learning now. Kneading, rubbing, deep pressure, stretching, cupping, and striking (tapotement) are all used in a traditional massage. Cherokee and other tribes use acupressure and acupuncture techniques similar to those of traditional Chinese medicine. They also use hot stone, herbal wraps, energetic bodywork, cryotherapy, and hydrotherapy, along with cranial manipulations to balance the spine. Cherokee healers are likely to use a homemade oil that is specific to the client's complaint and employ any and all methods to restore a client to health. Most Cherokee therapists today diversify their practice and may specialize in certain aspects of healing such as Reiki, healing touch, shamanism, or herbology (see chapter 16 for more information on Reiki).

Another main difference in the Cherokee approach to massage and healing is that the plan for the treatment may come from sources other than those traditionally accepted in a massage school. The therapist may consult a shaman who will use shamanic methods to determine the correct technique. The therapist may also use dream interpretation or talking stones and animal helpers to give them an idea of the problem. A Cherokee therapist always believes that there may be a reason other than physical, behind a muscle that continues to spasm and that the problem will not go away until the real issue is brought to light and corrected. For example, a continually sore throat that does not respond to usual treatment may be a sign that the client cannot speak the truth of something he or she has witnessed. This can happen to clients if a spouse or boss does not let them explain or speak their mind. Until they are able to say what they want to without fear, the sore throat will continue.

Most indigenous massage therapists, Cherokee and otherwise, take very seriously their commitment to helping their clients. They study and avail themselves of all the knowledge available to make them a better therapist.

Chapter Summary

Many types of health care techniques use how the mind speaks to the body as a basis of their healing. We are very fortunate to live in a time in which all of these wonderful techniques can be scientifically explained and easily added as a certification. To be a more balanced person and a better massage therapist because of such knowledge, take steps toward understanding the connection between your own body and mind. Do you speak words of affirmation to yourself, or are you your own worst enemy? When you have a balanced body and a focused mind, the world is full of possibilities for which you will be ready.

Applying Your Knowledge

Self-Testing

1. What field of science and method of treatment that understood the mind-body interaction emerged in the '70s?
   a) Psychopomp
   b) Immunology
   c) Neurology
   d) Psychoneuroimmunology

2. What are neuropeptides?
   a) Thinking cells
   b) Chemical messengers
   c) Rows of cells
   d) Nerves

3. What kind of changes trigger our body's fight-or-flight response?
   a) Planned and happy
   b) Dangerous or life-threatening
   c) Adrenal gland warnings
   d) Lethargic mood swings

4. What attitude is not a possible contributor to an unbalanced lifestyle?
   a) Get more
   b) Go more
   c) Relax more
   d) Work more

5. What you hold in your mind or thoughts can control how your _____ reacts.
   a) friend
   b) future
   c) body
   d) purpose

6. What is the state reached by having a calm mind?
   a) Relaxation response
   b) Alternate realities
   c) Biofeedback
   d) Chanting

7. Meditation can be as _____ as the person doing it.
   a) inappropriate
   b) relaxing
   c) ageless
   d) individual

8. What is a recording of the electrical currents of the brain called?

   a) Electroencephalogram

   b) MRI

   c) Skull x-ray

   d) Electrocardiogram

9. Between what parts of the body are the chakras a conduction system?

   a) Organs

   b) Muscles

   c) Bones

   d) Glands

10. What visualization technique takes the mind and body through a preplanned outcome or release of negativity?

    a) Qi

    b) Reiki

    c) Healing touch

    d) Guided imagery

Case Studies/Critical Thinking

A. *There have been many instances of lab animals placed in cages together that have transferred healing to one another. In fact, when five of 10 rats in a cage (all with cancer) were given a healing drug, the other five rats were healed as well. Is this the placebo effect? Faith of some sort? An energetic connection? What is your opinion?*

B. *You have seen the same doctor since you were a child; you feel that this doctor has always helped you to become well. After this trusted doctor retires, you become ill. You must see another doctor, one you have not met before. This new doctor wants you to try an experimental medication that could have some risks. How do you feel about your visit with the new doctor? How do you feel about following her suggestions? Will you trust her? In terms of your own practice, how will your clients feel about seeing you for the first time when you open your clinic? What can make for a trusting connection between the client and a newly graduated massage therapist? Can a person get well as quickly if they do not trust or feel comfortable with the health care provider?*

References for information in this chapter can be found in Quick Guide C at the end of the book.

CHAPTER 18

Nutrition and Wellness

LEARNING OUTCOMES

After completing this chapter, you will be able to:

- Discuss the relationship between food and health.

- List and discuss the classification of nutrients, including water, vitamins, minerals, carbohydrates, fats, and protein.

- Describe the processes of ingestion, digestion, absorption, and elimination.

- Discuss the process of metabolism.

- Identify amino acids and enzymes, and explain their functions within the body.

- Recognize nutritional imbalances and common eating disorders.

- Discuss how foods can affect us mentally and emotionally.

- Discuss alternative diets such as vegetarian and Latin American, Mediterranean, and Asian dietary plans.

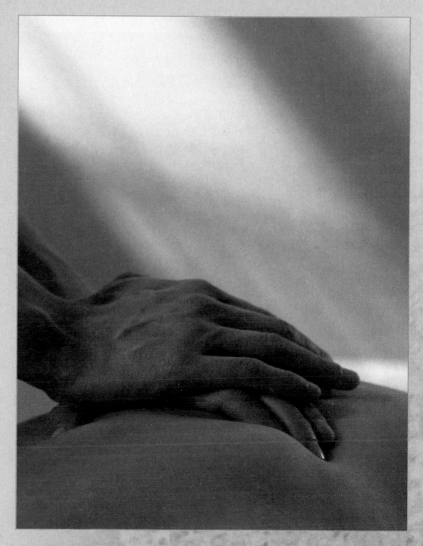

KEY TERMS

amino acids (p. 486)
bile (p. 488)
blood-brain barrier (p. 490)
carbohydrates (p. 484)
cellular edema (p. 480)
coenzymes (p. 481)
colon (p. 489)
complete proteins (p. 486)

dehydrated (p. 480)
digestion (p. 486)
electrolytes (p. 480)
enzymes (p. 481)
essential nutrients (p. 479)
fats (p. 485)
fiber (p. 484)
gallbladder (p. 488)

hypoglycemia (p. 488)
hypothalamus (p. 480)
liver (p. 488)
micronutrients (p. 481)
nutrients (p. 479)
pancreas (p. 488)
proteins (p. 486)

INTRODUCTION

The old saying "you are what you eat" has never been more on target than it is in today's society. With so many advances in science and medicine, we can not only prove that premise, but we can take it a step further and say, "you are what you eat, digest, absorb, metabolize, and then eliminate," and explain how some food habits can contribute to disease. You'll find that adopting (or maintaining) a healthful approach to eating and wellness will help you to optimize your on-the-job performance.

Table 18.1	Six Classes of Nutrients

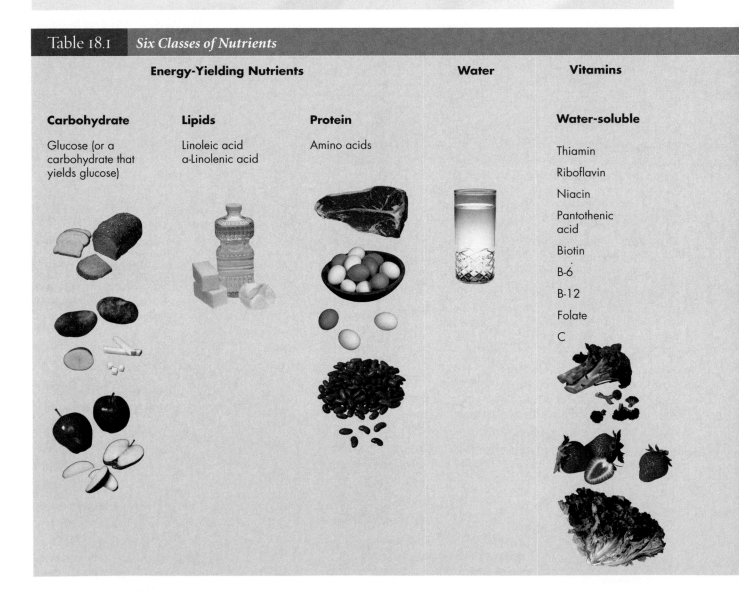

Energy-Yielding Nutrients

Water

Vitamins

Carbohydrate

Glucose (or a
carbohydrate that
yields glucose)

Lipids

Linoleic acid
a-Linolenic acid

Protein

Amino acids

Water-soluble

Thiamin

Riboflavin

Niacin

Pantothenic
acid

Biotin

B-6

B-12

Folate

C

As humans, we eat for two reasons: we are hungry, or we need to satisfy a psychological or physical craving. If we put food into our body that has the right amount of **nutrients**—chemical substances that are necessary to maintain life—we can provide the body with energy and the ability to build and repair tissue, and regulate the hormonal and other bodily processes. If we ingest a poor diet lacking in nutrients, the bodily processes will suffer. Fatigue and depression may become prevalent, and with continued nutritional imbalances, disease processes begin to take hold. Let us begin to study and understand how food substances can contribute to our wellness and longevity (table 18.1).

Parts of these nutrients can be made by the body. The nutrients that can only be made available by the food we ingest are called **essential nutrients.** These nutrient classes are divided further into organic nutrients containing carbon, hydrogen, oxygen, and inorganic nutrients. The organic nutrients must be broken down into smaller units to be used by the body; however, the inorganic nutrients are in their simplest forms when ingested—except for water.

Water

Water is essential for life. We may go for weeks without food, but death will occur after a few days without water. Our bodies are made up of 50 to 60% water. Muscle tissue has a higher content of water than fat tissue. The water in our body is divided into two types:

Vitamins		Minerals	
Fat-soluble	**Major**	**Trace**	**Questionable minerals**
A	Calcium	Chromium	Arsenic
D	Chloride	Copper	Boron
E	Magnesium	Fluoride	Nickel
K	Phosphorus	Lodide	Silicon
	Potassium	Iron	Vanadium
	Sodium	Manganese	
	Sulfur	Molybdenum	
		Selenium	
		Zinc	

intracellular, which is fluid within the cells; and extracellular, which is fluid outside the cells. The extracellular water is found in the blood, interstitial fluid, and glandular secretions.

Water acts as a solvent medium for nutrients, toxins, and waste products, and works to transport nutrients to and from cells via the bloodstream. Water transports toxins and waste products away from the cells and out of the body. Water is also used in digestive processes and as a lubricant for joints of the body. When we perspire, our bodies are using water to cool the body and eliminate some toxins through the skin. Water is also responsible for maintaining our acid-base balance. Excessive acids can lead to a condition of acidosis. Inadequate amounts of acid can lead to the condition of alkalosis. Both conditions can contribute to disease if unchecked.

If we fail to ingest enough water or when water is lost through diarrhea, vomiting, hemorrhage, or other health conditions, we become **dehydrated.** Some of the symptoms of dehydration are excessive thirst; hot, dry skin; fever; muscle weakness; and mental confusion. Dehydration can lead to death if not reversed. Sodium, chloride, and potassium are **electrolytes** that are part of the intracellular and extracellular fluids. When the electrolytes in the extracellular fluid are increased, the intracellular fluid moves to the extracellular fluid to try to achieve a balance. This movement triggers the **hypothalamus,** which is the regulator of thirst and hunger, to stimulate the pituitary gland to excrete antidiuretic hormone (ADH) whenever the electrolytes become concentrated in the blood and the blood volume or pressure is too low (figure 18.1). The antidiuretic hormone causes the kidneys to absorb water instead of excreting it; the healthy person feels thirsty.

When the sodium in the extracellular fluid is reduced, water flows from the extracellular fluid and into the cells, which causes **cellular edema.** When water is ingested, the fluid leaves the cells and the edema is reduced.

Figure 18.1

The hypothalamus, a region of the brain, regulates our desire to eat, find food when hungry, and the feeling of satisfaction (satiety) when we no longer desire to eat.

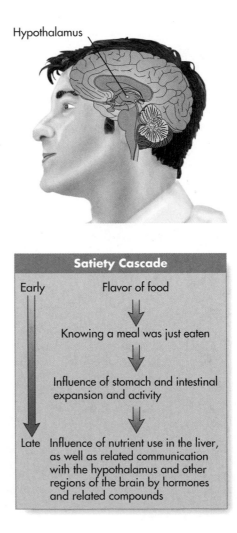

Hypothalamus

Satiety Cascade

Early

Flavor of food

Knowing a meal was just eaten

Influence of stomach and intestinal expansion and activity

Late · Influence of nutrient use in the liver, as well as related communication with the hypothalamus and other regions of the brain by hormones and related compounds

The amount of water that is necessary for optimal bodily function differs for each person, depending on age, activity level, environmental factors, and his or her health. A general rule to follow is to drink 1 milliliter of water for every kilogram calorie of food ingested. For most individuals, that is roughly eight glasses of fluid (four of pure water and four from other food sources) per day. Drinking enough water is especially important for those with physically demanding professions (such as massage therapists and bodyworkers) who exert a good deal of energy during their workday.

Vitamins and minerals are usually called the **micronutrients** of the body due to the small amounts needed. Vitamins are considered organic substances because they are naturally found in plants and animals. Vitamins are useful to the body as **coenzymes,** which means they work together with enzymes to activate chemical reactions that must occur for our bodies to function appropriately. **Enzymes** help us to digest our food by breaking down proteins into essential amino acids, and they help with nerve transmission. Vitamins also have specific functions that do not require enzymes; for example, vitamin E acts as an antioxidant and vitamin D functions as a hormone. Vitamins that have performed their task remain as part of the structure of the body. The B and C vitamins stay in the body for a short period of time and are called water-soluble vitamins. Vitamins A, D, E, and K belong to the fat-soluble vitamin group. These vitamins stay in the body and continue to work for longer periods of time. They are stored in the lipid or fat tissue and may be stored in the liver, other organs, and bones. Tables 18.2 and 18.3 list specific information on these vitamins, including the effects they have on the body.

Vitamins and Minerals

Table 18.2	**Water-Soluble Vitamins**				
Vitamin	**Major Functions**	**RDA or Adequate Intake**	**Dietary Sources**	**Deficiency Symptoms**	**Toxicity Symptoms**
Thiamin	■ Coenzyme of carbohydrate metabolism ■ Nerve function	1.1–1.2 milligrams	■ Sunflower seeds ■ Pork ■ Whole and enriched grains ■ Dried beans ■ Peas	■ Beriberi ■ Nervous tingling ■ Poor coordination ■ Edema ■ Heart changes ■ Weakness	None
Riboflavin	■ Coenzyme of energy metabolism	1.1–1.3 milligrams	■ Milk ■ Mushrooms ■ Spinach ■ Liver ■ Enriched grains	■ Inflammation of the mouth and tongue ■ Cracks at the corners of the mouth ■ Eye disorders	None
Niacin	■ Coenzyme of energy metabolism ■ Coenzyme of fat synthesis ■ Coenzyme of fat breakdown	14–16 milligrams (niacin equivalents)	■ Mushrooms ■ Bran ■ Tuna ■ Salmon ■ Chicken ■ Beef ■ Liver ■ Peanuts ■ Enriched grains	■ Pellagra ■ Diarrhea ■ Dermatitis ■ Dementia ■ Death	Upper level is 35 milligrams from supplements, based on flushing of skin.

(continued)

Table 18.2   *Water-Soluble Vitamins (Continued)*

Vitamin	Major Functions	RDA or Adequate Intake	Dietary Sources	Deficiency Symptoms	Toxicity Symptoms
Pantothenic acid	■ Coenzyme of energy metabolism ■ Coenzyme of fat synthesis ■ Coenzyme of fat breakdown	5 milligrams	■ Mushrooms ■ Liver ■ Broccoli ■ Eggs *Most foods have some.*	■ No natural deficiency disease or symptoms	None
Biotin	■ Coenzyme of glucose production ■ Coenzyme of fat synthesis	30 micrograms	■ Cheese ■ Egg yolks ■ Cauliflower ■ Peanut butter ■ Liver	■ Dermatitis ■ Tongue soreness ■ Anemia ■ Depression	Unknown
Vitamin B-6	■ Coenzyme of protein metabolism ■ Neurotransmitter synthesis ■ Hemoglobin synthesis *Many other functions*	1.3–1.7 milligrams	■ Animal protein foods ■ Spinach ■ Broccoli ■ Bananas ■ Salmon ■ Sunflower seeds	■ Headache ■ Anemia ■ Convulsions ■ Nausea ■ Vomiting ■ Flaky skin ■ Sore tongue	Upper level is 100 milligrams, based on nerve destruction.
Folate (folic acid)	■ Coenzyme involved in DNA synthesis *Many other functions*	400 micrograms (dietary folate equivalents)	■ Green leafy vegetables ■ Orange juice ■ Organ meats ■ Sprouts ■ Sunflower seeds	■ Megaloblastic anemia ■ Inflammation of tongue ■ Diarrhea ■ Poor growth ■ Depression	None likely; upper level for adults set at 1000 micrograms for synthetic folic acid (exclusive of food folate), based on masking of B-12 deficiency.
Vitamin B-12	■ Coenzyme of folate metabolism ■ Nerve function *Many other functions*	2.4 micrograms *Older adults should use fortified foods or supplements.*	■ Animal foods (not natural in plants) ■ Organ meats ■ Oysters ■ Clams ■ Fortified, ready-to-eat breakfast cereals	■ Macrocytic anemia ■ Poor nerve function	None
Vitamin C	■ Connective tissue synthesis ■ Hormone synthesis ■ Neurotransmitter synthesis ■ Possible antioxidant activity	75–90 milligrams *Smokers should add 35 milligrams.*	■ Citrus fruits ■ Strawberries ■ Broccoli ■ Greens	■ Scurvy ■ Poor wound healing ■ Pinpoint hemorrhages ■ Bleeding gums	Upper level is 2 grams, based on development of diarrhea; can also alter some diagnostic tests.
Choline	■ Neurotransmitter synthesis ■ Phospholipid synthesis	425–550 milligrams	Widely distributed in foods and self-synthesized	No natural deficiency	Upper level is 3.5 grams per day, based on development of fishy odor and reduced blood pressure.

Table 18.3   *Fat-Soluble Vitamins*

Vitamin	Major Functions	RDA or Adequate Intake	Dietary Sources	Deficiency Symptoms	Toxicity Symptoms
Vitamin A (preformed vitamin A and provitamin A)	▪ Promote vision: night and color ▪ Promote growth ▪ Prevent drying of skin and eyes ▪ Promote resistance to bacterial infection and overall immune system function	Females: 700 micrograms RAE Males: 900 micrograms RAE (2300–3000 IU if as preformed vitamin A)	Preformed vitamin A: ▪ Liver ▪ Fortified milk ▪ Fortified breakfast cereals Provitamin A: ▪ Sweet potatoes ▪ Spinach ▪ Greens ▪ Carrots ▪ Cantaloupe ▪ Apricots ▪ Broccoli	▪ Night blindness ▪ Xerophthalmia ▪ Poor growth ▪ Dry skin	▪ Fetal malformations ▪ Hair loss ▪ Skin changes ▪ Bone pain ▪ Fractures Upper level is 3000 micrograms of preformed vitamin A (10,000 IU), based on the risk of birth defects and liver toxicity.
Vitamin D	▪ Increase absorption of calcium and phosphorus ▪ Maintain optimal blood calcium and calcification of bone	5–15 micrograms (200–600 IU)	▪ Vitamin D-fortified milk ▪ Fortified breakfast cereals ▪ Fish oils ▪ Sardines ▪ Salmon	▪ Rickets in children ▪ Osteomalacia in adults	▪ Growth retardation ▪ Kidney damage ▪ Calcium deposits in soft tissues Upper level is 50 micrograms (2000 IU), based on the risk of elevated blood calcium.
Vitamin E	▪ Antioxidant: prevents breakdown of vitamin A and unsaturated fatty acids	15 milligrams alphatocopherol (22 IU natural form, 33 IU synthetic form)	▪ Plant oils ▪ Products made from plant oils ▪ Some greens ▪ Some fruit ▪ Nuts and seeds ▪ Fortified breakfast cereals	▪ Hemolysis of red blood cells ▪ Nerve degeneration	▪ Muscle weakness ▪ Headaches ▪ Nausea ▪ Inhibition of vitamin K metabolism Upper level is 1000 micrograms (1100 IU synthetic form, 1500 IU natural form), based on the risk of hemorrhage.
Vitamin K	▪ Activation of blood-clotting factors ▪ Activation of proteins involved in bone metabolism	90–120 micrograms	▪ Green vegetables ▪ Liver ▪ Some plant oils ▪ Some calcium supplements	▪ Hemorrhage ▪ Fractures	No upper level has been set.

Abbreviations: RAE=retinal activity equivalents; IU=international units

Minerals

Minerals are divided into two groups based on how much of the mineral is needed by the body. Trace (micro) minerals include iron, copper, zinc, manganese, chromium, selenium, potassium, iodine, and boron. Trace minerals are needed in relatively small amounts by the body. Bulk (macro) minerals are needed in a greater quantity and are calcium, magnesium, and phosphorus. Minerals are stored in many parts of the body, mostly in bone and muscle tissue.

Carbohydrates

Watching your "carbs" has become an extremely popular diet in our relatively new century. However, carbohydrate metabolism plays a big role in energy levels, digestive processes, and glycemic balance. **Carbohydrates** are found in plant foods such as fruits, vegetables, and grains. Our body breaks carbohydrates down into sugars, starches, cellulose, and gum.

Understanding the difference between good and bad carbohydrates can help you to plan a nutritious diet (figure 18.2). High-glycemic carbohydrates are in refined, highly processed foods. They are usually high in sugar and are digested quickly. The quick digestion and easy breakdown allows the sugars to enter the bloodstream at a jolting speed. Eating these refined carbohydrates too often can lead to a severe increase in blood sugar levels, which then triggers the release of insulin to compensate. This use of "bad" high-glycemic carbohydrates can put the body in a roller-coaster effect of too much energy followed by a quick drop to absolute fatigue. A snack of doughnuts and sugary coffee may be a quick energy fix. The surge of insulin your body will produce to correct the sugar levels, however, may actually cause you to feel more fatigued.

To keep energy levels stable, you should be eating "good" or low-glycemic foods such as vegetables, some fruits, and whole grains. These low-glycemic carbohydrates take longer to digest, so they are released slowly into the bloodstream, thus avoiding the roller-coaster ride. If you plan to watch your carbohydrates, you should go by a "glycemic index" that lists food sources and how they react when they reach the bloodstream. Product labels are not an effective way to accurately measure the physiological affects of carbohydrates. The US Food and Drug Administration (FDA) does not require manufacturers to list the total carbohydrate content on food packages. The FDA measures carbohydrates by their chemical makeup, not by their physiological effects on the consumer's body.

Fiber is a category of carbohydrate and is considered a "complex carbohydrate." It is the stringy and tough part of vegetables, fruits, and grains. Fiber does not supply the body with energy, but it serves the body by performing several important functions:

Figure 18.2
Carbohydrates should form the foundation of our diet.

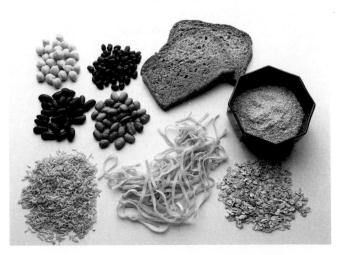

- Fiber increases and softens the stool to promote normal defecation.
- Fiber absorbs toxins and organic wastes so they can be removed from the body.
- Fiber decreases the rate of breakdown and absorption of carbohydrates.

Adding fiber to the diet can be of great help in treating constipation, hemorrhoids, diverticular disease, and especially irritable bowel syndrome. Adequate fiber intake can reduce blood cholesterol levels and aid in the control of certain types of diabetes. Fiber is found in two forms: soluble fiber (found in oats, beans, barley, and vegetables) and insoluble (found in wheat bran and brown rice). For fiber to do its job, adequate water intake is critical.

Fats and Lipids

The category of nutrients known as lipids is made up of fats, oils, and cholesterol. See examples in figure 18.3. The chemical makeup and role the substance plays in the body determine which category the lipid belongs to. Of these, **fats** are substances found in the food we eat. Fats are not water-soluble and can be stored indefinitely within the body. We all know that fats and especially the bad, low-density cholesterol (LDL) can contribute to arterial and cardiac disease, but fats do have a positive role within the body. Some of the benefits are:

- Fats include the essential fatty acids and provide the fat-soluble vitamins.
- Fats increase the flavor of our foods.
- Fats help us to feel full because they take longer to digest.
- Excess protein and carbohydrates are stored as fat to be used as the body needs extra nutrition.
- Estrogen and other hormones are stored in the fat of the body.
- The essential fatty acids (omega-3 and omega-6) are needed for energy, healthy skin, normal reproductive system functions, brain function, and blood pressure and clotting.

Cholesterol is a lipid that is found only in animal food products. Even lean meat has a large amount of cholesterol. In the past, cholesterol has been given a bad name because of its contribution to arterial and heart diseases, such as arteriosclerosis and hypertension. But cholesterol in moderated amounts plays a beneficial role in maintaining the health of our body. Cholesterol is found throughout the body and serves as the building block for estrogen, testosterone, and the vitamin D that is produced in the skin during exposure to sunlight. Cholesterol also contributes to brain and nerve function. Cutting all cholesterol from your diet can contribute to ill health and has been associated with symptoms of schizophrenia and other types of mental illness.

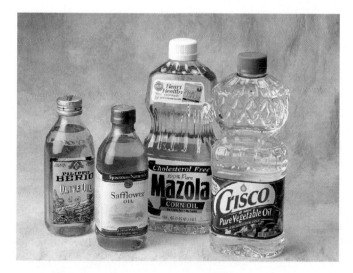

Figure 18.3
Plant oils vary in their fatty acid contents. Olive and canola oils are rich in monounsaturated fat.

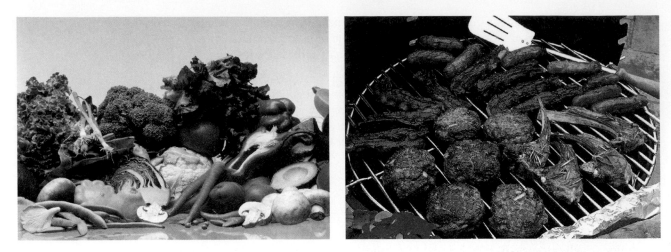

Figure 18.4
The body makes protein from amino acids that naturally occur in plants and animal foods.

Proteins

Proteins are vital to the growth and development of the human body. They are the building blocks for all bodily tissue. For healing of muscle and tissue injuries, it is very important that your diet includes enough protein.

The body makes protein from **amino acids,** which are naturally occurring organic compounds found in plant and animal foods. Figure 18.4 shows different sources of protein. These amino acids are used to build and maintain tissue. If other sources of energy are low, they may be used to supply energy. A gram of protein contains roughly 4 calories, and the excess protein in the body is broken down and stored as fat. A deficiency in protein can lead to weight loss and fatigue, malnutrition, dry skin, a lowered resistance to infection, and interference with cell division and normal growth processes.

There are 20 amino acids that are necessary to the body. The body can make 11 of them, but the remaining nine, called the essential amino acids, must be obtained through diet. Proteins that contain all nine essential amino acids are called **complete proteins.** Complete proteins are found in animal food products, such as fish, eggs, meat, poultry, and milk. Individual vegetables or fruits do not contain complete proteins and provide the incomplete proteins that lack one or more of the essential amino acids. However, combining different plant sources—such as beans and corn, or rice and beans—can provide all nine of the essential amino acids. These combinations can contribute to an adequate diet for vegetarians who eat no meat or animal products. A vegetarian diet allows the follower to eat more food and have a high fiber intake with less fat.

Digestion, Absorption, and Metabolism

Our body cannot receive the nutrients from food until the food that is eaten is digested. The process of **digestion**—the breakdown of food—can be very different for each person, depending on the efficiency the body maintains in completing it. Illnesses and age can change the body's ability to break down certain foods. If the food is not digested properly, then the nutrients remain locked away and the food substance may cause physical discomfort before it leaves the intestinal tract. See figure 18.5 for digestive functions.

Digestion begins in the mouth when we first begin to chew our food. This is known as ingestion. Food that is improperly chewed will remain as chunks as it passes through the intestines. This can cause severe gastrointestinal distress, such as bloating, gas, and abdominal cramping, along with diarrhea. When you chew your food until it is of paste consistency, you allow the digestive enzymes to break it down into tiny particles that can be digested.

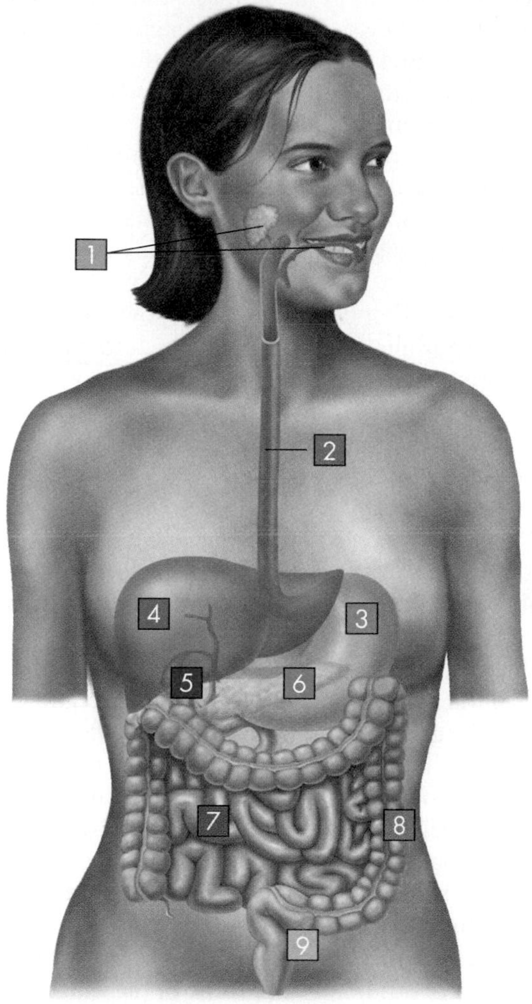

Organ	Digestive Functions
1 Mouth and salivary glands	Chewing begins
	Moisten food with saliva
	Lubrication with mucus
	Release of starch-digesting (amylase) enzyme
	Initiation of swallowing reflex
2 Esophagus	Lubrication with mucus
	Move food to stomach by peristaltic waves
3 Stomach	Store, mix, dissolve, and continue digestion of food
	Dissolve food particles with secretions
	Kill microorganisms with acid
	Release of protein-digesting (pepsin) enzyme
	Lubricate and protect stomach surface with mucus
	Regulate emptying of dissolved food into small intestine
4 Liver	Production of bile to aid in fat digestion and absorption
5 Gallbladder	Storage, concentration, and later release of bile into the small intestine
6 Pancreas	Secretion of sodium bicarbonate and carbohydrate-, fat-, and protein-digesting enzymes
7 Small intestine	Mixing and propulsion of contents
	Lubrication with mucus
	Digestion and absorption of most substances using enzymes made by the pancreas and small intestine
8 Large intestine	Mixing and propulsion of contents
	Absorption of sodium, potassium, and water
	Storage and concentration of undigested food
	Lubrication with mucus
	Formation of feces
9 Rectum	Store feces and expel via the anus

Figure 18.5
The organs of the digestive system work together to allow ingestion, digestion, absorption, and elimination.

In the mouth, saliva is secreted that contains the enzyme ptyalin. This enzyme is important in the digestion of starch. Since no starch-digesting enzymes are found in the stomach, the pancreas secretes an enzyme in the small intestine that continues the process to completion. The ptyalin in the mouth is also responsible for breaking down the starches and sugars that adhere to the teeth, helping to prevent periodontal disease and tooth decay.

When foods reach the stomach, hydrochloric acid and pepsin (an enzyme) begin the process of breaking down protein. Protein digestion is very slow, and a series of enzymes and stomach secretions work in a synchronized harmony to complete the process. At the same time as the secretions are emptying into the stomach, the stomach walls are moving in waves to "churn" or stir the mixture. If an antacid is taken before eating, the acid is not released and the process does not complete, leaving large chunks of protein to pass through the intestinal track and be of no nutritional value to the body.

Fruits and vegetables are processed more quickly and leave the stomach in a very short time. Their nutrients are more readily absorbed by the intestines, and very little of the body's energy is used to digest them. Fats remain in the stomach and require the longest time to process. You can understand how they sit heavy in the stomach by taking a look at bacon fat. The fat requires temperatures much higher than that produced by the body to become liquid, so as bacon fat passes through the stomach and intestines, it remains in the "glob" state that it becomes at room temperature.

The body is carefully choreographed to allow enzymes and mucus to balance the alkaline and acid of the stomach to produce the desired digestive effects. When this dance is not functioning normally, severe illness can occur. If the gastric juice, which is also known as hydrochloric acid, is deficient, then disorders such as pernicious anemia can occur.

The small intestine is where the absorption of food particles, now down to molecules, occurs. The small intestine is lined with millions of tiny villi, which themselves are covered with microvilli. These "hairy" projections filter the procession of molecules and absorb the nutrients, while preventing materials considered toxic, such as unhealthy bacteria and pollutants, from entering the bloodstream. This process can be weakened by continual ingestion of drugs, alcohol, and pesticides.

Pancreas and Liver

The **pancreas** lies in the center of the abdomen, at the solar plexus, and is only an organ of secretion. No food actually flows through the pancreas. This organ makes and secretes three enzymes. These enzymes break down proteins and act on fats and carbohydrates. If the food coming into the small intestine is too acid, then the pancreatic secretions, along with the **bile** secreted from the **gallbladder,** which are more alkaline in nature, help to break down the foods.

The **liver** is the chemical warehouse of the body. If the liver is not functioning properly, health and well-being, including mental health, cannot be possible. When food nutrients are absorbed through the walls of the small intestine, they go into the portal vein. All of the veins of the body go into the heart except for the portal vein. It goes into the liver and becomes tiny capillaries. The nutrient-laden blood flows around and through the liver cells and is then collected in the vena cava. This is where the liver works its magic. It releases nutrients into the bloodstream but holds back some of the nutrients, so as not to overload the body. The nutrients held in storage are released when the body needs them. If the liver is damaged by illness or abuse, the body can be poisoned by the release of unfiltered blood, and nutrients will not be sent when and where needed.

To complete the process for storage, the liver takes the many types of sugars, which come directly from ingested sugar or from starch chains that have been broken down, and hooks them together to make one huge storage molecule of glycogen. If the liver is healthy, it can pull a lot of sugar from the blood and convert it into glycogen to release later when little sugar is coming in. In that way, it controls the surge of sugar to the bloodstream. When the liver fails at this because it is diseased or weakened, the sugar is not filtered out and is carried throughout the body. When the sugar floods the bloodstream, the pancreas is stimulated to release more insulin to balance the blood sugar level. When the insulin is released, the cell walls become more permeable and the excess sugar is taken into the cells. The excess in insulin can cause the sudden drop in blood sugar due to the cells being saturated. This saturation of the cells can cause you to feel weak, irritable, and fatigued, and to experience muscle cramping and vision problems. This condition is called **hypoglycemia.** If there is a limited amount of stored sugar in the liver, you will reach for foods such as candy bars or pastries to give you quick energy. When this vicious cycle is a constant in your diet, the liver will begin to push excess sugar through the cell walls and into the fat lining of the stomach. The classic "beer belly" is a result of this syndrome. You become overweight very quickly when your consumption of sugars, carbohydrates, and starches is greater than the amount that the liver can process at any given time. Several small meals of complex foods keep the blood sugar steady and allow the liver to process and stop the storage, without you feeling a loss of energy or mood swings.

The processing of proteins is another amazing function in which the liver has as a major role. When protein is absorbed, the liver remakes the amino acids into new chemical forms. It then distributes them to the various cells in whatever form the cells need at that particular time.

The liver's role in processing fat depends on the presence of bile. Bile salts are formed in the liver from cholesterol. The bile passes from the liver into the gallbladder, where it is stored until it is needed. When food enters the small intestine, the gallbladder squirts the bile out to assist in the digestion of fats. After the bile salts have acted on the fats, they are removed by the body through the process of elimination. Most nutritionists agree that the faster the process of digestion and elimination, the less chance of cholesterol being stored in the body. When the process is slow due to poor diet or a compromised digestive system, the body has the time to reabsorb its own cholesterol and put it back into the bloodstream. When the bile contains a high concentration of cholesterol, it forms crystals. These crystals can become large enough to block the bile duct, which in turn backs up the bile. The crystals become gallstones, and if they block the duct, your body may be unable to digest fat, which can make you quite ill. Gallstones may be flushed from the body when small, but if they are too large, they must be surgically removed. They often damage the gallbladder, so it is removed as well.

Elimination

The digestive system is divided into two functional systems. The mouth, stomach, and small intestines—the upper system—work to digest and absorb. The lower part of the digestive system is made up of the colon or large intestine. The **colon** has one specific function, elimination. To help the colon further break down the waste material, quite a large number of microbes "live" within its walls. Some scientists who study these microorganisms feel that they are an organ of their own. New discoveries of how they function are occurring almost daily.

As food is passed through the upper digestive system, almost all of the nutrients are removed. The leftovers are in a semisolid mass that contains fiber and water. The water is absorbed to continue the solidifying process, and bacteria multiply and invade the material to turn it into feces, which passes. Along with bacteria, there are also fungi, yeasts, and viruses at work. Only certain microbes are suitable for this process, and if the balance is undone by antibiotics, toxins, or uncooked foods laden with outside bacteria, then irritation and illness can occur.

The amount of fiber that is eaten has the greatest influence on the number and type of intestinal microbes. Early humans had an abundance of fiber in their diet due to the natural aspects of the foods that were available for consumption. Modern humans, especially in the industrialized western nations, consume a mostly refined and overprocessed diet with little fiber. This constant lack of fiber plays havoc in the colon and can lead to chronic constipation and even colon cancer. For the body to operate efficiently, foods should take less than 72 hours to pass from mouth to colon. If the foods we ingest included the proper amount of fiber and were unrefined, our digestive systems could pass the food through in four to six hours. The less time spent processing food, the less time toxins, cholesterol, and unnatural bacteria will have to stay inside our bodies and do harm. Less time spent on digestion will also lead to a greater energy level and overall feeling of well-being.

As physicians, dieticians, and nutritionists study the nutritional factors involved in maintaining wellness, they are becoming more convinced and have the scientific evidence to link nearly all of our body's disease processes to the lack of proper nutrition. Even diseases you may feel have nothing to do with digestive processes, such as arthritis

Nutritional Pathology

Figure 18.6
Binge eating disorders occur in both men and women.

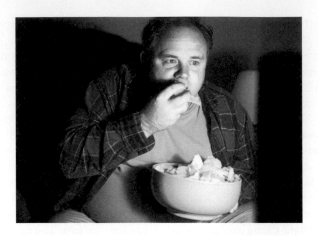

or kidney stones, are linked to the chemical and enzymatic processes that occur when we ingest foods.

Our food patterns begin when we are babies and set our body's eating habits. Such habits may contribute to the formation of a healthy, well-rounded, energetic, and bright individual, or they can lead to an illness-ridden, lethargic, and short-lived life (figure 18.6). Our food patterns usually imitate those of our parents, especially our mothers. Remember, 2-year-old children cannot drive to the fast-food restaurant, order, and pay for their own French fries; someone has to hand them the first one.

Many people today will stop at nothing to remain trim or athletic. The incidence of bulimia, which is a gorge-then-purge syndrome, and anorexia nervosa, a disease in which a person has an aversion to food, is at epidemic levels. The use of steroids and diet supplements to increase strength and endurance is contributing to the deaths of young people nationwide. We are fast becoming an obese and sick population. This could all change if a proper diet, with complete nutrition, is consumed and moderate exercise is practiced. Imagine a world in which many people over 50 years of age do not spend a quarter of their income on health concerns per year or miss, on the average, five workdays per month. Having the discipline and spending the time to maintain health and well-being is the path to a longer and better quality of life, with a stronger body and a sharper mind.

Food and the Mind

Our brains are nothing more than carbon-based computers. To work at maximum efficiency, the brain requires oxygen, glucose, and nutrients, which it does not manufacture. The process of "feeding the brain" is a highly complicated metabolic and physiological mechanism. All nutrients must pass through the **blood-brain barrier,** which is a protective barrier that occurs naturally and functions by allowing tight cell-to-cell contact within the capillaries to prevent harmful substances from leaving the blood and entering the brain tissue.

The nutrients that are sent to the brain come from the food that has been eaten, digested, and absorbed; from nutrients secreted or synthesized from organs and glands; and sometimes even from the intestinal microbes. So you can see that for the brain to work to its optimal level, there has to be a complex and complete nutritional system.

Many studies are being done that show the correlation between brain nutrition and mental distress, hyperactivity, depression, and criminal behavior. It has been found that young adults on a diet high in carbohydrates, with very little fiber or vitamin content, and food additives such as artificial sweeteners, flavors, and coloring tend to have lower grades in school, lack the ability to focus or remember, and exhibit violent, disruptive behavior. Most treatment centers for people with violent, uncontrollable behavior or debilitating phobias are now integrating a dietary program that will balance the brain chemistry and relax the neurological and glandular systems.

Natural health care practitioners have known for centuries that a properly balanced diet can lead to optimum health and even heal illnesses. Physicians also know through extensive research that infants who receive poor nutrition while in their mothers' wombs are born with developmental complications. Many of these complications are a result of the infants' brains not receiving the nutrients needed for growth. For instance, a lack of folic acid during gestation can lead to birth defects that include brain and neural dysfunction for the life of the child. Also, toxins such as alcohol, nicotine, or drugs passed from the mother to the fetus can also lead to impaired brain capacity and behavioral problems.

Alternative Diets

A wide variety of diets are popular today. Some diets are used primarily for weight loss. When planning a diet, you are more likely to be successful in losing weight if you choose a diet (eating plan) that includes proper nutrition and balances the blood sugar level. If your eating habits reflect good nutrition, the proper weight and muscle-to-body-fat ratio will be maintained. With good nutrition, you will also experience high energy levels and a feeling of mental clarity and lightheartedness that will spread into other areas of your life, such as relationships and work. A tired, irritable, often sick massage therapist will seldom have the level of practice that will ensure financial prosperity.

The type of diet you choose depends strictly on personal preference. We all remember the food pyramids we studied in school that gave us the choices of foods available for nutrition. Today, it has been proven that the Mediterranean pyramid plan, which uses whole grains, little meat, and an abundance of olive oil, can contribute to lower cholesterol and lessen the possibility of heart disease. The Latin American food pyramid gives a dietary plan that is high in fiber (beans and corn), which can lower blood pressure and the risk of colon cancer. It uses avocado in the same way that the Mediterranean dietary plan uses olives and olive oil to reduce cholesterol and give the brain the essential fatty acids it needs.

The Asian pyramid is a plan often adopted by menopausal women who choose soy protein, fish (omega acids), and phytoestrogens found in vegetables because they alleviate menopausal symptoms and can diminish the possibility of high blood pressure and breast cancer.

A vegetarian diet is one of the healthiest ways of eating. Vegetarians do not eat meat, poultry, or fish. Some vegetarians—those who follow a vegan diet—eat only vegetable, grain, or fruit products. Nonvegan vegetarians (lactovegetarians) do consume milk, yogurt, cheese, and other dairy products. Persons eating a strictly vegetarian diet have the lowest incidence of illness. Due to the antioxidants occurring naturally in fruits and vegetables, toxins are reduced that can contribute to premature aging. Although a vegetarian diet that does not include dairy products containing a high level of calcium may not seem likely to fight osteoporosis, broccoli, okra, and other vegetables provide ample calcium.

American Diet: Recommendations Versus Reality

The food pyramid accepted by the US Food and Drug Administration reflects American tastes. The US Department of Agriculture's (USDA) food guide pyramid is pictured in figure 18.7. Although it contains a high amount of meat products, it is primarily built around grains, fruits, and vegetables. It recommends three to five servings of vegetables daily to reduce cancer and heart disease, and six to 11 servings of grains (pasta, whole grain breads, rice, and cereal) to add fiber. The problem is not with the American dietary plan. We are a nation of many malnourished, obese people because we do not follow the plan as outlined. Most of us eat far less than the recommended portions of grains, and when we do eat grains, we choose hamburger buns full of salt, sugar, nondigestible fats, and empty calories. Many of us choose potatoes deep fried in heavy oils (French fries) for our vegetables or fruit packed in sugar syrup and preservatives. These are not

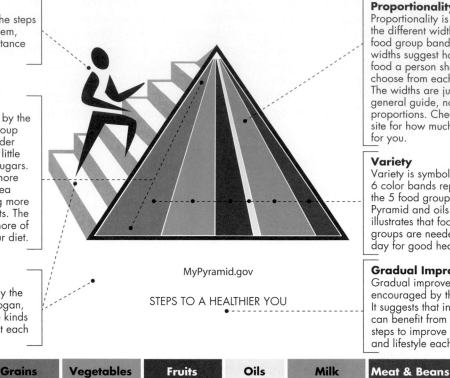

Activity
Activity is represented by the steps and the person climbing them, as a reminder of the importance of daily physical activity.

Moderation
Moderation is represented by the narrowing of each food group from bottom to top. The wider base stands for foods with little or no solid fats or added sugars. These should be selected more often. The narrower top area stands for foods containing more added sugars and solid fats. The more active you are, the more of these foods can fit into your diet.

Personalization
Personalization is shown by the person on the steps, the slogan, and the Web site. Find the kinds and amounts of food to eat each day at MyPyramid.gov.

Proportionality
Proportionality is shown by the different widths of the food group bands. The widths suggest how much food a person should choose from each group. The widths are just a general guide, not exact proportions. Check the Web site for how much is right for you.

Variety
Variety is symbolized by the 6 color bands representing the 5 food groups of the Pyramid and oils. This illustrates that foods from all groups are needed each day for good health.

Gradual Improvement
Gradual improvement is encouraged by the slogan. It suggests that individuals can benefit from taking small steps to improve their diet and lifestyle each day.

MyPyramid.gov

STEPS TO A HEALTHIER YOU

| Grains | Vegetables | Fruits | Oils | Milk | Meat & Beans |

Figure 18.7
The USDA's food guide pyramid uses a personalized approach to healthy eating and physical activity.

what the plan considers proper foods. The tendency to snack seems to plague even individuals who eat a balanced diet of nutritious meals. Many health-conscience people admit to consuming ice cream, candy bars, or the empty calories of carbohydrate snacks before going to bed at night or having pastries for breakfast instead of nutrient-rich, low-sugar grains. Our love of junk food snacking begins at an early age and often continues into adulthood. Many people, however, seek to break this cycle by advocating healthy snacking for children. The Children's Television Workshop's *Sesame Street* should be commended for suggesting that Cookie Monster reserve his cookies for special snacks and choose such things as bagels and fruits for his everyday snacks.

Chapter Summary

Good nutrition may take a little planning on your part, but its impact on your overall health is invaluable. When we eat the right foods and our body is able to digest and absorb nutrients efficiently, we maintain a level of health and energy that allows a quality of life that makes every aspect of living a joy. You will reap the benefits of working well-fueled in a profession that you enjoy. A massage therapist who eats a healthy, balanced diet is also a good example of someone who embraces the concept of wellness. The basic nutritional concepts presented here will help you to understand what you may need to do to remain healthy.

Box 18.1   Body Mass Index

The body mass index (BMI) is a method of measuring weight for height that provides a good estimate of body fat content. The ranges of BMI are used to define weights for height that correspond to underweight, normal weight, and obesity in adults. To calculate your BMI, divide your weight in pounds by your height in inches, then divide the result by height in inches again, and multiply that answer by 703.

Example:

Your weight is 140 pounds and your height is 5 feet, 3 inches.

Figure your height in inches: 5 feet =
60 inches + 3 inches =
63 inches

Divide your weight by your height: 140 ÷ 63 =
2.22

Divide the result by your height again: 2.22 ÷ 63 =
0.035

Multiply the answer by 703: 0.035 × 703 = 24.8

Your BMI is 24.8.

Where do you fall on the chart if your BMI is 24.8?

Underweight	Under 18.5
Normal	18.5–25
Overweight	25–30
Obese	30–35
Moderately obese	36–40
Severely obese	40+

Applying Your Knowledge

Self-Testing

1. Which of the following is not a benefit of fats in the body?

   a) Fats are needed for energy, healthy skin, and brain function.

   b) Fats increase the flavor of our foods.

   c) Essential fatty acids are needed for blood pressure and clotting.

   d) Fats keep bacteria away from our teeth.

2. What are lipids made of?

   a) Fats, oils, and bile

   b) Fats, lipids, and cholesterol

   c) Fats, oils, and cholesterol

   d) Omega 3, olive oil, and vitamin D

3. Which of the following choices represents the best way to lose weight?

   a) Not eating at bedtime

   b) Taking diet pills

   c) Eating fewer calories

   d) Eating empty calories

4. Which of the following substances in food is most often considered a contributor to high blood pressure?

   a) Cholesterol

   b) Sugar

   c) Salt (sodium)

   d) Calcium

5. Which of the following dietary conditions can lead to the development of osteoporosis?

   a) Not enough dietary fiber

   b) Low calcium intake

   c) Too much fat in the diet

   d) Eating too much salt

6. What eating disorder is characterized by extreme weight loss and an aversion to food?

   a) Amylophagia

   b) Anorexia nervosa

   c) Bulimia

   d) Atherosclerosis

7. What are the nutrients that can only be made available by the foods we eat called?

   a) Essential nutrients

   b) Organic food nutrients

   c) Lipids

   d) Nonessential nutrients

8. What is the layer of tight cell-to-cell walls used to protect the brain called?

   a) Bone calcium barrier

   b) Nonbrain barrier

   c) Blood toxin barrier

   d) Blood-brain barrier

9. When foods reach the stomach, what begins to break down protein?

   a) Hydrochloric acid and pepsin

   b) Potassium and phosphates

   c) Sodium and amylase

   d) Ptyalin and saliva

10. How many servings of grains per day does the American food pyramid recommend?

   a) 2 to 10

   b) 2 to 4

   c) 6 to 11

   d) 8 to 12

11. What does eating a balanced diet lead to?

   a) Better weight control

   b) High energy levels

   c) Healthy living

   d) All the above are correct.

Case Studies/Critical Thinking

A. Mary is a massage therapist working in an uptown spa. She often works extra hours by helping out the spa owner with paperwork after she has seen her clients for the day. Most days, she has so much to do that she skips lunch or grabs a candy bar from the vending machine next door. She recently has noticed that she feels weak and has little energy or strength when doing a massage on her 2 p.m. client. What may be her problem?

B. Garrett has been gaining weight consistently since he started to work as a therapist at a sports clinic. He is happy with his work and has continued to work out at least 30 minutes a day but has gained 25 pounds in the last two months. The only change he has made to his eating habits is that he eats lunch everyday—and sometimes grabs something for breakfast—from the fast-food restaurant across the street. While working at his old job, he usually ate at a nearby restaurant that served steamed seafood, vegetables, and fruit salads. What can Garrett do to change his eating habits and reduce his weight?

References for information in this chapter can be found in Quick Guide C at the end of the book.

CHAPTER 19

Eastern and Western Principles of Movement

LEARNING OUTCOMES

After completing this chapter, you will be able to:

- Recognize and be able to differentiate between Eastern and Western principles or philosophies of movement and stretching.

- Recognize the chakras and their locations, colors, and associated glands.

- Perform basic yoga asanas.

- Become acquainted with Qi Gong and T'ai Chi movements.

- Perform basic Western stretching exercises.

- Discuss the indications and contraindications to stretching.

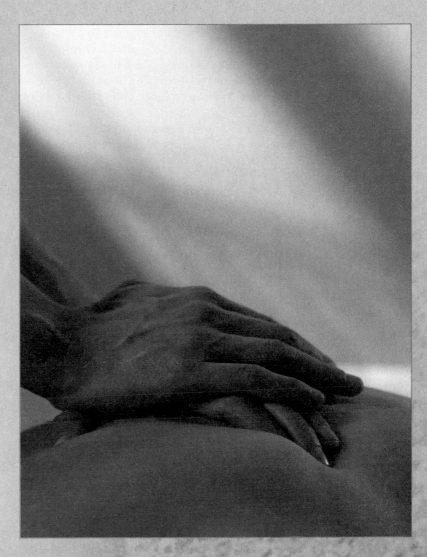

KEY TERMS

adaptation *(p. 514)*

asanas *(p. 497)*

chakras *(p. 498)*

elasticity *(p. 524)*

meditation *(p. 498)*

overload principle *(p. 514)*

plasticity *(p. 524)*

prana (p. 498)

Qi Gong *(p. 512)*

T'ai Chi *(p. 514)*

yoga *(p. 497)*

INTRODUCTION

Stretching should be an integral part of the massage therapist's self-care or wellness program. Chapters 15 and 16 illustrate the similarities and differences between the Eastern and Western approaches to massage and healing. In this chapter, we would like you to explore both Eastern and Western forms of movement and stretching.

Consider the focus of the Eastern health and wellness model: to view the body as a whole, closely intertwined with the mental and spiritual aspects of oneself. Eastern movements (exercises) are ones that involve the whole body, the breath, and the mental and spiritual components. Conversely, Western exercise tends to focus on one body part with each part (muscle or muscle group) being developed separately from others. The mental and spiritual aspects usually do not play a part other than to infuse stamina into the workout session, although the breath is employed during such movements as lifting and releasing weights.

A well-rounded health and wellness program will include both Eastern and Western principles of movement along with proper nutritional support (see chapter 18). We hope this chapter will encourage you to adopt a practice that will lead to greater control of your muscles, give you poise, and help you achieve mental and physical balance. Besides helping you deliver a memorable, well-choreographed massage, you may discover an additional direction in which to take your practice. Many massage therapists become certified in personal training or a discipline such as yoga so that they can instruct clients. Whether your personal tastes fall into the Eastern or Western genres and you enjoy the expressiveness of dance, the physicality of rollerblading, the strength of martial arts, or the equanimity of yoga, try to embrace an activity that helps you put it all together—full-body movements, rhythmic breathing, and focus on intent (figure 19.1).

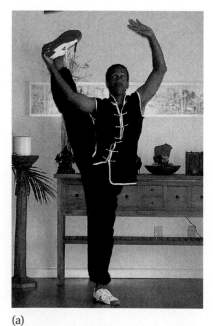 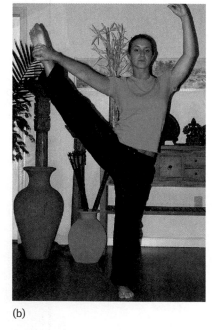 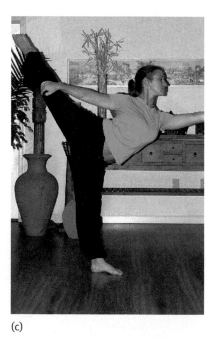

(a) (b) (c)

Figure 19.1

(*a*) The martial arts foster strength and flexibility.   (*b*) Dance develops poise.   (*c*) Expressiveness of dance.

Yoga originated over thousands of years ago with sages who were attuned to the workings of and movement of energy through their bodies. The most noted of these sages, Patanjali, wrote a treatise on medicine and yoga between 200 and 800 BCE that became known as *Patanjali's Yoga Sutra*. Although Patanjali brought together all known literature to form *The Eight Limbs of Ashtanga Yoga* (an eight-step path of living a balanced lifestyle), there exists today many types or paths of yoga, all of which originate from *Patanjali's Yoga Sutra*. Some forms of yoga focus on the physical or asana aspect (Hatha) while others emphasize meditation *(Raja)*, sound vibration *(Japa* or *Laya)*, or breathing techniques *(Pranayama)*.

The word *yoga* comes from the Sanskrit root word *yug*, meaning to join or unite.

EXAM POINT   Yoga is the union of mind, body, and spirit.

In India, the principle of health is based on these forces being in balance. In the Near and Far East, the philosophical basis for well-being is to look at the body as a whole. This "big picture" point of view strives to integrate all aspects of the human organism in an effort to prevent and treat *dis-ease*. In contrast, traditional Western ideology is "reductionist," or one that looks at parts of an individual. Treatment addresses each element separately, with prevention only having begun to enter into the Western medical model. Yoga encourages health through uniting these parts to be equal to a whole.

EXAM POINT   Chapter 15 introduced you to both *Ayurveda*, a system of health and well-being using diet, herbs, and massage, and the concept of yin and yang, or the dynamic balance of opposites.

Yoga, Qi Gong, and Tai Chi all encourage the entire body to move in balance with both strength and flexibility. Indeed, yoga is the only exercise that requires muscles to function in a contracted state (strength) with elongation (flexibility). In this chapter, we will explore both the meditative and physical aspects of yoga. Most yoga disciplines are based on Hatha yoga. The word *Hatha* represents the two polarities of yin and yang.

Today, numerous types of yoga exist, all to meet the needs of a wide variety of people and personality types. For example, hatha yoga, gentler in its approach to stretching and movement, is of interest to a laid-back person, while *Ashtanga* or Power Yoga fits well with the "Type-A" personality (usually the typical gym member). In fact, most yoga practiced in the Western Hemisphere is physical in nature with less emphasis on meditation and breathing. Several yogi gurus, or "personalities," have put together their own programs, which are known by their names. Two examples of popular yoga that carry the guru's name are Iyengar and Bik Ram.

Although many people think of yoga as merely convoluted twisted positions, it is so much more. Yoga serves as a source of connection to self and others, and makes even difficult tasks seem possible.

EXAM POINT   Breathing exercises, meditation, and gentle stretching postures **(asanas)** condition every muscle, tendon, and ligament to ensure a strong yet supple body.

Affirmations and mantras cultivate a positive attitude that helps to bring many hopes and desires to fruition.

In addition, an inverted posture, such as a head or shoulder stand, is beneficial to fostering a youthful appearance. A typical yoga session fulfills all of these requirements. Besides achieving optimal health through yoga, as a massage therapist, you will appreciate the balance, strength, and flexibility yoga practice has to offer. Indeed, asanas such as *Virabhadrasana* (the Warrior pose) are the same positions you will use at the side of the massage table. Further, yoga practice (or Tai Chi and Qi Gong) will encourage graceful movements, allowing you to "dance" around the table and harmoniously flow with your client.

If you are new to yoga, select a class that teaches basic Hatha yoga. This will give you an excellent introduction to yoga. Leave *Ashtanga* (power) or Bik Ram (done in a room heated to 104°F) yoga to those who are more experienced. Videotapes are helpful but should be used in conjunction with a class taught by a qualified yoga instructor. Look for an instructor who is a member of the Yoga Alliance (RYT). This group was formed to uphold the integrity of yoga and has strict critertia for registration.

The Three Bodies

In *Vedic* (ancient Indian writings) tradition, yogis view the body as three bodies made up of the physical body, the astral (ethereal) body, and the causal body, which together function as the vehicle through which we reach our inner self. The physical body is what we can feel, see, and touch: ligaments, tendons, muscles, skeletal structure, senses, and organ systems. In other words, the physical body is our waking state of consciousness. The astral body is the energetic body, which manifests as an aura or energy field. The causal body is even more subtle and represents the higher mind. We experience the causal body in **meditation.** Some yogis believe it is where our karmic path is stored.

Prana and Chakras

It is a subtle form of energy that is part of everything from air to food, water, and sunlight.

Pranayama is the practice of breath control that purifies the *nadis.* The central channel is *Sushumna,* which corresponds to the spinal cord in the physical body. On either side of this main channel are *Ida* and *Pingala,* which correspond to sympathetic ganglia of the spinal cord. For a more in-depth discussion of the physiological counterparts in the body, see the section on CerebroSpinal Fluid Technique Massage in chapter 16.

Table 19.1	The Chakras				
Chakra	Color	Location	Asana	Intention	Function
Seventh or crown chakra (*Sahasrara*)	White, amethyst, violet, gold, or silver	Crown/top of the head	Headstand	Cosmic consciousness	Upper brain, right eye, pineal gland
Sixth or Brow or Third Eye chakra (*Ajna*)	Indigo, violet	Between the eyebrows	Spinal Twist	Intuition, awareness	Lower brain, left eye, spine, ears, pituitary gland
Fifth or Throat chakra (*Vishuddha*)	Blue	Throat	Shoulder stand, Plow	Speaking truth and communication	Throat, upper lungs and arms, digestive tract, thyroid gland
Fourth or Heart chakra (*Anahata*)	Green	Heart	Fish, Camel	Unconditional love	Heart and lungs, circulation, thymus gland
Third or Solar Plexus chakra (*Manipura*)	Yellow	At the diaphragm or just above the navel	Bow, Boat	Strength and self-empowerment	Stomach, pancreas, digestive system, liver, gallbladder
Second or Sacral/Splenic chakra (*Svadisthana*)	Orange	Above the pubic bone	Cobra	Sensuality and creativity	Reproductive organs, kidneys, legs, gonads
First or Root/Base chakra (*Muladhara*)	Red	Perinium	Head to Knee Pose	Survival and existence	Bladder, genitals, spine, adrenal glands

(In Sanskrit, the "ch" is hard and pronounced as the "ch" of "church" in English.) These chakras are located along the *Sushumna* channel. See table 19.1 for the chakras, with their Sanskrit names and corresponding colors, locations, asana, intention (ethereal), and function (physical) counterparts. The locations and colors of the chakras are pictured in figure 19.2.

Practice chakra balancing by breathing into each chakra, beginning with the root chakra, *Muladhara*. Work your way up through each chakra, visualizing its corresponding color as a spinning vortex opening out in all directions from your body. During meditation, you can focus on the solar plexus chakra, *Manipura,* and create a word or phrase that is particular to you. It might be a quality you admire or a goal you would like to achieve. By centering your breath in the solar plexus and repeating this mantra, you will witness the manifestation of this affirmation.

Simple breathing exercises you will find useful for both yourself and your clients are the Complete Yogic Breath and *Nadi Sodhna* (alternate nostril breathing). The Complete Yogic Breath is performed as a three-part continuous breath. The diaphragm is filled first (lowest), followed by the lungs (middle), then by the upper bronchials (upper chest). Exhalation occurs from the diaphragm first, followed by the lungs, and then the upper chest. The breath may be counted (e.g., filling the diaphragm with a count of "1, 2, 3"; filling the lungs with another count of "1, 2, 3"; and filling the upper chest with a third count of "1, 2, 3"), or you can simply feel each of the three sections filling equally. Alternate nostril breathing uses the right-hand thumb and ring finger (the other three fingers are folded down against the palm). With the thumb placed against the right nostril inhalation occurs through the left nostril to a specific count. The ring finger is

Figure 19.2 Location of chakras

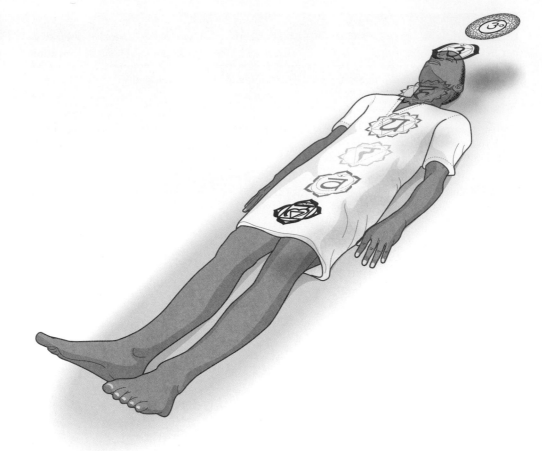

placed on the left nostril so both nostrils are held closed in retention for a specific count. The thumb is released from the right nostril, allowing exhalation for the same specific count. Inhalation occurs once again through the right nostril, both are closed in retention, and the left is released for exhalation. This is one round—from left to right and back to left. As a beginner, perform all inhalations and exhalations with equal counts. As you progress, exhalation should be twice as long as inhalation.

Basic Meditation

B. K. S. Iyengar states that yoga is a method that calms the restless mind. A Sanskrit adage holds "*Yogas chitta vritti nirodha,*" meaning yoga is a cessation of the mind. Meditation does not have to be mystical. Simply choose a convenient time and place. If possible, select an early-morning hour when the mind is still undisturbed by the day's activities. Also, try to use the same location, whether or not you set up a meditation-only room, where you will not be interrupted. You need not sit in a lotus or half-lotus position (cross-legged or "Indian style") and may sit in a straight-backed chair with your feet on the floor. It is more important to sit with a straight (but not rigid) spine, allowing the energy channels to be open. If you sit on the floor, sit on the edge of a pillow or folded blanket so that the pelvis tips slightly forward. Move into the Yogic Breath to help quiet the mind; concentrate on the sound and flow of the breath. Do not chastise yourself if your mind wanders a bit; gently bring it back to the breath. If you would like to chant, choose a word or sound that has significance for you. *Om* is the universal chant that represents the divine power in all of us. Inhale deeply, form the "O" and allow the exhale to happen. At the end of the exhale, close your lips for the "Mmm" sound (figure 19.3).

Another meditation that is uncomplicated and safe for a novice is a Tibetan meditation. This particular meditation draws on the Kundalini energy (powerful liberat-

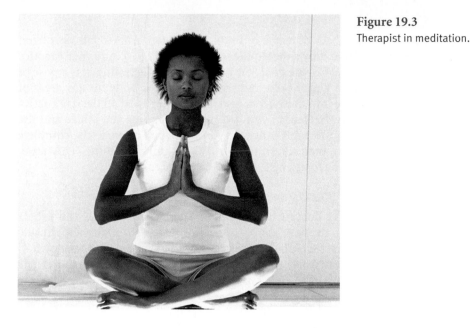

Figure 19.3
Therapist in meditation.

ing energy) housed in the base of the spine. Once again, sit with spine straight (not rigid) and move into a meditative state using one of the breathing techniques. Now visualize a ball of energy at the base of your spine. As you inhale, draw that ball of energy up your spine to the lower rib cage area, the twelfth or floating ribs, and breathe with it there. Inhale, drawing the energy up to the occipital ridge, the bony protrusion in the back of your skull, and breathe with the energy there. Now, take that energy diagonally through your head to the third eye (between your eyebrows) and breathe with it there. With practice, it is at this point that you may see things, feel things, or "know" things. Inhale once again and exhale, allowing the energy and breath to flow down the front of your spine, stopping at the heart to allow peace to enter the heart chakra. Pause and breathe until you feel ready to continue down the *sushumna* channel back to the base.

The Six Directions

In this section are simple asanas that will move your body in the six directions to achieve daily optimal health. Combine at least 20 minutes of yoga stretches with any of the Western strengthening exercises found later in this chapter to provide a total mind-body workout.

A few simple rules should be followed when performing any asana. First, always continue to breathe comfortably. If breathing is labored or you are holding your breath, back off in the pose to a comfortable position. Second, never lock your knees back in yoga; keep them "soft" so as to not hyperextend the knees. Third, always move within your body's comfort level. We all have different body types and have grown up in different environments. One person may be more flexible while another may possess more muscle strength; still others may have physical limitations, while others have absolutely none. Never try to look like the person in a video, book, or class. Remember to honor yourself by being mindful and respectful of your body.

You may find it helpful to use a yoga strap for some of the asanas. Yoga straps are made of woven canvas with a buckle on one end. They come in lengths of 8, 10, and 12 feet and in a variety of colors. Straps provide support and assistance in stretches. Do not use flexible straps; they will not give support. If you do not have a yoga strap, a belt or bathrobe tie will work well. It is also a good idea to perform asanas on a yoga mat to prevent slipping. Yoga mats can be purchased at department stores or through various yoga sites on the Web.

Corpse Pose (Savasana)

Begin with lying flat on your back on a mat or towel. Allow your arms to fall away from your sides with palms up. This allows the shoulder joint to roll open. Any yoga practice should begin and end with the Corpse pose *(Savasana)*. In the beginning, it is a pose of preparation; at the end, it is a pose of rest and repair. Scan your body for any areas of tightness and tension, breathe into these areas, and let it go. Let go of all the day's activities by focusing on your breath. Deepen your breath by extending the inhale and the exhale but keep it within a comfortable range. As you "settle in," move to the complete yogic breath for a few breaths, then return to normal, rhythmic breathing. This asana sets the stage for other poses by fostering focus and intent (figure 19.4).

Supine Big Toe/Hamstrings Stretch (Supta Padangusthasana)

From the Corpse pose, inhale, floating your arms up toward the ceiling, and exhale while lowering them to rest on the floor above your head. Stretch through the right side of your body, then through the left. Inhale once again and float the arms back down to your sides. Inhale, drawing both knees up and hugging them to your chest, and exhale while rocking back and forth (left to right). Inhale once again, exhale, and stretch the left leg out on the floor while keeping the right knee to your chest. Place a strap around the ball of the right foot or take a two-finger hold (using the index and middle fingers) on the big toe. Inhale and on the exhale, extend the right leg up toward the ceiling and breathe into the hamstring. Feel the hamstring release with each breath. (Remember to keep your spine flat on the floor, including the back of your neck.) Take the strap in your right hand, place the left hand on the left hip to keep it down on the floor, inhale, and on the exhale, open the right leg out to the right. Breathe into the adductor muscles on the inside of the thigh. Allow the strap to both facilitate the stretch and lend support so there is no straining in the groin. Inhale, drawing the leg up and switching hands so that you have the left hand holding the strap and the right hand on the right hip, then exhale, taking the right leg slightly over to the left until you feel a stretch in the IT band on the outside of the thigh. Breathe. Inhale, drawing the leg back up, and exhale, allowing the right leg to release back to the floor. Repeat this sequence with the left leg. This asana relaxes and stretches the hamstrings, adductors, and IT band/TFL (figure 19.5).

Easy Pose (Sukhasana)

Sit cross-legged with hands on your knees, palms down. Close your eyes and bring your focus to the base of your spine. Begin working your way up the spine, visualizing adding space between each vertebrae, and finishing with C1 and C2 and the crown of the head.

Figure 19.4
Savasana (Corpse pose).

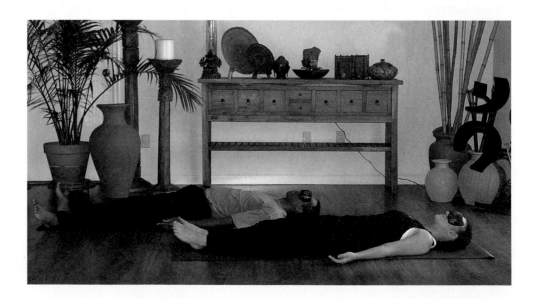

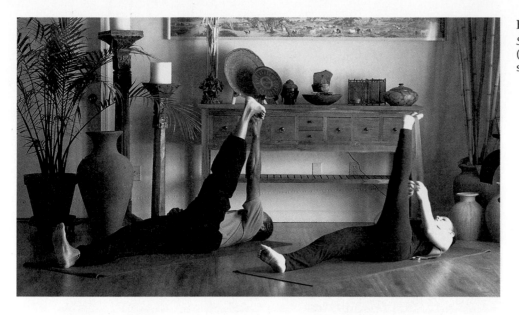

Figure 19.5
Supta Padangusthasana (supine big toe/hamstring stretch).

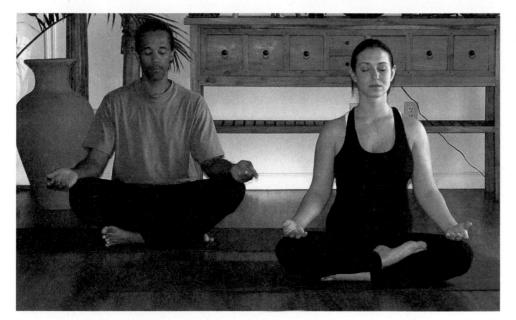

Figure 19.6
Sukhasana (Easy pose).

By visualizing space between the vertebrae, you will create length without rigidity or flattening the natural S curve in your spine. Inhale and on the exhale, fold forward from the hips, pulling on the knees for leverage, and go to a comfortable point and breathe. Feel the hips opening up and a gentle pull in the low back. Inhale, sitting back up, and exhale. Recross your legs in the other direction and repeat. This asana opens the hips and provides a gentle pull in the low back (figure 19.6)

Mountain Pose (Tadasana)

Stand with feet together or slightly apart. Imagine a triangle on the bottoms of the feet running from the ball of the foot over to the little-toe edge, down to the heel, and back up to the ball of the foot. Remain perfectly balanced on this triangle throughout. Legs are straight with knees "soft." Hip bones are open and straight ahead; tailbone points directly to the floor (but is not tucked under). Spine is comfortably straight. Arms are hanging loosely at your sides with shoulders relaxed and down. Neck is straight and

Figure 19.7
Tadasana (Mountain pose) with hands in *namasté*.

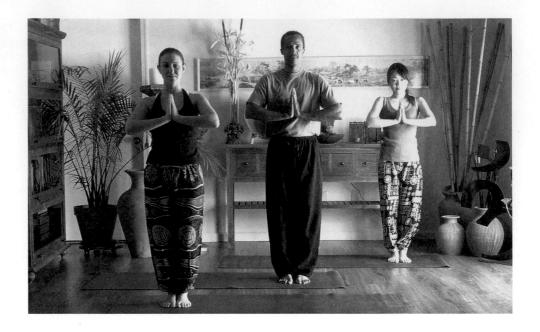

head is upright with chin lowered slightly and ears over the shoulders. Breathe. This asana encourages balance and poise (figure 19.7).

Lateral Bend (Parvatasana in Tadasana)

Standing in Mountain pose *(Tadasana)*, inhale, sweeping your arms out to the sides and up toward the ceiling; touch palms together. Exhale and drop the right arm down to your right thigh, palm facing the thigh; left arm remains up next to the left ear. Inhale, reach up with the left arm, then exhale and slide the right arm down the thigh. Inhale reaches up; exhale slides the hand down. Hips will flare to the left slightly. Go to a comfortable point and breathe. Inhale, coming up with the right arm and straightening the torso, palms touching once again, and exhale, dropping the left arm down. Repeat the lateral stretch. This asana allows for lateral flexibility in the spine.

Forward Bending Pose (Uttanasana)

From Mountain pose *(Tadasana),* place your hands in *namasté,* or prayer position, in front of your chest. Releasing your hands down to your sides, inhale, floating your arms out to the sides (with palms up) on up above your head, arms shoulder width apart with palms facing each other, and look up toward the ceiling (arms are pointing to the ceiling with shoulders relaxed and down), then exhale, folding forward from your hips, arms out to the sides or in front of you, all the way down and "hang" while holding your elbows. Release the elbows, contract your quadriceps, and use leg strength; inhale, coming up with flat back and arms out to the sides. Arms all the way up to the ceiling again, look up, and exhale, returning to starting position. Repeat several times. This asana releases the back and hamstrings (figure 19.8).

Mighty Stance (Utkatasana)

Standing in Mountain pose *(Tadasana),* extend your arms out in front of you at shoulder height, palms down. Inhale and on the exhale, bend your knees squatting down. Keep shoulders over hips and knees moving straight out. Hold. Inhale, and on the exhale, come up to standing position.

Maintaining the starting position with arms outstretched, raise up on your toes as high as you can. Inhale, and on the exhale, bend your knees squatting down once again. Hold. Inhale, and on the exhale, come up to standing position.

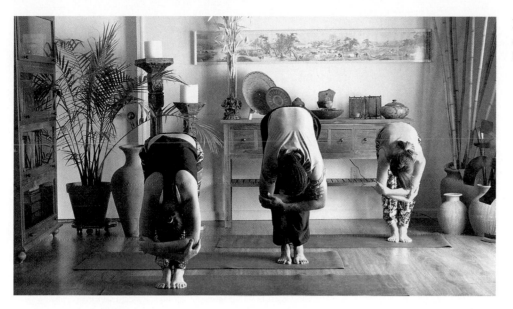

Figure 19.8
Uttanasana (Forward Bending pose).

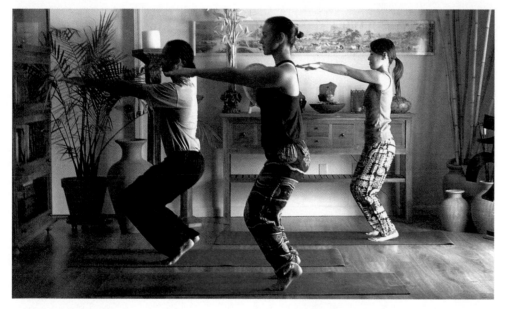

Figure 19.9
Utkatasana (Mighty Stance/quad strengthener).

Maintaining the starting position, stay on your toes (but not quite as high as before) and turn knees in and heels out. Inhale, and on the exhale, bend your knees squatting down. Hold. Inhale, and on the exhale, come up to standing. Release the arms. This asana strengthens your quadriceps, a much needed muscle group when performing massage (figure 19.9).

Warrior Pose (Virabhadrasana II)

From Mountain pose *(Tadasana)*, step out 3½ to 4 feet with your feet straight ahead. Keeping your right heel stationary, pick up your right toes and turn them out to the right 90 degrees. Keeping your left toes stationary, pick up the left heel and turn it out to the left slightly. Hold both arms out to the sides at shoulder height with palms down. Gaze over your right hand. Keep equal weight in both legs. Inhale, and on the exhale, bend the right knee to 90 degrees; exhale and glance down at your right big toe. If you cannot see the toe, draw your knee back until you can. Keep energy and

Figure 19.10
(*a*) *Virabhadrasana* II
(Warrior pose) position 1.
(*b*) *Virabhadrasana* II
(Warrior pose) position 2.
(*c*) *Virabhadrasana* II
(Warrior pose) position 3.

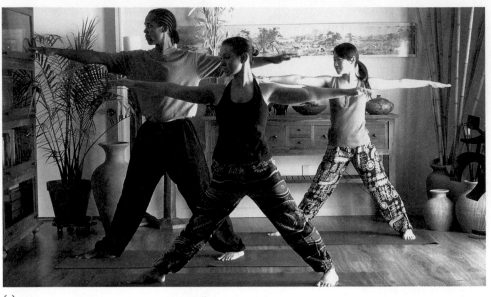

(a)

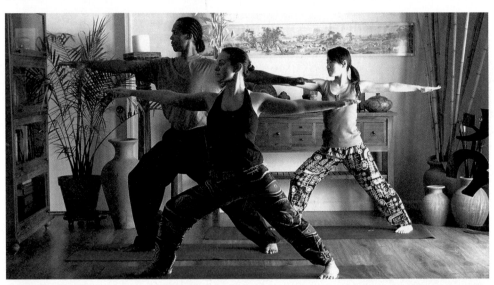

(b)

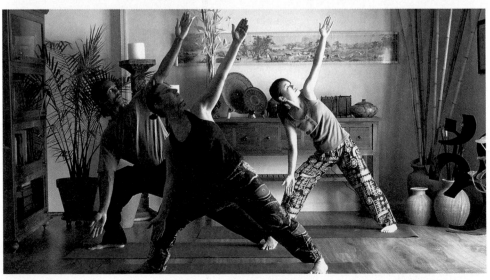

(c)

emphasis going down the right leg into the foot and press into the outside edge of the foot. Inhale once again, and on the exhale, place the right elbow on the right knee. Extend the left arm up toward the ceiling and look up at the left hand. Breathe. (You may extend the right arm down so the palm falls in front of the right ankle with palm facing out.) Inhale, coming up with the torso; exhale, straightening the right knee, with head and feet back to center. Repeat to the left. This asana helps you gain a sense of movement and balance when at the side of the massage table (figure 19.10).

Tree Pose (Vriksasana)

Standing in Mountain pose *(Tadasana)*, shift your weight over to the left. Draw the right foot up high on the inside of the left leg (thigh, calf, or ankle). Open your right knee to the side (without pulling your hips around). Place your hands in *namasté* at the chest. Inhale, and on the exhale, push your hands up above your head into steeple (fingers interlaced, index fingers pointing up). Stand tall out of the standing leg, tailbone pointing to the floor, shoulders relaxed and down, and breathe. This is a meditative pose and can be held for any length of time. Keep your eyes focused straight ahead on an object or point to help you maintain your balance. With breath and with control, lower your hands to *namasté*, lower your arms to the sides, and release the foot. Repeat on the other side. This asana promotes balance, equilibrium, and focus (figure 19.11).

Seated Spinal Twist (Bharadjasana)

Sit on the floor with legs extended. Make sure the sit bones are even. Bend the right knee and place the right foot on the floor on the outside of the left knee. Hug the knee with the left arm. Extend the right arm out in front of you at shoulder height with palm down. (Note: If one sit bone is higher than the other or off the floor, place a folded towel under the sit bone that is down to bring it up and the one up will come down. Never go into a spinal twist with an uneven pelvis.) Gaze over the right hand, and on the inhale, slowly follow it around to the right. As the arm comes slightly behind you, exhale, dropping the hand to the floor. Prop yourself up with the right hand as close to the body as possible (use a block or book under the hand if needed). Align your chin

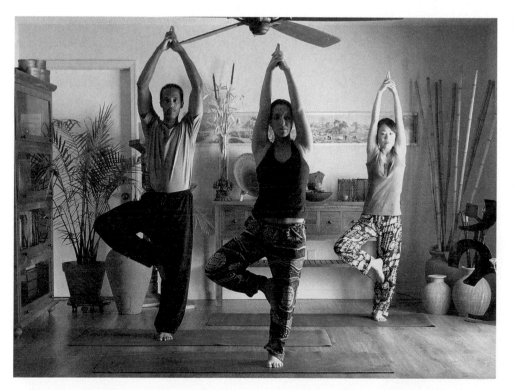

Figure 19.11
Vriksasana (Tree pose).

Figure 19.12
Bharadjasana (seated spinal twist).

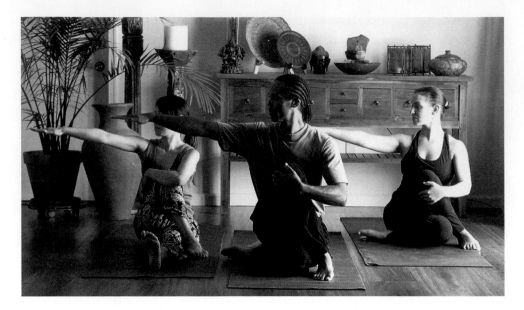

within the space between sternum and shoulder, inhale to create length, and on exhale, twist. Inhale creates length while exhale twists. Go to a comfortable point and breathe. Do not turn the head and look over the shoulder. To release, slowly pick the hand up and follow it back around to the front. Repeat to the left. This asana provides spinal rotation for flexibility (figure 19.12).

Knee/Head Pose (Janu Sirsasana)

Sit on the floor with legs stretched out in front of you; make sure your sit bones are even. Open the right leg out to the side and bend the left knee, drawing the left foot to the inside of the right thigh. Inhale, sweeping your arms out to the sides and up; exhale, turning and lining your sternum up with the right thigh. Inhale once again, and on the exhale, fold forward from your hips. Pause and inhale, getting length in the spine, and exhale, folding from the hips. Drop your hands and arms down to either side of your right leg. Looking out over the foot, breathe. If your back is strong, inhale and come up in reverse; otherwise, walk your hands up your legs and return to center. Return the right leg to the center and repeat to the left. This asana opens hips and stretches hamstrings (figure 19.13).

Boat Pose (Navasana)

Sit on the floor with legs outstretched. Draw knees up, place feet on floor, and hug knees. Rock back onto your sit bones, lifting feet from floor. Balance on sit bones, using abdominals to maintain posture. Inhale, and on the exhale, release the legs, stretching them out in front of you (off the floor). Arms are alongside legs with palms facing in. Hold and breathe. Bend knees, hug with arms, and return feet to floor. This asana strengthens the abdominals, obliques, and back muscles (figure 19.14).

Cobra (Bhujangasana)

Lie on your stomach, arms down at your sides with palms up, forehead on the mat. Contract your gluteus and leg muscles. Inhale, drawing your arms up until the palms fall under the shoulders and elbows are tucked into the body; shoulders are relaxed and down. Exhale. Inhale, brush the mat with your nose and chin; continue drawing the upper torso up off the floor using your back muscles (not your hands and arms) to a comfortable point. Exhale and breathe. Inhale once again, and on the exhale, slowly begin lowering your torso to the floor, returning to the starting position. Repeat. This asana encourages thoracic flexibility (figure 19.15).

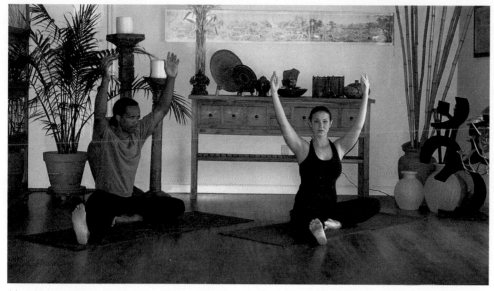

(a)

Figure 19.13
(*a*) *Janu Sirsasana*
(Knee/Head pose) position 1.
(*b*) *Janu Sirsasana*
(Knee/Head pose) position 2.

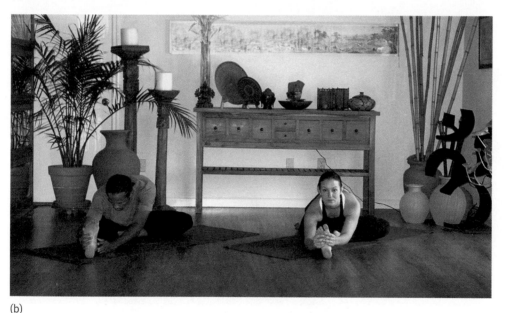

(b)

Bow (Dhanurasana)

Lying prone, stretch your arms out in front of you on the floor, shoulder width apart. Inhale, reaching out through the upper torso and arms and down through the lower torso and legs. Exhale, lifting both up. Inhale reaches out; exhale lifts up. Bend the knees, drawing the feet toward the head. Reach back and grab the feet, ankles, or shins. Inhale, pulling feet or shins up toward the ceiling; exhale, pushing feet back toward wall behind you. Breathe. Release slowly and rest. This asana is excellent for achieving full extension of the spine; it should not be performed if you have knee problems (figure 19.16).

Lying Spinal Twist (Bharadjasana)

Lie on your back. Inhale, drawing the right knee up to the chest, and hug it with an exhale. Extend the right arm out at shoulder height. Gaze is over the right hand. Inhale with the left hand on the right knee; exhale as the left hand takes the right knee to the left. Release and repeat to the left. This final asana releases all tension in preparation for *Savasana* (figure 19.17).

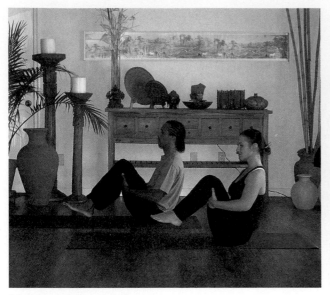

(a)

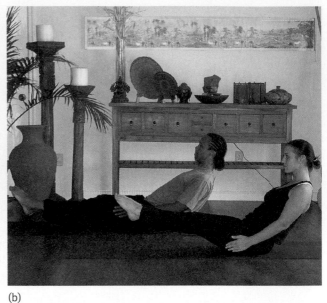

(b)

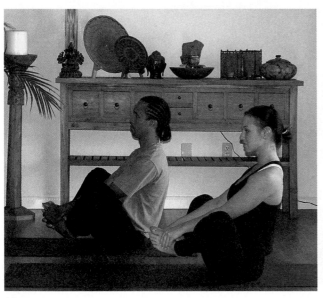

(c)

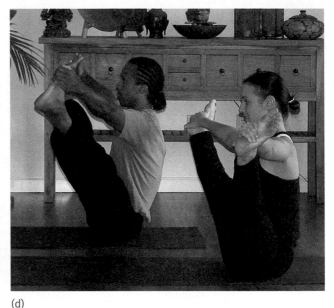

(d)

Figure 19.14

(*a*) *Navasana* (Boat pose) position 1. (*b*) *Navasana* (Boat pose) position 2. (*c*) Variation on *Navasana* (zero balancing point) position 1. (*d*) Variation on *Navasana* (zero balancing point) position 2.

Corpse Pose (Savasana)

Finish once again in the Corpse pose. Inhale, stretching the arms up and to the floor above your head; exhale with fingers interlocked and turned up. Release the arms back to the floor at your sides. Slowly roll your head from side to side to release the neck muscles. Open your jaw wide, stretching the facial muscles, and release. Focus on the breath once again and scan the body. Move into relaxation by focusing on or breathing into each body part, beginning with the feet. Practice a little chakra balancing (see section on "*Pranas* and Chakras" in this chapter). Bring your focus to the solar plexus and repeat an affirmation. This pose should be at least 10 to 15 minutes. The entire sequence should take approximately 40 minutes.

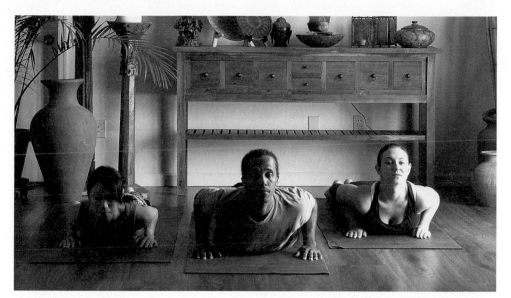

Figure 19.15
Bhujangasana (Cobra).

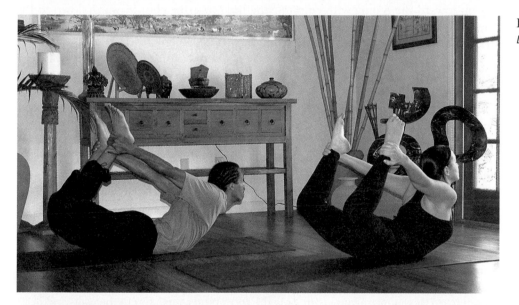

Figure 19.16
Dhanurasana (Bow).

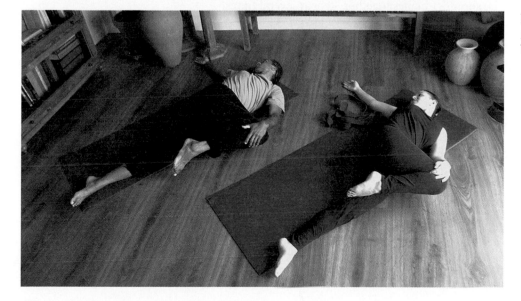

Figure 19.17
Bharadjasana (Lying Spinal Twist).

With these asanas, you have fulfilled the requirements of moving the body in six directions. Using a few of these asanas to fulfill the six directions requirements would take approximately 20 minutes to move through, making it an excellent way to start your day. Performing the sequence in its entirety will take approximately 40 minutes. Consult a yoga teacher, video, or book to add poses.

Since clients enjoy taking part in their own health or rehabilitation, you may recommend some of the asanas if you are a certified teacher; otherwise, refer them to a qualified instructor or class.

Qi Gong for the Massage Therapist

Qi Gong is a Chinese "exercise" that is similar in focus and intent to yoga. *Qi* (pronounced "chee") means energy, and *Gong* means movement (see chapter 15). Many therapists can benefit from a few Qi Gong exercises to keep the joints of the shoulders, arms, and hands healthy.

Movement 1: Crane's Neck

Standing erect with relaxed shoulders, visualize adding space between each vertebrae in your neck, creating length. Keeping that length, very slowly drop the head back, looking up toward the ceiling with chin moving up. Move the chin forward, down to the chest, up along the chest, and upright to head in starting position. Perform several times in this direction and then reverse direction by dropping chin down first. Crane's Neck is an excellent way to stretch the neck muscles (levator scapulae, SCM, scalenes).

Movement 2: Dragon's Head

Standing erect with relaxed shoulders, slowly lower the left ear to the left shoulder without twisting the neck. "Push" the ear up, move the head back upright, and slowly lower the right ear to the right shoulder. "Push" the right ear up. It may be helpful to hold the chin in place while lowering the ear from one side to the other to ensure no twisting of the neck. You can also visualize the infinity symbol with the chin held in place being the center. Dragon's Head is a safe way to stretch the neck. Rolling the head around is extremely harmful to the cervical vertebrae.

Movement 3

This exercise focuses on the rhomboids. Extend arms out to the sides at shoulder height, and place wrists in extension (palms facing out to the walls). Push out to "touch" the walls; using the rhomboids, draw the shoulder blades together (allow the elbows to soften to do this). Once again, using only the rhomboids, push out to the walls and draw the shoulder blades together. Repeat several times.

Movement 4

With arms extended out to the sides at shoulder height, flex the wrists, drawing the fingertips and thumbs together. Extend the wrists (palms up) and open the fingers one joint at a time. Repeat several times.

Movement 5

With arms out to the sides at shoulder height, wrists are in extension with palms up and fingers together. Simultaneously, open the thumb and little finger, index and ring finger; close thumb and little finger, index and ring finger. Repeat several times (figure 19.18).

> You are what your deep driving desire is
>> As your deep, driving desire is,
>> So is your will;
>> As your will is, so is your deed
>> As your deed is, so is your destiny.
>> *The Upanishad*

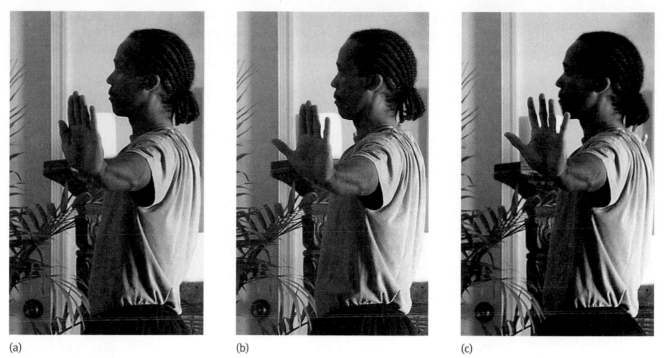

(a) (b) (c)

Figure 19.18

(*a*) Qi gong movement 5 position 1. (*b*) Qi gong movement 5 position 2. (*c*) Qi gong movement 5 position 3.

Since the beginning of time, humans have practiced and used martial arts (in one form or another) for the purpose of self-preservation or conquest. The Chinese are no different in this respect. For centuries, the Chinese people developed and continue to refine a diverse array of martial arts systems to suit the environmental, geological, and social needs of the day. Chinese martial arts, or *Wu Shu* (as it is more aptly described), could be generally characterized as internal or external systems. Further classification may define systems as hard hard, soft hard, soft soft, and so forth; these classifications are indicative of the way in which energy is generated. Regardless of the system, however, there are certain principles inherent in all Chinese martial arts; these include the concepts of yin and yang and Qi (Chi).

Yin and Yang Symbol

The yin and yang symbol is represented by a circle with an S-shaped curve down the middle. The curve separates the circle into two opposing dewdrops, with one traditionally black and the other clear or white. Each dewdrop has an eye of the opposite color (black eye on white drop, white eye on black drop). The symbol is a common fixture among many martial arts schools as well as institutes of Eastern medicine. It represents the comingling of opposing forces (weak-strong, soft-hard, in-out, feminine-masculine). Ultimately, the yin and yang symbol is a metaphor for life and portrays the concept of harmony in the universe. The philosophy dictates that when there is imbalance among opposing forces, the resulting combination is disharmony. A perfect example would be the blockage of Qi due to the imbalance of yin and yang in the human body.

Qi

The human body uses a signaling network of nerves and bioelectrical energy to communicate internally and to maneuver the environment. Chinese culture has known of this bioelectrical energy for centuries and describes it as an internal life force continuously

T'ai Chi

circulating throughout the human body and necessary to sustain life. Qi travels through various channels and vessels in the body and can manifest itself as physical energy used in martial combat or healing. This life force (Qi) can be difficult to understand and may prove elusive to harness. The martial artist seeks to channel this force in a display of physical energy.

Internal and External Systems

The philosophy governing the acquisition and utilization of Qi is what defines a martial system as being either internal or external. External martial arts systems emphasize an aggressive display of energy generation (rigid postures, static muscular postures). Internal martial arts systems advocate just the opposite. They are characteristically soft in posture, with relaxed muscles approximately 95% of the time and static explosive energy 5% of the time.

T'ai Chi Chuan is one of three such internal systems, the other two being *Ba Gua Zhang* and *hsing yi chuan*. *T'ai Chi Chaun* could be roughly translated as "mind form boxing." The system uses meditation and internal concentration to channel the Qi and manifest it physically. These mental exercises have been coupled with a predetermined routine of physical movements to create forms; these forms are practiced to teach the student correct posture, proper technique, and control. T'ai Chi movements are pictured in figure 19.19; martial arts movements are featured in figure 19.20. Although these martial arts systems were originally designed to develop fighters of the highest caliber, they have become synonymous with good physical health and well-being. It is for these physical and mental health benefits that Westerners have embraced T'ai Chi. The Chinese have had a national obsession with health, and at given times of the day, citizens of all ages assemble in various courtyards in China to practice their T'ai Chi forms.

Traditional Western Stretching Exercises

A physically fit person is generally energetic, healthy, confident, and mentally alert. A regularly practiced plan of physical activity can also aid in weight loss, firm and tone the body, and reduce mental or emotional stress with its wear on the body's structures.

Therapeutic exercise is defined as any exercise plan or program done with the single intent of improving the physical condition of the body. The goals for therapeutic exercise can include to maintain weight, build muscle, improve posture, and increase strength, flexibility, and mobility. The following section will focus on gaining flexibility through stretching. We do recommend, however, that you add periods of cardio work and weight lifting to a stretching routine (figure 19.21).

Strength, Mobility, and Flexibility

Physiological changes in the body take place when an exercise program is begun at just above the maximum levels of strength, flexibility, and mobility, and then the number of repetitions are gradually increased at a carefully controlled level of higher endurance. An effective exercise program is based on what a physiologist (a specialist in the functions and activities of organs, tissues, or cells) calls the **overload principle.**

During the training program, the body goes through an acceptance of the stresses placed on its systems called **adaptation.** In other words, the body changes physiologically to meet the new standard. This special ability of adaptation can work for the body or against it.

Muscle Strength

The strength of a muscle or muscle group is measured as the ability of a muscle to contract to produce a maximum force. The cross-sectional size of a muscle is associated with the overall strength of that muscle or the group of muscles that work together for

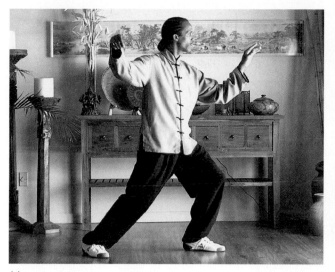

(a)

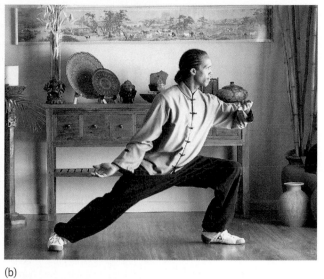

(b)

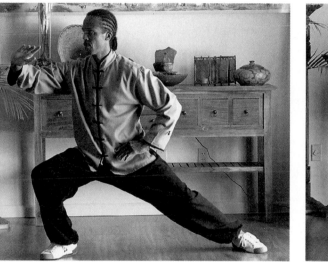

(c)

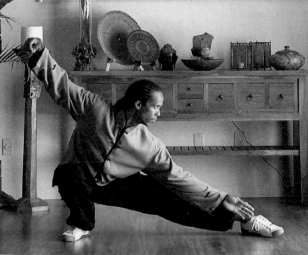

(d)

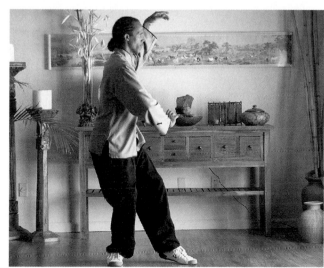

(e)

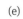

(f)

Figure 19.19 Tai chi movements

(*a*) Push forward. (*b*) Advancing forward. (*c*) Transition (wave to the right). (*d*) Snake creeps down. (*e*) Transition to white crane spreads its wings. (*f*) Grasp sparrow's tail.

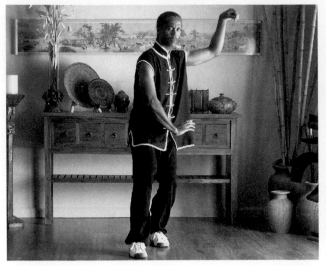

(a)

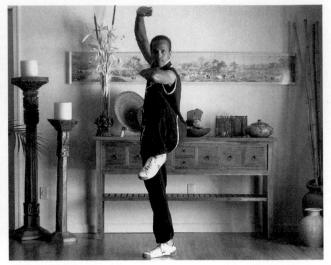

(b)

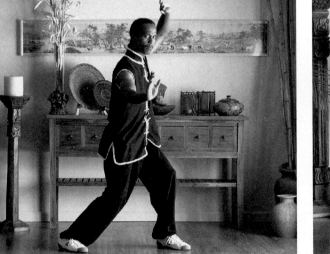

(c)

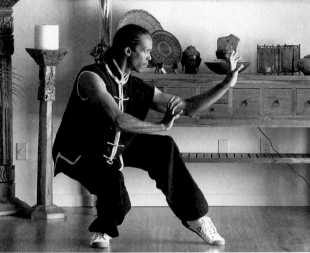

(d)

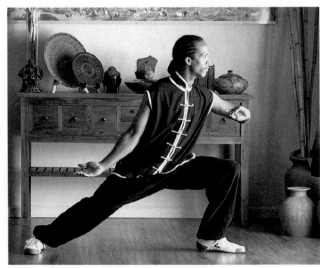

(e)

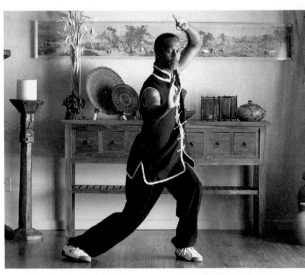

(f)

Figure 19.20 Martial arts movements

(*a*) Tiger opens up (cat stance).   (*b*) Transition.   (*c*) Transition.   (*d*) Transition.   (*e*) Strike the tiger.   (*f*) Tiger opens up (scissors stance).

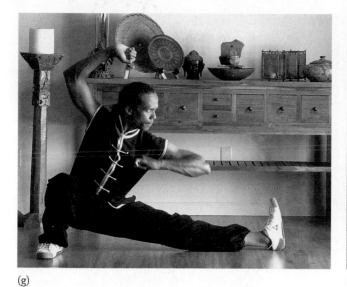
(g)

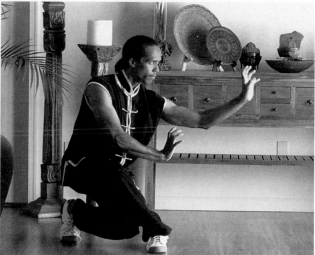
(h)

Figure 19.20 Martial arts movements (Continued)
(*g*) One leg crane stance. (*h*) Transition.

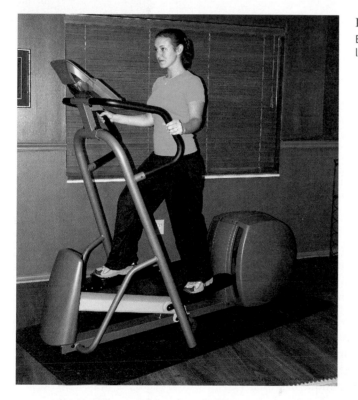

Figure 19.21
Elliptical training provides low-impact range of motion.

a specific task. When weight lifters "bulk up," they have increased the bulk of their muscles. The increase in size is due to the thickness of myofibrils (the actin and myosin filaments in the fiber of the muscle) and in the amount of capillary density within the muscle (figure 19.22).

Muscle strength is also determined by the force of contractions controlled by a motor unit, which is a group of muscle fibers controlled by a single motor neuron. When a motor neuron fires, the muscle fibers affected by that neuron contract. The more motor neurons that fire at the same instant, the greater the force of the contraction.

Figure 19.22
Weight lifting develops muscle strength.

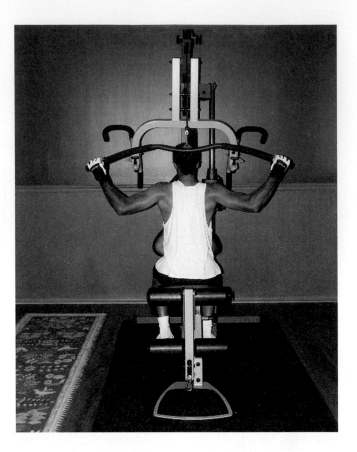

Stretching

The soft tissues that surround a joint (muscles, connective tissue, and skin), together with adequate joint mobility and flexibility, are necessary for a normal range of motion. Pain-free range of motion is required to perform daily living tasks as well as occupational or recreational activities. If our joints do not move in an unrestricted fashion, we are much more susceptible to injury and reinjury.

Therapeutic Stretching Methods

To elongate the musculotendinous unit, you can use one of three methods: manually applied passive stretching, active inhibition, and self-stretching. All therapeutic stretching procedures should be preceded by heat to warm up the tissue involved. Ice may be applied in some cases after a rigorous workout.

- Passive range of motion technique involves working with a partner and applying an external force to control the direction, speed, and duration of the stretch, resulting in tissues being elongated beyond their usual resting length.
- Active inhibition is a technique in which a client would relax the muscle to be elongated during the stretching procedure. When a muscle is relaxed, there is minimal resistance to the elongation process. Since the active inhibition method relaxes only the contractile structure and not the connective tissue of the muscle, this type of elongation of the muscle must be done with the muscle under control. It cannot be used for clients who have paralysis or other neuromuscular conditions.
- Self-stretching techniques are flexibility exercises that you can perform on your own. In this method, you passively stretch out your contractures by using your own body weight as a force. Self-stretching techniques can enhance an exercise program and acquire a sufficient range of motion much more quickly.

Benefits of Stretching

1. Regain a normal range of motion of joints and mobility of soft tissue.

2. Increase the general flexibility of a body part in conjunction with strengthening exercises.

3. Prevent or minimize the risk of musculotendinous injuries related to activity specific to the client.

Muscle Maintenance Program for Massage Therapists

One of the prerequisites to becoming a successful massage therapist is adherence to a comprehensive muscle maintenance program. This is advisable to ensure longevity in your career.

There are, however, other very important reasons for these toning practices. Therapists who fail to take care of themselves run the risk of transferring any tension and anxiety they are experiencing to their clients (see chapter 17). They also run the risk of developing repetitive motion-related diseases such as carpal tunnel syndrome; as a result, therapists may see their enthusiasm for the profession wane and their clientele dwindle.

With respect to potential injury, it would be misleading to assume that only the upper body is involved. During a massage, the therapist must engage a wide range of muscle groups. Proper massage technique diffuses the contact force with the client throughout the therapist's body, thus avoiding concentrated pressure on any one body part. In this manner, the potential for injury is greatly diminished.

In designing a comprehensive muscle maintenance program it is helpful for the therapist to review the range of motion involved during a massage session and isolate those muscle groups that most frequently come into play. More often than not, these muscle groups include the shoulder, wrists, hands, lower back, thighs, and ankles.

Western Stretching Exercises

Following is a list of exercises that may prove useful in maintaining muscle tone and elasticity. You will also find them helpful in increasing range of motion. Remember to warm and relax the area before beginning a stretch procedure. Please note that these exercises should be performed slowly and on both sides; hold the stretch for about 15 seconds and repeat three times.

Shoulder shrugs: Stand in functional position. Rotate the shoulder girdles upward and back at least three times, then reverse direction to work all muscles of the shoulder area, chest, and upper back (figures 19.23).

Shoulder stretch: Elevate the right arm above the head then flex the elbow so that the palm of the hand touches the back of the neck. Place the left hand on the right elbow and pull gently to traction the right shoulder (stretches the triceps as well). In the horizontal version (figure 19.24) of this exercise, bring the right arm horizontally across the body, grasp the right elbow with the left hand and pull gently (stretches the deltoids as well).

Finger and wrist stretch: Standing 2½ to 3 feet away from a wall, place the right hand on the wall below chest height and gently lean into the wall to stretch ligaments and tendons (wrist extension) (figure 19.25).
Secondly grasp the outer side of the right hand with the left hand and gently flex the right wrist (wrist flexion).
Thirdly, grasp the right hand with the left hand and gently rotate the right wrist (figure 19.26).

Knee flexion/calf stretch: Flex the right knee and grab hold of the instep with both hands, then gently pull to stretch quadriceps muscles. This also has the effect of forcefully plantar flexing the right foot. Conversely, place the sole of the right foot

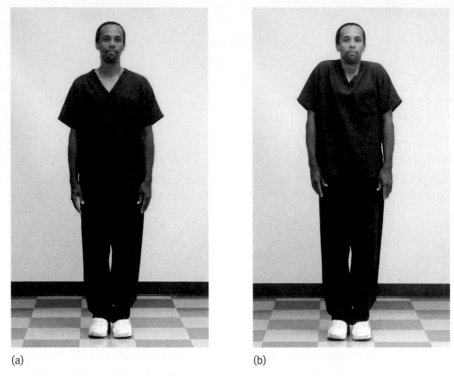

(a)   (b)

Figure 19.23

(*a*) Beginning position for shoulder shrugs. (*b*) Elevated shoulders position.

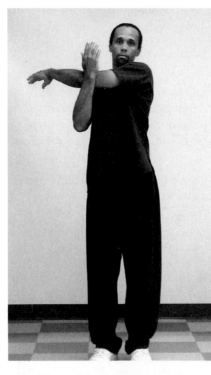

Figure 19.24

The horizontal version of shoulder traction.

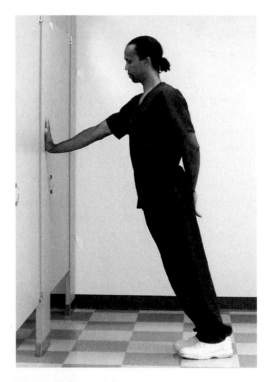

Figure 19.25

Wrist extension.

on the wall so that only the heel is on the floor, then, keeping the right knee straight, lean into the wall to stretch gastrocnemius, soleus, and hamstring muscles (figure 19.27).

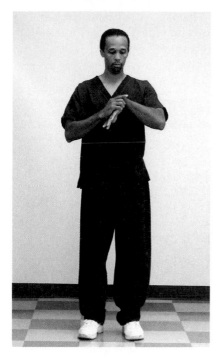

Figure 19.26
Wrist flexion.

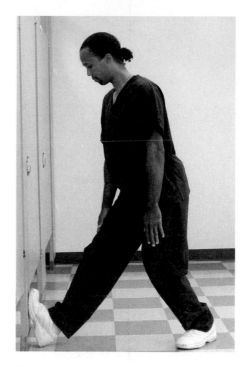

Figure 19.27
Calf stretch.

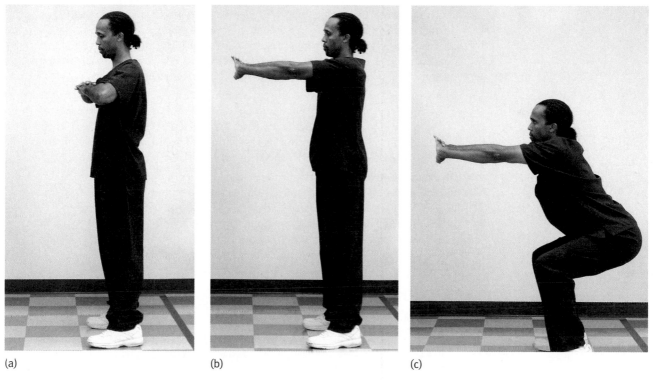

(a)   (b)   (c)

Figure 19.28
(*a*) Beginning position for half squats.   (*b*) Middle position for half squats.   (*c*) Ending position for half squats.

Half squats: Stand with feet shoulder-width apart and hands clasped in front of
you (palms facing away from the body); push palms forward, extending arms.
Keep your back straight and squat down until you can no longer see your toes
covered by your knees (figure 19.28). Stand upright and repeat seven to 10 times.

Ankle circumduction: Sit on the floor with feet in front of you. Create circular patterns with pointed toes, then reverse direction and repeat exercise. You should do at least seven or eight repetitions in each direction.

Think About It | Terms Related to Stretching

- **Flexibility** is the ability to move a single joint or series of joints through an unrestricted, pain-free range of motion. It depends on the extensibility of muscles, which allows muscles that cross a joint to relax, lengthen, and yield to a stretch force. Often the term *flexibility* is used to refer to the musculotendinous elongation as the body part moves through the range of motion. *Dynamic flexibility* refers to the active range of motion of a joint. *Passive flexibility* is the degree to which a joint can be passively moved through the available range of motion.

- **Stretching** is a general term used to describe any therapeutic maneuver designed to elongate a pathologically shortened soft tissue structure and increase range of motion. *Passive stretching* is done by using an external force, applied either manually or mechanically, to lengthen shortened muscles. *Active inhibition* is when the client participates in the stretching maneuver to inhibit tonus in a tight muscle. *Selective stretching* is a process whereby the overall function of a client may be improved by applying stretching techniques selectively to some muscles and joints while simultaneously allowing limitation of motion to develop in other muscles or joints. An example of this may be to correct the posture by strengthening certain muscle groups in a person who has scoliosis or cerebral palsy.

- **Overstretch** is a stretch well beyond the normal range of motion of a joint and the surrounding soft tissues. This may be used by athletes who require a greater-than-normal range of flexibility to prevent injury. Overstretching can become a contraindication when the supporting structures of a joint and the strength of the muscles around a joint are not sufficient and cannot hold a joint in a stable position during activity. This condition is often referred to as a *stretch weakness.*

- **Contracture** is defined as the adaptive shortening of muscle or other soft tissues that cross a joint, which results in a limitation of range of motion. *Contractures* are described by identifying the tight muscle action. The term *contraction* is the process of tension developing in a muscle during shortening or lengthening. These terms are not the same and should not be used interchangeably.

- **Myostatic contracture** occurs when there is no specific tissue disease or injury, but the musculotendinous unit has adaptively shortened and there is a significant loss of range of motion. *Tightness* is a nonspecific term referring to a mild shortening of an otherwise healthy musculotendinous unit. Tightness is more likely to develop after unusual activity, such as painting your house or jumping over a hole, in the two-joint muscles such as the hamstrings, rectus femoris, or gastrocnemius.

Adapting Stretches for a Client

As mentioned earlier, many massage therapists broaden their practice to include therapeutic exercise for clients by being trained in personal training or physical therapy. There are precautions you should take when working with clients on a stretching program. Following is an approach for such a program.

Initial Client Consultation

As wonderful as exercise is for the body, it can cause harm if done improperly or if the exercise requirements are not specifically based on a client's current medical condition and physical limitations. An exercise consultation form (figure 19.29) should be used to gather (and keep on file) physical fitness information, medical conditions, type of exercise program, and the client's progress. Always make sure you give a complete client assessment and have the client sign and date a statement such as the one at the bottom of the form. A signed form can protect you if a situation or a problem arises during the client's period of care. Always have clients visit their physicians before beginning any exercise program

Common Client Issues

The conditions that contribute to an adaptive shortening of soft tissues around a joint and subsequent loss of unrestricted range of motion can include prolonged immobilization, restricted mobility, connective tissue or neurological disease, tissue pathology due to trauma, and congenital deformities.

EXERCISE CONSULTATION FORM

Name _____ Date _____

Address _____ Telephone _____

Birthdate _____ Height _____ Weight _____

Referred by _____ Telephone _____

Posture _____ Physical limitations _____

Desired results _____

Exercises recommended _____

General goals _____

Progress notes _____

Restrictions/contraindications _____

***Statement of health

I have no health problems that prevent normal exercising with or without machines or apparatus.

I hereby release (business name or therapist name) and its/their employees from responsibility

for injuries I may incur as the result of participation in a program of health-related exercises.

Client's signature _____ Date _____

Figure 19.29 Sample exercise consultation form

(continued)

Prolonged immobilization occurs when a client wears a cast or splint for a period of time after a fracture or surgical repair. The muscles often atrophy (shrink), and the circulation decreases. The joints often "freeze in place," and physical therapy or range of motion exercise and strength training are needed to bring the affected area back to a normal condition. Bed rest or extended wheelchair or crutch use can cause problems in areas other than the injury site.

Neurological diseases that affect the muscle or joint tissue can lead to paralysis, weakness, muscle imbalance, and pain, which can make it difficult to maintain a normal range of motion. Connective tissue disease such as scleroderma and joint diseases such as rheumatoid arthritis and osteoarthritis can cause pain, muscle weakness, spasm, and inflammation. Such diseases may scar the tissue surrounding a joint and make movement all but impossible.

When tissue is damaged by injury (such as from a sports activity or automobile accident), the individual may face a lifelong battle to regain mobility. For professional athletes, these injuries often result in the loss of their career; they are likewise left with the residual effects of scarring and inflammation. When these injuries heal, the body replaces the damaged tissue with a more rigid, fibrous tissue that causes the soft tissue to lose its **elasticity** and **plasticity,** which leads to a loss of normal range of motion. Muscle strength is always affected with a loss of range of motion due to the shortening of the muscle. When the muscle shortens, it can no longer produce a peak tension. This condition is often referred to as tight weakness of the muscles.

Beginning Stretching Exercises

There are normally indications as to when treatment through therapeutic exercise is warranted. The client must have limited range of motion as a result of contractures, adhesions, and scar tissue formation that leads to a shortening of muscles, connective tissue, or skin. When these contractures interfere with daily living tasks and may lead to structural deformity such as poor posture or to muscle weakness, you may choose to begin passive stretching. Remember to assess your client and to set specific goals.

Steps for Passive Stretching

1. Assess the client and identify specific range of motion and mobility functions. Consider the possibility of contractures, adhesions, or scar tissue being involved.

2. Assess the strength of muscles in which motion is limited.

3. Explain your findings and the goals of the stretching procedures to the client.

4. Position the client in a stable setting, apply heat to the treatment area, and employ relaxation techniques to prepare the client.

Applying the Stretch

1. Move the extremity slowly through the free range of motion to the point of restriction.

2. Grasp proximally and distally to the joint in which motion is to occur. Use a firm but not uncomfortable grip. Use padding to prevent bruising or tearing of skin and underlying tissue. Use the broad surface of the hands to apply force.

3. Firmly stabilize the proximal segment and move the distal segment. To stretch a multijoint muscle, move the muscle over one joint at a time, then over all joints simultaneously. Avoid joint compression by applying gentle traction to the moving joint.

4. Apply the stretch force in a gentle, controlled, and sustained manner. Take the restricted soft tissues to the point of tightness and then move just beyond.

5. Hold the client in the stretched position for 15 to 30 seconds. The client should feel pulling but not pain. When the tension decreases, move the extremity or joint a little farther. Then gradually release the force; allow the client to relax before beginning the maneuver again.

After Stretching Procedure

1. Apply cold to the tissues that have been stretched and allow these structures to cool in a lengthened position.

2. Have the client perform exercises and functional activity that use the gained range of motion. Increasing flexibility is a gradual process and may take several weeks of treatment to see significant results.

3. Develop a balance in strengthened muscles in the new range so that there is control as flexibility increases.

Inhibition and Relaxation Techniques

Inhibition and relaxation procedures are used to relieve pain and muscle tension. Using these techniques can be a successful way to reduce tension headaches, high blood pressure, and respiratory distress seen in asthmatic and emphysemic conditions (see chapter 13 for discussion of PNF techniques).

Procedure for Active Inhibition Applications

1. Begin with the tight muscle in a lengthened position.

2. Ask the client to isometrically contract the tight muscle for 10 seconds until the muscle begins to fatigue, then relax the muscle.

3. Passively lengthen the muscle by moving the extremity through the new range and repeat after a short rest period.

Precautions and Contraindications of Stretching

1. Never force a joint beyond a normal range of motion, which can vary for each client.

2. Newly healed fractures should be stabilized between the fracture site and the joint in which the motion is taking place.

3. Do not perform on clients who may have osteoporosis, have had prolonged bed rest, or may be taking steroids.

4. If a client has joint pain or muscle soreness lasting more than 24 hours after the exercise, too much force may have been used and no additional stress should be applied until the affected sites have returned to their normal state and the pain is completely absent.

5. Avoid stretching of inflamed or swollen tissue, or areas showing broken veins or severe bruising.

6. Never perform stretching exercises if there has been a recent fracture, blood clot, or evidence of an infectious element.

7. Stop the procedure immediately if a bony block limits movement or if sharp or severe pain is felt with joint movement.

8. It is imperative that the scapula be stabilized when force is used to stretch the muscles in the area of the chest or shoulder girdle.

Chapter Summary

To maintain good health and enjoy a long career as a massage therapist, you must partake in some form of exercise. This chapter has provided you with several possibilities for achieving this goal. You will benefit not only physically but also mentally from any or all of the movements or exercises mentioned.

Applying Your Knowledge

Self-Testing

1. What is the color of the heart chakra?
   a) Blue
   b) Green
   c) Yellow
   d) Violet

2. What gland does the heart chakra govern or influence?
   a) Pituitary
   b) Pineal
   c) Gonads
   d) Thymus

3. Where is the *Ajna* or third eye chakra located?
   a) Between the brows
   b) In the throat
   c) At the crown of the head
   d) At the navel

4. In yoga, what is the vital life force called?
   a) Chi
   b) Qi
   c) *Ki*
   d) *Prana*

5. What is the definition of a chakra?
   a) Light form
   b) Electrical current
   c) Energy wheel or center
   d) Sound wave

6. What does *Qi Gong* mean?
   a) Energy movement
   b) Energy balance
   c) Energy sound
   d) Energy food

7. Traditionally, what were the martial arts used for?
   a) Conquest
   b) Self-preservation
   c) Competition
   d) a and b

8. Besides increasing range of motion and increasing flexibility, what is the third benefit of stretching?
   a) Developing muscle strength
   b) Preventing musculotendinous injury
   c) Increasing bulk
   d) Decreasing atrophy

9. Before beginning an exercise program with your client, what should you always do?
   a) Obtain a full assessment of your client's physical condition.
   b) Make sure the room is warm.
   c) Write out your plan before you see the client.
   d) Change into a jogging suit.

10. What are the soft tissues that surround a joint?
    a) Bones, hair, and collagen
    b) Blood, nails, and hair
    c) Muscles, connective tissue, and skin
    d) Fluid and skin

11. What does a normal range of motion rely on?
    a) Treatment of injury
    b) Age of the client
    c) Actin and myosin filaments
    d) Adequate mobility and flexibility

12. Some of the conditions that contribute to loss of range of motion can include prolonged immobilization, restricted mobility, and _____.
    a) connective tissue or neurological disease
    b) tissue pathology due to trauma
    c) congenital deformities
    d) All of the above.

Case Studies/Critical Thinking

A. A client has an appointment with you. During the client assessment, the client tells you that she has been having severe tension headaches, and pain and tightness between her shoulders. The client is 23 years old and has a very stressful job as a receptionist. Her job duties include holding a phone to her ear and filling orders by typing information into a computer. What plan of treatment do you feel would bring about the relief of symptoms in the client? What method of exercise or stretching could be used to keep the problem from occurring? What might you instruct the client to do to avoid pain and injury in the future?

B. A client has extremely tight IT Bands and asks you for an exercise to help stretch this area that is so difficult to relax. She would like to try some yoga positions (asanas). Which yoga exercises would you recommend?

References for information in this chapter can be found in Quick Guide C at the end of the book.

PART VI

Ethics and Professional Business Practices

CHAPTER 20   Law, Ethics, and Professionalism

CHAPTER 21   Business Development, Marketing
Success, and Community Education

Law, Ethics, and Professionalism

LEARNING OUTCOMES

After completing this chapter, you will be able to:

- Recognize the importance of ethical and professional standards.

- Discuss basic rules and regulations governing massage and the scope of practice.

- Recognize the difference between licensing and regulating massage therapists.

- Identify appropriate forms of touch and client boundaries.

- Identify and comply with Health Insurance Portability and Accountability Act (HIPAA) regulations.

- Recognize the role of the therapist in professional relationships.

- Practice role-playing in scenarios involving ethical and other real-life situations.

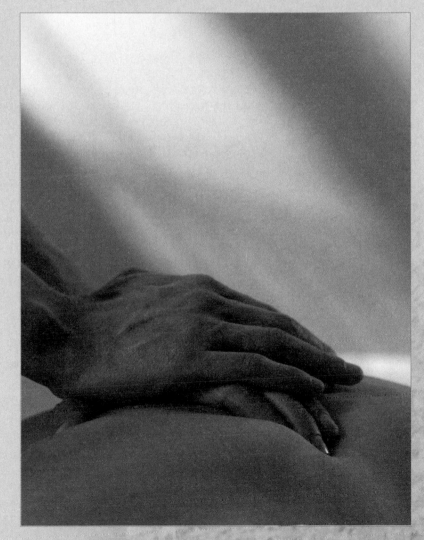

codes of ethics *(p. 532)*
countertransference *(p. 544)*
Health Insurance Portability
    and Accountability Act
    (HIPAA) *(p. 538)*

multidimensional or dual
    relationships *(p. 544)*
personal boundaries *(p. 543)*
professional boundaries *(p. 543)*

right to privacy *(p. 538)*
right of refusal *(p. 540)*
scope of practice *(p. 535)*
transference *(p. 544)*

INTRODUCTION

All massage therapists, whether or not they work in a state that licenses or regulates the profession, need to be well-versed in the laws governing health care workers, including Health Insurance Portability and Accountability Act (HIPAA) regulations. Complete knowledge, understanding, and compliance with guidelines on professional conduct issued by professional organizations in the field of massage therapy, such as the American Massage Therapy Association (AMTA), the Associated Bodywork & Massage Professionals (ABMP), and the International Massage Association (IMA), are crucial to be an exemplary member of the profession. You will further need to be able to identify what working within your scope of practice or training means and how to recognize red flags in the course of your practice.

Codes of Ethics and Laws

Most professional organizations have established sets of standards, known as **codes of ethics,** to serve as guidelines for professional conduct. A member's adherence to a specified code of ethics ensures quality service as well as speaks to the personal character of the professional. Simply put, a professional code of ethics is a reflection of the personal standards of the individual members of the larger group. Included here are examples of codes of ethics of four massage professional organizations. Whether or not you become (or perhaps already are) a member of AMTA, ABMP, or IMA and have taken the certification exam of the National Certification Board for Therapeutic Massage and Bodywork or your state's exam, as a massage therapist you should strive to uphold the principles set forth by these and similar organizations. Keep in mind that these organizations offer more than codes of ethics; they also lend support to their members in numerous ways, from marketing techniques to networking opportunities to group rates for insurance. Please take the time to request printed information from or view information offered on the websites of these organizations, listed in Quick Guide A. One of these groups may meet your needs better than the others: you may simply be looking for insurance coverage, you may be interested in learning new marketing approaches and acquiring help with establishing good business practices, or you may be looking for an organization that will be your voice in current issues affecting the profession. It is important to join an organization that resonates with you and your massage therapy practice.

Laws Governing Massage

The laws governing massage and massage therapists vary widely from state to state.

★ **EXAM POINT** Some states license massage therapists (LMT) and massage practitioners (LMP), while others regulate them (regulated massage therapist or RMT).

Although the majority of people practicing in the massage profession call themselves "massage therapists," a growing number refer to themselves as "massage practi-

Therapeutic Massage and Bodywork Codes of Ethics

AMTA Code of Ethics

Founded in 1943, the American Massage Therapy Association (AMTA) is the oldest and largest international, member-driven organization representing the massage therapy profession. On an ongoing basis, the AMTA develops and reexamines guidelines for the ethical practice of massage to keep such guidelines current and to advance the profession through ethics and professional standards, certification, school accreditation, continuing education, professional publications, legislative efforts, and public education.

Massage therapists shall:

1. Demonstrate commitment to provide the highest quality massage therapy/bodywork to those who seek their professional service.

2. Acknowledge the inherent worth and individuality of each person by not discriminating or behaving in any prejudicial manner with clients and/or colleagues.

3. Demonstrate professional excellence through regular self-assessment of strengths, limitations, and effectiveness by continued education and training.

4. Acknowledge the confidential nature of the professional relationship with clients and respect each client's right to privacy.

5. Conduct all business and professional activities within their scope of practice, the law of the land, and project a professional image.

6. Refrain from engaging in any sexual conduct or sexual activities involving their clients.

7. Accept responsibility to do no harm to the physical, mental, and emotional well-being of self, clients, and associates.

Associated Bodywork & Massage Professionals

Associated Bodywork & Massage Professionals (ABMP) is a membership organization that includes a wide range of massage, bodywork, somatic, and skin care professionals. ABMP offers liability insurance, business support, educational materials, and legislative advocacy and updates.

As a member of Associated Bodywork & Massage Professionals, I hereby pledge to abide by the ABMP Code of Ethics as outlined below.

Client Relationships

- I shall endeavor to serve the best interests of my clients at all times and to provide the highest quality service possible.

- I shall maintain clear and honest communications with my clients and shall keep client communications confidential.

- I shall acknowledge the limitations of my skills and, when necessary, refer clients to the appropriate qualified health care professional.

- I shall in no way instigate or tolerate any kind of sexual advance while acting in the capacity of a massage, bodywork, somatic therapy, or esthetic practitioner.

Professionalism

- I shall maintain the highest standards of professional conduct, providing services in an ethical and professional manner in relation to my clientele, business associates, health care professionals, and the general public.

- I shall respect the rights of all ethical practitioners and will cooperate with all health care professionals in a friendly and professional manner.

- I shall refrain from the use of any mind-altering drugs, alcohol, or intoxicants prior to or during professional sessions.

- I shall always dress in a professional manner, proper dress being defined as attire suitable and consistent with accepted business and professional practice.

- I shall not be affiliated with or employed by any business that utilizes any form of sexual suggestiveness or explicit sexuality in its advertising or promotion of services, or in the actual practice of its services.

Scope of Practice/Appropriate Techniques

- I shall provide services within the scope of the ABMP definition of massage, bodywork, somatic therapies, and skin care, and the limits of my training. I will not employ those massage, bodywork, or skin care techniques for which I have not had adequate training and shall represent my education, training, qualifications, and abilities honestly.

- I shall be conscious of the intent of the services that I am providing and shall be aware of and practice good judgment regarding the application of massage, bodywork, or somatic techniques utilized.

- I shall not perform manipulations or adjustments of the human skeletal structure, diagnose, prescribe, or provide any other service, procedure, or therapy, which requires a license to practice chiropractic, osteopathy, physical therapy, podiatry, orthopedics, psychotherapy, acupuncture, dermatology, cosmetology, or any other profession or branch of medicine unless specifically licensed to do so.

(continued)

Therapeutic Massage and Bodywork Codes of Ethics (Continued)

■ I shall be thoroughly educated and understand the physiological effects of the specific massage, bodywork, somatic, or skin care techniques utilized in order to determine whether such application is contraindicated and/or to determine the most beneficial techniques to apply to a given individual. I shall not apply massage, bodywork, somatic, or skin care techniques in those cases where they may be contraindicated without a written referral from the client's primary care provider.

Image/Advertising Claims

■ I shall strive to project a professional image for myself, my business or place of employment, and the profession in general.

■ I shall actively participate in educating the public regarding the actual benefits of massage, bodywork, somatic therapies, and skin care.

■ I shall practice honesty in advertising, promote my services ethically and in good taste, and practice and/or advertise only those techniques for which I have received adequate training and/or certification. I shall not make false claims regarding the potential benefits of the techniques rendered.

International Massage Association

Formed in 1994, the International Massage Association (IMA) includes practitioners of various massage and bodywork modalities as well as estheticians and dance and yoga instructors.

As an IMA Group member, you agree to abide by the following standards of professional and ethical behavior in your field:

To put my clients' well being first and foremost.

To conduct myself professionally and responsibly.

To uphold the integrity of my profession.

To acknowledge, respect, and cooperate with my colleagues and peers in order to advance our profession and ensure that the highest level of excellence is available to the consuming public.

I shall promote myself, the IMA Group, and my profession honestly, tactfully, and with the aim of educating both my peers and the public, so that they may be empowered to demand and receive all the benefits that my profession provides.

To acknowledge the limitations of my skills and scope of practice and refer clients, when necessary, to other health professionals to provide the most appropriate care.

To maintain a safe and comfortable working environment, paying particular attention to avoidable hazards and respecting personal boundaries.

To ascertain and comply with the requirements of all governing laws and abide by them to the best of my ability. Where laws are unjust, I will labor with my association to change them.

To communicate responsibly, truthfully, and respectfully with clients, and to hold their communications in strict confidence.

Any member failing to abide by the Code of Ethics shall be answerable to the board of directors for "peer review."

National Certification Board for Therapeutic Massage and Bodywork

The National Certification Board for Therapeutic Massage and Bodywork (NCBTMB) is a not-for-profit organization that certifies massage and bodywork practitioners by offering exams in therapeutic massage, and therapeutic massage & bodywork. Certificants are required to abide by professional standards to protect the integrity of the profession. Those practitioners who have been awarded national certification by the NCBTMB will:

■ Have a sincere commitment to provide the highest quality of care to those that seek their professional services.

■ Represent their qualifications honestly, including their educational achievements and professional affiliations, and will provide only those services, which they are qualified to perform.

■ Accurately inform clients, other health care practitioners, and the public of the scope and limitations of their discipline.

■ Acknowledge the limitations of and contraindications for massage and bodywork and refer clients to appropriate health professionals.

■ Provide treatment only where there is reasonable expectation that it will be advantageous to the client.

■ Consistently maintain and improve professional knowledge and competence, striving for professional excellence through regular assessment of personal and professional strengths and weaknesses and through continued education training.

■ Conduct their business and professional activities with honesty and integrity, and respect the inherent worth of all persons.

■ Refuse to unjustly discriminate against clients or other health professionals.

■ Safeguard the confidentiality of all client information, unless disclosure is required by law, court order, or is absolutely necessary for the protection of the public.

■ Respect the client's right to treatment with informed and voluntary consent. The NCBTMB practitioner will

- obtain and record the informed consent of the client, or client's advocate, before providing treatment. This consent may be written or verbal.
- Respect the client's right to refuse, modify, or terminate treatment regardless of prior consent given.
- Provide draping and treatment in a way that ensures the safety, comfort, and privacy of the client.
- Exercise the right to refuse to treat any person or part of the body for just and reasonable cause.
- Refrain, under all circumstances, from initiating or engaging in any sexual conduct, sexual activities, or sexualizing behavior involving a client, even if the client attempts to sexualize the relationship.
- Avoid any interest, activity, or influence, which might be in conflict with the practitioner's obligation to act in the best interests of the client or the profession.

- Respect the client's boundaries with regard to privacy, disclosure, exposure, emotional expression, beliefs, and the client's reasonable expectations of professional behavior. Practitioners will respect the client's autonomy.
- Refuse any gifts or benefits, which are intended to influence a referral, decision, or treatment that are purely for personal gain and not for the good of the client.
- Follow all policies, procedures, guidelines, regulations, codes, and requirements promulgated by the National Certification Board for Therapeutic Massage and Bodywork.

tioners." For some, it may be a matter of semantics, while for others, being called a "practitioner" is a way to differentiate themselves from the "therapy" field, which denotes training in psychology. States that do not license massage therapists regulate them by requiring proof of education, training, or competency. Currently, 36 states and the District of Columbia license or regulate the profession of massage therapy and bodywork, with some of those states having multiple levels based on education and training or dual (massage and esthetician) licensing.

There are several common denominators, however, such as a specific definition of massage (scope of practice), formal education, code of ethics, professional standards, and local laws or regulations. For example, Florida state law—Chapter 480, the Massage Practice Act—defines what massage is and the formal education required, and details the continuing educational requirements for renewal. This law also specifies prohibited actions, both sexual and licensure violations, and lists fines for such infractions. As mentioned in the Overview, a new organization—the Federation of State Massage Therapy Boards—may very well accomplish many therapists' and practitioners' long-term goals of creating consistency across the nation for massage education, standards, and regulations.

You will find a list of the states that license massage therapists and detailed contact information in appendix A. Because laws governing the profession are continually defined and updated, check your state's website for the most current information. If your state regulates rather than licenses massage therapists and is not on this list, please check with your state commerce or health department, or the local massage therapy organization for requirements and contact information.

⭐ **EXAM POINT** The massage therapist's **scope of practice**—or the parameters within which a therapist may work—is based on the governing state's laws.

Scope of Practice

Again, there are differences from state to state, with the common denominator being completion of a specified number of educational hours and strict adherence to the ethical and professional standards. The laws also clearly define work that a massage therapist cannot perform. A specific example is direct manipulation of the spine: this work is performed by chiropractors and is therefore outside of the scope of practice for therapeutic massage and bodywork (figure 20.1). Massage therapists are qualified to manipulate soft

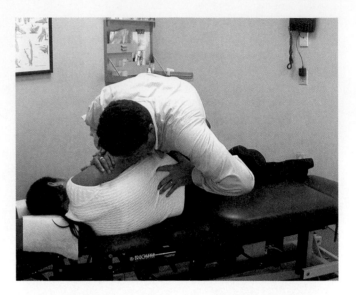

Figure 20.1
Chiropractors are trained in the manipulation of the spine.

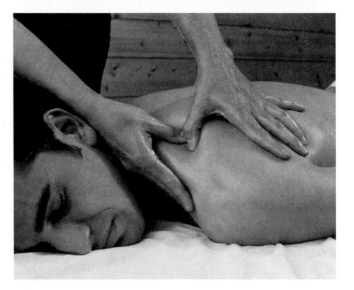

Figure 20.2
Massage therapists work with soft tissue, which includes muscle, tendon, fascia, and skin.

tissue (muscle, tendon, and fascia), which may indirectly affect structural alignment, but cannot under any circumstances "adjust" clients (figure 20.2).

Working Within the Scope of Practice

Taking the scope of practice one step further, massage therapists may perform only those modalities in which they are trained. Therapists trained only in basic Swedish massage may not ethically perform an advanced modality such as neuromuscular massage, nor can they represent themselves as a certified Neuromuscular Therapist (NMT) without specific training and certification. Remember to operate within the parameters of your training; do not let a client talk you into attempting to perform a massage modality in which you are not trained. Clients who travel a great deal often boast of the great work they receive from a therapist in another area of the country and attempt to convince other therapists to achieve similar results. Ego needs to remain at the door and does not belong in the massage room. Do not believe yourself to be any less of a therapist because you work differently than someone else.

In the aforementioned scenario, you may find yourself in a Catch-22 situation. Always do the best job you can with what you know and are capable of; let your work stand for itself. By the end of the session, you may surprise him by meeting or exceeding his standards, or you simply may not be able to do anything to please the client even though you have tried your best. Remember the old adage, "You can please some of the people some of the time, but you can't please all of the people all of the time."

Outside the Scope of Practice

Another area of potential liability falls in the realm of diagnosing. Massage therapists are not medical professionals who are qualified to diagnosis or treat disease. Again, a forceful client may press you for your opinion and take that to heart as an official diagnosis. Stand your ground and recommend that your client see the appropriate medical professional. Remember, however, that it is not necessary for a client to have a prescription from a physician to receive massage unless you are filing an insurance claim.

A growing number of clients are interested in and may inquire about adjunct alternative healing modalities (figure 20.3). Handle these questions the same way as you would more traditional medical questions: refer out. For example, unless you have had training in the use of herbal preparations, do not recommend or advise but rather keep on hand a list of qualified practitioners to whom you can refer clients. In fact, it is an excellent business tool to build a referral list of persons who are experts in their field. This list can be drawn from personal experience, feedback from clients, or recommendations from professional organizations. Often, the same professionals will then continually refer to each other and can be a great resource for building a client list.

Medical Massage within the Scope of Practice

Currently, debate within the industry is heated concerning the use of the term *medical massage*. The term is a bit of a misnomer and often misunderstood by the public. The misconception is that medical massage is massage performed by a therapist who has attended medical school. It is more correct to say medical massage is clinical massage and bodywork that involves neuromuscular therapy and myofascial release and is performed by a licensed or regulated massage therapist, often under the tutelage of a physician or other health care provider and in a health care setting. All massage therapists who have successfully completed their state's requirements for massage practice and are licensed or registered within that state may deliver massage therapy as a service. Additionally, all licensed or registered massage therapists may treat clients and file for reimbursement through insurance with a prescription from a physician *if* they are a provider and the insurance company approves

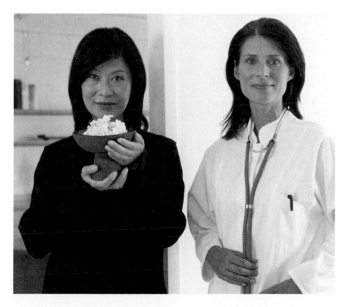

Figure 20.3
Any question from a client concerning therapies outside of massage, such as about herbal remedies or traditional medical treatments, should be referred to the appropriate professional.

the service. All licensed or regulated massage therapists may perform "medical massage" or therapeutic massage. Although additional training, specialized education in specific modalities, and certifications are beneficial, it is not necessary to acquire a *certification* in medical massage to deliver therapeutic or medical massage.

Right to Privacy

All clients have the **right to privacy.** You may not share any information about a client with other clients, a client's friends and relatives, or even with other medical professionals *unless you have written consent to do so* (figure 20.4). Keep this in mind as you build your client list if some of your clients come out of your associations with other medical professionals.

Health Insurance Portability and Accountability Act

On April 14, 2003, the first federal health care privacy protection standard was put into law. This law, the **Health Insurance Portability and Accountability Act (HIPAA)** was designed to protect the privacy of patients and clients and confidentiality of health records from insurance companies, doctors, hospitals, and other health care individuals. As a massage therapist, you will document information about a client's past medical history, current health status, prescription use, and any other aspects regarding the health of your client that will also fall under this law.

HIPAA regulations were developed by the U.S. Department of Health and Human Services (HHS). They represent a uniform federal privacy standard across the United States. Individual state laws that provide additional protections to consumers are not affected by HIPAA.

These regulations protect identifiable health information, whether in a computer, on paper, or communicated orally. Some of the key provisions affecting massage therapy are:

WRITTEN CONSENT FORM

I, _____, allow _____
           (client's name)   (therapist's name)

to disclose information pertaining to the massage therapy sessions with

the following: _____
                       (physician's name, etc.)

_____
(signature)

Print Name: _____

Address: _____

_____

_____ (date)

Figure 20.4
Sample consent form for the client to sign in order to share personal information.

- *Access to medical records.* Clients should be able to see and obtain copies of their medical records and request corrections if they identify an error. The health care provider has 30 days in which to turn over records. You must always keep the original record, but the cost of making copies can be charged to the client.
- *Limits on use of personal records.* The client must be provided with a release of information form to sign that designates what part of the records that have been requested by another health provider can be shared. For example, if a client has a massage weekly for a previous back injury and the orthopedic surgeon wants a copy of the client's progress notes, you would not send the client's history form that might include information about an abortion or a drinking problem.
- *Prohibition on marketing.* The regulations address the selling of patient information (such as addresses and phone numbers) to companies involved in marketing. You may not sell a photograph or image of a client using your facility or include it in your own marketing brochures unless you have the written permission of the client.
- *State laws.* When reporting a communicable disease or information about a possible crime involving a client, state laws covering such claims override the federal HIPAA regulations.
- *Confidential communications.* Under the privacy rule, clients can request that you not call their homes to confirm appointments or pass information about visits to family, coworkers, or friends.
- *Complaints.* Clients may file a formal complaint regarding privacy practices to the HHS office for Civil Rights.
- *Health care insurance.* If you file insurance reimbursement claims for massage therapy procedures, you may be responsible for following the medical HIPAA regulations as well as the nonmedical practice rules and regulations.
- *Civil and criminal penalties.* Complaints are investigated by the Department of Justice. Penalties for civil violations, *including honest mistakes*, are up to $100 per violation, up to a total of $25,000 per year, for each rule violated. Criminal penalties can range up to $50,000 in fines and one year in prison, and up to $100,000 in fines and five years in prison if the offenses are committed under false pretenses. Penalties are up to $250,000 in fines and up to 10 years in prison if the offenses are committed to take advantage of a client or for personal gain and with intent to harm.

Think About It | **Massage Therapy Clinic Checklist for HIPAA**

1. Do staff members discuss confidential patient information (CPI) among themselves or with clients or family in public areas?

2. Is CPI ever announced over intercoms, pagers, or cell phones?

3. Are progress or SOAP notes completed in a private area?

4. Are computer monitors positioned away from public areas?

5. Are all paper records and client charts stored in a private area that is inaccessible to visitors, clients, and unauthorized staff?

6. Is CPI on paper shredded?

7. Are answering services and answering machines accessible only to staff with a "need to know"?

8. Is a client sign-in list visible to other clients or visitors?

9. Are computer records—financial and others—protected with a password to prevent access by unauthorized staff, clients, or visitors?

10. Are fax machines monitored to ensure material with CPI is not left unattended?

Written consent must be obtained from the client before any information is given out, and clients have the right to see a copy of their records, request corrections, and receive copies. Clients also have the right to request information as to whom or what organization may have requested information.

Right of Refusal and Informed Consent

Both the therapist and the client maintain the right to discontinue treatment. The reasons may vary and may or may not have anything to do with the massage itself.

However, if the client is willing to discuss it, it can be helpful to the therapist to learn whether or not the quality of service or interpersonal relationship skills are involved in the client's decision to stop treatment.

This is called "informed consent" and refers to the educational process a client goes through to make an informed decision on whether or not to get massage or a particular type of massage (see chapter 3).

Working Smart, Working Safely

If you choose to be a sole proprietor, you must give careful consideration to the location of your business (see chapter 21). Chances are that you will be working alone at times if you rent office space or operate a business out of your home (if zoning permits). To lessen the potential for problems, try to schedule massage appointments when other people are in adjacent offices or when family members are in the house. Most health care workers follow these guidelines; in fact, many male doctors will not see a female patient without a female nurse or attendant present. Therefore, office location will dictate the manner in which you acquire clients.

Marketing and advertising are essential to your success. If you take clients on a referral-only basis, you may lessen the likelihood of finding yourself in an inappropriate or dangerous situation (provided you are upholding the ethics and standards of your profession). This manner of working, however, decreases the size of the pool of prospective clients.

If you advertise in the local paper or yellow pages, prospective clients are usually unknown to you. Consider where and how you want to work. Are you primarily making out-calls (home visits)? Or are you working in rented office space or out of your home? To reiterate, it is best to always have other people around, especially when you are working on a new client. Having a new client referred to you by a friend or coworker does not necessarily ensure your personal safety but does lessen the likelihood of problematic clients.

If you are making out-calls, common sense and gut reaction prevail. First, get adequate information in the phone call to make the appointment. Ask callers how they got your name. Find out what kind of massage the caller is looking for. Does it fall within your scope of training? Is the caller asking for a reasonable time slot, or is he looking for a late-night appointment? Learn to identify red flags by role-playing with fellow students or work through "what if" scenarios in your own mind.

Take into consideration the location to which you will be driving. Do you know it to be a safe area, a development housing mostly families, or is it a rural location without neighboring houses close by? If at any time you are uncomfortable driving into a certain area, trust your gut instincts and refuse the appointment.

Regardless of whether you are working in an office or on an out-call, if a client begins to show signs of arousal but you do not believe it to be intentional (an expected physiological effect) (see chapter 5), you may do one of several things to change the situation: change to a different modality, perhaps with a lot of stretching; change the lighting or the music to be less soft and relaxing; or alter the tactile sense and pressure by switching to working with your elbows and forearms instead of your hands.

Questionable Outcalls

You have accepted the appointment, are dressed appropriately (including no jewelry), and have your table packed up. Upon entering the residence, place your car keys and cell phone in a conspicuous place where they are easy to grab if need be. Do not take anything into the appointment, such as a purse, that may get left behind if you have to leave quickly. Set up the table, take a client history, and perform your massage with a professional attitude. If at any time you feel you are in danger or are approached inappropriately either verbally or physically, end the massage immediately. Pack up and leave if you are not in immediate danger; grab your car keys and cell phone and leave immediately if you are. As soon as you are safely in your car, dial 911 and alert the authorities. This may seem like a drastic measure, but we will not eliminate this scenario until the public realizes that unseemly behavior will not be tolerated under any circumstances. You can always return with the appropriate authorities to collect your table and supplies. (*Although this scenario is directed toward female therapists, it applies equally to male therapists.*)

Male Therapists

Unfortunately, massage can be a tough business for male therapists at times. Men who choose to enter the massage profession often find themselves having to place more emphasis on professional appearance and conduct so as to not be accused of inappropriate touch. Learn to recognize red flags here as well. Refer a female client to another therapist, preferably a female therapist, if she becomes too attached to you or exhibits what you deem to be inappropriate behavior toward you, such as asking for a date (see the section on relationships in this chapter). Be extremely careful with draping; ask permission to work on areas such as the gluteal muscles *over* the draping, and obtain

Practice Realities

Be Prepared

One of my first jobs as a massage therapist was at my local fitness center. The gym did not have room for a separate "massage-only" room; therefore, I agreed to work on clients on an out-call basis. Since I lived not far from the gym, some clients came to me for their massage immediately after working out. The first couple of clients were bodybuilders who were preparing for competition. I was comfortable knowing that they were referred by the gym but uncomfortable working on strong men I did not know personally. It was not possible to have another person in the vicinity during the first couple of massages, but I did make arrangements to have a friend standing by her phone. With her number on speed dial, I felt a little safer knowing I could hit the speed dial and run if anything untoward developed and she would follow with help.

written permission to work on gluteal or pectoralis muscles with limited or no draping. (This pertains to both male and female clients.)

Dress must always be appropriate: no "muscle shirts" or tight jeans (see the section on professional appearance in this chapter).

Female Therapists

It goes without saying that female therapists also need to dress appropriately. That means no tight shirts, short skirts, or other clothing that could be misconstrued as provocative. I am not suggesting that women (or men for that matter) cannot choose to wear whatever clothing they like. We would like to believe that sexism no longer exists, but the fact of the matter is there are people who still view such attire as provocative. There is a time and place for certain attire; the massage session is definitely not the place for unprofessional clothing. Perfumes and aftershaves are also not acceptable to wear while giving a massage because some clients may be sensitive or allergic to scents used in them.

Professional Appearance

Traditional typical dress that is professional in nature for both male and female massage therapists are scrubs, lightweight slacks and short-sleeve shirts, or khakis and polo shirts (figure 20.5). Shorts, even those that are midthigh or knee length, are inappropriate unless you are working at a spa that requires you to wear them. Comfortable lightweight slacks (of a cotton or rayon blend) and a pressed cotton shirt are excellent choices. This material allows for ease of movement and a loose-fitting cut helps keep you cool; you do work up a sweat while giving a massage. Appropriate footwear such as athletic shoes, sneakers, or other flat shoes should be worn. Long hair is to be tied back. Wear only minimal jewelry and keep it simple.

Appropriate dress and professional demeanor will speak volumes for you as a therapist and for all of us in this noble profession. A professional demeanor is illustrated by body language. Appropriate body language is also dictated by culture. In the West,

Figure 20.5
Appropriate attire for the massage professional is khakis and polo shirt, lightweight slacks and shirt, or neatly pressed scrubs.

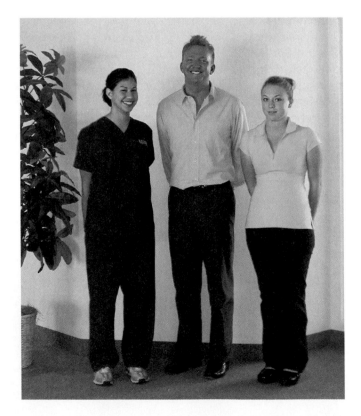

specifically North America, we tend to place at least a foot of space between ourselves and another person to whom we are not related. An out-stretched hand offered to greet clients or a hand gently placed on the shoulder to direct them toward the massage room is proper. Once in the massage room, remember to give clear, concise instructions about the massage process before exiting the room (see chapter 4). Most clients pay for services after the massage. This bookkeeping matter allows for a short period of time to transition from the massage itself, which invariably involves close contact, to a more distant salutation. The session finishes with the fee being paid, another appointment scheduled, and a wave good-bye.

Professional Demeanor

The massage therapist's professional demeanor is as important as dress or appearance. As a member of the health care field, you will no doubt be working with other professionals, including (but not limited to) medical doctors, chiropractors, and physical therapists. It is imperative that you not only speak the medical language but also pronounce and spell the medical terms correctly. Especially if English is your second language, you must work extremely hard at being articulate. Along with adhering to the code of ethics, being able to speak clearly and understandably reflects well on the profession in general and you in particular. Remember that many references may come to you from other medical professionals; being able to converse with these professionals will keep those referrals coming your way.

All massage therapists must work within personal and professional boundaries. These boundaries exist for the benefit of all parties. Our lives are often fast-paced and complicated. With many things going on at once, there tends to be some overlap; work may push its way into our home life, and personal issues may find their way into work if we are not careful to clearly define boundaries.

A boundary is defined as "something that indicates a border or limit." Personal and professional boundaries are defined as the areas or parameters within which you work, live, and play.

Boundaries and Professional Relationships

Professional Boundaries

Professional boundaries are based on legal and societal rules. They are conscious decisions that we make each and every day. The codes of ethics mentioned earlier in this chapter are examples of documents that have been formulated by people who have a consensus of opinion regarding massage as a profession. Asking all massage therapists to abide by the same code of ethics ensures consistency throughout the profession.

More obvious examples of professional boundaries are using proper draping, respecting a client's privacy, and not forming a personal (dating) relationship with a client. With any question involving boundaries, besides referring to the massage therapist's code of ethics, a good litmus test is to ask yourself if a potential action may have a detrimental affect on your client-therapist relationship.

Personal Boundaries

Personal boundaries are a protection of self: you consciously and deliberately decide whom you let into your "inner circle" and whom you keep at arm's length. This holds true for situations as well. Some situations you are comfortable in and others you are not.

Keep in mind that you have a right to privacy also. You will not want clients to have knowledge of personal issues, positive or negative. Make sure the client respects your "personal space."

Some clients may have different personal boundaries from yours. They may not want certain areas worked on, for example, the inner thighs or feet if ticklish. The boundaries or limits may be defined by subjects that are taboo as far as the client is concerned. Always respect their boundaries and work within their comfort level.

Multidimensional Relationships

Multidimensional or dual relationships are relationships in which the therapist plays more than one role in a client's life. The therapist may also be a relative or friend, or have a previous connection with the client.

Personalization

Psychologists refer the phenomenon of personalization as embracing or transferring emotions between one's self and another.

Transference occurs when the client personalizes the professional therapeutic relationship. For example, a long-time client believes it proper to ask very personal questions or suggest an evening out.

Countertransference is the inability on the part of the therapist to keep the therapist-client relationship separate and professional. For example, a massage therapist begins to have intimate feelings for the client and gives him or her extra time or attention during the massage. Countertransference may lead to inappropriate actions on the part of the therapist, such as asking the client for a date.

One more important issue is that of working with friends or acquaintances. Many texts currently state emphatically that you cannot work on friends or date clients. Although on the surface, this is a valid statement, in reality, many therapists do work on friends. In this practical, real-world text, the approach is to ask you to take appropriate measures to ensure that there will not be a detrimental effect on your friendship or professional relationship. Clearly spell out, in writing if necessary, massage is your job for which you rightfully receive payment. Consider a written agreement similar to a prenuptial marriage agreement partners sometimes make before the wedding. As long as you and your friend abide by that agreement, you should be able to keep a professional and platonic relationship separate.

Dating, on the other hand, is an entirely different issue. Your options are to refer the person to another therapist if he or she is under specific treatment, or to not accept payment. Take it out of the confines of a professional relationship and place it within a very personal one. Several husband-and-wife massage therapist teams who worked on each other while dating have continued to have a successful practice together.

Emotional Release

Occasionally, a client may experience an emotional release during the massage. It often happens with, but is not limited to, a client who has suffered from some form of inappropriate touch, or was emotionally, verbally, physically, or sexually abused as a child. Clients who have suffered a separation from a divorce, death of a spouse, or breakup of a relationship may exhibit signs of being emotionally distraught. Loss of a job and financial problems can create an enormous amount of stress that can erupt at any time and in many forms. A chronic illness, pain, or anxiety can take its toll and manifest as many other issues.

An emotional release may happen for quite complex reasons. Suffice to say, we call this "muscle having memory" (see chapters 5 and 17). As the body is worked on, old memories from the past or relatively new negative experiences rise to the surface and become insurmountable. The result can manifest as uncontrollable crying, shaking, and even nervous laughing. Not all emotional releases are overt and immediate. Some may manifest later in the day or evening as flashbacks or dreams. Feelings of helplessness or anxiety may manifest as withdrawal or being unresponsive or restlessness while on the table. It is important for the massage therapist to not *react* but rather *respect* the person's experience by quietly discontinuing the massage and waiting for an indication from the client of what the next step should be. That next step may be ending the session or lending support. A compassionate therapist can offer support by placing a hand on the client's shoulder, offering tissues, or even simply allowing the person space by being present but not obtrusive. Resume the massage only if and when the client asks you to. Chapter 12 discusses working with abuse victims and offers a protocol to follow. This information can be adapted to many situations where trauma has occurred in a client's life—regardless of whether the trauma was physical, verbal, emotional, or sexual abuse, or a type of loss.

Chapter Summary

As massage therapy and bodywork grows and gains recognition, it becomes even more important to recognize, internalize, and display the strength of character that allows one to operate as a *professional* in the health care field. A good way to prepare for putting ethical principles into action is to practice such scenarios using role-playing with fellow students, such as those provided in the case studies section of this chapter. Keep in mind that any action, positive or negative, on any one therapist's part is a reflection on all therapists. Be acquainted with the laws of your state and uphold the codes of ethics of local and national massage organizations.

Applying Your Knowledge

Self-Testing

1. What is the definition of *scope of practice?*
   a) Parameters the massage professional works within
   b) Fee schedule allowed
   c) Extensive training needed to practice
   d) All of the above are correct.

2. What is the right of refusal?
   a) Right of the therapist to refuse to treat a client
   b) Right of the state to not license a professional
   c) Right of the client to stop or refuse further treatment
   d) a and c

3. What is an emotional release by a client on the table?
   a) Experiencing past or recent unpleasant memories
   b) A sexual release
   c) Both a and b
   d) None of the above is correct.

4. Besides changing strokes and changing the music, name another way to diffuse sexual arousal during a massage.
   a) Use another body part such as elbows or forearms
   b) Switch to another modality such as stretching
   c) Turn the lights up
   d) All of the above are correct.

5. Tricky situations tend to develop due to a lack of what factor?
   a) Ethical standards
   b) Business practices
   c) Common sense
   d) All of the above are correct.

6. What factor is important to setting boundaries?
   a) Respecting personal space
   b) Respecting the client's comfort zone
   c) Upholding ethical standards
   d) All of the above are correct.

7. What is the definition of *disclosure?*
   a) The client's right to refuse treatment
   b) The therapist's declaration of their reason for invoking the right of refusal to work on someone
   c) The requirement to fully and truthfully fill out the client intake form
   d) The law that specifies all therapists must declare all monies earned

8. In reference to client records, CPI is an acronym for what?
   a) Cardiopulmonary infarction
   b) Coronary pulse interference
   c) Confidential patient information
   d) Covert patient intent

9. Under what conditions can you use a photograph of a client at your facility?
   a) Written consent of the client
   b) Oral consent of the client
   c) Do not need consent because it's your business
   d) Cannot ever use it

10. Privacy rules pertain to *all* forms of communication.
    a) True
    b) False

Case Studies/Critical Thinking

A. A female client in her early forties is receiving her weekly massage. This is her third visit to you. Twenty minutes into the massage, she appears to experience an emotional release (shaking, crying, etc.). As a trained therapist, you recognize this phenomenon and understand that it is not a provoked reaction but rather is a result of "muscle having memory." How do you handle this situation?

B. You are a massage therapist located in an area that is a seasonal vacation hot spot. A first-time vacationing client proceeds to tell you about his wonderful massage therapist at home. This therapist had specialized training in a certain type or modality of massage that you are acquainted with but not qualified to perform. You don't want to disappoint this client and would like to have him as a return client. Do you do your regular massage or try to do what the other therapist does?

C. You go out to dinner and take several of your clients' charts with you to finish your SOAP notes. Since you're eating dinner, you leave the charts on the front seat of your car. Your car is burglarized. You are relieved because it appears the thief took only your new CD. You return the charts to your clinic without realizing that the thief also took the patient information sheet from each chart. Later in the month, two of the clients report to you that they were victims of identity theft. Do you think that you contributed to this crime? How? What should you have done?

D. You are thrilled that you have moved into a larger space for your massage practice. You want everything to be state of the art so you get a new computer and sell your old one to a client who works for a bank. You downloaded and installed your clients' records on the new computer but failed to delete the files from the old one. On the old computer is a reference to a client, Mr. Jones, being under stress because of a separation from his wife. The banker reads all the information on your old computer. Mr. Jones applies for a new-home loan using his wife as the coborrower and listing himself and his wife as living together. Will the banker believe Mr. Jones' statement? Will Mr. Jones receive the loan? What role did you play in the outcome of Mr. Jones' loan application?

References for information in this chapter can be found in Quick Guide C at the end of the book.

21

Business Development, Marketing Success, and Community Education

LEARNING OUTCOMES

After completing this chapter, you will be able to:

- Identify your attitude toward and attraction quotient for money.

- Determine strategies required for developing, marketing, and creating a massage practice.

- Recognize pitfalls of starting a business and how to avoid them.

- Write a draft of a business plan that includes goals.

- Know what questions to ask yourself before starting your own business.

- Design a business card and brochure for your business.

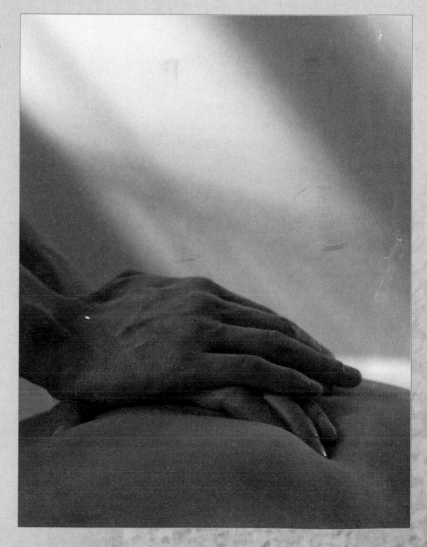

KEY TERMS

business plan (*p. 550*)

C Corporation (*p. 559*)

corporation (*p. 559*)

DBA (doing business as) (*p. 560*)

entrepreneur (*p. 548*)

general partnership (*p. 559*)

limited liability corporation
  (LLC) (*p. 559*)

limited partnership (*p. 559*)

networking (*p. 558*)

professional corporation (*p. 560*)

Schedule C (*p. 559*)

Schedule K-1 (form 1065) (*p. 559*)

Schedule SE (*p. 559*)

S corporation (Subchapter S
  corporation) (*p. 560*)

sole proprietorship (*p. 559*)

INTRODUCTION

Many massage practitioners choose to be self-employed; the balance of therapists work within chiropractic and medical clinics, health clubs, and spas. Although the nature of caregivers generally implies gentle and intuitive people who work well in a less-structured environment, it is discipline and organization that will separate the successful therapist from one who struggles in this admirable career. This chapter will give you insight into the type of employment that will work best for you as well as offer the necessary tools to establish and manage your business. Also included in this chapter is a discussion of corporate (or chair) massage; many practitioners choose to focus on this service as a complement to their table massage clients and to market their new business.

Keys to Success

The principles of a successful business and those of a healing arts practice often seem at odds with one another. We often think we cannot do good work and make money at the same time. This stems from a historical view that helping or charity work is altruistic and meant to embrace poverty or at the least a lower standard of living. (People in religious orders such as monks or individuals like Mother Theresa come to mind.) Remember, however, that you can incorporate into your business plan those general rules of operation for a successful business that match your personal philosophy and ideology. In fact, these qualities, which originate from your intent, set you apart from others in practice.

Most people who are successful hold a good sense of self. In other words, they know who they are and where they want to go. Additionally, successful people are knowledgeable and well-acquainted with every aspect concerning their business, from accounting to marketing. Their attitude toward money is appropriate. If you don't respect money, it doesn't respect you. The universe has a funny way of handling attraction. Positive attitudes attract; negative do not. If you hold a negative view of money, whether it be fear of handling it or believing everyone else has it and takes it from you, it will never come to you.

Financial planners have pointed out that our relationship with money is related to our attitude toward it. There are several indicators of your attitude toward money, such as the manner in which you physically handle your money. Are all of the bills (paper currency) in your wallet in order from least denomination to highest? Are the bills all "face up"? Or do you wad up the bills and stuff them in your pocket or purse? Do you have excess debt or obligation that burdens every thought? If you respect money, it respects you.

Entrepreneur or Employee

Is entrepreneurial management for you? Not all of us possess the personality and skills required for entrepreneurial work. The term **entrepreneur** has many meanings, but it usually refers to one who is ideologically a capitalist or industrialist, has a high tolerance for risk, and enjoys being his or her own boss. Any business venture has risk. According to the Small Business Administration, only two out of six small businesses survive for at least six years. All business owners need to follow one basic edict of life: "Know thy self!" First and foremost, you must decide what type of business you want to run or work in. As a massage therapist, you have many options, such as a spa, massage center, chiropractic office, physical therapy facility, gym, airport staff room, professional office, health food store, or home-based business with out-calls.

What is the difference between a person who runs a lemonade stand and a massage therapist who sets up shop in the neighborhood? When life gives you lemons, make lemonade. When life becomes stressful, get a massage. In both, the fundamental product is squeezed, then essential elements are added to enhance the flavor and texture for the end user. If you are the lemonade stand owner and your product is equal in flavor and texture to that of your competitors, what sets you apart from the other lemonade stands on any given day on any given corner in the marketplace? The analogy remains true as the owner/operator of a massage practice in Anywhere, USA. If the marketplace follows the model of free and open competition, what separates your massage products and services from the rest of the pack?

The massage therapist is a unique being who makes the statement "We won't rub you the wrong way." If this is true, the therapist must examine all aspects of the customer's needs. Not unlike lemonade stand owners, owner/operators of massage practices must ask crucial questions such as what is the quality, service, and cleanliness value of their business? Consistent, day-in-day-out delivery of quality service is the best yardstick for this equation.

Many therapists starting out wondering what they should charge for their services. The answer to most pricing objectives is what the market will bear. Take the time to do research in your area. Find out what other therapists are charging for *comparable* services and set your fees accordingly. Also, consider the socioeconomic level of your area: a neighborhood with a high standard of living (above-average income level) may accept a higher price structure than a working- or middle-class area.

Another question you should ask is what kind of environment would your clients find pleasing or comfortable? Some clients prefer intimate rooms that are warm, with soft light and candles, aromatherapy, and relaxing "new age" music, while others prefer a more clinical setting for therapeutic massage. Injury and rehabilitation facilities may appear sterile by comparison, but they serve the community and can be very lucrative (see chapter 2).

Questions to Ask Yourself

You will need answers to many detail-oriented questions. Ask yourself the following questions to ensure you cover all bases:

- What credentials and licenses will you need (federal, state, municipal, etc.)?
- What form of payment will you accept (cash, credit card, checks, insurance, barter)?
- What system of accounting will you use (computer-based or traditional accounting ledger), and how will you report income?
- What forms will you need to track finances and client information (client intake, SOAP notes, etc.)?
- What will be the structure of your business (corporation, sole proprietorship, partnership, etc.)?
- What knowledge and skills do you need to successfully administer the day-to-day operations of the business (scheduling, hiring, purchasing, marketing, and bookkeeping)?

The external communication model you choose will be a key component of your massage business. If you choose a simple model, all you have to do is list your phone (cell or landline) number on your business card and you're in business. More complex models may include e-mail or a website and multiple phone lines for networking personal computers with DSL. You will have so many choices, but so little time and resources when you first start out. You can always grow into the business—if flexibility and tenacity are characteristics you possess. When cash to start a business is low, you must rely on strong communication and negotiating skills.

The Business Plan

If you choose to open your own business, you must create and write a business plan. Before getting to the business plan, consider your personal and professional goals. Success in anything doesn't just happen. Even if you have not yet written out your desires, chances are you have thought often, or daydreamed, of how it will be. This is a good start. Manifestation begins in the mind and in the solar plexus; an affirmation brings it to fruition (see chapter 19).

The **business plan** is the map you need for setting up your massage business. It will identify the goals that will provide direction and landmarks for your massage achievements. Further, the business plan will help you identify the opportunities and obstacles you may encounter. Development of a business plan can start at school, using your instructors, peers, and school library to help you chart your course and explore career options. Visiting existing institutions such as a day spa, chiropractic clinic, and private massage establishment will give you a snapshot of those markets. Focusing on only those markets that appeal to you will help you follow your dream from the onset. Learning to recognize what you resonate with allows you to manifest it as reality. Remember, belief in yourself and your ideals dictates your uniqueness in this field, which in turn translates into success.

Anatomy of a Business Plan

Whether you are writing a business plan strictly for yourself or for potential investors, consider it both a sales pitch and something that will hold you to your dreams. The business plan document should be typewritten, double-spaced, and placed in a cover. It should include the following:

- Title page (with business name and your name, address, and phone number)
- Description page (with a description and details of the business)
- Goals page (with projected outcomes and reasons for believing the business will succeed)
- Marketing page (with a description of your clientele or who you expect to reach and acquire as clients). Specify what makes your business different from others in your area. Spell out what your marketing strategy will be for achieving this.
- Financial analysis page (with a description of your income potential and current financial status)

Goal-Setting

Think about and write down in positive "I am" terms what you want to achieve. Don't be afraid of deciding on a time frame. Life—and success—is an ongoing process: you will frequently review, revise, or completely alter your goals. It does not mean you are wishy-washy or a failure. Writing out your goals gives them a sense of validity and more weight. It gives you something concrete to look at when you find yourself saying, "Why am I doing this?" Keep goal writing simple and to the point. It is easy to be overwhelmed by goals. Five or 10 life-altering points are not what you are going for here but rather a step-by-step approach to creating the business you see in your mind's eye. The Small Business Administration is an excellent source for general information and prospects for loans. An accountant or financial planner will also be a valuable source of information.

Goal-setting becomes easier when the steps to creating your business are defined. Think of setting and attaining goals as part of your life's voyage. Make the goals attainable and realistic. As with any voyage, plan for stops and rest periods to maintain a fresh and positive outlook for you and your client base. These stops may include educational seminars for synergy purposes. Designate some "ports of call" for recreation and reenergizing, and others for revamping or re-creating your business and changing crews! Planning these aspects of the voyage kindles the financial spark required to determine start-up costs.

Start-Up Costs

Start-up costs for a massage business would consist mainly of the basic equipment and facilities.

A portable massage table (used or new) can range from $300 to $900 (see chapter 2). Administration forms, business cards, brochures, client intake forms, and other necessary items will cost $300 to $500. Communication devices such as landline, cell phone, fax, photocopier, and personal computer with a scanner can total from $1000 to $2500. Membership in a professional association that provides liability insurance will be approximately $300.

Renting office space can be quite costly, ranging from $500 to $1000 per month, depending on location and size. For example, in South Florida a C class building is approximately $10-$12 sq/ft, in a B class building $15-$20 sq/ft, and in an A class building $22-$27 sq/ft. Common area and maintenance fees can differ greatly for a new building versus an older one. Do not lock in the lease for more than one year unless your business plan calls for long-term growth in *that* specific market. In conclusion, total start-up costs can range from $2100 to $7100 monthly. This also implies the business owner has access to transportation for out-calls.

When renting or leasing a facility, it is important to secure a facilities and service agreement that outlines the terms between you as the tenant and the landlord. Remember, you must ensure the unit is yours and know what the cost of operating out of that unit will be in the short- and long-terms. Who is responsible for leasing improvements? Is it a one- or two-year agreement? Are utilities and water covered in the fee, or must you pay those separately? What is the common area cost if the space is part of strip mall or other complex? Does the rental agreement include a "no compete" clause to ensure you are the only massage therapist in the complex? Please consider all these factors, and, if necessary, consult a business associate or attorney before you commit money or time to the facility. Figure 21.1 is an example of such an agreement.

Insurance

In some states, the individual business owner, proprietor, or independent contractor is required to have liability insurance and sometimes workers' compensation insurance. The amount of insurance depends on your level of risk, but often a minimum amount is required by state law. Again, seek out the information through your local health department before purchasing insurance. Many professional organizations, such as American Massage Therapy Association, Associated Massage & Bodywork Professionals, International Myomassetics Federation, and International Massage Association, offer lower group rates. Another avenue to explore for reduced rates is through your local state chapter, such as the FSMTSA (Florida State Massage Therapy Association).

★ **EXAM POINT** Depending on state law, massage therapists may be required to have insurance before they can work for or with any employer. Even if you are an independent contractor and self-employed, in most states you must have your Establishment insurance and license displayed in the office or with you when practicing massage.

Sample Contract:

FACILITIES AND SERVICES AGREEMENT

Agreement, made this _____ day of _____, 20 _____, by and between _____,
Massage Therapist and (ABC Massage Therapist Group, This City, USA).

Whereas, _____, Massage Therapist is an independent contractor wishing to
use the facilities and services of _____(ABC Massage Therapist Group)_____ located
_____(New York, NY)_____ for the express purpose of the rendition of therapeutic massage services or
activities related to massage therapy.

TERMS OF AGREEMENT

1) Fee for a 1 hour massage is $60.00
   Massage therapist receives 60% of massage fees and _____(tips, etc.)_____.

2) Fees may be adjusted only upon agreement by both parties.

3) This contract is in effect through (date). At that time either party may cancel or modify the agreement. A
   new contract would be drawn from _____(date)_____.

**The following *facilities and services* will be provided by the
_____(chiropractor/therapist office)_____ for massage therapist:**

A. Storage for all massage supplies (e.g., linens, oils, etc.).

B. Use of the facility and its services (e.g., telephone, bathroom, microwave, refrigerator).

C. Booking and confirmation of all massage therapy appointments.

D. Collection of money, whether cash, credit card, or insurance.

E. A room for massage therapist use in the rendition of the therapeutic massage services or activities
   related to massage therapy, and also electricity, heat, and cleaning for this room.

F. Promote therapeutic massage as an enhancement to (chiropractic/therapy) care.

Massage Therapist will:

A. Bring all necessary supplies associated with the therapy.

B. Launder all sheets.

C. Pay any or all costs associated with being an independent contractor (e.g., liability insurance,
   professional memberships, or association fees).

D. Control own hours and schedule.

E. Not be held accountable for any expenses incurred by facilities or services not included in this
   agreement.

F. Keep all tips.

G. Keep all client information confidential.

H. Work at facility by appointment only.

I. Reconcile all accounts and pay proper percentage to chiropractor/massage therapist office at end of
   each said term (e.g., weekly, monthly, etc.)

*Cancellation of use of facilities and services is to be in writing, giving at least 30 days' notice, thereafter
releasing each party from all financial and legal obligations with the other party.*

Having read the terms of this agreement does hereby agree to terms and by signing does agree to use
_____ facilities and services to begin on _____(date)_____.

Date: _____   Date: _____

Figure 21.1 Sample facilities and service agreement
This agreement can be customized based on your needs.

The employment status of each massage therapist is directly related to his or her motivation, passion, and commitment to excellence. Your résumé is a snapshot for potential employers, investors, or partners. The résumé (figure 21.2) should reflect your previous jobs and educational accomplishments. Experience in related fields such as physical therapy and personal training is important; however, the emphasis should be on your hands-on experience with specific massage modalities. Continuing education units (CEUs) you have earned illustrate your experience with advanced classes and should be included.

Cards and Brochures

Design and produce a business card or brochure or both advertising your skills and services. Use a professional graphic artist and printing company if you do not have an "eye" for marketing materials or are not proficient in using a personal computer. These professional services are not necessarily cost-prohibitive. Check with local print shops and quick print shops such as Kinko's. If you use a personal computer, there are many publisher programs that have templates for business cards and brochures.

For the brochure and card, a high-quality paper stock will accommodate the wear and tear of daily storage and handling of these vital links to the outside world. A full-color (four-color) brochure is desirable when economically feasible. If you can afford only a black-and-white (two-color) brochure, consider using a color instead of black with the white. White space is very important, and less is more when making an impression on potential clients. When giving out business cards, always give the clients two cards, one for the client and one for their associate or friend.

The back of a business card is another marketing tool that is often overlooked. Use it to record subsequent appointments by adding lines for date and time. It can offer a discount on the next visit or a free consultation for the recipient. Albert Einstein once said, "Imagination is more important than knowledge!" Get creative and let the left and right sides of your brain play with the format, color, font style and size, and logos. All of these elements are important when designing a business card or stationery for your business. Refer to the sample business card in figure 21.3 for an idea.

The brochure (figure 21.4) should maintain continuity by following the same design established by the business card. This primary tool to educate the public and potential clients should include the following five main elements:

1. The nature of the services you offer

2. Description of all services offered

3. Credentials and qualifications of the practitioner

4. Client fees and relevant times associated with each modality

5. Address, phone number, fax number, e-mail address, and website, if applicable, plus hours and days of operation

Marketing Yourself Through Chair Massage

One of the best ways to market your services is through chair massage. Whether you perform pro bono (free) work or make visits to company offices, chair massage is a great way to break up the routine of the normal work week for both you and the recipient.

Corporate offices throughout North America are awakening to the rewards of chair massage in the workplace. Companies are looking for ways they can better serve their employees as well as their customers. One way is by giving employees the rewards of a 15-minute chair massage in the office (figure 21.5). Whether the chair massage is an occasional thank you to staff or part of a weekly wellness program, clinical tests have shown that massage increases alertness and productivity.

Astral Being

1234 This Street

Someplace, USA

(123) 456-7890

myaddress@web.com

OBJECTIVE   To develop a professional, ethical, client-oriented, and therapeutic massage career.

QUALIFICATIONS   AMTA Professional Member.
Proficient in Microsoft Word; 60 wpm.
Education from School of Natural Health massage therapy school.

- Proficiency is SOAP charting and documentation
- Knowledge of massage indications and contraindications
- Understanding of physiological developmental stages
- Current Red Cross certification in CPR and First Aid Safety

EXPERIENCE   SCHOOL OF NATURAL HEALTH, Anywhere, US
Student – 1/98 to 6/99
- 300 hours classroom/coursework
- 300 hours of clinical practice in student clinic

GO AWAY TRAVEL, Someplace, US
Sales Representative – 6/94 to 12/98
- Escorted groups to destinations in Europe and Asia
- Obtained and secured loyal corporate travel organizations
- Responsible for marketing travel specials
- Served as backup office manager

BEND OVER BACKWARDS CHIROPRATIC, This-place, US
Receptionist and Administrative – 1/92 to 6/94
- Responsible for scheduling appointments
- Processed medical billing for insurance
- Managed accounts payable and receivable
- Assisted chiropractor with patients

EDUCATION   School of Natural Health, Anywhere, US
600-hour Massage Therapy Program - graduated 1999

Our Community University, This-place, US
B.S., Marketing – graduated 1994

REFERENCES   Available upon request

Figure 21.2 Sample resume

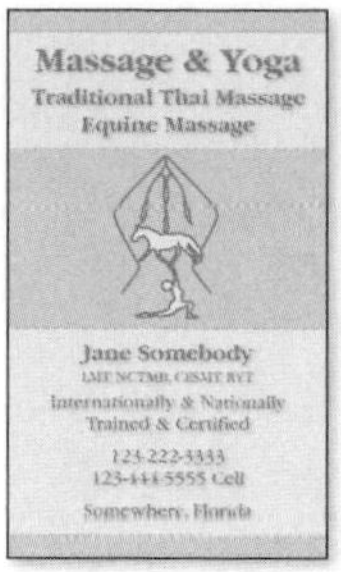

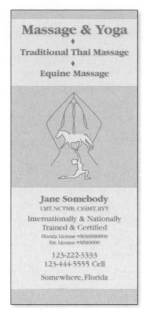

Figure 21.3 Sample business card

Figure 21.4 Sample brochure

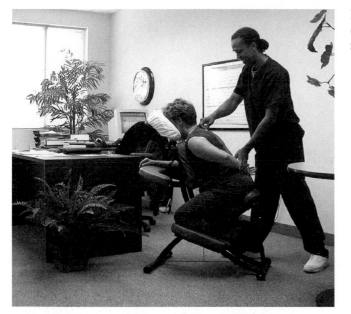

Figure 21.5
Corporate chair massage is a great marketing tool.

Corporate Stress Management

A key point to include when marketing chair massage to potential corporate clients is the prospect of more alert, productive, healthy, and happy employees with less absenteeism through stress management. Of utmost importance is showing employees that they are genuinely valued as human beings with top-of-the-line treatment. The following suggested wording could work as you market this service: "In less time than it would take for the average coffee break, show your employees how valued they are. What a difference 15 minutes can make!"

The use of chair massage has been a staple in the massage therapy program for many years. This unique modality incorporates Swedish, deep tissue, shiatsu, and a myriad of stretching techniques associated with relaxing the neck and back. The body mechanics for chair massage need to be emphasized more so than for any other form of massage.

Box 21.1   Personal Care

As a therapist, you will be on your feet for a minimum of two hours during a chair massage session, if the session is to be profitable. Proper posture will save your lower back and upper trapezius, and reduce cervical strain. Individual massage therapists have been known to do three to four hours of intense chair massage without exhaustion to their hands, legs, neck, and back by utilizing proper mechanics and deep-breathing techniques.

Plan for the break times between massages to be approximately two to three minutes, and stretch the appropriate muscle groups to ensure a healthy session for you and an enjoyable experience for your clients.

Benefits of Chair Massage

Chair massage serves many purposes in the workplace.
Benefits to the employer include:

- More productivity
- Less absenteeism
- Better employee-employer relations
- Lower health care costs
- Lower turnover
- Reduce desk rage

Benefits for employees are:

- Renewed alertness
- Greater vitality
- More creativity
- Better decision making
- Boost in morale

Chair Massage Tutorial

The art of chair massage can be summed up in a single phrase: "Less is more!" Unlike in full-body massage, clients do not need to disrobe, be concerned with sheets, or decide on the type of oil, lotion, or cream they would like for the massage. Clients simply climb on the seat, fold their arms onto the arm rest, and lean forward into the face cradle. They are then ready for a relaxing neck, back, arm, hand, or even leg massage.

The practitioner needs to be aware of the basic contraindications that apply to all clients: major injury to the back, neck, and spine may be a red flag. Do a verbal client intake and proceed with caution. Refrain from unorthodox techniques and stick to basic Swedish massage techniques—kneading, effleurage, vibration, hacking, and rocking—to ensure a great massage. Some basic arm and hand stretching with specific range of motion not to exceed the client's pain threshold will add greater relaxation to the massage.

Back rollers and magnetic rollers are effective in reducing the tension on the erector spinae, rhomboids, mutifidi, and trapezius. After two to three minutes of a mid-pressure roll-out, apply slight pressure with the palms and work from distal to proximal the entire lateral muscle groups of the lumber, thoracic, and lower cervical muscle groups.

Kneading of the deltoids, triceps, and biceps will relieve tension in the arms. Proceed down to the forearms, wrist, and eventually hands and fingers. Thoroughly massage left and right appendicular regions, and continue your routine to the kneading of the neck and lower skull.

For a minimum of two hours, a massage therapist will come directly to your workplace for the convenience of you and your employees. The results are immediate and guaranteed! So start or add to your wellness program by introducing chair massage to your employees. Our professional therapists bring quality massage chairs to your location and work on fully clothed clients. All you need to do is arrange a time and provide a space. The massage chair can be set up quickly in almost any location: a quiet boardroom or office is ideal.

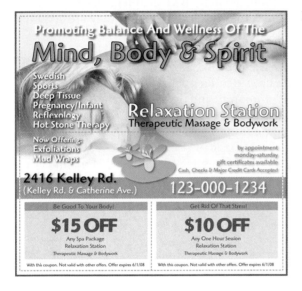

Figure 21.6 Massage coupon samples

Marketing Via Local Media

The print media can be a very effective means of marketing yourself within a specific time frame, especially during your grand opening. Local papers enjoy running stories about a new business or service being offered in their community. Often, a local paper will accept a piece you have written in a news release format for publication.

One of the most effective and least costly means of advertising is to perform chair (or table) massage pro bono at charity walks or runs. These events get you in front of the public while reaping the benefit of contributing to the community.

Make use of gift certificates and coupons. These can be printed separately from or along with your brochure for distribution in neighboring locations (figure 21.6).

Mailings can take the form of many different offerings for various reasons. A postcard introducing you and your massage services to the neighborhood is a very inexpensive and effective way of getting your name and face out to the community. Include a black-and-white photo and brief list of your credentials. Be sure to specify "free consultation" or "limited time offer" to spur a "call to action" for the consumer.

Any and all materials sent via mail or published in a newspaper are considered advertising and should be budgeted in the initial start-up costs.

EXAM POINT In most states, the law requires the therapist to have a license, or at least be registered, and therefore, a license number must be included on all advertising materials that are circulated to the public.

If you have a place of business, an establishment number is also required. Check the requirements of your state, municipality, and county before going to print any advertising for your business.

Networking

Networking has become the key element to marketing yourself in any business. Joining the local Chamber of Commerce, Rotary Club, massage association chapter, or other professional associations will enhance your image and directly increase the revenue of your business. The Business Network International (BNI) has many chapters throughout the United States and Canada, and around the world. This well-structured networking group is an excellent resource for getting, tracking, and following up on referrals for your massage business. Unfortunately, BNI chapters usually require owner/operators to be in business a minimum of two years before they are accepted into the chapter.

In the BNI philosophy, you are gifted with a code of ethics and the relationship management idea of "givers, gain." The more you give, the more you gain. All relationships are founded on trust. Just as each client requires your confidentiality and trust, your word is your bond in the business community, and the integrity of the actions you take and display dictates your success.

Other networking opportunities come from involvement in religious, sports, or other social groups. Look to your immediate circle of friends and acquaintances as a great place to start getting your name out to the public. Remember that volunteering time doing chair massage at the local senior assisted-living center or charity events benefits others in your community as well as yourself.

Type of Business

Now that you have your résumé, business cards and brochures, stationery, appropriate license, insurance, and networking group in place, you are ready to embark on this noble career. Hold on, captain! Before you set sail, consult those charts and maps so that you'll be able to navigate through unknown waters. Be sure to have plenty of supplies on hand for the voyage. Is the ship a one-person sailboat or cruise liner? In other words, is it a sole proprietorship or a corporation with stockholders?

You must decide how you want to work—whether as an employee, a sole proprietor, or a co-owner. As an employee, everything is done for you—all the marketing, cleaning, booking, and so on. As a sole proprietor, you can set your own schedule, work as much as you want, take off when you want, answer to no one but yourself, and have simple governmental regulations to follow. However, the disadvantages of a sole proprietorship are long hours, no one to share the workload with, and bearing the full financial burden. As a co-owner of a business, you will have someone with whom to share the responsibilities and workload.

As an employee, you will not have to worry about setting up a practice, acquiring clientele, or paying business expenses.

EXAM POINT You will probably work as an independent contractor; as such, you will be responsible for paying your own taxes, health insurance, and workers' compensation insurance.

The simplicity of forming a sole proprietorship versus a corporation has many advantages and disadvantages, depending on the level of risk you want to take with personal liability.

Sole Proprietorship

 EXAM POINT In a **sole proprietorship**, one person has ownership and liability of the business.

Most self-employed massage therapists operate as independent contractors and own their business as sole proprietors. This is the simplest form of business organization. In some states, you can be a single member (sole proprietorship) limited liability corporation (LLC). A LLC may offer you corporate-type protection. You must check with your state for details.

EXAM POINT As a sole proprietor, you will file a **Schedule C** tax form to report business losses or profits and a **Schedule SE** form to report self-employment tax if there are net earnings.

Partnership

EXAM POINT A **general partnership** has partners that share ownership and liability, whereas a **limited partnership** has partners who are invested in the business but do not play an active role.

Limited partners have a liability only up to the amount of their investment. General limited partners play an active role and have unlimited liability.

EXAM POINT Often seen today is the **limited liability corporation (LLC)**, which is permitted in most states and generally must have at least two owners. The owners are taxed as a partnership, while their liability is limited as in a corporation.

Forming any type of partnership allows therapists to build a larger practice. An agreement is signed or corporation papers are drawn up by an attorney, and the business's name is registered with the proper authorities. A business license is obtained if required by law.

EXAM POINT If you are a partner in a business, you will file a **Schedule K-1 (form 1065)** to report your share as a partner of income, deductions, credits, and other items.

Corporation

A **corporation** is a legal organization whose assets and liabilities are separate from those of its owners. Each state has different laws and requirements. These requirements include filing papers called articles of incorporation, electing officers, and obtaining an employer identification number from the Internal Revenue Service (IRS).

A **C corporation** is a separate entity from its owners or stockholders formed in accordance with state regulations. The corporation pays income tax, and the owners pay tax on any dividends.

EXAM POINT You will file a C corporation form 1120.

An **S corporation (Subchapter S corporation)** is a corporation that meets IRS size and stock ownership requirements. If the corporation qualifies, the shareholders may request S corporation status. This type of corporation pays no taxes. The profit or loss is passed on to the shareholders, who pay taxes on their individual tax returns but retain the advantages of a corporation.

 EXAM POINT You will file an S corporation form K-1 (1120S).

A **professional corporation** is a C corporation that is taxed at a higher rate than other corporations and has limited liability for its owners.

 EXAM POINT This type of corporation files like a partnership.

If you find it necessary to go after venture capital, meaning you will have investors' money for which you will be responsible, make sure all expectations are spelled out in a contract. Additionally, make sure to include an "exit clause" or exit strategies for both parties, should you need to end the business relationship.

You may also buy an existing practice. Make sure it is a practice comparable to what you would offer. If the existing business and your particular talents do not blend well together, the client base will not stay with you. It could be an expensive lesson to learn that you have bought equipment and assumed rental space for more than you would have paid for starting new.

Selecting a Business Name

In choosing a name for your business, select one that represents your profession but is not too "far out." You can do a name search online with the state agency that registers corporations (often the secretary of state's office). If the name is not currently in use or has not been used within the past year, it is up for grabs. You can also trademark your business name for a hefty fee of $325.

 EXAM POINT Most states require that you file a **DBA (doing business as)** name if the business name is different from your own name.

A DBA is also known as a fictitious name. Contact the agency that registers corporations in your state.

Chapter Summary

Whether you choose to open your own business or work for someone else, launching your career as a massage professional is an exciting time in your life (both personally and professionally). There are benefits and complications that go hand-in-hand with any type of business. Weigh each question and concern, as well as anticipated hopes, carefully and give yourself honest responses to all. Intent paired with knowledge and expertise will ensure success.

Applying Your Knowledge

Self-Testing

1. What is the definition of an entrepreneur?
   a) One who takes risks
   b) One who enjoys being his or her own boss
   c) One who is inherently wealthy
   d) a and b

2. What agencies should you check with pertaining to licensure?
   a) Federal
   b) State
   c) Municipal
   d) All of the above are correct.

3. What is the most important thing you can do before starting a business?
   a) Print a card and brochure
   b) Obtain office space
   c) Write a business plan
   d) Purchase office equipment

4. If you work for someone else but are not an employee, what is your status?
   a) Independent contractor
   b) Self-employed
   c) Consultant
   d) Part-time help

5. What do you take into account before setting a fee schedule?
   a) The amount you would like to make
   b) The amount you need to make to cover expenses
   c) The going rate in the area
   d) All of the above are correct.

6. What is the simplest form of business organization?
   a) Partnership
   b) Sole proprietorship
   c) Limited liability corporation
   d) S corporation

7. Who assigns the employer identification number?
   a) State
   b) City
   c) IRS
   d) Bank where you have your business account

8. What is another term for DBA?
   a) *Also known as*
   b) Your name
   c) A fictitious name
   d) None of the above is correct.

9. Which corporation is a separate entity from its stockholders?
   a) S corporation
   b) C corporation
   c) Professional corporation
   d) LLC

10. According to the Small Business Administration, how many businesses survive past six years?
    a) Five out of six
    b) Three out of six
    c) Two out of six
    d) One out of six

Case Studies/Critical Thinking

A. *Although you want to open your own massage center, you are low on funds. An acquaintance expresses interest in investing in your business. What documents or statements do you and your acquaintance need to sign before going into business? What are the pros and cons of entering into such an arrangement?*

B. *You have found an ideal location for your day spa. What considerations need to be fully explored before you enter into a lease for the space?*

References for information in this chapter can be found in Quick Guide C at the end of the book.

PART VII

Pharmacology and Specific Pathology Routines

CHAPTER 22   **Common Medications and Effects in Clients**

CHAPTER 23   **Special Massage Routines for Common Pathologies**

Common Medications and Effects in Clients

LEARNING OUTCOMES

After completing this chapter, you will be able to:

- Recognize common medications and herbal preparations.

- Understand the effects of common medications on clients.

- Alter the client care plan according to medication guidelines.

- Understand drug classifications and categories.

- Describe how medications/drugs are absorbed and metabolized by the body.

- Review possible basic pharmacology questions that may appear on the national exam.

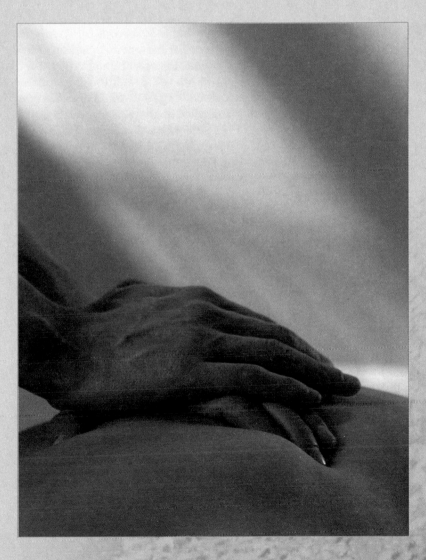

KEY TERMS

chemical name *(p. 569)*

depression *(p. 577)*

drug *(p. 573)*

excretion *(p. 573)*

generic (nonproprietary)
 name *(p. 569)*

micronutrients *(p. 579)*

noncontrolled drugs *(p. 573)*

over-the-counter (OTC)
 medications *(p. 567)*

pharmacodynamics *(p. 567)*

pharmacognosy *(p. 567)*

pharmacokinetics *(p. 567)*

pharmacology *(p. 567)*

pharmacotherapeutics *(p. 567)*

phytoceuticals *(p. 580)*

psychotropic drugs *(p. 577)*

standardized *(p. 581)*

topical administration *(p. 572)*

toxicology *(p. 567)*

trade (brand) name *(p. 569)*

INTRODUCTION

The purpose of this chapter is to provide you with information on medications, herbal preparations, and supplements that may be a part of your client's health care practices. With so much of our population over the age of 65, it stands to reason that you will encounter a number of clients who may daily take several forms of medications (figure 22.1). It is of prime importance that you realize you have a responsibility to your clients to have a basic knowledge of common medications and how they may possibly affect or enhance your massage applications.

All clients are required to fill out a client intake/history form (figure 22.2), regardless of the setting in which they are seeking massage therapy services; this includes physician's offices, chiropractor's offices, wellness centers, spas, and private home visits (out-calls). An extremely important part of this form is the section in which a client lists his or her current medications and supplements. For geriatric clients, this list may be as long as their arm and include several medications for high blood pressure, high cholesterol, diuretics, heart conditions, and so on. For a middle-aged, overweight client, this may include insulin and other medications related to controlling adult-onset diabetes. Even young, physically fit clients may be taking a wide range of medications such as analgesics or inhaled steroids for exercise-induced asthma. An entirely different segment of the population may be taking antidepressants or antianxiety medications, not to mention recreational drugs including, but not limited to, alcohol and tobacco.

With the ever-increasing interest in alternative health care, many clients turn to herbal remedies and natural supplements to address their particular health issues. Often these are taken in conjunction with other pharmaceuticals. Rather than consulting a trained herbalist, many people dangerously rely on the advice of a sales clerk at their local health food store. As a result, they may be either taking incorrect doses or improper herbs for their condition, a situation that may be magnified by massage.

As we have seen in chapter 5 and indeed throughout this text, circulatory (Swedish or therapeutic) massage, which improves blood flow and thereby possibly intensifies a medication's effect, as well as other massage modalities, can have a dramatic effect on or interaction with medications, herbal preparations, and natural supplements. Even the time at which a medication, herb, or supplement is consumed must be taken into account when scheduling a massage; for some clients, this will mean refraining from an early morning or late evening massage session that coincides with when they take their medications.

Keeping in mind that a massage therapist can neither diagnosis nor prescribe, a responsible therapist will be well acquainted with medications, herbs, and supplements, and their effects on clients. At any given time, a decision may have to be made whether to stop massage therapy treatment or, at the very least, alter the modality so as not to cause an adverse reaction for the client. In this chapter, we provide the massage therapy student, as well as practicing therapists, an overview of common pharmaceuticals, herbal preparations, and natural supplements they may encounter in their practice. As a massage therapist or bodyworker, it is not within your scope of practice to diagnose or treat. This includes giving advice, suggestions, or personal preferences to clients regarding the medications or supplements they are taking. You merely need the knowledge to help you better understand your client's health issues and how you can achieve through massage and bodywork results that are in the best interest of your client.

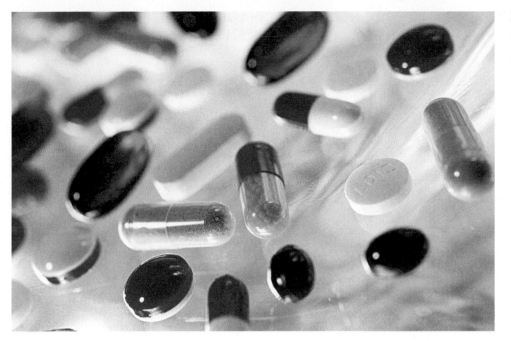

Figure 22.1
Massage clients may take many medications on a regular basis.

Pharmacology Basics

Pharmacology is defined as the study of drugs, their origins, nature, properties, and effects on living organisms. The five branches of pharmacology are:

- **Pharmacokinetics**—deals with the activity or fate of drugs in the body; includes absorption, distribution, metabolism, and excretion
- **Pharmacodynamics**—the study of the biochemical and physiological effects of drugs and the mechanisms of their actions
- **Pharmacotherapeutics**—the study of the uses of drugs in the treatment of disease
- **Toxicology**—the study of poisons and their actions, detection, and treatment of the conditions produced by them
- **Pharmacognosy**—deals with natural drugs and their constituents derived from plants, animals, and minerals

★ **EXAM POINT** In pharmacology, the word *drug* really means any chemical substance that changes normal body function and so includes medicines as well as poisons and drugs of abuse.

It may be assumed that the prescribing provider is keeping track of the client's medications and that any problems or contraindications have been communicated to any other health care personnel from whom the client seeks care. But in today's society, the reality is that no one health care provider can adequately maintain all the information regarding a client's prescribed medications as well as self-prescribed use of **over-the-counter (OTC) medications,** vitamins and minerals, and herbs, as well as medications obtained via the Internet. As you can see, the subject of pharmacology is immensely broad and covers large areas of physiology, biochemistry, and toxicology, all of which are concerned with the effects of chemicals on living organisms.

EVERYDAY GOODFEELING MASSAGE CLINIC
CLIENT INFORMATION/INTAKE FORM

Name: _____ Birth date: _____

Address: _____ Home phone: _____

_____ Cell phone: _____

Occupation: _____ Work phone: _____

General health condition: _____ Usual blood pressure: _____

Have you had any serious or chronic illnesses, operations, infections, or trauma?

_____

_____

_____

Are you in recovery for addictions, emotional issues, or abuse? _____

Are you under a doctor's, chiropractor's, or other health practitioner's care? _____

If so, for what conditions? _____

Please list any medications, vitamins/minerals, or herbal supplements you may be taking, and what it is for.

_____

_____

_____

_____

Do you have any allergies? _____

Do I have permission to contact your doctor/practitioner/therapist? _____

Names of doctors/practitioners/therapists:

_____ phone # _____

_____ phone # _____

Why did you come in for our service? _____

What results would you like to achieve? _____

Is this your first massage/treatment? _____

How did you find out about our services? _____

In case of emergency, notify _____ Phone # _____

I have completed this information form to the best of my knowledge. I understand the massage services are designed to be a health aid and are in no way to take the place of a doctor's care when it is indicated. Information exchanged during any massage session is educational in nature and is intended to help me become more familiar and conscious of my own health status and is to be used at my own discretion. I agree to notify this clinic 24 hours in advance of any cancellation.

Date: _____ Signature: _____

Figure 22.2

Medications should be listed on the client's intake form, and questions should be asked of the client to give the massage therapist a broader understanding of the medications.

The Body's Response to Chemicals

Most of the communication systems in the body are chemical in nature. Cells (such as nerve cells, gland cells, or blood cells) communicate with each other mainly by chemical substances produced and released by one particular type of cell and to which others are highly and specifically sensitive. Every cell in the body is continually responding to chemical messengers. This intricate communication system is vital for coordinated function, and most types of drug action mimic, change, or disrupt this communication system.

Understanding Pharmacology Terminology

There are many terms related to pharmacology that a massage therapist or bodyworker may encounter. Many of these terms have already been discussed or explained in previous chapters, and this section will review those terms as they pertain to pharmacology. It is important when reviewing a client's intake or history forms to mentally review the indications, contraindication, and adverse reactions as you would with any condition or disease before providing a massage or bodywork. Most clients will have very limited knowledge concerning their medications. They may say they take a "heart pill" two times a day, but it is important that you know if the medication is for fluid that affects the heart, cholesterol problems that affect the vessels to the heart, or conditions that affect the rhythm of the heart itself. A number of publications can give you specific information. These are easily found at a bookstore or online and can be kept at your clinic for easy reference; however, they are intended for giving you information that may affect how you proceed with the client and are not to be shared with the client. Medication questions that the client may have need to be addressed by the prescribing physician. Following are some of the terms that are listed in the reference material.

- *Indications*—describes what diseases or conditions a drug is commonly used to treat
- *Contraindications*—describes diseases or conditions for which a drug should *not* be used
- *Adverse reactions and side effects*—describes the body's reaction to a drug in an unexpected way, causing secondary effects that may be unpleasant or endanger the client.
- *Toxic effect*—describes what occurs when too much drug has accumulated. It may be due to an acute high dose of a drug, chronic buildup over time, or increased sensitivity to the standard dose of a drug.
- *Drug allergy (hypersensitivity)*—describes the body's reaction when it sees the drug as an antigen and establishes an immune response against the drug. This response may be immediate or delayed.

Thousands of drug products are already on the market with varying names, and each week, many new formulas become available to the public (figure 22.3). Each drug has a **chemical name** that is used by the manufacturer during the development and production phases. The chemical name describes the chemical formula and molecular structure of the product. After the drug is perfected, it is then sold to the marketing company with a **generic (nonproprietary) name,** which must appear on the label of the medication. The generic name is the official name that is listed with the government agencies that control drug patents. The drug is then given a **trade (brand) name** when it is produced to be sold to the public. The company that markets the drug chooses this name so the average individual can readily recognize the product. The trade name is registered with the US Patent and Trademark Office as the property of the drug company. For example:

Chemical name	Alpha-4 dimethylamino-3 methyl-1-2,2-diphyenyl-2 butanol, proprionate hydrochloride
Generic name	propoxyphene hydrochloride
Trade name	Darvon® (Eli Lilly Company)

Figure 22.3
Thousands of drug products are sold everyday in this country.

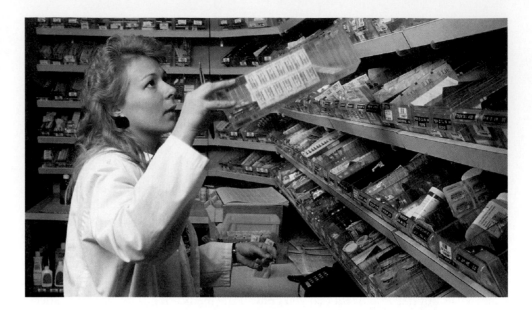

Sources of Drugs

Medicinal agents have been around for hundreds of years. Generations in every culture have passed on teachings and stories of how substances such as plants, leaves, herbs, roots, and bark found in nature, either alone or combined, can aid in healing. Many of the drugs used today were developed by identifying the active properties found in nature and then reproducing those properties by synthetic means in a chemistry lab. As technology progressed, research led to the use of substances from animals such as hogs and cows as effective drugs. Substances that are lacking in the human body can be replaced with substances from the glands, organs, and tissues of animals.

Beginning in the 1930s, synthetic drugs gradually replaced the herbals that had lined the shelves of apothecary shops throughout the United States. Laboratories have now replaced nature to allow for mass production. Because synthetic drugs are produced in the laboratory, this allows for improved standardization and purity of the drug over what is derived in nature (table 22.1).

How Drugs Are Processed by the Body

Routes of Administration

Drugs can be administered in a variety of ways (figure 22.4.)

Table 22.1	*Drug Sources*		
Source	**Example**	**Drug**	**Classification**
Plants	cinchona bark	quinidine	antiarrhythmic
	purple fox glove	digitalis	cardiotonic
Minerals	magnesium	milk of magnesia	antacid, laxative
	gold	solganal; nuranofin	anti-inflammatory (rheumatoid arthritis)
Animals	pancreas of hog or cow	insulin	antidiabetic
	thyroid gland of animals	thyroid	hormone
Synthetics	meperidine	Demerol	analgesic
	dipheoxylate	Lomotil	antidiarrheal

Figure 22.4
Common routes of medication administration.

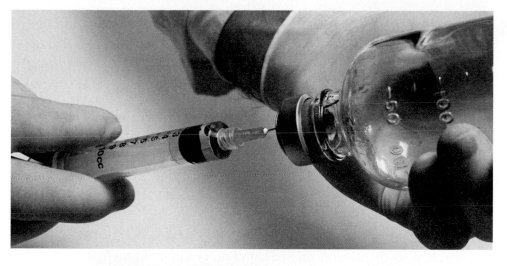

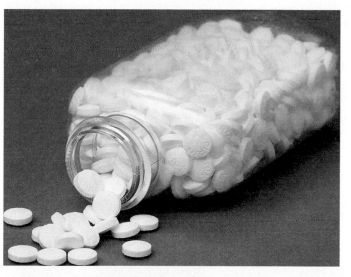

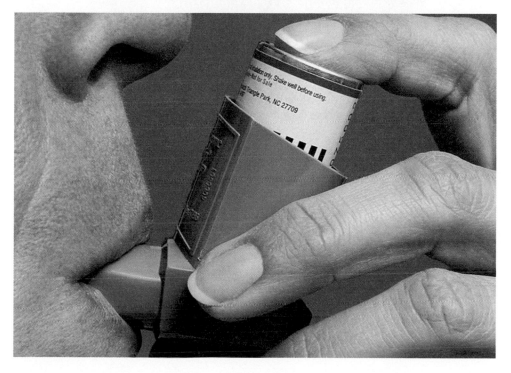

Chapter 22 Common Medications and Effects in Clients

Locally implies that the effects of the drug are confined to a specific area, as with **topical administration.** Topical preparations may be applied to the skin, mouth, nose, oropharynx, cornea, ear, urethra, vagina, or rectum. *Systemically* means that the drug has to enter the vascular and lymphatic systems for delivery to body tissues when administered orally or parenterally. Parenteral administration of a drug refers to the giving of a preparation by any route other than the gastrointestinal tract, such as through an injection, skin patch, or inhaled treatment. Drugs applied topically can have a local effect, as when applied to an injured muscle, or a systemic effect, as when a hormone is rubbed onto the skin. Table 22.2 lists the most common routes by which drugs are administered.

Pharmacokinetics

Pharmacokinetics considers the movement of drugs within the body and the way in which the body affects drugs with time. Once a drug has been administered by one of the routes previously described, it undergoes four basic processes:

- Absorption
- Distribution
- Metabolism
- Excretion

Primary factors affecting pharmacokinetics include:

- Rate of drug absorption
- Amount absorbed in body
- Distribution of drug throughout body
- Process and timing of drug metabolism
- Rate and route of drug excretion from the body

Table 22.2	*Common Routes of Drug Administration*

Primarily for Local Effects

- Topical—mucous membrane or skin
- Intraarticular—within the cavity of a joint
- Intradermal or intracutaneous—into the skin
- Inhalation—sprayed into the respiratory tract
- Intrathecal—into the spinal column

Primarily for Systemic Effects

Via the gastrointestinal tract

- Buccal— placed in the cheek
- Oral—by mouth
- Sublingual—under the tongue
- Rectal—suppository absorbed in the rectum

Via injection

- Intramuscular—into the muscle
- Intravenous—into a vein
- Subcutaneous—into the tissue below the skin

Via skin

- Transdermal—applied to unbroken skin

Other factors such as the dose of drug, the client's condition, and other therapeutic and environmental issues may also have an impact on the effectiveness of these processes.

Drug Excretion

Drugs and their metabolites may be eliminated from the body in several ways. The most significant route is through the kidneys. Some drugs may be secreted by the liver into bile and excreted in the feces. Additional routes of **excretion** include the respiratory tract, breast milk, saliva, and sweat. Herbal wraps, heat treatments, and certain massage manipulations can contribute to drug excretion through the skin and result in a loss of the level of a medication in the client's bloodstream or fat storage cells.

> ★ **EXAM POINT** Alcohol and nicotine can be eliminated from the skin during a massage, contributing to a detoxification of the bodily tissues.

Drug Classifications

The definition of a **drug**—as far as legal agencies classify them—is any chemical substance that has an effect on living tissue but is not used for food. Herbal substances and vitamin supplements come under the food division of the U.S. Food and Drug Administration. Drug classification categorizes drugs by how they affect the body in similar ways or by their therapeutic effects. Drugs that have several therapeutic effects can fit under multiple classifications. An example is aspirin, which acts as an analgesic to relieve pain, an antipyretic to reduce fever, and an anti-inflammatory to reduce inflammation to tissues. A number of medication categories are important to the massage therapist (table 22.3).

Examples of drug classifications include general, chemical, and therapeutic.

- *General:* Drugs are grouped according to their source, whether animal, vegetable, mineral, or synthetic.
- *Chemical:* Medications are grouped by their chemical characteristics. Examples are acids, bases, or salts.
- *Therapeutic* (pharmacological): Drugs are classified according to their action on the body. A drug may have more than one action.

The drug classifications can be further divided into two groups: noncontrolled and controlled drugs.

Noncontrolled Drugs

Noncontrolled drugs are nonprescription or over-the-counter drugs (figure 22.5).

Controlled Drugs

All prescription drugs are to be treated with respect; certain groups considered to have a potential for abuse, such as narcotics, stimulants, and sedatives, require special handling and security measures. Controlled substances are those drugs listed in the Controlled Substance Act of 1970, which is administered by the Drug Enforcement Administration of the Justice Department. Controlled drugs are categorized into five schedules, as indicated in table 22.4.

Topical Medications

The many topical medications available today, both OTC and prescription, are too numerous to list. They run the list of reasons for application, from analgesic, capillary dilatation,

Table 22.3 *Common Drugs Categories (Contraindications to massage, in italics, refers to medication group, not individual medications.)*

Category	Example/*Generic (trade) name*	Action/*Contraindications*
Analgesic	acetaminophen (Tylenol®) acetylsalicylic acid, or aspirin tramadol HCl (Ultram®) hydromorphone HCl (Dilaudid®) morphine sulfate (MS Contin®) Oxycodone HCl (Percoset®, Oxycontin®)	Relieves pain, discomfort *Client may not feel pain; stretching may contribute to injury.*
Anesthetic	lidocaine HCl (Xylocaine®) tetracaine HCl (pontocaine)	Prevents sensation of pain (topical application) *Client may not feel pain; prolonged massage may send topical anesthetic into deeper tissues.*
Antacid	calcium carbonate (Tums®) magaldrate (Riopan®)	Neutralizes stomach acid *Client should not be placed flat on the table and may need to be elevated at the head.*
Antiarrhythmic	verapamil (Isoptin®, Calan®) amiodarone (Cordarone®) disopyramide (Norpace®) propanolol HCl (Inderal®)	Normalizes heartbeat *Get a complete history on client to determine actual condition.*
Antibiotic	cefaclor (Ceclor®) erythromycin (E-Mycin®) penicillin V potassium (Pen Vee K®) tetracycline HCl (Tetracap®) vancomycin (Vancocin®)	Kills microorganisms or inhibits their growth *Due to the way antibiotics work, a client may be sensitive to light, heat, and touch, have joint pain and rashes; review medications and use caution; may need to wait to massage until the antibiotics have left the client's system.*
Anticoagulant	warfarin sodium (Coumadin®) enoxaparin sodium (Lovenox®)	Thins blood to prevent clotting *These medications can lead to extensive bruising; clots may be moved when deep massage of extremities is applied; heat or cold can cause blood pressure issues.*
Anticonvulsant	clonazepam (Klonopin®) phenytoin (Dilantin®)	Controls seizures *Extreme changes in heat or cold; depending on condition, client may not be left alone.*
Antidepressant	amitriptylie HCl (Elavil®) fluoxetine HCl (Prozac®) sertraline HCl (Zoloft®)	Relieves depression
Antihistamine	cetirizine HCl (Zyrtec®) diphenhydramine HCl (Benedryl®) loratadine (Claritin®)	Relieves allergic symptoms
Antihypertensive	atenolol (Tenormin®) metoprolol (Lopressor®) captopril (Capoten®)	Reduces blood pressure *Observe caution in the use of heat or cold; extreme or excitable activity.*
Anti-inflammatory (two types)		Reduces inflammation
Nonsterioid (NSAIDs)	ibuprophren (Advil®, Motrin®)	*Client may not feel pain; stretch may cause injury.*
Steroids	dexamethasone (Decadron®) methylprednisolone (Medrol®) prednisone (Deltasone®)	*Bruising possible; swelling and edema usually present; skin integrity may be compromised.*

Category	Example/*Generic (trade) name*	Action/*Contraindications*
Bronchodilator	albuterol (Proventil®, Ventolin®) theophylline (Theo-dur®)	Dilates bronchi *Shorten duration of massage; release of endorphins can bring changes quickly; heat or cold can trigger problems.*
Decongestant	oxymetazeline (Afrin®) pseudophedrine HCl (Sudafed®)	Relieves nasal congestion *Use caution when placing client face down; blood pressure and heart rhythm changes can occur with prolonged activity.*
Diuretic	hydrochlorothiazide (Hydrodiuril®) furosemide (Lasix®)	Increases urine output, reduces blood pressure *Skin integrity may be compromised; blood pressure and bruising are concerns.*
Hormone replacements	insulin (Humulin®)	Used by diabetics *Avoid injection sites; massage for short duration; deep tissue massage can cause injury; skin integrity is of major concern.*
	levothyroxine sodium (Synthroid®)	Thyroid deficiency *Avoid sudden heat and cold changes.*
Muscle relaxant	carisoprodol (Rela® or Soma®) cyclobenzaprine HCl (Flexeril®) diazepam (Valium®)	Relaxes skeletal muscles *Can greatly change client responses to massage; stretch may lead to injury; heat and cold effect is modified.*
Statin	simvastatin (Zocor®)	Inhibits synthesis of cholesterol *Client may exhibit muscle weakness; statin group is often taken with blood thinners that cause bruising.*
Vasoconstrictor	dopamine HCl (Intropin®) norepinephrine bitartrate (Levophed®)	Constricts blood vessels and increases blood pressure *Massage can change blood pressure and blood flow dramatically; cryotherapy should not be used.*
Vasodilator	nitroglycerine (Nitrostat®) reserpine (Serpasil®)	Dilates blood vessels and decreases blood pressure *Get a complete history; take precautions when using heat or cold, depending on condition; do not place client's torso on flat surface or elevate extremities for long periods of time; do not press on medication patches or get them wet.*

bacteriostatic, antiviral, and antifungal to hormonal delivery. When a client gives the name of a topically applied medication, check to see what it is used to treat. If it is for a contagious type of rash, make sure you do not come in contact with the treated area.

⭐ **EXAM POINT** The medication will in no way protect you from exposure.

Many older clients or clients with sports injuries may use a topical analgesic such as Biofreeze® or Ben Gay®; you may need to request that this or other topical applications be applied after the massage. Your sports massage or orthopedic massage instructor should be able to explain under what circumstances it is within your scope of practice to apply this type of product along with your massage. Always be aware that the pharmacokinetics of a topically applied product can be greatly affected by the action of massage on the body.

Figure 22.5

A person with a cold usually takes several over-the-counter medications.

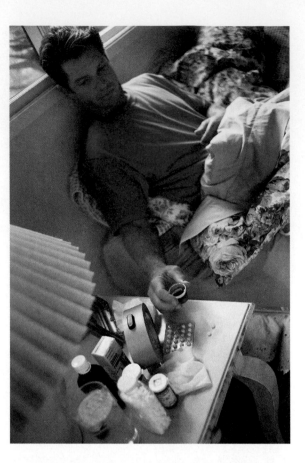

Table 22.4	**Drug Schedules**	
Drug Schedule	**Description**	**Example**
I	■ *Not* considered to be legitimate for medical use ■ Research only ■ High risk of abuse	LSD, heroin, marijuana
II	■ Accepted medical use ■ High risk of abuse ■ New written prescription for each fill	Morphine, cocaine, codeine, demerol, dilaudid
III	■ Moderate potential for abuse or addiction; low potential for physical dependence ■ Written or phone prescription expires in six months ■ No more than five refills in six months	Tylenol with codeine, butisol, hycodan
IV	■ Less potential for abuse or addiction; limited physical dependence ■ Written or phoned prescription expires in six months ■ Can be fill up to five times in six months	Librium, valium, darvon, equanil
V	■ Small potential for abuse or addiction ■ Written or phoned prescription ■ No limit on refills ■ Some may not need a prescription	Robitussin A-C, donnagel-PG, lomotil

Make sure you do not come in contact with a product that has been applied to the skin to which you may be allergic. Many products may have a penicillin, iodine, or sulfa base that could cause your hands to itch or swell.

Psychotropic Medications

Medications that act on the mind by causing therapeutic effects are classed as **psychotropic drugs.** Many of the sedative, hypnotic, and analgesic medications also affect the mind, but the psychotropic medications either react to stimulate the central nervous system or work to restore balance by controlling the chemical neurotransmitters dopamine, serotonin, and norepinephrine. **Depression** is considered a condition of a shortage of the neurotransmitters. There are four main categories of antidepressants:

- Tricyclics have possible side effects of dehydrated skin, cardiac palpitations, confusion, and hypotension.
- MAO (monamine oxidase) inhibitors increase the concentrations of the neurotransmitters and have possible side effects of nervousness, headache, stiff neck, muscle spasms, and hypertension that can rise to fatal levels.
- Selective serotonin reuptake inhibitors (SSRIs) have possible side effects of headache, tremors, fatigue, and profuse sweating.
- Heterocyclics alter dopamine, norepinephrine, and serotonin and have as possible side effects drowsiness, cardiac problems, seizures, and insomnia.

These have been included here because some of your clients may be coming in for massage to help with these side effects. The side effects must be dealt with as a "condition," and the appropriate massage plan should be incorporated.

EXAM POINT Massage may help the symptoms of the side effects; however, these side effects will not go away as long as the medication is taken.

Recreational Drugs

EXAM POINT Alcohol is classified as a psychotropic drug and a depressant.

It acts on the central nervous system and affects the brain to impair control over judgment and memory. It first acts to cause excitement and then leads to sedation before a complete central nervous system (CNS) shutdown as anesthesia. Clients affected by alcohol will produce an unsteady gait, slurred speech, and incoordination of movement. Prolonged use will cause permanent CNS damage and peripheral neuritis. Liver damage will contribute to bruising and blood loss under the skin. Dehydration will cause a lack of skin integrity and muscle wasting. Alcoholics are not clients to be considered for massage.

EXAM POINT Recovering alcoholics who have been clean long enough to overcome the minor symptoms of alcohol abuse may be considered. Keep in mind, however, that with some clients, the effects of long-term alcohol abuse will not be reversed.

Amphetamines, "meth," and cocaine are stimulants. The side effects that go along with use are teeth grinding, temporomandibular joint dysfunction, malnutrition, decaying teeth, ulcers on skin, and a sensitivity to heat and light. Cardiac malfunctions are common, as well as hypertension and circulatory collapse.

Clients who abuse amphetamines are not to be massaged due to the instability of their body's condition.

Marijuana, or tetrahydrocannabinol (THC) as it is medically known, is classified as a central nervous depressant. It creates euphoria, sedation, and hallucinations.

The active agent is stored in the fat of the body and can be redistributed with deep massage techniques.

The bodies of clients who use marijuana store the THC for four to six weeks. It contributes to lethargy, muscle weakness, and impaired reflex action of the skeletal muscles. Persons actively smoking marijuana or inhaling the second-hand smoke are not likely to benefit from massage.

Tobacco's active ingredient is nicotine.

Nicotine is a poison to the body and contributes to vasoconstriction, respiratory problems, and fluctuations in blood pressure and cardiac rhythms (figure 22.6).

Studies are now being done to see if regular massage can help with smoking cessation by releasing the neurotransmitters that control anxiety and cravings. Since nicotine is stored in the tissues, a tobacco smell may be experienced when a client who smokes is massaged. One way the body gets rid of toxins is through the skin.

General Contraindications

With proper precautions, massage is a viable tool in the health care of clients. However, caution should be observed with certain clients. Massage has proven a useful tool in regulating blood sugar levels.

Figure 22.6
Nicotine and tar residue from smoking tobacco contribute to many forms of disease.

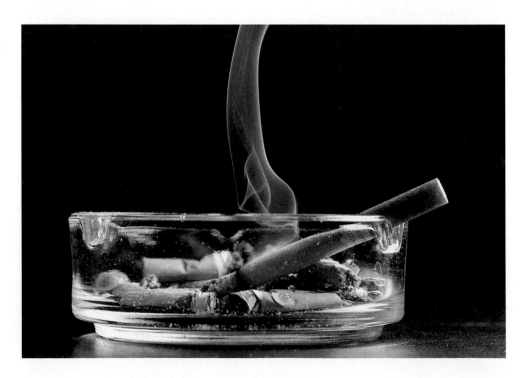

EXAM POINT Diabetic clients should check their blood sugar levels immediately after a massage and again an hour later to make sure the level is not too low.

You should reconsider or use extreme caution when massaging clients with congestive heart failure, kidney failure, infection of the veins or soft tissue (phlebitis, cellulites), blood clots, bleeding disorders, or contagious skin conditions. Clients undergoing chemotherapy will have fragile tissue and skin conditions. Clients taking medication for osteoporosis may have severely fragile bones, and clients with leukemia may be targets for skin tears that lead to infection.

Check with your clients at the beginning of each session to see if they have started any new medications. Remember: a client does not receive a prescription or buy something over the counter unless symptoms have been happening. A client with a stent, liver damage, or a gastric bypass can have problems if the area of concern is vigorously manipulated. Being aware can help you safely perform massage that will benefit your clients in every way.

Vitamins and minerals are necessary in small but steady amounts for maintaining optimal functioning of the body.

Vitamins and Minerals

EXAM POINT Together, vitamins and minerals are called **micronutrients.**

Found in nature and acquired through diet, vitamins and minerals are needed for a variety of biologic processes; among them are growth, digestion, mental alertness, and resistance to infection. Your body cannot make most micronutrients, so you must get them from the foods you eat or, in some cases, from supplements. Whole foods—such as fruits, vegetables, and whole grains—provide a complex combination of vitamins, minerals, fiber, and other substances that promote health. Whole foods are your best sources of vitamins and minerals (figure 22.7). They contain not just one but a

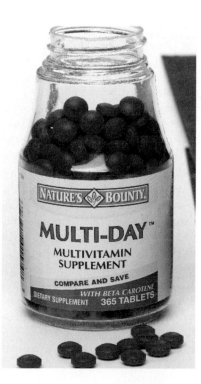

Figure 22.7
Vitamins, minerals, and herbal supplements are taken by many health-conscious individuals.

complement of the micronutrients your body needs. An orange, for example, provides vitamin C but also contains beta carotene, calcium, and other nutrients. A vitamin C supplement lacks these other micronutrients. If you depend on using supplements rather than eating a variety of whole foods, you may miss the potential benefits of these other substances. (See chapter 18.)

Vitamins are classified as to whether they are fat-soluble or water-soluble.

Water-soluble vitamins: Vitamin C, biotin, and the seven B vitamins—thiamin (B-1), riboflavin (B-2), niacin (B-3), pantothenic acid (B-5), pyridoxine (B-6), folic acid (B-9), and cobalamin (B-12)—dissolve in water (water-soluble) and are not stored in your body in any significant amounts. Excess water-soluble vitamins are simply excreted in your urine.

Fat-soluble vitamins: Excess vitamin A, D, E, or K not utilized by your body right after ingestion is stored in your body fat and liver. Accumulation of fat-soluble vitamins can lead to toxicity. You are especially sensitive to excess amounts of vitamins A and D. Because vitamins E and K affect blood clotting, caution must be observed in taking these when blood thinners such as warfarin (Coumadin) are prescribed.

Minerals are the main components in your teeth and bones, and they serve as building blocks for other cells and enzymes. Minerals also help regulate the balance of fluids in your body and control the movement of nerve impulses and muscle contractions. Some minerals also help deliver oxygen to cells and help carry away carbon dioxide. Minerals have two categories:

Major minerals: Calcium, phosphorus, magnesium, sodium, potassium, sulfur, and chloride are considered major minerals because adults need them in larger amounts—more than 250 milligrams a day.

Trace minerals: Chromium, copper, fluoride, iodine, iron, manganese, molybdenum, selenium, and zinc are considered trace minerals because adults need them in smaller amounts—fewer than 20 milligrams a day.

Herbs

 EXAM POINT Herbal medicine is also known as botanical medicine, phytotherapy, or phytomedicine.

Many modern-day herbal preparations that are processed and packaged to sell are called **phytoceuticals.** The herbal part of a remedy may have come from the leaf, flower, stem, seed, root, fruit, or bark of the plant and may be used to treat wounds, abrasions, cuts, and a number of conditions (figure 22.8). Herbal medicine is considered to be the most ancient form of healing. Herbs have been used in most traditional cultures and have had an extraordinary influence on many systems of medicine, with many prescription drugs still derived from trees, shrubs, or herbs.

An estimated 250,000 to 500,000 plants are known today, but only about 5000 of these have been studied or used medicinally. Many researchers believe that there are plants as yet unrecognized for their healing powers. We may find in the future that some herbs may replace some types of antibiotics and prescription drugs as widespread treatments.

Plants were used for medicinal purposes long before recorded history. Ancient Chinese and Egyptian papyrus writings describe medicinal plant uses. Indigenous cultures (such as African and Native American) used herbs in their healing rituals, while others developed traditional medical systems (such as *Ayurveda* and traditional Chinese medicine) in which herbal therapies were used systematically. During their research, scientists found that people in different parts of the globe tended to use the same or similar plants for the same purposes.

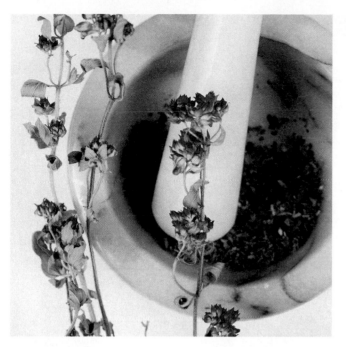

Figure 22.8
Herbs being prepared for use.

Although it is classed as "alternative" or "complementary" in most Western countries, herbal medicine still remains the only form of medicine widely available to most of the world's population.

⭐ **EXAM POINT** The herbs available in most stores come in several different forms: teas, syrups, oils, liquid extracts, tinctures, and dry extracts (pills or capsules) (figure 22.9).

Teas are simply dried herbs left to soak for a few minutes in boiling water. Syrups, made from concentrated extracts and added to sweet-tasting preparations, are frequently used for sore throats and coughs. Oils are extracted from plants and often used as rubs for massage, either alone or as part of an ointment or cream. Tinctures and liquid extracts are solvents (usually water, alcohol, or glycerol) that contain the active ingredients of the herbs. Tinctures are typically a 1:5 or 1:10 concentration, meaning that one part of the herbal material is prepared with five to 10 parts (by weight) of the liquid. Liquid extracts are more concentrated than tinctures and are typically a 1:1 concentration. A dry extract form is the most concentrated form of an herbal product (typically, 2:1 to 8:1) and is sold as a tablet, capsule, or lozenge.

Currently, no organization or governmental body in the United States regulates the manufacture or certifies the labeling of herbal preparations. In Europe, however, a group known as Commission E regulates herbal products. Some herbal preparations are **standardized,** meaning that they are *guaranteed* to contain a specific amount of the active ingredients of the herb.

Herbs contain a large number of naturally occurring chemicals (constituents) that have some type of biological activity. Herbs work in a similar fashion to many pharmaceutical preparations, and this is what causes the most debate between conventional and alternative medicine practitioners. Because our metabolism is well-suited to digesting plants and herbal medicines have a gentle, cumulative effect, they have no side effects for most people. However, like all medications, dosage instructions should be followed, and you should consult your doctor before taking them if you are pregnant, breast-feeding, or regularly taking other prescribed medicines. Herbal medicine has shown to be of most benefit when it is used to treat chronic, ongoing conditions.

Figure 22.9
Many forms of alternative and
herbal products are available.

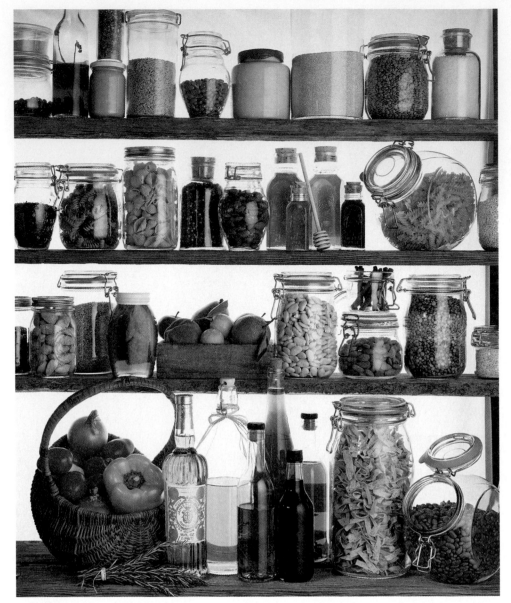

However, this is not the case with all herbs—especially if they are taken in large
quantities.

Many words are used to describe herbs and their actions on the body. Understanding terms or words commonly used in herbal literature provides a foundation for understanding herbal preparations and reinforces the basics for those with some experience with herbal medicine. Table 22.5 presents herbal terminology used for the many types of herbal preparations. Table 22.6 lists the categories used to classify herbal properties.

Table 22.5 *Herbal Preparations*

Decoction: A tea made from boiling plant material, usually the bark, rhizomes, roots, or other woody parts, in water.

Infusion: A tea made by pouring water over plant material (usually dried flowers, fruit, leaves, and other parts, though fresh plant material may also be used), then allowing it to steep. The water is usually boiling, but cold infusions are also an option.

Tincture: An extract of a plant made by soaking herbs in a dark place with a desired amount of either glycerine, alcohol, or vinegar for two to six weeks. The liquid is strained from the plant material.

Liniment: Extract of a plant added to either alcohol or vinegar and applied topically.

Poultice: A topical application of a soft, moist mass of plant material (such as bruised fresh herbs), usually wrapped in a fine, woven cloth.

Essential oils: Aromatic volatile oils extracted from the leaves, stems, flowers, and other parts of plants. Therapeutic use generally includes dilution of the highly concentrated oil.

Herbal infused oils: A process of extraction in which the volatile oils of a plant substance are obtained by soaking the plant in carrier oil for approximately two weeks and then straining the oil. The resulting oil is used and may contain the plant's aromatic characteristic.

Percolation: A process to extract the soluble constituents of a plant with the assistance of gravity. The material is moistened and evenly packed into a tall, slightly conical vessel; the liquid (menstruum) is then poured onto the material and allowed to steep for a certain length of time. A small opening is then made in the bottom, which allows the extract to slowly flow out of the vessel. The remaining plant material (the marc) may be discarded. Many tinctures and liquid extracts are prepared this way.

Practice Realities

Using a Drug/Medication Guide

Many very good drug guides on the market today will give you information concerning your client's medication. Most are easy to use and have a "how to use" section in their preface. The guides usually list drugs alphabetically by the generic name. An index will give the brand name and tell you where to find the drug under its generic name. Compounds of more than one medication will be found in the brand name index. After finding the medication, you will find the following sections under its name (sections of importance to massage are in italics):

- Pregnancy category

- Controlled substance schedule number

- Availability (how it comes: tablet, capsule, injection, cream, etc.)

- *Actions and therapeutic effects (This information helps you understand how the drug works in the body.)*

- Uses

- Contraindications and cautions

- Route and dosage

- *Adverse effects (side effects, such as easily bruised, skin dryness, muscle weakness, etc.)*

- *Pharmacokinetics (absorption, distribution, metabolism, and elimination)*

There are programs and websites that also provide excellent information. If ever in doubt, you can call a pharmacist or the nurse at the physician's office that prescribed the medication. New medications and new names for old ones are constantly being added to the market.

Table 22.6	**Common Herbs and Supplements**
Herb	**Uses**
Aloe vera	Topical use for minor burns, irritation
Black cohosh	PMS, menopause symptoms
Capsaicin	Topical use for pain, neuralgia, arthritis
Chamomile	Used as a tea for insomnia, anxiety, nausea
Echinacea	Helps strengthen immune system, relieves cold/flu symptoms
Ephedra	Nasal congestion
Evening primrose oil	Hormone balance, irritable bowel syndrome
Flaxseed oil	Constipation, colon cleansing
Feverfew	Migraines, fever reducer
Garlic	Lowers blood pressure, reduces cholesterol, boosts immunity
Ginger	Nausea, migraines, stomach inflammation, flu
Gingko	Alzheimer's (improves memory), tinnitus
Ginseng	Stress and anxiety; improves stamina
Glucosamine	Anti-inflammatory for arthritis
Kava kava	Anxiety and insomnia
Licorice	Menopause, colds and cough, peptic ulcers
Melatonin	Insomnia, jet lag, boosts immune system
Saw palmetto	Benign prostatic disease
Slippery elm	Colds, cough, chest congestion
Soy	Menopause symptoms, cancer prevention
St. John's wort	Depression
Valerian	Anxiety, insomnia

Chapter Summary

As a massage therapist, you have a great responsibility toward your clients—as well as to the profession—to maintain the highest standards of practice. One of these standards is to "do no harm" to your clients. By acquiring knowledge and using good judgment concerning a client's medications, you are taking steps to securing a therapeutic massage practice that is safe and effective.

General Safety Advisory

- The information in this chapter does not replace medical advice.
- Before taking a supplement, herb, or botanical, consult a doctor or other health care provider—especially if you have a disease or medical condition, are taking any medications, are pregnant or nursing, or are planning to have surgery.
- Before treating a child with a supplement, herb, or botanical, consult with a doctor or other health care provider.
- Like drugs, supplements and herbal or botanical preparations have chemical and biological activity. They may have side effects. They may interact with certain medications. These interactions can cause problems and can even be dangerous.
- If you have any unexpected reactions to a supplement, herbal, or botanical preparation, inform your doctor or other health care provider.

Applying Your Knowledge

Self-Testing

1. What is defined as the study of drugs?
   a) Pharmacodynamics
   b) Herbology
   c) Pharmaceutical
   d) Pharmacology

2. *Over-the-counter medications* refers to the drugs you buy where?
   a) At the grocery store
   b) With a prescription
   c) Self-prescribed
   d) Online

3. What is toxicology the study of?
   a) The uses of drugs to treat disease
   b) Poisons and their actions
   c) Chemical analysis
   d) Tissue damage

4. Most of the body's communication systems are what in nature?
   a) Chemical
   b) Biological
   c) Electrical
   d) Receptors

5. What is the source of digitalis?
   a) Animal
   b) Plant
   c) Mineral
   d) Synthetic

6. Insulin is considered an anti- _____ medication.
   a) thyroid
   b) ciabetic
   c) Cardiotonic
   d) decongestant

7. What is a common route for administration of a drug that is applied to the skin?
   a) Topical
   b) Intradermal
   c) Intrathecal
   d) Buccal

8. What are injections into the cavity of a joint considered?
   a) Intracutaneous
   b) Inhalation
   c) Intraarticular
   d) Subcutaneous

9. What is a primary factor of pharmacokinetics that is of importance to a massage therapist?
   a) Amount absorbed into the body
   b) Gut motility
   c) Rate and route of excretion
   d) Metabolic rate

10. Which category of medications is used to relieve pain?
    a) Antacid
    b) Anticoagulant
    c) Muscle relaxant
    d) Analgesic

11. In the naming process of steroids, what are the usual last three letters of the drug?
    a) Arre
    b) One
    c) Rhy
    d) Ate

12. What are noncontrolled drugs also listed as?
    a) At the drugstore
    b) Controlled drugs
    c) Over-the-counter (OTC)
    d) Substances

13. What is another name for plant-derived drugs?
    a) Phytoceutical
    b) Nutraceutical
    c) Pharmaceutical
    d) Apothecary

14. Which plant extract is used topically for minor skin discomforts?
    a) Chamomile
    b) Valerian
    c) Licorice
    d) Aloe vera

15. Which supplement is used to reduce inflammation from arthritis?
    a) Gingko
    b) Glucosamine
    c) Capsaicin
    d) Melatonin

Case Studies/Critical Thinking

A. *A 67-year-old male becomes a new client at your clinic. He is requesting deep tissue massage. On his client intake/history form, he lists "Coumadin®" as a medication. You know that this is primarily a blood thinner used to keep blood from clotting. He has not listed* any health issues related to heart disease or blood clots. Should you ask additional questions about why the client is taking this medication? Should you ask questions that will give you a more in-depth look at the client's health history before proceeding with the massage? How should you perform the massage if you find that the client has a history of several blood clots in his extremities?

B. A 45-year-old woman has scheduled an appointment in your spa. She is requesting a sauna and maybe hydrotherapy. She has listed on her intake form that she injects "Humulin®" twice a day. Should heat be a factor in her care that you should be concerned about? Why or why not?

References for information in this chapter can be found in Quick Guide C at the end of the book.

CHAPTER 23

Special Massage Routines for Common Pathologies

LEARNING OUTCOMES

After completing this chapter, you will be able to:

- Recognize certain pathological conditions that benefit from massage.

- Implement massage routines for carpal tunnel syndrome, thoracic outlet syndrome, torticollis, temporomandibular joint dysfunction, and fibromyalgia syndrome.

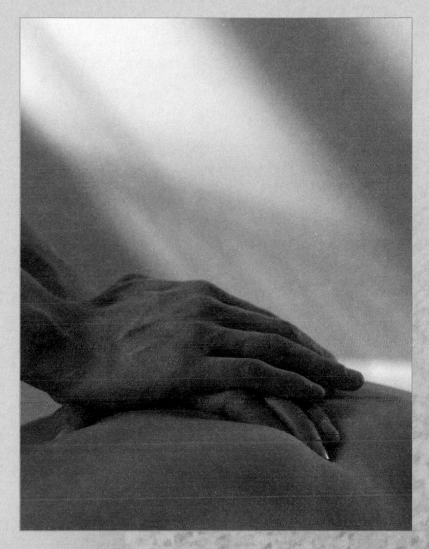

KEY TERMS

Adson's test/Allen's test *(p. 590)*
bilaterally *(p. 588)*
bruxism *(p. 593)*
malocclusion *(p. 593)*

paresthesia *(p. 588)*
Phalen's test *(p. 588)*
radicular *(p. 590)*
retinaculum *(p. 590)*

Tinel's test *(p. 588)*
unilaterally *(p. 588)*
Wright's test *(p. 590)*

INTRODUCTION

Although any massage therapist who desires to perform highly specific therapeutic work (such as neuromuscular therapy) will be required to take advanced courses in such work, we include massage routines for five common pathologies. During the course of a normal workday, most massage therapists will encounter clients with complaints of carpal tunnel syndrome, thoracic outlet syndrome, torticollis (wryneck), temporomandibular joint dysfunction, and fibromyalgia syndrome.

If you have clients who have been diagnosed by their physician as having one of these five pathologies, you may choose—under the guidance of the physician—to use one of these routines to address the client's chief complaint. And, since massage therapists are prone to injuries such as carpal tunnel syndrome, learning these routines to use in exchange with another therapist will benefit both of you. Since these routines use more advanced techniques such as those found in sports massage, please see chapter 13 for an explanation of the strokes.

As already mentioned, if this work interests you, attend the appropriate classes in your area to advance your studies and become fully proficient in these routines.

Carpal Tunnel Syndrome

⭐ **EXAM POINT** Carpal Tunnel Syndrome (CTS) is also known as Nerve Entrapment Syndrome affecting the median nerve.

⭐ **EXAM POINT** Nine flexor tendons and the median nerve pass through a "tunnel" formed by the "roof" or transverse carpal ligament; the "floor" is formed by the eight carpal bones.

These tendon sheaths become inflamed and press on the median nerve.

⭐ **EXAM POINT** Symptoms are burning, numbness, and **paresthesia** (tingling) in the thumb, index finger, middle finger, and half of the ring finger.

These symptoms worsen at night. CTS usually presents **unilaterally** (on one side) but can occur **bilaterally** (both sides).

The client's physician may have performed a **Phalen's Test,** in which the wrists are held in forced flexion for 60 seconds, eliciting pain, or a **Tinel's Test,** in which finger-tapping over the nerve elicits symptoms (figures 23.1 and 23.2).

Treatment includes rest or splinting, cold packs to reduce edema, and massage. In extreme cases, surgical intervention is required. The transverse ligament is incised to release the pressure.

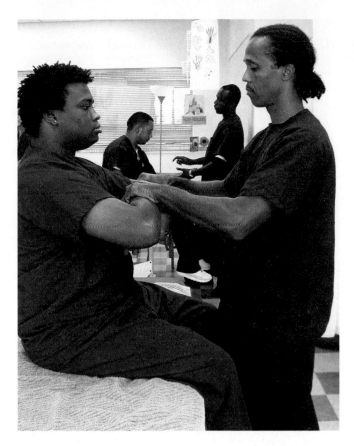

Figure 23.1
Phalen's test for carpal tunnel syndrome.

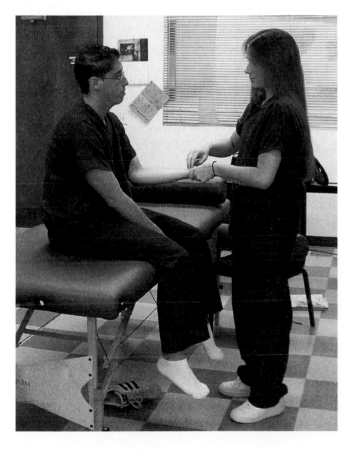

Figure 23.2
Tinel's test for carpal tunnel syndrome.

PROCEDURE 23.1 Performing a Massage Routine for Carpal Tunnel Syndrome

Objective: **To give your client a massage focusing on relief from carpal tunnel syndrome**

Routine steps:

1. No lubricant is used until step 5. With the client supine, begin with a mild torque to 360 degrees and traction of the arm.

2. With palms or fists, compress the anterior and posterior aspects of the arm.

3. Use skin rolling on the entire arm, especially the **retinaculum,** from wrist to elbow.

4. Use a compression-torque with thumbs ("hedge clipper") stroke anterior and posterior wrist to elbow.

5. Using a small amount of lubricant, perform deep effleurage followed by thumb stripping.

6. With fingertips, apply "tuck and friction" under the medial border of the radius and ulna.

7. Hold trigger points on tendon at the medial epicondyle of the humerus.

8. Perform traction on the wrist by positioning the client's arm at 90 degrees and placing your elbow on client's bicep to stabilize the arm; both hands grasp the client's hand and perform traction.

9. Apply effleurage and friction between each metacarpal.

10. Supinate the hand and use thumb glide on the palm. Apply friction to the pollicis muscle.

11. Use compression-broadening on the biceps.

12. Apply compression to the pectoralis muscle followed by pincher palpation ("money sign") on the pectorals.

13. Position the client prone and use compression-broadening on the triceps; follow with skin rolling, effleurage, and strip.

14. Use effleurage to finish.

This routine is performed every other day for severe CTS. Follow with ice therapy for 15 minutes immediately after treatment every two hours.

Thoracic Outlet Syndrome

★ **EXAM POINT** Thoracic outlet syndrome (TOS), also known as cervical rib syndrome, is a neurovascular compression of the shoulder girdle; specifically, the subclavian vessels and vertebral nerve (**radicular**) of the brachial plexus are compressed.

Compression is the result of outgrowths of the transverse process ("extra rib") or spasms in the anterior scalenes and pectoralis muscles. The brachial plexus transverses through the middle and anterior scalenes and under the clavicle, and continues under the coracoid process of the scapula and down the arm. Movements that deviate from correct posture can cause tension, compression, and entrapment.

★ **EXAM POINT** The median and ulnar nerves also transverse through this region and are responsible for the arm, forearm, and little and ring fingers.

For this reason, TOS symptoms can be confused with those of CTS.

The client's physician may have performed an **Adson's Test or Allen's Test,** which requires the client to look up and over the affected shoulder while the tester feels for changes in the radial pulse, or a **Wright's test** in which diminished radial pulse is felt when the arm is abducted. Adson's test is being performed on a client in figure 23.3.

Treatment involves instruction in proper posture, neck flexibility exercises, manual traction, and massage. Some clients report exacerbated symptoms at night because they sleep with one arm raised above their head.

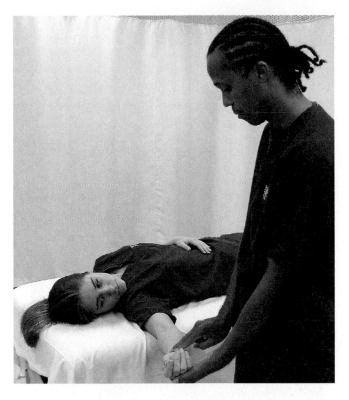

Figure 23.3
Adson's test for Thoracic Outlet Syndrome.

PROCEDURE 23.2   Performing a Massage Routine for Thoracic Outlet Syndrome

Objective: **To give your client a massage focusing on relief from thoracic outlet syndrome**

Routine steps:

Supine

1. Use petrissage on the trapezius followed by rolling the trapezius over your thumbs.

2. Apply thumb strip from occipital ridge to acromion process medial to lateral.

3. Repeat stripping with frictioning.

4. Position client's head toward the working side and apply effleurage and friction to the scalenes. Follow with effleurage on the scalenes using the "web" of hand.

5. Supporting the head with the opposite hand, use stripping from C1 to C7.

6. Traction the neck using either a towel under the occipital ridge and drawn up over the ears and sides of head or place your forearm under the occipital ridge and your other hand on the forehead, "pinning" the head between forearm and hand (figure 23.4).

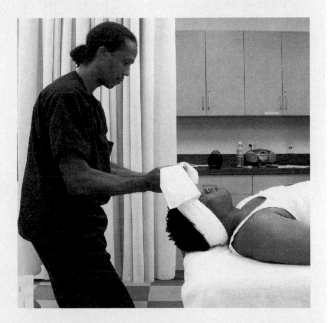

Figure 23.4
Neck traction with a towel.

7. Perform lateral flexion (ear to shoulder) on both sides. While holding the head in one hand, rotate the head to one side and flex the neck

Continued next page—

slightly; with the other hand, gently depress the shoulder. Repeat to the other side.

8. Use "scoop and friction" (with braced index or middle finger) on the insertions on the clavicle and subclavius muscle.

9. Release the pectorals with palm or fist compressions medial to lateral and back.

10. Apply thumb stripping to pectorals superior to inferior.

11. Use stripping on the pectorals between ribs laterally (from sternum to shoulder).

12. Apply pincher palpation ("money sign") on the pectorals.

Side-lying

1. Position clients toward the edge of the table (stand directly behind them so they feel secure); place a pillow under the client's head.

2. With a small amount of lubricant, use effleurage on the neck and trapezius.

3. With one hand stabilizing the shoulder (cupping), use thumb stripping with the other hand from shoulder up the trapezius and neck.

4. With the ulnar side of the hand, scoop down the neck and trapezius.

5. Remove pillow and repeat steps 3 and 4.

6. Use pincher palpation ("money sign") on the trapezius (figure 23.5).

7. Apply effleurage to finish.

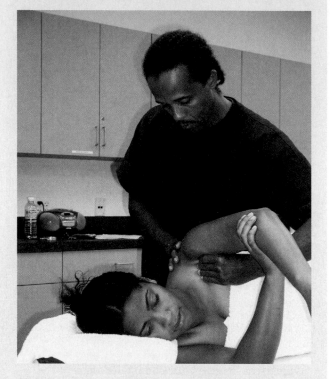

Figure 23.5
Pincer palpation on the pectoralis muscle in side-lying position.

TECHNIQUE EMPHASIS One client with TOS once reported that he strapped his arm down to his side when going to bed and had great relief!

Torticollis

★ **EXAM POINT** Torticollis, also known as wryneck, is a tonic or intermittent spasm in the neck muscles and sternocleidomastoid (SCM), causing rotation of the head to one side.

It is unilateral and a result of an injury or sleeping in the "wrong" position.

Symptoms are obvious in that clients cannot turn their heads to one side and report "sleeping funny" or "just woke up like this." Treatment includes physician-prescribed muscle relaxants and massage. This routine works well on whiplash when it is appropriate to do so according to a physician. Ice only in acute phase; perform light work when allowed.

PROCEDURE 23.3 Performing a Massage Routine for Torticollis (Wryneck)

Objective: To give your client a massage focusing on relief from torticollis

Routine steps:

1. With the client supine, apply effleurage followed by thumb stripping from occiput to acromion process.

2. Rotate the head onto a braced thumb; begin medially just off the cervical spine and move out laterally along occipital ridge (figure 23.6).

3. Apply friction along the occipital ridge.

4. Apply friction along the occipital ridge rotating head away and use stripping down with movement of the head.

5. Placing your fingertips against the occipital ridge (back of the hands on the table), balance the head on your fingertips and perform "picket fence" (a movement performed with the therapist's fingertips positioned on the occipital ridge then straightened; as the neck muscles relax, the head drops back).

6. Place your index finger under the sternocleidomastoid (SCM) just below the mastoid process and thumb on top to apply pincher palpation ("money sign"), asking the client to take a deep breath (figure 23.7).

7. Apply friction to the mastoid and sternum attachments.

8. Use scooping on the SCM and platysma, turning head away from the working side.

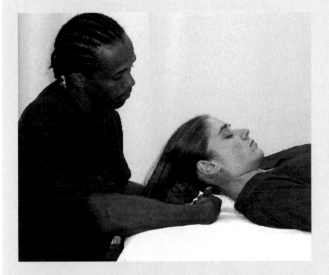

Figure 23.6
Rotate head onto a braced thumb.

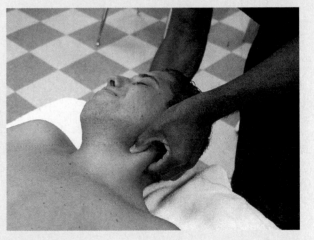

Figure 23.7
Pincer palpation on the sternocleidomastoid.

The area involved in TMJ occurs at the articulations of the temporal bone, mandible, temporalis muscle, masseter, pterygoids, ligaments, and the articular disc, which acts like a shock absorber. Pain can result when there is a **malocclusion** (poor alignment), tension, jaw clenching, **bruxism** (teeth grinding) during sleep, and arthritis.

Temporo-mandibular Joint Dysfunction

⭐ **EXAM POINT** TMJ occurs more frequently in women than men.

Either a dentist or physician can diagnose TMJ. Treatment can include massage and a special device made by the dentist for the client to wear at night that prohibits clenching of the teeth.

PROCEDURE 23.4 Performing a Massage Routine for Temporomandibular Joint Dysfuction

Objective: **To give your client a massage focusing on relief from Temporomandibular Joint Dysfunction (TMJ)**

Routine steps:

1. With the client supine, treat the temporal area:
   a. With fingers interlocked, apply lateral glide to the temporalis.
   b. With palms, use compression and circular friction on the temporalis (figure 23.8).
   c. With fingertips or thumbs, apply circular friction to the temporalis.
   d. Use a hair pull with twist counterclockwise (if client has short or no hair, use thumbs in an S shape).
   e. Use ear pull on the lobe and ear twist.

2. Treat masseter area:
   a. Use skin rolling to the zygomatic arch.
   b. With braced finger, apply friction to the origin.
   c. Use thumb glide to lengthen.
   d. With braced finger, apply parallel friction, then cross-fiber friction under the arch to the mandible.

3. Treat posterior neck:
   a. Use thumb stripping on the occipital ridge out over the trapezius.

   b. With braced thumb, rotate the occiput onto the thumb.

4. Treat SCM:
   a. Use thumb stripping from insertion to origin (mastoid down the SCM to clavicle).
   b. Apply pincher palpation ("money sign") all the way down the SCM.
   c. Use friction under the mandible followed by ulnar scoop.

5. Perform intraoral with gloved hand (figure 23.9). Note: in some states, either special training and licensure or written consent is required for this type of work.
   a. With index finger and thumb, apply compression and pincher palpation ("money sign") to the obicularis oris and buccinator.
   b. With index finger and thumb under the cheekbone, apply compression.
   c. With index finger, sweep under the tongue.

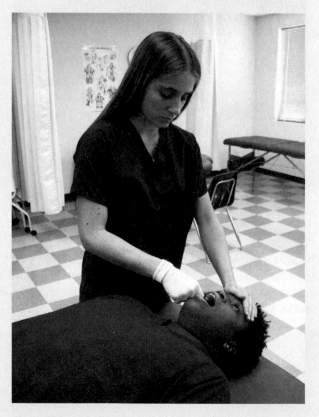

Figure 23.9
Intraoral work with gloved hand.

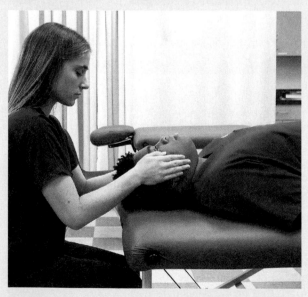

Figure 23.8
Compression and circular friction on the temporalis muscle.

⭐ **EXAM POINT** Fibromyalgia Syndrome (FMS) is diffuse chronic pain in soft tissues (muscles, tendons, and ligaments) and is closely associated with chronic fatigue syndrome, myofascial pain syndrome, irritable bowel syndrome, and sleep disorders.

FMS occurs mostly in women.

⭐ **EXAM POINT** Although there is no definitive test for FMS, a positive reaction is tenderness in 11 out of 18 specific points located throughout the body.

These 18 specific points (nine pairs) are illustrated in figure 23.10. Fibromyalgia clients experience pain on a daily basis. Treatment includes massage, although FMS clients may not be able to endure a prolonged massage. Therefore, it is best to perform the routine in Procedure 23.5 in combination with gentle effleurage for no more than 30 minutes. Points can be held singularly (while working on the extremities) or simultaneously (while working along the occipital ridge). FMS clients will not be able to tolerate a cold environment or any ice therapy. It is particularly important to be attentive to the client and listen to feedback while working. Points should be held within the client's tolerance or comfort level (pressure approximately the weight of a nickel is a good analogy to keep in mind).

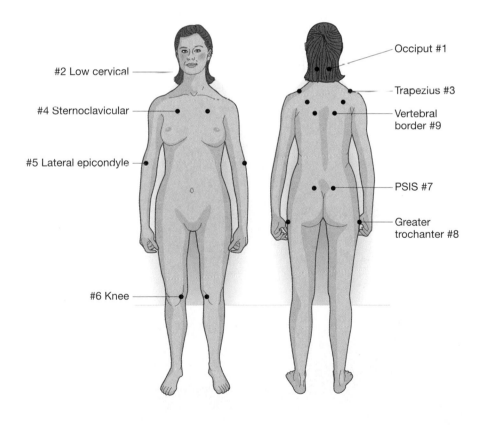

Figure 23.10
The 18 fibromyalgia points.

#2 Low cervical

#4 Sternoclavicular

#5 Lateral epicondyle

#6 Knee

Occiput #1

Trapezius #3

Vertebral border #9

PSIS #7

Greater trochanter #8

Objective: **To give your client a massage focusing a relief from Fibromyalgia Syndrome**

Routine steps:

1. With the client supine, apply traction to the neck, holding point 1 along occipital ridge.

2. Gently massage the face with long, slow strokes accompanied by circles at the TMJ and a mild stretch of the masseter.

3. Hold point 2 on the SCM posterior to the mandible.

4. Cup shoulders with hands and gently depress shoulders, holding for several seconds.

5. Hold point 3 midway on the upper trapezius.

6. Hold point 4 of the SCM at the sternoclavicular.

7. Move to the client's side and perform gentle range of motion with gentle traction of the arm.

8. Hold point 5 at the lateral epicondyle of the elbow.

9. Gently massage the hand.

10. Hold *hoku* point (an acupoint located between thumb and index finger).

11. Apply nerve stroke from shoulder to hand.

12. Perform steps 7 to 11 on the other arm.

13. Move to the feet and perform gentle traction on both legs.

14. Gently massage one foot.

15. Place hands over the knee and gently rock.

16. Hold point 6 at the medial aspect of the knee.

17. Apply nerve stroke from hip to foot.

18. Perform steps 14 to 17 on the other leg.

19. Perform gentle rocking by placing a hand on the client's diaphragm and the other hand on the client's forehead (figure 23.11).

20. Position the client prone and move to the client's side. On one leg, stretch the Achilles tendon by dorsiflexing the foot.

21. Bend the knee to 90 degrees and gently shake.

22. Hold point 7 at the PSIS (Posterior Superior Iliac Spine) and 8 at greater trochanter.

23. Apply nerve stroke from buttocks to foot.

24. Perform a lateral lumbar stretch with palms at shoulder and pelvis.

25. Perform steps 20 to 24 on the other side.

26. Move to the client's head and slowly stroke from low back to shoulders and out the arms.

27. Gently squeeze the trapezius.

28. Hold point 9 at the midvertebral border of scapula (rhomboid attachments).

29. With the ulna side of hand, apply friction down along the side of the spine.

30. Gently squeeze the back of the neck.

31. Apply traction with palms over the sacrum.

32. Apply nerve stroke from shoulders to feet.

33. Perform gentle rocking with one hand on the upper back and one hand on the low back.

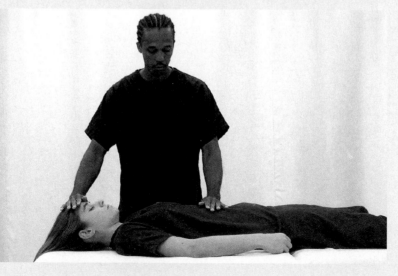

Figure 23.11
Calming hand on diaphragm and forehead.

Applying Your Knowledge

Self-Testing

1. Fibromyalgia Syndrome is closely linked to what other syndrome?
   - a) CTS
   - b) TOS
   - c) CFS
   - d) MPS

2. Where are FMS patients affected?
   - a) Head and neck
   - b) Shoulders
   - c) Low back
   - d) All of the above are correct.

3. Torticollis is also known as wryneck.
   - a) True
   - b) False

4. What is whiplash also known as?
   - a) CAD
   - b) Cervical acceration-decleration
   - c) a and b
   - d) Torticollis

5. Carpal tunnel syndrome (CTS) involves entrapment of which nerve?
   - a) Ulnar
   - b) Radial
   - c) Median
   - d) Brachial

6. Thoracic outlet syndrome (TOS) involves entrapment of nerves in the brachial plexus. What is it also known as?
   - a) Brachialitis
   - b) Neurovascular entrapment
   - c) Pectoralis entrapment
   - d) None of the above is correct.

7. In TOS, the transverse processes of the cervical vertebrae grow longer than normal, extending into territory where they do not belong.
   - a) True
   - b) False

8. Tests for TOS are Wright's test and which other?
   - a) Tinnel's test
   - b) Phalen's test
   - c) Adson's test
   - d) None of the above is correct.

9. Pain resulting from a malocclusion (poor alignment) is indicative of which disease?
   - a) TMJ
   - b) FMS
   - c) TOS
   - d) None of the above is correct.

10. Which two maladies are more common in women?
    - a) TMJ and FMS
    - b) CTS and TMJ
    - c) TOS and FMS
    - d) TMJ and torticollis

Case Studies/Critical Thinking

A. A client comes in for a massage complaining of neck pain on the left side only. She reports no recent injury but believes she slept very hard and "funny" after a long day at work. On which areas of her body would you focus your work?

B. A client comes in for a massage and tells you that she believes she has Carpal Tunnel Syndrome. Her assumption is based mostly on the commonality of this condition today. On further questioning, you learn that she has numbness and tingling in the little finger and on the ulnar side of her hand rather than in the thumb and first two fingers. What do you suspect she is really suffering from (for which you refer her to a physician)?

References for information in this chapter can be found in Quick Guide C at the end of the book.

Quick Guide A *State-by-State Requirements*

Note: State requirements for curriculum hours, licensure, and registration or certification are constantly changing. For this reason, we ask that you check with your individual state and the AMTA or NCBTMB for current data. The information listed below can be found on individual state, AMTA, or NCBTMB websites.

Alabama Massage Therapy Board
610 S. McDonough St.
Montgomery, AL 36104
Ph: (334) 269-9990
www.almtbd.state.al.us
Educational requirements: 1000 (or 650) hours from accredited massage therapy school
Fees: application, $25.00; licensing, $100.00; renewal, $100.00; exam, $160.00
Reciprocity: On a state-by-state basis
Continuing education: 16 hours biennially
Exam: NCETMB

Arizona
http://MassageTherapy.az.gov or massageboard.az.gov
Educational requirements: 500 hours from an accredited massage therapy school
Fees: renewal fee, $180.00 biennially
Continuing education: 25 hours biennially
Exam: NCETMB

Arkansas State Board of Massage Therapy
103 Airways
Hot Springs, AR 71903-0739
Ph: (501) 623-0444
www.state.ar.us or arkansasmassagetherapy.com
Educational requirements: 500 hours from an accredited massage therapy school
Fees: renewal, $30 a year
Reciprocity: On a state-by-state basis
Continuing education: 6 hours a year
Exam: NCETMB

California
www.californiahealthfreedom.com
Freedom of Access

Connecticut
Massage Therapy Licensure
Department of Public Health
410 Capitol Ave.—MS#12APP
P.O. Box 340308
Hartford, CT 06134-0308
Ph: (860) 509-7573
www.dph.state.ct.us
Educational requirements: 500 hours at a COMTA-approved school
Fees: application, $300.00; renewal, $200.00
Reciprocity: No
Continuing education: 24 every four years
Exam: NCETMB

Delaware Board of Massage and Bodywork
Cannon Building
861 Silver Lake Blvd. #203
Dover, DE 19904
Ph: (302) 744-4506
www.state.de.us or professional licensing.state.de.us
Educational requirements: 300 hours plus CPR for CMT, 500 hours for LMT
Fees: application, $25.00; renewal, $82.00 annually
Reciprocity: Yes
Continuing education: 24 hours biennially for CMT, 12 hours biennially for LMT
Exam: NCETMB

District of Columbia Massage Therapy Board
Occupational and Professional
Licensing Administration
941 N. Capitol St. N.E., 7th floor
Washington, DC 20002
Ph: (202) 727-7185
www.dcra.org/main.shtm or www.doh.dc.gov
Educational requirements: 500 hours from board-approved school
Fees: application, $50.00; License, $45.00; renewal, $100.00
Reciprocity: No
Continuing education: 12 hours biennially
Exam: NCETMB

Florida Board of Massage Therapy
Department of Health
2020 Capital Cir. S.E.
Bin #C09
Tallahassee, FL 32399-3259
Ph: (850) 488-0595
www.doh.state.fl.us/mqa/massage/ma_home.html
Educational requirements: 500 hours from board-approved school plus 3 hours
    HIV/AIDS
Fees: application, $155.00
Reciprocity: No
Continuing education: 24 hours biennially
Exam: NCETMB

Georgia
As of December 2007 Georgia will accept the NCTMB exam for licensure.

Hawaii Board of Massage Therapy
DCCA
P.O. Box 3469
Honolulu, HI 96801
Ph: (808) 586-2699
www.state.hi.us or hawaii.gov
Educational requirements: 570 hours—must spend a minimum of 6 months at an
    AMTA or Rolf Institute school
Fees: application, $50.00; exam, $120.00; renewal (biennial), $20.00
Reciprocity: No
Continuing education: No
Exam: State exam

Idaho
freedom of access

Illinois
Ph: (217) 782-8556
www.ildpr.com
Educational requirements: 500 hours from an accredited school
Fees: renewal, $175.00
Continuing education: 24 hours biennially

Iowa Department of Health
Board of Massage Therapy
321 E. 12th St.
Des Moines, IA 50319
Ph: (515) 281-6959
www.idph.state.ia.us/licensure
Educational requirements: 500 hours from accredited school
Fees: application, $100.00; renewal, $60.00
Reciprocity: Yes
Continuing education: 24 hours biennially
Exam: NCETMB

Kentucky
www.finance.ky.gov
Educational requirements: 500 hours from an accredited school
Fees: renewal, $100.00
Continuing education: 24 hours biennially

Louisiana Board of Massage Therapy
P.O. Box 1279
Zachary, LA 70791
Ph: (504) 658-8964
www.lsbmt.org
Educational requirements: 500 hours from accredited school
Fees: renewal, $125.00
Reciprocity: Yes
Continuing education: 12 hours annually
Exam: NCETMB plus written and oral exam

Maine Board of Massage Therapy
Department of Professional and Financial Regulation
35 State House Station
Augusta, ME 04333-0035
Ph: (207) 624-8612
www.state.me.us/pfr/led/massage or www.maineprofessionalreg.org
Educational requirements: 500 hours from an accredited school plus CPR
    and first aid
Fees: application, $25.00; registration, $100.00; license and annual renewal, $50.00;
    criminal record check, $8.00
Reciprocity: Yes
Continuing education: No
Exam: NCETMB *or* diploma from a COMTA training program

Maryland Board of Chiropractic Examiners
Massage Therapy Advisory Committee
4201 Patterson Ave., 5th floor
Baltimore, MD 21215-2299
Ph: (410) 764-4738
www.mdmassage.org
Educational requirements: 500 hours from COMTA school plus 60 hours of college
    and CPR for RMT or 500 hours and 60 college credits for CMT
Fees: application, $100.00; certification, $200.00; state exam, $275.00; renewal
    (biennial), $200.00
Reciprocity: Yes
Continuing education: 24 hours biennially
Exam: NCETMB and state exam

Minnesota
800-657-3957
Freedom of access

Mississippi State Board of Massage Therapy
P.O. Box 12489
Jackson, MS 39236-2489
Ph: (601) 856-6127
www.msbmt.state.ms.us
Educational requirements: 700 hours from an accredited school plus CPR and first aid
Fees: application, $50.00; certification, $125.00; renewal, $62.50
Reciprocity: Yes
Continuing education: 12 hours CEU board-approved program and CPR annually
Exam: NCETMB

Missouri Massage Therapy Board
3605 Missouri Blvd.
Jefferson City, MO 65102
Ph: (573) 522-6277
www.ecodev.state.mo.us/pr or www.pr.mo.gov/massage.asp
Educational requirements: 500 hours from a board-approved school
Fees: application, $150.00; renewal, $200.00
Reciprocity: Yes
Continuing education: 12 hours biennially
Exam: NCETMB

Nebraska Massage Therapy Board
Health and Human Services Credentialing Division
301 Centennial Mall South, 3rd floor
Lincoln, NE 68509
Ph: (402) 471-2115
www.state.ne.us or www.hhs.state.ne.us
Educational requirements: 1000 hours
Fees: certification, $25.00; license, $101.00, renewal, $25.00
Reciprocity: Yes
Continuing education: 24 hours biennially approved by state board
Exam: NCETMB

New Hampshire Office of Program Support
Board of Massage Therapy
Health Facilities Administration
129 Pleasant St.
Concord, NH 03301-6527
Ph: (603) 271-5127
www.dhhs.state.nh.us or www.dhhs.nh.gov
Educational requirements: 750 hours plus CPR
Fees: application, $125.00; renewal, $100.00
Reciprocity: Yes
Continuing education: 12 hours biennially
Exam: NCETMB *or* state exam

New Jersey Board of Nursing
Massage, Bodywork & Somatic Therapy Examining Committee
P.O. Box 45010
Newark, NJ 07101
Fax: (973) 648-3481
www.state.nj.us
Educational requirements: 500 hours
Fees: renewal, $120 biennially
Continuing education: 20 hours biennially

New Mexico Board of Massage Therapy
2055 Pacheco St. #400
Santa Fe, NM 87504
Ph: (505) 476-7090
www.rld.state.nm.us/b&c/massage
Educational requirements: 650 hours
Fees: application, $25.00; renewal (annual), $125.00
Reciprocity: No
Continuing education: 16 hours biennially, approved by board
Exam: NCETMB *and* state exam (take-home)

New York State Board of Massage Therapy
Cultural Education Center #3041
Albany, NY 12230
Ph: (518) 473-1417
www.op.nysed.gov/massage.htm
Educational requirements: 1000 hours from New York school program or equivalent
Fees: application, $100.00; exam, $195.00; renewal, $55/3 yr
Reciprocity: Yes
Continuing education: No
Exam: State exam

North Carolina Board of Massage and Bodywork Therapy
P.O. Box 2539
Raleigh, NC 27602
Ph: (919) 546-0050
www.bmbt.org
Educational requirements: 500 hours from a board-approved school
Fees: application, $20.00; licensure, $150.00; renewal, $100.00
Reciprocity: Yes
Continuing education: 25 hours biennially
Exam: NCETMB

North Dakota Massage Board
119 Victoria Ct.
Grand Forks, ND 58201
Ph: (701) 772-0000
www.health.state.nd.us or www.ndboardofmassage.com
Educational requirements: 750 hours from a COMTA school
Fees: application, $150.00; renewal (annual), $50.00
Reciprocity: Yes
Continuing education: 18 hours per year
Exam: State exam

Ohio Massage Therapy Board
77 South High St., 17th floor
Columbus, OH 43266-0315
Ph: (614) 466-3934
www.state.oh.us/med or www.med.ohio.gov
Educational requirements: 750 hours from board-approved school
Fees: application, $35.00; exam, $250.00; renewal, $50.00
Reciprocity: Case-by-case
Continuing education: No
Exam: State exam

Oregon Board of Massage Technicians
State Office Building
3218 Pringle Rd. S.E. #250
Salem, OR 97302-1596
Ph: (503) 365-8657
www.oregonmassage.org
Educational requirements: 500 hours
Fees: application, $80.00; exam, $100.00; renewal, $100.00
Reciprocity: Certain states
Continuing education: 25 hours biennial plus current CPR
Exam: NCETMB

Rhode Island Department of Health
Professional Regulation
3 Capitol Hill, Room 104
Providence, RI 02908-5097
Ph: (401) 222-2827
www.health.state.ri.us
Educational requirements: 500 hours from a COMTA school
Fees: licensing, $37.50
Reciprocity: Endorsement-approved
Continuing education: No
Exam: NCETMB

South Carolina Department of Labor Licensing and Regulation
P.O. Box 11329
Columbia, SC 29211-1329
Ph: (803) 896-4588
www.myscgov.com or www.llr.state.sc.us
Educational requirements: 500 hours from an accredited school
Fees: application, $50.00; licensing, $100.00; renewal, $200.00
Reciprocity: Yes
Continuing education: 12 hours biennially
Exam: NCETMB

South Dakota Department of Health
Ph: 800-738-2301
www.state.sd.us/doh/massage
Educational requirements: 500 hours
Continuing education: No

Tennessee Massage Licensure Board
Cordell Hull Building, 1st floor
425 Fifth Ave. N.
Nashville, TN 37247-1010
Ph: (615) 532-3202
www.state.tn.us/hh.html
Educational requirements: 500 hours from a state-approved school
Fees: application, $75.00; license, $200.00; state registration, $10.00; renewal, $200.00
Reciprociity: Yes
Continuing education: 25 hours biennially
Exam: NCETMB

Texas Department of State Health Services
1100 West 49th St.
Austin, TX 78756
Ph: (512) 834-6616
www.dshs.state.tx.us/massage/default.shtm
Educational requirements: 300 hours from a state-approved school
Fees: application: $117.00; written exam: $87.00; practical: $100.00;
    renewal: $106.00/bi-annually
Reciprocity: No
Continuing education: 6 hours annually
Exam: State exam (written is offered in specific cities throughout Texas and practical
    only offered in Austin)

State of Utah Department of Commerce
Board of Massage Therapy
P.O. Box 146741
Salt Lake City, UT 84144-6741
Ph: (801) 530-6964
www.commerce.state.ut.us/dopl/wpapp.htm or www.dopl.utah.gov
Educational requirements: 600 hours from a COMTA-approved school for LMT and
    1000 hours for AMT
Fees: application, $50.00; FBI fingerprint, $24.00; renewal (biennial), $52.00
Reciprocity: Yes
Continuing education: No
Exam: NCETMB *and* Utah Massage Law and Rule Examination

Virginia Board of Nursing
6606 W. Broadway St., 4th floor
Richmond, VA 23230-1717
Ph: (804) 662-9909
www.vdh.state.va.us or www.dhp.virginia.gov
Educational requirements: 500 hours from a board-approved school
Fees: application and certification (biennial), $105.00; renewal, $70.00
Reciprocity: Yes
Continuing education: 25 hours biennially
Exam: NCETMB

State of Washington Department of Health
1300 S.W. Quince St.
P.O. Box 47867
Olympia, WA 98504-7867
Ph: (360) 236-4700
www.don.wa.gov
Educational requirements: 500 hours from a board-approved school
Fees: license, $55.00; exam, $150.00; renewal (annual), $40.00
Reciprocity: Yes
Continuing education: 16 hours biennially
Exam: NCETMB

State of West Virginia Board of Massage Therapy
200 Davis St. #1
Princeton, WV 24740
Ph: (304) 487-1400
www.state.wv.us/massage or www.wvmassage.org
Educational requirements: 500 hours from a COMTA-approved school
Fees: application, $25.00; license, $200.00; renewal, $100.00
Reciprocity: Yes
Continuing education: 25 CEUs biennially
Exam: NCETMB

Wisconsin Department of Regulation and Licensing
Massage Therapy Board
1400 E. Washington Ave.
Madison, WI 53703
Ph: (608) 266-0145 or drl.wi.gov
www.state.wi.us/regulation
Educational requirements: 600 hours
Fees: initial credential, $53.00; exam, $57.00; renewal (biennial), $53.00
Reciprocity: Yes
Exam: No state exam *and* NCETMB
Footnote—www.amtamassage.org/about/Regulated%20Chart.pdf

Quick Guide B *Resource List*

Canadian Federation of Aromatherapists
(519) 475-9038
www.cfacanada.com

International Aromatherapy and Herb Association
(602) 938-4439

National Association for Holistic Aromatherapy
(888) 275-6242
www.naha.org

The Flower Essence Society
(800) 736-9222
www.flowersociety.org

American Association for Teachers of Oriental Medicine
(512) 451-2866

American Association of Oriental Medicine
(610) 266-1433
www.aaom.org

American Organization for Bodywork Therapies of Asia
(856) 782-1616
www.aobta.org

British Columbia Acupressure Therapists' Association
(250) 920-9986
www.islandnet.com/-bcata

Canadian Practitioners' Association of Asian Medicine
(416) 410-6419
www.cpaam.ca

International Thai Therapists Association
(773) 792-4121
www.thaimassage.com

International Tao Shiatsu Society
(808) 257-4663
www.taoshiatsu.com

Hawaiian Lomilomi Association
(808) 965-8917
www.lomilomi.org

Shiatsu Therapists Alliance
Canada
(416) 410-0174

CranioSacral Therapy

American CranioSacral Therapy Association
(877) 942-2782
www.acsta.com

Craniosacral Therapy Association/North America Canada
(416) 755-7734
www.craniosacraltherapy.org

The Upledger Institute
(800) 233-5880
www.upledger.com

Energy Therapies

International Society for the Study of Subtle Energies and Energy Medicine
(303) 425-4625
www.issseem.org

American Polarity Therapy Association
(303) 545-2080

American Reiki Masters Association
(904) 755-9638

Canadian Reiki Association
(416) 783-9904
www.reiki.ca

International Reiki Foundation
(810) 249-3402

Reiki Alliance
(208) 783-3535

Reiki Council
(630) 926-5891
www.reikicouncil.com

Healing Touch

Healing Touch International
(303)989-7982
www.healingtouch.net

Healing Touch Canada, Inc.
(705) 652-0506
www.axxent.ca/-htcanada/

Hospice and Geriatric Massage

Hospice-Based Massage/Nursing American Holistic Medical Association
(703) 556-9728
www.ahmaholistic.com

American Holistic Nurses Association
(800) 278-2462
www.ahna.org

National Association of Nurse Massage Therapists
(800) 262-4017
www.nanmt.org

American Massage Therapy Association
(847) 864-0123
www.amtamassage.org

Ancient Healing Arts Association
(866) 843-2422
www.ancienthealingarts.org

Associated Bodywork & Massage Professionals
(800) 458-2267
www.abmp.com

Association of Massage Therapists and Wholistic Practitioners Canada
(888) 711-7701
www.amtwp.org

Canadian Massage Therapists Alliance
(905) 849-7606
www.cmta.ca

Federation of State Massage Therapy Boards
(336) 851-2345
www.fsmtb.org

International Massage Association
(540) 351-0800
www.imagroup.com

Massage Therapists Association of British Columbia
(604) 873-4467
www.massagetherapy.bc.ca

National Certification Board for Therapeutic Massage and Bodywork
(800) 296-0664

Professional Association of Traditional Healers
(303) 478-5847

Massage and Bodywork Associations

American Medical Massage Association
(888) 375-7245
www.americanmedicalmassage.com

National Integrative Medicine Council
(520) 571-1110
www.nimc.org

Orthopedic Massage Education & Research Institute
(888) 340-1614

Medical Massage

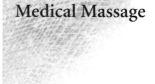

National Association of Pregnancy Massage Therapy
(888) 451-4945

International Association of Infant Massage
(805) 644-8524
www.iaim-us.com

Pediatric and Pregnancy Massage

Reflexology	American Reflexology Certification Board (303) 933-6921 www.arch.net International Council of Reflexologists (905) 770-2464 Reflexology Association of America (702) 971-9522 www.reflexology-USA.org
Spa Associations	The Day Spa Association (201) 865-2065 www.dayspaassociation.com International Spa Association (888) 651-4772 www.experiencespa.com SPA Association (970) 226-6145 www.thespaassociation.com
Sports Massage Associations	US Sports Massage Federation/International Sports Massage Federation (949) 642-0735 Canadian Sport Massage Therapists Association (416) 488-4414
Structural Integration Associations	Guild for Structural Integration (800) 447-0122 www.rolfguild.org Rolf Institute of Structural Integration (800) 530-8875 www.rolf.org International Association of Structural Integrators www.theiasi.org
Therapeutic Touch and Touch Research Associations	Canadian Touch Research Center (514) 272-2254 www.ccrt-crtc.org Nurse Healers Professional Association, Inc. (801) 273-3399 www.therapeutic-touch.org The Therapeutic Touch Network Canada (416) 658-6824 www.therapeutictouchnetwork.com

Touch for Health Kinesiology Association
(800) 466-8342
www.tfh.org

Touch Research Institute, University of Miami
(305) 243-6781
www.miami.edu/touch-research/

Trager International
(216) 896-9383
www.trager.com

Trager® Work

Zero Balancing Association
(434) 244-2458
www.zerobalancing.com

Zero Balancing

Below is a list of organizations that accredit various vocational schools, colleges, and training programs. Make sure your school is accredited by one of these organizations.

Accrediting Organizations

ACCET: Accrediting Commission for Continuing Education and Training

ACCSCT: Accrediting Commission of Career Schools and Colleges of Technology

COE: Commission on Occupational Education

COMTA: Commission on Massage Therapy Accreditation

NATTS: National Association of Trade and Technical Schools

SACS: Southern Association of Colleges and Schools

www.massageresource.com

www.massagemag.com has a link to check laws and regulations

www.healingandlaw.com/Massage_Law_Newsletter.html

Regulations/ Laws Resource Websites

www.massagemag.com

www.massageresource.com

www.nationalschooldirectory.com

School Locator Resource Websites

American Red Cross National Headquarters
2025 E Street, NW
Washington, DC 20006
(202) 303-4498
(800) 435-7669

Other Resources

American Heart Association
National Center
7272 Greenville Avenue
Dallas, TX 75231
(800) 242-8721

American Massage Therapy Association
500 Davis Street, Suite 900
Evanston, IL 60201-4695
(877) 905-2700
Fax: (847) 864-1178

Centers for Disease Control
1600 Clifton Road, N.E.
Atlanta, GA 30333
(404) 639-3311
Public inquiries: (800) 311-3435

National Certification Board for Therapeutic Massage and Bodywork (NCBTMB)
8201 Greensboro Drive, Suite 300
McLean, VA 22102
(800) 296-0664
(703) 610-9015
Fax: (703) 610-9005

National Safety Council
1121 Spring Lake Drive
Itasca, IL 60143-3201
(630) 285-1121

US Department of Agriculture Agricultural Research Service
George Washington Carver Center
5601 Sunnyside Avenue
Beltsville, MD 20705

US Department of Agriculture Food and Nutrition Service
3101 Park Center Drive, Room 926
Alexandria, VA 22303
(703) 305-2062

Quick Guide C *Reference List*

American Massage Therapy Association, 500 Davis Street, Suite 900, Evanston, IL 60201-4695; (877) 905-2700; fax: (847)864-1178.

American Psychiatric Association. *Diagnostic and Statistical Manual of Mental Disorders,* 4th ed. Arlington, VA: ©2000.

Antoni, M. H., L. Baggett, G. Ironsen, A. LaPerriere, S. August, N. Klimas.

Australian Unani Medicine Society, Inc. *Introduction to Unani Medicine.* Elizabeth, South Australia, 2000.

Benjamin, Patricia J., and Scott P. Lamp. *Understanding Sports Massage.* Champaign, IL: Human Kinetics Publishers, 1996.

Berkman, L. F., and S. L. Syme. "Social networks, host resistance, and mortality: A nine-year follow-up study of Alameda County residents," *American Journal of Epidemiology,* 109 (1979).

Bigelow, Mark. "The Effects of Repetitive Movement on a Muscle," CMT, Bigelow Seminars, 2004.

Bower, J., M. E. Kemeny, S. E. Taylor, and J. L. Fahey. "Cognitive processing, discovery of meaning, CD 4 decline and AIDS-related mortality among bereaved HIV seropositive men." *Journal of Consulting and Clinical Psychology,* 65 (1998).

California Coalition Against Sexual Assault. *2002 Report: Research on Rape and Violence.*

California Department of Justice. *Crime and Delinquency in California 2000.* Department of Justice, Division of Criminal Justice Information Services, Sacramento, 2000.

Calvert, Robert Noah. *The History of Massage.* Rochester, VT: Healing Arts Press, 2002.

Cantu, R., and A. Grodin. *Myofascial Manipulation: Theory and Clinical Application.* Gaithersburg, MD: Aspen, 1992.

Cassileth, B. R., and A. J. Vickers. "Massage therapy for symptom control: Outcome study at a major cancer center." *Journal of Pain and Symptom Management,* 2004.

Dallam, S. J. *The Hidden Effects of Childhood Maltreatment on Adult Health.* New York: Putnam, 1998.

Erickson, Signeg, DC, CST-D, "Subtle Palpation," Upledger Institute, Inc., Palm Beach Gardens, FL, 2005.

Esterling, B. A., M. H. Antoni, M. Kumar, and N. Schneiderman. "Emotional repression, stress disclosure responses and Epstein-Barr viral capsid antigen titers." *Psychosomatic Medicine,* 52 (1990).

Federal Bureau of Investigations, *Uniform Crime Reports for the United States 2000.* Washington, D.C.: U.S. Department of Justice, 2000.

Feuerstein, George. *Tantra: The Path of Ecstasy.* Boston: Shambhala Publications, Inc., 1998.

Florida College of Natural Health. *FCNH Handbook for Advanced Tissue Therapeutics.* Pompano, FL, 1998.

Frawley, David. *Tantric Yoga and the Wisdom Goddesses.* Salt Lake City: Passage Press, 1996.

Ganong, William F., *Review of Medical Physiology* (Lange Basic Science Series), 22nd ed. New York: McGraw-Hill Medical, 2005.

Gillespie, Barry R. *Healing Your Child.* Philadelphia: Dr. Barry R. Gillespie, 1999.

Graham, Douglas. *Manual Therapeutics, A Treatise on Massage: Its History, Mode of Application, and Effects.* Philadelphia; London: J.B. Lippincott, 1902.

Greenman, Philip E. *Principles of Manual Medicine.* 3rd ed., Philadelphia: Lippincott, Williams, & Wilkins, 2003.

Griffith, Winter H., *The Complete Guide to Sports Injuries,* 3rd ed., New York: Berkley Publishing Group, Division of Penguin, 2004.

Guyton, Arthur C., and John E. Hall. *Textbook of Medical Physiology,* 10th ed., W.B. Saunders, Philadelphia: 2000

Hall, S., *Basic Biomechanics.* St. Louis: Mosby, 1991.

Hamwee, John. *Zero Balancing, Touching the Energy of Bone.* London: Frances Lincoln Ltd., 1999.

Herman, Judith. *Trauma and Recovery.* New York: Basic Books, 1992.

Hislop, Helen J., and Jacqueline Montgomery. *Daniels and Worthingham's Muscle Testing Techniques of Manual Examination,* 7th ed. Philadelphia: W.B. Saunders Co., 2002.

Honervogt, Tanmaya. *The Power of Reiki.* New York: Henry Holt and Company, 1998.

Hoppenfeld, S. *Physical Examination of the Spine and Extremities.* New York: Appleton-Century-Crofts, 1976.

Hudson, John. *Instant Meditation for Stress Relief.* New York: Lorenz Books, 1996.

Johns Hopkins School of Public Heath and Center for Healthcare Gender Equality Population Information Program, Center for Communications Programs. *Population Reports: Ending Violence Against Women.* Baltimore, 1999

Kamenetz, Herman L., "History of Massage." In *Manipulation, Traction, and Massage,* ed. by Joseph P. Rogoff. Baltimore: Williams and Wilkins, 1980.

Karow, J. "Biology—stressed for life," *Scientific American,* 2000.

Kellogg, J. H. *The Art of Massage,* Battle Creek, MI: Modern Medicine Publishing, 1929.

Kilpatrick, D., and B. Saunders. *The Prevalence and Consequences of Child Victimization: Summary of a Research Study.* Washington, DC: U.S. Department of Justice, National Institute of Justice, 1997.

King, Robert K. *Performance Massage.* Champaign, IL: Human Kinetics Publishers, 1993.

Komisar, Randy. *The Monk and the Riddle.* Boston: Harvard Business School Press, 2001.

Krager, Dan, and Carole Krager. *HIPAA for Medical Office Personnel.* Clifton Park, NY: Thomson, Delmar Learning, 2005.

Levangie, P., and C. Norkin. *Joint Structure and Function: A Comprehensive Analysis,* 3rd ed. Philadelphia: F. A. Davis, 1992.

Love, Patricia. *The Emotional Incest Syndrome.* New York: Bantam Books, 1990.

Mehta, Silva, Mira, and Shyam, *Yoga the Iyengar Way.* New York: Alfred A. Knopf, Inc., 1999.

Mindell, Arnold. *Working with the Dreaming Body.* London: Routledge & Kegan Paul, 1985.

Murrell, William. *Massage as a Mode of Treatment.* London: H. K. Lewis, 1886.

National Certification Board for Therapeutic Massage and Bodywork (NCBTMB), 8201 Greensboro Drive, Suite 300, McLean, VA 22102; (800) 296-0664; (703) 610-9015; fax: (703) 610-9005.

Neumann, D. *Kinesiology of the Musculoskeletal System, Foundation for Physical Rehabilitation.* St. Louis: Evolve Mosby, 2002.

Norton, K., and T. Olds. *Anthropometrica.* Sydney, Australia: UNSW Press, 1996.

Orman, Suze. *The 9 Steps to Financial Freedom.* New York: Crown Publishers, Inc., 1997.

Pelletier, Kenneth R. *Mind as Healer, Mind as Slayer.* New York: Dell Publishing, 1992.

Pincus, Harold Alan, and Thomas A. Widiger. *Diagnostic Criteria from DSM-IV™.* Washington, DC: American Psychiatric Association, 1994.

Raheem, Aminah. *Soul Return, Integrating Body, Psyche and Spirit.* Fairfield, CT: Aslan Publishing, 1987.

Raheem, Aminah. *Soul Lightning: Awakening Soul Consciousness.* New York: iUniverse, Inc., 2005.

Raheem, Aminah. *Soul Lightning: Psychological Considerations for Working with Clients and Students* New York: Universe, Inc.

Ramutkowski, Barbara. *Medical Assisting: Administrative and Clinical Competencies,* 2nd ed. New York: McGraw-Hill, 2005.

Rattray, Fiona S. *Massage Therapy: An Approach to Treatments,* 2nd ed. Toronto: Massage Therapy Texts and Maverick Consultants, 1995.

Rice, R. "Neurophysiological development in premature infants following stimulation." *Developmental Psychology,* 13 (1977).

Saladin, Kenneth. *Anatomy and Physiology: The Unity of Form and Function,* 3rd ed., New York: McGraw-Hill, 2004.

Schneiderman, N., and M. A. Fletcher. "Cognitive-behavioral stress management intervention buffers, distress responses and immunologic changes following notification of HIV-1 seroscopy," *Journal of Consulting and Clinical Psychology,* 59 (1991).

Shannon, Margaret T. *Health Professional's Drug Guide.* Upper Saddle River, NJ: Prentice Hall, 2005.

Shier, David. *Hole's Essentials of Anatomy,* 8th ed., New York: McGraw-Hill, 2003.

Smith, Fritz Frederick. *Inner Bridges—A Guide to Energy Movement and Body Structure.* Atlanta: Humanics New Age, 1986.

Sohnen-Moe, Cherie. *Business Mastery,* 3rd ed. Rochester, VT: Healing Arts Press, 1997.

Spiegel, D., J. R. Bloom, H. C. Kraemer, and E. Gottheim. "Effect of psychosocial treatment on survival of patients with metastatic breast cancer." *Lancet 2,* 8668 (1989).

Strouhal, Eugen. *Life of the Ancient Egyptians.* Norman, OK: University of Oklahoma: Press with Opus Publishing Ltd., London: 1992.

Swerdlow, J. L., *Nature's Medicine: Plants That Heal.* Washington, DC: National Geographic, 2000.

Taylor, S. E. *Positive Illusions: Creative Self-Deception and the Healthy Mind.* New York: McGraw-Hill, 1999.

Taylor, Stacy, MSW. *Living Well with a Hidden Disability.* Oakland, CA: New Harbinger Publications, 1999.

Teeguarden, Iona Marsaa, MA. *The Complete Guide to Acupressure.* Tokyo: Japan Publications, Inc., 1996.

Thibodeau, Gary A. *Anatomy and Physiology.* St. Louis: Times Mirror/Mosby College, 1987.

Thibodeau, Gary A. *Structure and Function,* 12th ed., St. Louis, Mosby, 2004.

Thibodeau, Gary and Kevin Patton, *The Human Body in Health and Disease,* 2nd ed., St. Louis: Mosby Publishing, 1997.

Thomas, C. L. (ed). *Taber's Cyclopedic Medical Dictionary.* Philadelphia: F.A. Davis Company, 1997.

Tjaden, P., and Nancy Thoennes. *Prevalence, Incidence, and Consequences of Violence Against Women: Findings from the National Violence Against Women Survey Series: Research in Brief.* National Institute of Justice, Centers for Disease Control and Prevention, November 1998.

Travell, J., and D. Simons. *Myofascial Pain and Dysfunction: The Trigger Point Manual.* Baltimore: Williams & Wilkins, 1983.

USDA Agricultural Research Service, George Washington Carver Center, 5601 Sunnyside Avenue, Beltsville, MD 20705.

US Department of Agriculture Food and Nutrition Service, 3101 Park Center Drive, Room 926, Alexandria, VA 22303; (703) 305-2062.

US Department of Health and Human Services, Fact Sheet, *Protecting the Privacy of Patients: Health Information.* Washington, DC: 2004.

Vanderbilt, Heidi. "Incest: A Chilling Report," *Lears Magazine,* February 1992.

Wang, Ching-Tang, and Deborah Daro. *Current Trends in Child Abuse Reporting and Fatalities: The Results of the 1997 Annual Fifty State Survey.* Chicago: National Center on Child Abuse Prevention Research, National Committee to Prevent Child Abuse, 1998.

Werner, Ruth, *A Massage Therapist's Guide to Pathology,* 3rd ed. Baltimore: Lippincott Williams & Wilkins, 2005.

Massage for Maternity, Infant, Pediatric, and Special Needs

Auckett, Amelia D. *Baby Massage.* New York: Newmarket Press, 1989.

Awiakta, Marilou. *Selu: Seeking the Corn-Mother's Wisdom.* Colorado: Fulcrum Publishing, 1993.

Beck, Mark F., *Milady's Theory and Practice of Therapeutic Massage,* 3rd edition, Milady Publishing Company, Albany, NY, 1999.

Beers, Mark H. *The Merck Manual of Medical Information.* New Jersey: Merck & Co., Inc., 2003.

Cox, Connie A. *Maternity Massage.* Scottsdale, Arizona: Stress Less Publishing, Inc., 1994. Listed on pg: 267: "Historically .. form the cells."; Listed on pg 267: "Massage promoted . . . remove toxins."; Listed on page 269: "Prolonged . . . by indicated,"; Listed on pg 271: "During the first trimester . . . anemia."; Listed on pg 274: "Research shows . . . fight off infection."; Listed on pg 278: "Only gentle . . . weak connection."

Field, Tiffany M. *Touch in Early Development.* New Jersey: Lawrence Erlbaum Associates, 1995. Listed on pg 295: "The Touch Research . . . per infant."

Gellis and Kegan. Current Pediatric Therapy. W.B. Saunders Company: Philadelphia, London, Toronto, 1971. Listed on pg 298: "Down's syndrome . . . of the muscles."

Guyer, Evelyn A. *Family Bonding.* New York: Evelyn A. Guyer, 1997. Listed on pg 280: "National statistics . . . in our society."; Listed on pg 280: "An important dynamic . . . needs of the child."; Listed on pg 281: "Psychologists . . . raise children."

Johnson, Denny. *Touch Starvation in America.* Santa Barbara, California: Rayid, 1985. Listed on page 279: "Nutrition touch . . . coordination."

Jordan, Kate. *Bodywork for the Childbearing Year.* California: Kate Jordan Seminars, 1998. Listed on pg 266: "While massage . . . physical and emotional benefits"; Listed on pg 267: "Increase in heart rate . . . low birth weight"; Listed on pg 268: "Increased parasympathic . . . blood pressure"; Listed on pg 274: "A pregnant woman's body . . . systemic levels."; Listed on pg 274: "The endocrine system . . . blood supply,"; Listed on page 276: "The rib cage . . . pectoral girdle anteriorly."

Klaus, M., & Kennell, J. H. Parent Infant Bonding 2nd Ed., St. Louis, MO: Mosby, 1982. Listed on pg 280: "a unique relationship . . . through time."

Mabrey, R. *The New Age Herbalist.* New York, 1988, Simon & Shuster, 1988.

Magid, K., & Mckelvey, C. *High Risk: Children Without a Conscience.* Bantam Books: New York, NY, 1989. Listed on pg 280: "Parent-infant bonding…and spiritually."

McClure, Vimala. *Infant Massage.* New York: Bantam Books, 2000. Listed on pg 281: "Some of our basic…consumerism."; Listed on pg 281: "Infant massage presents…breathing."; Listed on pg 282: "These continually…and sounds."; Listed on pg 283: "Next, the caregiver…to proceed." Listed on pg 291: "The colic routine…repeat step 2."

Mones, Paul (1991), *When a Child Kills.* Pocket Star Books, 1991.

Montague, Ashley. *Touching.* New York: Harper & Row, 1986. Listed on pg 280: "As we discussed…and war."; Listed on pg 280: "Cross-cultural studies…compassionate."

Noble, Elizabeth. *Essentials for the Childbearing Year.* Fourth Edition. New Life Images: Harwich, MA, 1995. Listed on pg 276: "A passive tilt…spine erect."

Osborne-Sheets, Carole. *Pre- and Perinatal Massage Therapy.* California: Body Therapy Associates, 1998.; Listed on pg 266: "Massage therapy…rewards to the therapist."; Listed on pg 266: "It is important…changes."; Listed on pg 275: "Fibrinolysis…third trimester and postpartum."; Listed on pg 275: "Increased pressure…smooth muscle walls."

Powers, Michael D. *Children with Autism: A Parents' Guide.* Bethesda: Woodbine House, 2000.

Prescott, J. "Pleasure/violence reciprocity theory: The distribution of 49 cultures, relating infant physical affection to adult physical violence." *Futurist,* April 1975.

Samuels, Mike and Nancy. *The New Well Pregnancy Book.* New York: Simon & Schuster, 1996. Listed on pg 267: "Relaxation…removal of waste."; Listed on pg 274: "In one day…in three years."

Sinclair, Marybetts. *Massage for Healthier Children.* California: Wingbow Press, 1992. Listed on pg 290: "Massage…and movement."; Listed on pg 294: "The bonding process…channels of communication."

Sinclair, Marybetts. *Pediatric Massage Therapy.* Philadelphia, Maryland: Lippincott Williams & Wilkins, 2005. Listed on pg 293: "Specific development…varying symptoms."; Listed on pg 294: "Treatment…ritalin."; Listed on pg 295: "Children with Down's…stretching."; Listed on pg 295: "Asthma…past 10 years."

Thibodeau, Gary A. *Anatomy and Physiology.* St. Louis: Missouri: Times Mirror/Mosby College, 1987.

Thibodeau, Gary A. *Structure and Function,* 12th ed., St. Louis, Mosby, 2004.

Thomas, C. L. (1997). *Taber's Cyclopedic Medical Dictionary* (editor), F.A. Davis Company: Philadelphia.

Werner, Ruth. "Working with clients who have Cerebral Palsy." *Massage Today,* August 2002. Listed on pg 292: "Cerebral Palsy…in the United States."; Listed on pg 292: "Much of the damage…within the brain."; Listed on pg 293: "This is done…the reflex."

Massage for Hospice and Palliative Care

Cassileth, B. R., and A. J. Vickers "Massage therapy for symptom control: Outcome study at a major cancer center." *Journal of Pain and Symptom Management*, 2004. Listed on pg 301: "At the Hospice . . . diagnosed with cancer."

Gillespie, Barry R. *Healing Your Child.* Philadelphia: Dr. Barry R. Gillespie, 1999.

Lynn, Joanne, MD, and Joan Harold, MD. *Handbook for Mortals—Guidance for People Facing Serious Illness.* New York: Oxford University Press, 1999. Listed on pg 302: "Many people . . . can be helped."; Listed on pg 303: "Grief is one . . . our own grief."

MacDonald, Gayle. " Massage as an alternative respite intravention for primary caregivers of the terminally ill." Journal of Alternative Therapies in Clinical Practice, May/June 1997. Listed on pg 308: "A project in Portland . . . hospice agencies."

National Hospice and Palliative Care Organization, 1700 Diagonal Road, Suite 625, Alexandria, VA 22314; 703-837-1500 (phone); 703-837-1233 (fax)

Polubinski, Joseph P., and Laurie West. "Implementation of a Massage Therapy Program in the Home Hospice Setting." *Journal of Pain and Symptom Management,* July 2005. Listed on pg 301: "Patients reported . . . anxiety and peacefulness."

Rice, R. "Neurophysiological development in premature infants following stimulation." *Developmental Psychology 13* (1977).

Williams, Mary E. *Terminal Illness.* San Diego: Greenhaven Press, Inc., 2001. Listed on pg 299: "Dying can be . . . family members and friends."

Wright, L. D. "Complementary and alternative medicine for hospice and palliative care." *American Journal of Hospice and Palliative Medicine,* 2004. Lised on pg 300: "Massage Therapy . . . appropriately administered."

Working with Survivors of Sexual Abuse

American Psychiatric Association. *Diagnostic and Statistical Manual of Mental Disorders,* 4th ed. Washington, DC: 2000.

Antoni, M. H., L. Baggett, G. Ironsen, A. LaPerriere, S. August, N. Klimas, N. Schneiderman, and M. A. Fletcher. "Cognitive-behavioral stress management intervention buffers, distress responses and immunologic changes following notification of HIV-1 seroscopy," *Journal of Consulting and Clinical Psychology,* 59 (1991).

Beers, Mark H., MD, and Robert Berkow, MD, ed. *The Merck Manual.* Whitehouse Station, NJ: Merck Research Laboratories, 1999.

Berkman, L. F., and S. L. Syme. "Social networks, host resistance, and mortality: A nine-year follow-up study of Alameda County residents," *American Journal of Epidemiology,* 109 (1979).

Bower, J., M. E. Kemeny, S. E. Taylor, and J. L. Fahey. "Cognitive processing, discovery of meaning, CD 4 decline and AIDS-related mortality among bereaved HIV seropositive men." *Journal of Consulting and Clinical Psychology,* 65 (1998).

California Coalition Against Sexual Assault, 2002. *2002 Report: Research on Rape and Violence.*

California Department of Justice. *Crime and Delinquency in California 2000.* Sacramento: Department of Justice, Division of Criminal Justice Information Services, 2000.

Cerio, Donna C., "Zero balancing with survivors of sexual abuse," *Interface,* Newsletter of the Zero Balancing Association, 2003.

Cerio, Donna C. "The wounded client: Massage with survivors of sexual abuse," *Massage Magazine,* November/December 2003.

Cerio, Donna C. "Dealing with traumatic touch," *Health and Fitness Connection,* October 1994.

Cerio, Donna C. "Touch—The unspoken language: Healing from sexual abuse," *Skinship Journal,* January, April, July, October 2004.

Cerio, Donna C. "Therapeutic report on touch," *AMTA Florida Journal,* Summer Issue 34 (2005).

Cerio, Donna C. *Zero Balancing with Survivors of Sexual Trauma.* Santa Cruz, CA: 2004.

Cerio, Donna C. *Bodywork Therapy with Survivors of Sexual Abuse,* 3rd ed. Santa Cruz, CA: 2004.

Dallam, S. J. *The Hidden Effects of Childhood Maltreatment on Adult Health.* New York: Putnam, 1998.

Esterling, B. A., M. H. Antoni, M. H. M. Kumar, and N. Schneiderman. "Emotional repression, stress disclosure responses and Epstein-Barr viral capsid antigen titers." *Psychosomatic Medicine,* 52 (1990).

Federal Bureau of Investigations. *Uniform Crime Reports for the United States 2000.* Washington, DC: U.S. Department of Justice, 2000.

Hamwee, John. *Zero Balancing, Touching the Energy of Bone.* London: Frances Lincoln Limited, 1999.

Herman, Judith. *Trauma and Recovery.* New York: Basic Books, 1992.

Karow, J. 10/01/00 "Biology—Stressed for life," *Scientific American* (2000).

Kilpatrick, D., and B. Saunders. *The Prevalence and Consequences of Child Victimization: Summary of a Research Study,* Washington DC: US Department of Justice, National Institute of Justice, 1997.

Love, Patricia. *The Emotional Incest Syndrome.* New York: Bantam Books, 1990.

Mindell, Arnold. *Working with the Dreaming Body.* London: Routledge & Kegan Paul, 1985.

Mones, Paul. *When a Child Kills.* New York: Pocket Star Books, 1991.

Pincus, Harold Alan, and Thomas A. Widiger, *Diagnostic Criteria from DSM-IV™.* Washington, DC: American Psychiatric Association. 1994.

Population Information Program, Center for Communications Programs. *Population Reports: Ending Violence Against Women.* Baltimore: Johns Hopkins School of Public Health and Center for Healthcare Gender Equality, 1999

Raheem, Aminah. *Soul Return, Integrating Body, Psyche and Spirit.* Fairfield, CT: Aslan Publishing, 1987.

Raheem, Aminah. *Soul Lightning: Awakening Soul Consciousness.* New York: iUniverse, Inc., 2005.

Raheem, Aminah. *Soul Lightning: Psychological Considerations for Working with Clients and Students.* New York: iUniverse.

Smith, Fritz Frederick. *Inner Bridges—A Guide to Energy Movement and Body Structure.* Atlanta: Humanics New Age, 1986.

Spiegel, D., J. R. Bloom, H. C. Kraemer, and E. Gottheim. "Effect of psychosocial treatment on survival of patients with metastatic breast cancer." *Lancet 2* 8668 (1989).

Taylor, S. E. *Positive Illusions: Creative Self-Deception and the Healthy Mind.* New York: McGraw-Hill, 1999.

Taylor, Stacy, MSW. *Living Well with a Hidden Disability.* Oakland, CA: New Harbinger Publications, 1999.

Teeguarden, Iona Marsaa, MA. *The Complete Guide to Acupressure.* Tokyo: Japan Publications, Inc., 1996.

Thomas, C. L., ed. *Taber's Cyclopedic Medical Dictionary.* Philadelphia: F. A. Davis Company, 1997.

Tjaden, P., and Nancy Thoennes. *Prevalence, Incidence, and Consequences of Violence Against Women: Findings from the National Violence Against Women Survey Series: Research in Brief,* National Institute of Justice, Centers for Disease Control and Prevention, November 1998.

Vanderbilt, Heidi. "Incest: A Chilling Report," *Lears Magazine,* February 1992.

Wang, Ching-Tang, and Deborah Daro. *Current Trends in Child Abuse Reporting and Fatalities: The Results of the 1997 Annual Fifty State Survey.* Chicago: National Center on Child Abuse Prevention Research, National Committee to Prevent Child Abuse, 1998.

Werner, Ruth, and Ben E. Benjamin. *A Massage Therapist's Guide to Pathology.* Baltimore: Lippincott, Williams & Wilkins, 1998.

Philosophical Foundation of Massage

Calvert, Robert Noah. *The History of Massage.* Rochester, VT: Healing Arts Press, 2002.

Carlson, Richard, and Benjamin Shield, eds. *Healers on Healing.* Los Angeles: Jeremy P. Tarcher, Inc., 1989.

Dubos, Rene. *A God Within.* Woodbridge, CT: Charles Scribner's Sons, 1972.

Epstein, Donald, DC. *The Vitalistic Practitioner.* Innate Intelligence Inc., 1989.

Garrison, Fielding H., AB, MD. *History of Medicine,* 4th ed. Philadelphia: W. B. Saunders, 1929.

Equipment and Environment

Cox, Kathleen. *The Power of Vastu Living.* New York: Fireside, Simon and Schuster, 2002.

Ouseley, S. G. J. *Colour Meditations with a Guide to Colour Healing,* 15th ed. L. N. Fowler & Co., Ltd., 1986.

Pegrum, Juliet. *The Vastu Home.* Berkeley, CA: Ulysses Press, 2002.

Safety First in the Massage Environment

American Heart Association National Center, 7272 Greenville Avenue, Dallas, TX 75231; (800)-242-8721.

American Red Cross National Headquarters, 2025 E Street, NW, Washington, DC 20006; (202) 303-4498; (800) 435-7669.

Centers for Disease Control, 1600 Clifton Road, N.E., Atlanta, GA 30333 (404) 639-3311; public inquiries, (800) 311-3435.

Groust-Lakomia, L., and E. Fong. *Microbiology for Health Careers,* Clifton Park, NY.

National Safety Council. *Standard First Aid, CPR, and AED.* New York: McGraw-Hill, 2005.

National Safety Council, 1121 Spring Lake Drive, Itasca, IL 60143-3201; (630) 285-1121.

Chinese Medicine, Meridians, and Acupressure

Cho, H. *Oriental Medicine.* Compton, CA: Yuin University Press, Number 12, 1996.

Deadman, P. K. Baker, and M. Al-khafaji. *A Manual of Acupuncture.* Eastland Press: Vista, CA, 1998.

Hammer, L. *Chinese Pulse Diagnosis: A Contemporary Approach.* Eastland Press: Vista, CA, 2003.

Jarmey, C., and J. Tindall. *Acupressure for Common Ailments.* New York: Simon & Schuster, 1991.

Macioccia, G. *The Foundations of Chinese Medicine.* New York: Churchill Livingstone, 2003.

Tappan, F., and P. Benjamin. *Healing Massage Techniques.* Stamford, CT: Appleton & Lange, 1998.

Toguchi, M. and F. Warren. *The Complete Guide to Acupuncture and Acupressure.* New York: Grammercy Publishing, 1976.

Young, J. *Acupressure Step by Step.* London: Thorsons, 1994.

Ayurveda

Lad, Vasant. Ayurveda—*The Science of Self-Healing.* Sante Fe, NM: Lotus Press, 1984.

Svoboda, Robert E., *Your Ayurvedic Constitution.* Albuquerque: Geocom, 1988.

Thai Massage

International Training Massage (ITM) Institute, Chiang Mai, Thailand, phone (053) 218632.

Mercati, Maria. *Thai Massage.* London: Marshall Publishing, 1998.

Old Medicine Hospital, Chiang Mai, Thailand, phone (053) 275085.

Lomi lomi

Hawaiian Lomilomi Association, P.O. Box 2356, Kealakekua, Hawaii, 96750-2356; www.lomilomi.org.

Reiki

Global Reiki Association, www.thegra.org

International Association of Reiki Professionals, www.iarp.org (603) 881-8838

Reiki Alliance, www.reikialliance.com, 204 N. Chestnut Street, Kellogg, ID 83837 (828) 628-1706

Stein, Diane *Essential Reiki.* Trumansburg, NY: The Crossing Press, 1948.

Reflexology

Reflexology World Magazine, www.reflexologyworld.com
P.O. Box 1032, Bondi Junction
NSW 2022 Australia
Tel: +61 (0) 2 9300 9391

Reflexology Association of America
4012 Rainbow, Ste. K-PMB #585
Las Vegas, NV 89103-2059

Polarity Therapy

American Polarity Association, www.polaritytherapy.org
P.O. Box 19858, Boulder, CO 80308
(303)545-2080

Trigger Point Therapy

Travell, M. D., Janet G. and David G. Simons. *Myofascial Pain and Dysfunction: The Trigger Point Manual*, Vol. 1 and 2. Baltimore: Williams & Wilkins, 1983.

Myofascial Release

Barnes, J. F. *Myofascial Release: The Search for Excellence.* Paoli, PA: MFR Seminars, 1990.

Bohm, D. *Causality and Chance in Modern Physics.* Philadelphia, University of Pennsylvania Press, 1957.

Bohm, D. *The Special Theory of Relativity.* Boston: Addison Wesley, 1988.

Chaitow, L. *Neuro-Muscular Technique: A Practitioner's Guide to Soft Tissue Mobilization.* New York: Thorsons, 1985.

Davis, C. *Complementary Therapies in Rehabilitation.* Thorofare, NJ: Slack, Inc., 2004.

Hameroff, S. R. "Quantum coherence in microtubules: A neural basis of emergent consciousness." *Journal of Consciousness Studies,* Summer 1994, 1(1):91-118.

Hawkins, R., and E. Kandel. "Steps toward a cell-biological alphabet for elementary forms of learning." In *Neurobiology of Learning and Memory,* ed. by G. Lynch, J. McCaugh, and N. Weinberger (383-404). New York: Guilford Press, 1991.

Juhan, D. *Job's Body,* Barrytown, NY: Station Hill Press, 1987.

Katake, K. "The strength for tension and bursting of human fasciae," *Journal of Kyoto Pref. Med. Univ.,* 69 (1961): 484-88.

Korb, K. B. "Stage effects in the Cartesian theater: A review of Daniel Dermetts 'Consicousness Explained.'" *Psyche,* 1 (December 1993): 1.

Kuhn, T. S. *The Structure of Scientific Revolutions.* Chicago: University of Chicago Press, 1970.

Kurtz, R. *Body Centered Psychotherapy: The Hakomi Therapy.* Ashland, OR: Hakomi Institute, 1988.

Lynch, G., J. McCaugh, and N. Weinberger, eds. *Neurobiology of Learning and Memory.* New York: Guilford Press, June 15, 1998.

Oschman, J. L. *Energy Medicine—The Scientific Basis.* New York: Churchill Livingstone, 2000.

Oschman, J. L. *Energy Medicine in Therapeutics and Human Performance.* Edinburgh: Butterworth-Heinemann, 2003.

Popper K. R., and J. C. Eccles. *The Self and Its Brain.* Berlin: Springer, 1977.

Rosenzweig, M., and E. Bennett. "Basic processes and modulatory influences in the stages of memory formation". In, edited by G. Lynch, J. McCaugh and N. Weinberger

Rossi E. "From mind to molecule: A state-dependent memory, learning, and behavior theory of mind-body healing." *Advance,* 2 (April 1987):46-60.

Scott, J. "Molecules that keep you in shape." *New Scientist,* (1986):11149–53.

Searle, J. R. "Minds, brains and programs." *Behavioral and Brain Sciences,* 3 (1980):417-24.

Selye, H. *The Stress of Life.* New York: McGraw-Hill, 1976.

Selye H. History and Present Status of the Stress Concept. In *Handbook of Stress,* (7-20) L. Goldberger and S. Breznitz, eds. New York: Macmillan, 1982:7-20.

Siegel, B. *Love, Medicine and Miracles.* New York: Harper & Row, 1986.

Taylor, J. G. "Towards a neural network model of the mind." *Neural Network World.* 6 (1992):797-812.

Upledger, J., and J. Vredevoogd. *Craniosacral Therapy.* Seattle: Eastland Press, 1983.

Rolf, I. *Rolfing: The Integration of Human Structures.* New York: Harper & Row, 1977.

Rolfing

Cohen, Don. *An introduction to Craniosacral Therapy.* Berkeley: North Atlantic Books, 1996.

Magoun, Harold Ives. *Osteopathy in the Cranial Field.* Boise, ID: Northwest Printing, Inc., 1966.

Manheim, Carol J., and Diane K. Lavett. *Craniosacral Therapy and Somato-Emotional Release.* Thorofare, NJ: Slack, Inc., 1989.

Milne, Hugh. *The Heart of Listening.* Berkeley: North Atlantic Books, 1995.

Still, A.T. *Osteopathy, Research and Practice.* Seattle: Eastland Press, 1992.

Sutherland, William G. *Contributions of Thought.* Portland, Oregon: Rudra Press, 1971.

The Upledger Institute, 11211 Prosperity Farms Road, Palm Beach Gardens, Florida. Phone (800) 233-5880, extension 4528.

Upledger, John E. *A Brain Is Born.* Berkeley: North Atlantic Books, 1995.

Upledger, John E. *Your Inner Physician and You.* Berkeley: North Atlantic Books, 1997.

Upledger, John E., and Jon D. Vredevoogd. *Craniosacral Therapy.* Seattle: Eastland Press, 1983.

CranioSacral Therapy

Fulford, Robert C., with Gene Stone. *Dr. Fulford's Touch of Life.* New York: Pocket Books, 1996.

Guyton, Arthur, and John Hall. *Guytan's Textbook of Physiology.* New York: Saunders Co., 2000.

Juhan, Dean. *Job's Body—A Handbook for Body Work,* expanded edition. Barrytown Station Hill Press: Tarrytown, NY, 1998.

Pert, Candace. *Molecules of Emotion.* New York: Scribner, 1997.

Upledger, John E. *Cerebrospinal Fluid—What It Is and Where to Find It.* Palm Beach, FL: Upledger Institute, 1998.

Upledger, John E. *The Expanding Role of Cerebrospinal Fluid in Health and Disease.* Palm Beach, FL: Upledger Institute, 2000.

Whedon, James. "Clinical Anatomy and Physiology of the CSF for Body Workers." Cerebrospinal Fluid Technique Seminars, Feasterville, PA, 1997.

Cerebrospinal Fluid Massage

Aselli G, *De Lactibus Seu Lactis Venis, Quarto Vasorum Mesaraicorum Genere Novo Inventa,* Dissertatio Mediolan, 1627.

Chikly B. *Silent Waves: Theory and Practice of Lymph Drainage Therapy with Applications for Edema, Chronic Pain and Inflammation.* Scottsdale: IHH Publishers, 2001.

Chikly, B. "Who discovered the Lymphatic System?" *Lymphology,* December 1997, 30, No. 4, p. 186.

Chikly, B. "Applications of pre- and post-surgical—lymph drainage therapy." *Massage and Bodywork,* Summer/Fall 1997, 12, 3, p. 64-67.

Lymphatic Drainage Therapy

Millard, F. P. "Applied anatomy of the lymphatic." A. G. Walmstey, ed., International Lymphatic Research Society, 1922.

Miller, C. E. "Osteopathic treatment of acute infections by means of the lymphatics," *Journal of American Osteopath Association,* 1920, (19):494-499.

Olszewski, W. L., and A. Engeset. "Intrinsic Contractility of Prenodal Lymph Vessels and Lymph Flow in Human Leg, *American Journal of Physiology,* 1980, (2390): 775-783

Vodder, E. "Le Drainage Lymphatique, Une Nouvelle Méthode Thérapeutique," Santé Pour Tous, Paris, 1936.

Quick Guide D   *Medical Terminology*
and Anatomical Abbreviations for Massage and Bodywork

Medical terminology consists of several components:

- Prefix—the word beginning
- Suffix—the word ending
- Root word—the basis of a word
- Combining vowel—a vowel (a, e, i, o, u, or y): usually "o" that connects a root word to a suffix or a root word to another root word
- Combining form—the combination of a root word and a combining vowel

There are four rules for medical terminology:

1. Words are read with the ending suffix first, then the prefix, and then across to the root word.
2. The combining vowel is dropped before a suffix that begins with a vowel.
3. Keep the combining vowel before the suffix if the suffix begins with a consonant.
4. Keep the combining vowel between two root words even if the second root word begins with a vowel.

Forming Plurals

1. When the word ends in an **a,** retain the *a* and add *e* (vertebra/vertebrae).
2. When the word ends in **is,** drop the *is* and add *es* (diagnosis/diagnoses).
3. When the word ends in **ex** or **ix,** drop the *ex* or *ix* and add *ices* (apex/apices).
4. When the word ends in **on,** drop the *on* and add *a* (ganglion/ganglia).
5. When words end in **um,** drop the *um* and add *a* (bacterium/bacteria).
6. When words end in **us,** drop the *us* and add *i* (bronchus/bronchi).

Prefixes	Meaning	Example
A		
a-	without, not	atypical—not typical
ab-	away from	abduction—away from the body
ad-	to, toward	adhere—to stick together
adeno-	gland	adenosis—disease of a gland
ambi-	on both sides	ambidextrous—using both hands
an-	not, without	anoxia—without oxygen

(continued)

Prefixes	Meaning	Example
ana-	up, apart, absence	anaphia—loss of touch sensation
ante-	before	anteflexion—bending forward
anti-	against	antibody—against microorganisms
arteri-/o-	arteries	arteriosclerosis—hardening of arteries
arthr-	joint	arthritis—inflammation of a joint
aur-/o-	ear	auricle—external ear
auto-	self	autoinfection—reinfecting yourself

B

bi-	two	biarticular—pertaining to two joints
brady-	slow	bradycardia—slow heartbeat
bronch-/o-	bronchial tube	bronchitis—inflammation of the bronchi

C

cata-	down	cataphoria—downward-turned eyes
co-	with, together	cojoined—joined together
con-	with, together	confluent—merged
contra-	against, opposite	contraindication—not indicated

D

de-	lack of	dehydrated—lack of water
di-	two, twice	diplopia—double vision
dia-	complete, thorough	diarrhea—complete discharge
dis-	reversal, separation	dislocate—separate from the site
dys-	painful, difficult	dyspnea—difficult breathing

E

ecto-	outside	ectopic—out of the usual place
en-	within	encephalitis—within the brain
endo-	within	endocardium—within the heart
epi-	above, upon	epidermis—top layer of skin
eu-	good, easy	euphoric—happy
ex-	outside, out	excision—remove, take out
exo-	outside, outward	exorenal—outside the kidney

H

hemi-	half	hemiplegia—paralysis of one side of body
hyper-	above, excess	hyperglycemia—high blood sugar
hypo-	low, deficient	hypoglycemia—low blood sugar

I

in-	not	insoluble—not soluble
infra-	below, inferior	infrasternal—below the sternum
inter-	between	intervertebral—between the vertebra
intra-	within	intracutaneous—within the skin

L

lei-	smooth	leiomyoma—smooth muscle tumor
leu-	white	leukocyte—white blood cell
lipo-	fatty tissue	lipoma—fatty tumor

Prefixes	Meaning	Example
M		
macro-	large	macrocephalic—large head
mal-	bad, odd	malformed—not normal shape
meso-	middle	mesorenal—middle of the kidney
meta-	beyond, changing	metastasis—moving beyond the original tissue
micro-	small	microscopic—unseen with the naked eye
N		
necro-	dead	necrosis—death of cells
neo-	new	neonatal—newborn
P		
pan-	all, every	pandemic—affecting everyone
para-	beside	parathyroid—glands beside the thyroid
per-	through	percutaneous—through the skin
peri-	around	pericardium—around the heart
poly-	many	polyneuritis—inflammation of many nerves
post-	after, behind	postpartum—after birth
pre-	before	prenatal—before birth
pro-	before	prognosis—before knowledge
R		
re-	back, again	relapse—return of a disease or condition
retro-	behind	retrogastric—behide the stomach
S		
semi-	half, part of	semiprone—lying face downward
sub-	below, under	subcostal—below the ribs
supra-	above, over	suprarenal—over the kidney
sym-	together, with	sympodia—fused lower extremity
syn-	together, with	syndromatic—syndromes occurring together
T		
tachy-	fast, rapid	tachycardia—rapid heart rate
trans-	across, through	transdermal—through the skin

Combining Forms	Meaning	Example
A		
aden/o-	gland	adenitis—gland inflammation
angio-	vessel	angioplasty—repair of a vessel
arteri/o-	artery	arterial flow—flow in an artery
arthr/o-	joint	arthritis—inflammation of a joint

(continued)

Combining Forms	Meaning	Example
B		
blephar/o-	eyelid	blepharitis—infection of the eyelid
brachi/o-	arm	brachiocubital—arm and elbow
bronchi-	bronchi	bronchial—pertaining to bronchus
bucc/o-	cheek	buccolingual—cheek and tongue
burs/a-	bursa	bursitis—inflammation of the bursa
C		
carcin/o-	cancer	carcinoma—malignant neoplasm
cardi/o-	heart	cardiodynia—pain in the heart
cephal/o-	head	cephalad—toward the head
cerebr/o-	brain	cerebrospinal—brain and spine
cervic/o-	neck	cervicodynia—neck pain
coccyg/o-	coccyx	coccyxgodynia—pain in the coccyx
cost/o-	ribs	costalgia—rib pain
crani/o-	skull	craniosclerosis—thickening of the skull
cric/o-	cricoid	cricothyroid—cricoid and thyroid cartilage
cutane/o-	skin	transcutaneous—through the skin
cyst/o-	urinary bladder	cystoplegia—paralysis of the bladder
D		
dactyl/o-	finger, toe	polydactyl—abnormal number of fingers
dent/i-	tooth	denture—artificial teeth
dips/o-	thirst	dipsomania—compulsion to drink
dors/o-	back	dorsal—toward the back
E		
electr/o-	electricity	electrolysis—destruction of hair follicles
encephal/o-	brain	encephalopathy—brain disorder
enter/o-	intestine	enterosepsis—intestinal sepsis
esophag/o-	esophagus	esophagitis—inflammation of the esophagus
F		
fasci/o-	fascia	faciitis—inflammation of the fascia
femor/o-	femur	femorocele—herniation of the thigh
fibul/o-	fibula	fibular—pertaining to the fibula
G		
gastr/o-	stomach	gastrocele—herniated stomach
gingiv/o-	gums	gingivitis—inflamed gums
gloss/o-	tongue	glossocele—swollen tongue
gynec/o-	female	gynecic—pertaining to women
H		
hemat/o-	blood	hematherm—warm blood
hepat/o-	liver	hepatoma—liver tumor
hist/o-	tissue	histolysis—destruction of tissue
hypn/o-	sleep	hypnosis—induced trancelike state
hyster/o-	uterus	hysterectomy—removal of the uterus

Combining Forms	Meaning	Example
I		
idi/o-	individual	idiophobia—morbid fear of new ideas
ile/o-	ileum	ileocecal—illeum and cecum
ili/o-	ilium	iliocostal—pertaining to the ilium and ribs
J		
jejun/o-	jejunum	jejunitis—inflammation of the jejunum
K		
kerat/o-	cornea	keratectomy—operation on the cornea
kinesi/o-	movement	kinesiology—study of movement
L		
labi/o-	lip	labionasal—upper lip and nose
laryng/o-	larynx	laryngismus—narrowing of the larynx
later/o-	side	lateral—on the side
lip/o-	fat	lipocardial—fatty heart
lith/o-	stone	lithiasis—formation of stones
M		
mamm/o-	breast	mammectomy—breast removal
mast/o-	breast	mastography—making breast x-rays
my/o-	muscle	myocardial—muscle of the heart
myel/o-	spinal cord Bone marrow	myelopoiesis—formation of bone marrow
N		
nas/o-	nose	nasogastric—from nose to stomach
nephr/o-	kidney	nephrorragia—hemorrhage from the kidney
noct/i-	night	noctiphobia—fear of darkness or night
norm/o-	normal	normocytosis—normal state of blood
O		
onc/o-	mass	oncogenesis—production of tumors
oo/o-	egg/ovum	oocyte—an immature egg
ophthalm/o-	eye	ophthalmology—study of the eye
orchid/o-	testis	orchidectomy—removal of a testicle
or/o-	mouth	oral—taken by mouth
osteo/o-	bone	osteomalacia—softening of the bones
ot/o-	ear	otodynia—earache
ov/o-	egg	ovoid—having an egg shape
P		
pachy-	thick	pachyderm—thick skin
path/o-	disease	pathology—study of disease processes
poster/o-	back	posterolateral—behind and to the side
pseud/o-	false	pseudipsia—false thirst
psych/o-	mind	psychosis—condition of the mind

(continued)

Combining Forms	Meaning	Example
R		
radi/o-	radiation	radiothermic—heat from a radiant source
ren/o-	kidney	renal—of the kidney
rhin/o-	nose	rhinoplasty—nose repair
S		
sacr/o-	sacrum	sacroiliac—sacral and iliac junction
sarc/o-	flesh/muscle	sarcolemma—membrane of muscle fiber
sect/i-	dissection	To cut into sections
T		
thorac/o-	chest	thoracic—area of the chest
tibi/o-	tibia	tibialgia—pain in the shin area
top/o-	location	ectopic—located away from normal position
tox/o-	poison	toxic—poisonous
trache/o-	trachea	tracheotomy—incision in the trachea
U		
ur/o-	urinary tract	urology—study of the urinary system
uter/o-	uterus	uterolith—uterine stones (calculi)
V		
vas/o-	vessel	vasodilation—widening of the lumen in blood vessels
ven/o-	vein	venopuncture—puncturing the vein
viscer/o-	internal organs	viscerad—toward the viscera (organs)
X		
xanth/o-	yellow	xanthophobia—fear of the color yellow
xer/o-	dry	xerosis—abnormal dryness

Suffixes	Meaning	Example
A		
-ac	pertaining to	cardiac—pertaining to the heart
-al	pertaining to	renal—pertaining to the kidney
-algia	pain	neuralgia—pain originating in the nerves
-asthenia	lack of strength	myasthenia—lack of muscle strength
C		
-cele	hernia	cystocele—hernial protrusion into the bladder
-centesis	surgical puncture	amniocentesis—puncture to remove amnionic fluid
-cidal	killing	germicidal—kills germs
-coccus	bacterial cell	staphylococcus—infectious microorganism
-cyte	cell	erythrocyte—red blood cell

Suffixes	Meaning	Example
D		
-desis	binding	arthrodesis—surgical fixation of a joint
E		
-ectasis	stretching	angiectasis—lengthening of a blood vessel
-ectomy	removal	myomectomy—removal of a myoma
-emesis	vomiting	hyperemesis—excessive vomiting
-emia	blood condition	anemia—lack of red blood cells
G		
-genesis	originating	blastogenesis—reproduction by budding
-gram	record	myelogram—spinal cord x-ray
-graphy	process of recording	sonography—recording of sound waves
I		
-ia	condition	dyspepsia—bad digestion
-ic	pertaining to	thoracic—pertaining to the chest area
-ist	specialist	oncologist—tumor specialist
-itis	inflammation	bronchitis—inflammation of the bronchi
L		
-logy	study of	neurology—study of nerves
-lysis	destruction	hemolysis—destruction of blood cells
M		
-malacia	softening	osteomalacia—softening of the bones
-megaly	enlargement	cephalomegaly—enlarged head
O		
-odynia	pain	gastrodynia—pain in the stomach
-ole	little, small	arteriole—small arterial branch
-oma	tumor	myoma—tumor of the muscle
-opia	vision	diplopia—double vision
-osis	condition	scoliosis—curvature of the spine
-ostomy	new opening	colostomy—surgical opening of the colon
P		
-pepsia	digestion	dyspepsia—bad digestion
-phagia	eating	polyphagia—excessive eating
-phobia	fear	xenophobia—fear of strangers
-plasia	formation	chondroplasia—formation of cartilage
-plegia	paralysis	hemiplagia—paralysis of one side of the body
-pnea	breathing, air	dyspnea—difficult breathing
-ptosis	drooping	blepharoptosis—drooping of the eyelid
-ptysis	spitting	hemoptysis—spitting blood
S		
-sclerosis	hardening	arteriosclerosis—hardening of the arteries
-stasis	control	hemostasis—stopping the flow of blood
-stenosis	narrowing	angiostenosis—narrowing of a blood vessel

(continued)

Suffixes	Meaning	Example
T		
-therapy	treatment	hydrotherapy—treatment with water
-tomy	incision	tracheotomy—incision of the trachea
-trophy	development	hypertrophy—excessive development
U		
-ule	little, small	venule—small vein
-uria	urine	polyuria—excessive urination

Anatomical Abbreviations Common to Massage and Bodywork

abs	abdominals
AC	acromioclavicular
ACL	anterior crutiate ligament
AIIS	anterior inferior iliac spine
ASIS	anterior superior iliac spine
ATFL	anterior talofibular ligament
AW	abdominal wall
BBB	blood brain barrier
BEF	bioenergetic field
bi	biceps
BJM	bones, joints, and muscles
BR	breath
C, C 1-7	cervical vertebrae
CN 1-8	cervical nerves
CrN 1-12	cranial nerves
CSF	cerebral spinal fluid
ch	chest
Cl	clavicle
CM	carpometacarpal
CNS	central nervous system
coc	coccygeal
Cr	cranium
delt	deltoid
DH	dominant hand
dia	diaphragm
elb	elbow
ES	erector spinae muscle
FE	fémur
gastroc	gastrocnemius
GHL	glenohumeral ligament
gluts	gluteal muscle group
GT	greater trochanter
hams	hamstring muscles
he	heart
hd	head

H & N	head and neck
hum	humerus
IC	ileocecal
IF	iliofemoral
IP	ilio-psoas
ISF	interstitial fluid
ITB	illiotibial band
IT	ischial tuberosity
IVD	intervertebral disk
IVDJ	intervertebral joint complex
J, jt	joint
L, L 1-5	lumbar vertebrae
LC	lymph capillaries
LCL	lateral collateral ligament
lats	latissimus dorsi
lev sca	levator scapula
LN	lymph node
mas	masseter
meta	metacarpal
mm	muscles
nn	nerves
NR	nerve root
NS	nervous system
os	bone
pecs	pectoralis major and minor
PNS	parasympathetic nervous system
PSIS	posterior sacroiliac spine
QL	quadratus lumborum
quads	muscles
RC	rib case
rhomb	rhomboids
SB	sternal border
SC	sternoclavicular, sternocostal
SCM	sternocleidomastoid
ScM	scalene muscle group
SI	sacroiliac
sh	shoulder
sol	soleus
ST	soft tissue
st	sternum
T, T 1-12	thoracic vertebrae
TC	thoracic cage
TFA	tibiofemoral angle
TFL	tensor fascia lata
tib	tibialis
TMJ	temporomandibular joint
traps	trapezius
tri	triceps
UN	ulnar nerve
vert	vertebrae

Quick Guide E

Muscular System Tables with Origin,
Insertion, Innervation, and Actions

Table E1	*Muscles of Facial Expression*	

O = origin, I = insertion, N = innervation (n. = nerve), A = action

Occipitofrontalis (oc-SIP-ih-toe-frun-TAY-lis)

Occipitalis

A: Retracts scalp; fixes galea aponeurotica

O: superior nuchal line	I: galea aponeurotica	N: facial n. (VII)

Frontalis

A: Raises eyebrows and creates wrinkles in forehead when occipitalis is contracted; draws scalp forward when occipitalis is relaxed

O: galea aponeurotica	I: skin of forehead	N: facial n. (VII)

Orbicularis oculi (or-BIC-you-LERR-iss OC-you-lye)

A: Closes eye; compresses lacrimal gland to promote flow of tears

O: medial wall of orbit	I: eyelid	N: facial n. (VII)

Levator palpebrae (leh-VAY-tur pal-PEE-bree) **superioris**

A: Opens eye; raises upper eyelid

O: roof of orbit	I: upper eyelid	N: oculomotor n. (III)

Corrugator supercilii (COR-oo-GAY-tur SOO-per-SIL-ee-eye)

A: Medially depresses eyebrows and draws them closer together; wrinkles skin between eyebrows

O: superciliary ridge	I: skin of eyebrow	N: facial n. (VII)

Procerus (pro-SER-us)

A: Wrinkles skin between eyebrows; draws skin of forehead down

O: skin on bridge of nose	I: skin of forehead	N: facial n. (VII)

Nasalis (nay-SAY-liss)

A: One part widens nostrils; another part depresses nasal cartilages and compresses nostrils

O: maxilla and nasal cartilages	I: bridge and alae of nose	N: facial n. (VII)

Orbicularis oris (or-BIC-you-LERR-iss OR-iss)

A: Closes lips; protrudes lips as in kissing; aids in speech

O: muscle fibers around mouth	I: mucous membrane of lips	N: facial n. (VII)

Levator labii superioris

A: Elevates upper lip

O: zygomatic bone, maxilla	I: upper lip	N: facial n. (VII)

(continued)

Levator anguli (ANG-you-lye) **oris**

A: Elevates corners of mouth, as in smiling and laughing

| O: maxilla | I: superior corner of mouth | N: facial n. (VII) |

Zygomaticus (ZY-go-MAT-ih-cus) **major and zygomaticus minor**

A: Draw corners of mouth laterally and upward, as in smiling and laughing

| O: zygomatic bone | I: superolateral corner of mouth | N: facial n. (VII) |

Risorius (rih-SOR-ee-us)

A: Draws corner of mouth literally, as in grimacing

| O: fascia near ear | I: corner of mouth | N: facial n. (VII) |

Depressor anguli oris, or triangularis

A: Depresses corner of mouth, as in frowning

| O: mandible | I: inferolateral corner of mouth | N: facial n. (VII) |

Depressor labii inferioris

A: Depresses lower lip

| O: near mental protuberance | I: lower lip | N: facial n. (VII) |

Mentalis (men-TAY-lis)

A: Pulls skin of chin upward; elevates and protrudes lower lip, as in pouting

| O: near mental protuberance | I: skin of chin | N: facial n. (VII) |

Buccinator (BUCK-sin-AY-tur)

A: Compresses cheek; pushes food between teeth; expels air or liquid from mouth; creates suction

| O: lateral aspects of maxilla and mandible | I: orbicularis oris | N: facial n. (VII) |

Platysma (plah-TIZ-muh)

A: Depresses mandible; opens and widens mouth; tenses skin of neck

| O: fasciae of deltoid and pectoralis major muscles | I: mandible, skin of lower face, muscles at corners of mouth | N: facial n. (VII) |

| Table E2 | Muscles Acting on the Head |

O = origin, I = insertion, N = innervation (n. = nerve, nn. = nerves), A = action

Flexors of the Neck

Sternocleidomastoid (STIR-no-CLY-doe-MASS-toyd)

A: Contraction of either one draws head down and toward the side opposite the contracting muscle; contraction of both draws head forward and down, as in looking between the feet

| O: clavicle, manubrium | I: mastoid process | N: accessory n. (XI) |

Scalenes (SCAY-leens) (three muscles)

A: Flex neck laterally; elevate ribs 1 and 2 in inspiration

| O: vertebrae C2-C6 | I: ribs 1-2 | N: C5-C8 |

(continued)

Table E2 — Muscles Acting on the Head (Continued)

Extensors of the Neck

Trapezius (tra-PEE-zee-us)

A: Abducts and extends neck

O: external occipital protuberance, nuchal ligament, spinous processes of vertebrae C7-T12	I: clavicle, acromion, scapular spine	N: accessory n. (XI), C3-C4

Splenius capitis (SPLEE-nee-us CAP-ih-tis) **and splenius cervicis** (SIR-vih-sis)

A: Rotate head, extend neck

O: *capitis*—spinous processes of vertebrae C7-T3 or T4; *cervicis*—spinous processes of T3-T6	I: *capitis*—mastoid process, superior nuchal line; *cervicis*—transverse processes of C1-C2 or C3	N: dorsal rami of middle and lower cervical nn.

Semispinalis (SEM-ee-spy-NAY-liss) **capitis**

A: Rotates and extends head

O: transverse processes of vertebrae T1-T6, articular processes of C4-C7	I: occipital bone	N: dorsal rami of cervical nn.

Table E3 — Muscles of Chewing and Swallowing

O = origin, I = insertion, N = innervation (n. = nerve), A = action

Geniohyoid (JEE-nee-oh-HY-oyd)

A: Elevates and protracts hyoid; dilates pharynx to receive food; opens mouth when hyoid is fixed

O: inner aspect of mental protuberance	I: hyoid	N: hypoglossal n. (XII)

Mylohyoid

A: Forms floor of mouth; elevates hyoid; opens mouth when hyoid is fixed

O: inferior margin of mandible	I: hyoid	N: trigeminal n. (V)

Hyoid Muscles—Infrahyoid Group

Omohyoid

A: Depresses hyoid; fixes hyoid during opening of mouth

O: superior border of scapula	I: hyoid	N: ansa cervicalis

Sternohyoid

A: Depresses hyoid; fixes hyoid during opening of mouth

O: manubrium, coastal cartilage 1	I: hyoid	N: ansa cervicalis

Thyrohyoid

A: Depresses hyoid; elevates larynx; fixes hyoid during opening of mouth

O: thyroid cartilage of larynx	I: hyoid	N: hypoglossal n. (XII)

Sternothyroid

A: Depresses larynx; fixes hyoid during opening of mouth

O: manubruim, coastal cartilage 1 or 2	I: thyroid cartilage of larynx	N: ansa cervicalis

(continued)

Extrinsic Muscles of the Tongue

Genioglossus (JEE-nee-oh-GLOSS-us)

A: Depresses and protrudes the tongue; creates dorsal groove in the tongue that enables infants to grasp nipple and channel milk to pharynx

| O: hyoid bone | I: hyoid bone, lateral aspect of tongue | N: hypoglossal n. (XII) |

Hyoglossus

A: Depresses sides of the tongue

| O: hyoid bone | I: hyoid bone, lateral aspect of tongue | N: hypoglossal n. (XII) |

Styloglossus

A: Elevates and retracts tongue

| O: styloid process | I: lateral aspect of tongue | N: hypoglossal n. (XII) |

Palatoglossus

A: Elevates posterior part of tongue; constricts entry to pharynx

| O: soft palate | I: lateral aspect of tongue | N: accessory n. (XI) |

Muscles of Mastication

Temporalis (TEM-po-RAY-liss)

A: Elevates mandible for biting and chewing; retracts mandible

| O: temporal lines | I: coronoid process of mandible | N: trigeminal n. (V) |

Masseter (ma-SEE-tur)

A: Elevates mandible for biting and chewing; causes some lateral excursion of mandible

| O: zygomatic arch | I: lateral aspect of mandibular | N: trigeminal n. (V) |

Medial pterygoid (TERR-ih-goyd)

A: Elevates mandible; produces lateral excursion

| O: pterygoid process of sphenoid bone | I: medial aspect of mandibular angle | N: trigeminal n. (V) |

Lateral pterygoid (TERR-ih-goyd)

A: Protracts mandible; produces lateral excursion

| O: pterygoid process of sphenoid bone | I: slightly anterior to mandibular condyle | N: trigeminal n. (V) |

Muscles of the Pharynx

Pharyngeal constrictors (three muscles)

A: Constricts pharynx to force food into esophagus

| O: mandible, medial pterygoid plate, hyoid bone, larynx | I: posterior median raphe (fibrous seam) of pharynx | N: glossopharyngeal n. (IX), vagus n. (X) |

Hyoid Muscles—Suprahyoid Group

Digastric

A: Retracts mandible; elevates and fixes hyoid; depresses mandible when hyoid is fixed

| O: mastoid notch and inner aspect of mandible near protuberance | I: hyoid, via fascial sling | N: trigeminal n. (V), facial n. (VII) |

O = origin, I = insertion, N = innervation (n. = nerve, nn. = nerves), A = action

Diaphragm (DY-uh-fram)

A: Prime mover of inspiration; compresses abdominal viscera to aid in such processes as defecation, urination, and childbirth

O: xiphoid process, ribs 10-12, costal cartilages 5-9, lumbar vertebrae   I: central tendon   N: phrenic n.

External intercostals (IN-tur-COSS-tulz)

A: When scalenes fix rib 1, external intercostals draw ribs 2-12 upward and outward to expand thoracic cavity and inflate lungs

O: inferior margins of ribs 1-11   I: superior margins of ribs 2-12   N: intercostal nn.

Internal intercostals

A: When quadratus lumborum and other muscles fix rib 12, internal intercostals draw ribs downward and inward to compress thoracic cavity and force air from lungs; not needed for relaxed expiration

O: inferior margins of ribs 1-11   I: superior margins of ribs 2-12   N: intercostal nn.

O = origin, I = insertion, N = innervation (n. = nerve, nn. = nerves), A = action

Rectus abdominis (ab-DOM-ih-niss)

A: Supports abdominal viscera; flexes waist as in sit-ups; depresses ribs; stabilizes pelvis during walking; increases intra-abdominal pressure to aid in urination, defecation, and childbirth

O: pubis   I: xiphoid process, costal cartilages 5-7   N: intercostal nn. 7-12

External abdominal oblique

A: Flexes waist as in sit-ups; flexes and rotates vertebral column

O: ribs 5-12   I: xiphoid process, linea alba   N: intercostals nn. 8-12, iliohypogastric n., ilioinguinal n.

Internal abdominal oblique

A: Similar to external oblique

O: inguinal ligament, iliac crest, thorocolumbar fascia   I: xiphoid process, linea alba, ribs 10-12   N: same as external oblique

Transversus abdominus

A: Compresses abdomen, increases intra-abdominal pressure, flexes vertebral column

O: inguinal ligament, iliac crest, thoracolumbar fascia, costal cartilages 7-12   I: xiphoid process, linea alba, pubis, inguinal ligament   N: intercostal nn. 8-12, iliohypogastric n., ilioinguinal n.

O = origin, I = insertion, N = innervation, (n. = nerve, nn. = nerves), A = action

Superficial Group—Erector Spinae (ee-RECK-tur SPY-nee)

Iliocostalis cervicis (ILL-ee-oh-coss-TAH-liss SIR-vih-sis), **iliocostalis thoracis** (tho-RA-sis), and **iliocostalis lumborum** (lum-BORE-um)

A: Extend and laterally flex vertebral column; thoracis and lumborum rotate ribs during forceful inspiration

O: angles of ribs, sacrum, iliac crest	I: *cervicis*—vertebrae C4-C6; *thoracis*—vertebra C7, angles of ribs 1-6; lumborum—angles of ribs 7-12	N: dorsal rami of spinal nn.

Longissimus (lawn-JISS-ih-muss) **cervicis and longissimus thoracis**

A: Extend and laterally flex vertebral column

O: *cervicis*—vertebrae T1 = T4 or T5; *thoracis*—sacrum, iliac crest, vertebrae T1-L5	I: *cervicis*—vertebrae C2-C6; *thoracis*—vertebrae T1-T12, ribs 3 or 4 to 12	N: dorsal rami of spinal nn.

Spinalis (spy-NAY-liss) **cervicis and spinalis thoracis**

A: Extend vertebral column

O: *cervicis*—nuchal ligament, spinous process of vertebra C7; *thoracis*—spinous processes of T11-L2	I: *cervicis*—spinous process of axis; *thoracis*—spinous processes of upper thoracic vertebrae	N: dorsal rim of spinal nn.

Superficial Group—Serratus Posterior Muscles

Serratus (she-RAY-tus) **posterior superior**

A: Elevates ribs 2-5 during inspiration

O: spines of vertebrae C7-T3	I: ribs 2-5	N: intercostal nn. 2-5

Serratus posterior inferior

A: Depresses ribs 9-12 during inspiration

O: spines of vertebrae T10-L2	I: ribs 9-12	N: ventral rami of T9-T12

Deep Group

Semispinalis cervicis (SEM-ee-spy-NAY-liss SUR-vih-sis) and **semispinalis thoracis** (tho-RA-sis)

A: Extend neck; extend and rotate vertebral column

O: transverse processes of vertebrae T1-T10	I: spinous processes of vertebrae C2-T5	N: dorsal rami of spinal nn.

Quadratus lumborum (quad-RAY-tus lum-BORE-um)

A: Laterally flexes vertebral column; depresses rib 12

O: iliac crest, lower lumbar vertebrae, thoracolumbar fascia	I: upper lumbar vertebrae, rib 12	N: ventral rami of L1-L3

Multifidus (mul-TIFF-ih-dus)

A: Extends and rotates vertebral column

O: sacrum, iliac crest, vertebrae C4-L5	I: laminae and spinous processes of vertebrae above origins	N: dorsal rami of spinal nn.

O = origin, I = insertion, N = innervation, (n. = nerve, nn. = nerves), A = action

Pectoralis (PECK-toe-RAY-liss) **major**

A: Prime mover of the shoulder flexion, abducts and medially rotates humerus; depresses pectoral girdle; elevates ribs; aids in climbing, pushing, and throwing

| O: clavicle, sternum, costal cartilages 1-6 | I: intertubercular groove of humerus | N: medial and lateral pectoral nn. |

Latissimus dorsi (la-TISS-ih-muss DOR-sye)

A: Adducts and medially rotates humerus; extends shoulder joint; produces strong downward strokes of arm, as in hammering or swimming ("swimmer's muscle"); pulls body upward in climbing

| O: vertebrae T7-L5, lower three or four ribs, thoracolumbar fascia, iliac crest, inferior angle of scapula | I: intertubercular groove of humerus | N: thoracodorsal n. |

Deltoid

A: Lateral fibers abduct humerus; anterior fibers flex and medially rotate it; posterior fibers extend and laterally rotate it

| O: clavicle, scapular spine, acromion | I: deltoid tuberosity of humerus | N: axillary n. |

Teres (TERR eez) **major**

A: Adducts and medially rotates humerus; extends shoulder joint

| O: from inferior angle to lateral border of scapula | I: medial aspect of proximal shaft of humerous | N: subscapular n. |

Coracobrachialis (COR-uh-co-BRAY-kee-AL-iss)

A: Adducts arm; flexes shoulder joint

| O: coracoid process | I: medial aspect of shaft of humerus | N: musculocutaneous n. |

Rotator Cuff

A: All rotator cuff muscles hold head of humerus in glenoid cavity and stabilize shoulder joint in addition to performing the functions below.

Infraspinatus (IN-fra-spy-NAY-tus)

A: Extends and laterally rotates humerus

| O: infraspinous fossa of scapula | I: greater tubercle of humerus | N: suprascapular n. |

Supraspinatus (SOO-pra-spy-NAY-tus)

A: Abducts humerus; resists downward displacement when carrying heavy weight

| O: supraspinous fossa of scapula | I: greater tubercle of humerus | N: suprascapular n. |

Subscapularis (SUB-SCAP-you-LERR-iss)

A: Medially rotates humerus

| O: subscapular fossa of scapula | I: lesser tubercle of humerus | N: subscapular n. |

Teres minor

A: Adducts and laterally rotates humerus

| O: lateral border of scapula | I: greater tubercle of humerus | N: axillary n. |

Table E8	Actions of the Forearm

Boldface indicates prime movers; others are synergists. Parentheses indicate only a slight effect.

Flexion	Extension
Biceps brachii	**Triceps brachii**
Brachialis	Anconeus
Brachioradialis	
Flexor carpi radialis	
(Pronator teres)	
Pronation	**Supination**
Pronator teres	**Supinator**
Pronator quadratus	Biceps brachii

Table E9	Muscles Acting on the Forearm

O = origin, I = insertion, N = innervation, (n. = nerve, nn. = nerves), A = action

Muscles with Bellies in the Arm (Brachium)

Biceps brachii (BY-seps BRAY-kee-eye)

A: Flexes elbow; abducts arm; supinates forearm; holds head of humerus in glenoid cavity

O: *long head*—supraglenoid tubercle of scapula; *short head*—coracoid process of scapula   I: radial tuberosity   N: musculocutaneous n.

Brachialis (BRAY-kee-AL-iss)

A: Flexes elbow

O: anterior distal shaft of humerus   I: coronoid process of ulna, capsule of elbow joint   N: musculocutaneous n., radial n.

Triceps brachii (TRI-seps BRAY-kee-eye)

A: Extends elbow; long hand adducts humerus

O: *long head*—infraglenoid tubercle of scapula; *lateral head*—proximal posterior shaft of humerus; *medial head*—posterior shaft of humerus   I: olecranon of ulna   N: radial n.

Muscles with Bellies in the Forearm (Antebrachium)

Brachioradialis (BRAY-kee-oh-RAY-dee-AL-iss)

A: Flexes elbow

O: lateral supracondylar ridge humerus   I: styloid process of radius   N: radial n.

Anconeus (an-CO-nee-us)

A: Extends elbow

O: lateral supracondylar ridge of humerus   I: styloid process of radius   N: radial n.

Pronator teres (PRO-nay-tur TERR-eez)

A: Pronates forearm

O: medial epicondyle of humerus, coronoid process of ulna   I: lateral midshaft of radius   N: median n.

(continued)

Pronator quadratus (PRO-nay-tur quad-RAY-tus)

A: Pronates forearm

O: anterior distal shaft of ulna	I: anterior distal shaft of radius	N: median n.

Supinator (SOO-pih-NAY-tur)

A: Supinates forearm

O: lateral epicondyle of humerus, proximal shaft of ulna	I: proximal shaft of radius	N: radial n.

| Table E10 | *Muscles Acting on the Wrist and Hand* |

Anterior Compartment—Deep Layer

Flexor digitorum profundus

A: Flexes wrist and distal interphalangeal joints

O: shaft of ulna, interosseous membrane	I: four tendons to distal phalanges II-V	N: median and ulnar nn.

Flexor pollicis (PHAL-ih-sis) longus

A: Flexes interphalangeal joint of thumb, weakly flexes wrist

O: radius, interosseous membrane	I: distal phalanx I	N: median n.

Posterior Compartment—Superficial Layer

Extensor carpi radialis longus

A: Extends and abducts wrist

O: lateral epicondyle of humerus	I: base of metacarpal II	N: radial n.

Extensor carpi radialis brevis

A: Extends and abducts wrist; fixes wrist during finger flexion

O: lateral epicondyle of humerus	I: base of metacarpal III	N: radial n.

Extensor carpi ulnaris

A: Extends and abducts wrist

O: lateral epicondyle of humerus, posterior shaft of ulna	I: base of metacarpal V	N: radial n.

Extensor digitorum (DIDJ-ih-TOE-rum)

A: Extends fingers II-V at metacarpophalangeal joints

O: lateral epicondyle of humerus	I: dorsal aspect of phalanges II-V	N: radial n.

Extensor digiti minimi (DIDJ-ih-ty MIN-in-my)

A: Extends metacarpophalangeal joint of little finger; sometimes considered to be a detached portion of extensor digitorum

O: lateral epicondyle of humerus	I: distal and middle phalanges V	N: radial n.

Posterior Compartment—Deep Layer

Abductor pollicis longus

A: Abducts and extends thumb; abducts wrist

O: posterior aspect of radius and ulna, interosseous membrane	I: trapezium, base of metacarpal I	N: radial n.

(continued)

Table E10 — *Muscles Acting on the Wrist and Hand (Continued)*

Extendor indicis (IN-dih-sis)

A: Extends index finger at metacarpophalangeal joint

O: shaft of ulna, interosseous membrane	I: middle and distal phalanges II	N: radial n.

Extensor pollicis longus

A: Extends thumb at metacarpophalangeal joint

O: shaft of ulna, interosseous membrane	I: distal phalanx I	N: radial n.

Extensor pollicis brevis

A: Extends thumb at metacarpophalangeal joint

O: shaft of radius, interosseous membrane	I: proximal phalanx I	N: radial n.

Table E11 — *Actions of the Wrist and Hand*

Boldface indicates prime movers; others are synergists. Parentheses indicate only a slight effect

Wrist flexion	Wrist extension
Flexor carpi radialis	**Extensor digitorum**
Flexor carpi ulnaris	Extensor carpi radialis longus
Extensor digitorum superficialis	Extensor carpi radialis brevis
(Palmaris longus)	Extensor carpi ulnaris
(Flexor pollicis longus)	

Wrist abduction	Wrist adduction
Flexor carpi radialis	Flexor carpi ulnaris
Extensor carpi radialis brevis	Extensor carpi ulnaris
Abductor pollicis longus	

Finger flexion	Finger extension	Thumb opposition
Flexor digitorum superficialis	Extensor pollicis longus	Opponens pollicis
Flexor digitorum profundus	Extensor pollicis brevis	Opponens digiti minimi
Flexor pollicis longus	Extensor digitorum	
	Extensor indicis	

O = origin, I = insertion, N = innervation, (n. = nerve, nn. = nerves), A = action

Thenar Group

Abductor pollicis (PAHL-ih-sis) **brevis**

A: Abducts thumb

O: scaphoid, trapezium, flexor retinaculum	I: lateral aspect of proximal phalanx I	N: medial n.

Adductor pollicis

A: Adducts thumb and opposes it to the fingers

O: trapezium, trapezoid, capitate, metacarpals II-IV	I: medial aspect of proximal phalanx I	N: ulnar n.

Flexor pollicis brevis

A: Flexes thumb at metacarpophalangeal joint

O: trapezium, flexor retinaculum	I: proximal phalanx I	N: median n.

Opponens (op-OH-nens) **pollicis**

A: Opposes thumb to fingers

O: trapezium, flexor retinaculum	I: metacarpal I	N: median n.

Hypothenar Group

Abductor digiti minimi

A: Abducts little finger

O: pisiform, tendon of flexor carpi ulnaris	I: medial aspect of proximal phalanx V	N: ulnar n.

Flexor digiti minimi brevis

A: Flexes little finger at metacarpophalangeal joint

O: hamulus of hamate, flexor retinaculum	I: medial aspect of proximal phalanx V	N: ulnar n.

Opponens digiti minimi

A: Opposes little finger to thumb; deepens pit of palm

O: hamulus of hamate, flexor retinaculum	I: medial aspect of metacarpal V	N: ulnar n.

Midpalmar Group

Dorsal interosseous (IN-tur-OSS-ee-us) **muscles (four muscles)**

A: Abduct digits II-IV

O: two heads on facing sides of adjacent metacarpals	I: proximal phalanges II-IV	N: ulnar n.

Palmar interosseous muscles (three muscles)

A: Adduct digits II, IV, and V

O: metacarpals II, IV, V	I: proximal phalanges II, IV, and V	N: ulnar n.

Lumbricals (four muscles)

A: Flex metacarpophalangeal joints; extend interphalangeal joints

O: tendons of flexor digitorum profundus	I: proximal phalanges II-V	N: median and ulnar nn.

O = origin, I = insertion, N = innervation, (n. = nerve, nn. = nerves), A = action

Anterior Muscles of the Hip (Ilio-psoas)

Iliacus (ih-LY-uh-cus)

A: Flexes hip joint; medially rotates femur

O: iliac fossa	I: lesser trochanter of femur, capsule of coxal joint	N: femoral n.

Psoas (SO-ass) **major**

A: Flexes hip joint; medially rotates femur

O: vertebral bodies T12-L5	I: lesser trochanter of femur	N: lumbar plexus

Lateral and Posterior Muscles of the Hip

Tensor fasciae latae (TEN-sor FASH-ee-ee LAY-tee)

A: Flexes hip joint; abducts and medially rotates femur; tenses fascia lata and braces knee when opposite foot is lifted from the ground

O: iliac crest near anterior superior spine	I: lateral condyle of tibia	N: superior gluteal n.

Gluteus maximus

A: Extends hip joint; abducts and laterally rotates femur; important in the backswing of the stride

O: ilium and sacrum	I: gluteal tuberosity of femur, fascia lata	N: inferior gluteal n.

Gluteus medius and gluteus minimus

A: Abduct and medially rotate femur; maintain balance by shifting body weight during walking

O: ilium	I: greater trochanter of femur	N: superior gluteal n.

Lateral Rotators

Gemellus (jeh-MEL-us) **superior and gemellus inferior**

A: Laterally rotate femur

O: body of ischium	I: obturator internus tendon	N: sacral plexus

Obturator (OB-too-RAY-tur) **externus**

A: Laterally rotates femur

O: anterior margin of obturator foramen	I: greater trochanter of femur	N: obturator n.

Obturator internus

A: Abducts and laterally rotates femur

O: posterior margin of obturator foramen	I: greater trochanter of femur	N: sacral plexus

Piriformis (PIR-ih-FOR-miss)

A: Abducts and laterally rotates femur

O: anterolateral aspect of sacroiliac region	I: greater trochanter of femur	N: ventral rami of S1-S2

Quadratus femoris (quad-RAY-tus FEM-oh-riss)

A: Adducts and laterally rotates femur

O: ischial tuberosity	I: intertrochanteric ridge of femur	N: sacral plexus

Medial (Adductor) Compartment of the Thigh

Adductor longus and adductor brevis

A: Adduct and laterally rotate femur; flex hip joint

O: pubis	I: posterior shaft of femur	N: obturator n.

O = origin, I = insertion, N = innervation, (n. = nerve), A = action

Anterior (Extensor) Compartment of Thigh

Quadriceps femoris (QUAD-rih-seps FEM-oh-riss)

A: Extends knee; rectus femoris also flexes hip

O: *rectus femoris*—anterior spine of ilium; *vastus lateralis*—posterolateral shaft of ilium; *vastus medialis*—linea aspera of femur; *vastus intermedius*—anterior shaft of femur

I: tibial tuberosity

N: femoral n.

Sartorius

A: Flexes hip and knee; rotates femur medially; rotates tibia laterally; used in crossing legs

O: anterior superior spine of ilium

I: medial aspect of tibial tuberosity

N: femoral n.

Posterior (Flexor) Compartment of Thigh (Hamstring Group)

Biceps femoris

A: Flexes knee; extend hip; laterally rotates leg

O: *long head*—ischial tuberosity; *short head*—posterior midshaft of femur

I: head of fibula

N: *long head*—tibial n.; *short head*—common peroneal n.

Semimembranosus (SEM-ee-MEM-bran-OH-sis)

A: Flexes knee; extends hip; medially rotates tibia; tenses joint capsule of knee

O: ischial tuberosity

I: medial condyle of tibia, collateral ligament of knee

N: tibial n.

Semitendinosus

A: Flexes knee; extend hip; medially rotates tibia

O: ischial tuberosity

I: near tibial tuberosity

N: tibial n.

Posterior Compartment of Leg

Popliteus (pop-LIT-ee-us)

A: Unlocks knee to allow flexion; flexes knee; medially rotates tibia

O: lateral condyle of femur

I: posterior proximal tibia

N: tibia n.

O = origin, I = insertion, N = innervation, (n. = nerve, nn. = nerves), A = action

Dorsal Aspect of Foot

Extensor digitorum (DIDJ-ih-TOE-rum) **brevis**

A: Extends toe

| O: dorsal aspect of calcaneus | I: tendons of extensor digitorum longus | N: deep peroneal n. |

Ventral Layer 1 (Most Superficial)

Flexor digitorum brevis

A: Flexes toes II–V

| O: calcaneus, plantar aponeurosis | I: middle phalanges II–V | N: medial plantar n. |

Abductor digiti minimi

A: Abducts and flexes little toe; supports lateral longitudinal arch

| O: calcaneus, plantar aponeurosis | I: proximal phalanx V | N: lateral plantar n. |

Abductor hallucis (hal-oo-sis)

A: Flexes hallux (great toe); supports medial longitudinal arch

| O: calcaneus, plantar aponeurosis | I: proximal phalanx I | N: medial plantar n. |

Ventral Layer 2

Quadratus plantae (quad-RAY-tus PLAN-tee)

A: Flexes toes

| O: calcaneus, plantar aponeurosis | I: tendons of flexor digitorum | N: lateral plantar n. |

Lumbricals (four muscles)

A: Flex metatarsophalangeal joints; extend interphalangeal joints

| O: tendon of flexor digitorum longus | I: extensor tendons to digits II–V | N: lateral and medial plantar nn. |

Ventral Layer 3

Adductor hallucis

A: Adducts hallux

| O: metatarsals II–IV | I: proximal phalanx I | N: medial plantar n. |

Flexor digiti minimi brevis

A: Flexes little toe

| O: metatarsal V; plantar aponeurosis | I: proximal phalanx V | N: lateral plantar n. |

Flexor hallucis brevis

A: Flexes hallux

| O: cuboid, plantar aponeurosis | I: proximal phalanx I | N: medial plantar n. |

Ventral Layer 4 (Deepest)

Dorsal interosseous muscles (four muscles)

A: Abduct toes II–V

| O: each with two heads arising from adjacent metatarsals | I: proximal phalanges II–IV | N: lateral plantar n. |

Plantar interosseous muscles (three muscles)

A: Adduct toes III–V

| O: medial aspect of metatarsals III–V | I: proximal phalanges III–V | N: lateral plantar n. |

Quick Guide F *Aromatherapy and Herbal Preparations*

Base Oils

almond oil

borage seed oil

carrot oil

corn oil

evening primrose oil

grapeseed oil

jojoba oil

olive oil

safflower oil

sunflower oil

Essential Oils

cedarwood (men are fond of this one)

chamomile German (mild enough for children)

chamomile Roman

cinnamon (use sparingly, very strong)

clary sage

clove (very, very strong)

eucalyptus, lemon or peppermint (too strong for children, does not blend well with other scents)

geranium (women like this)

grapefruit

jasmine (use purest form)

juniper (great for hands and feet, tones cellulite)

lavender (older women consider this a favorite)

lemon (careful around the eyes, works well with foot massage)

lime (very similar to lemon)

mandarin (spicy orange)

myrrh (very spiritual experience)

neroli (great fragrance and wonderful for sensitive skin)

orange (children love this)

patchouli (this oil can both relax with a strong blend or energize with a small amount)

peppermint (energizing fragrance, too bold for large amounts)

rose (most loved by all ages, very relaxing)

Essential Oils for Aromatherapy

sandalwood

spearmint (energizes the spirit)

ylang-ylang (similar to jasmine)

Remember to check with your client as to which fragrance may be acceptable to her. Always check for allergies.

Essential Oils That Should Not Be Used

arnica

bitter almond

camphor (should not be used during pregnancy)

elecampane

fennel (never use during pregnancy)

horseradish

origanum

pennyroyal (very dangerous during pregnancy or with children)

rue

sage

sassafras

savory

tansy

thuja

wintergreen

wormwood

Be extra careful with all herbs used in cooking; they may be too strong for the skin.

Herbal Preparations

Essential Oil Blends

(Use sparingly—formulas are strong.)

General stress reduction

sweet almond oil (base oil)

4 drops lavender

2 drops ylang-ylang

Place a drop on forehead and at temples; massage with gentle, soothing strokes.

Situational high blood pressure or high stress issues
Footbath
In a bowl of hot water, add:

2 drops rose

2 drops ylang-ylang

3 drops lavender

Mix with wooden spoon; let cool to a comfortable warmth; and soak feet for 5 minutes. Make sure feet are dry before you walk to avoid slipping.

Headache soother

sweet almond oil (base oil)

4 drops peppermint

4 drops chamomile

In a darkened room, with recipient lying down, place 1 drop on forehead and gently massage forehead, back of neck, and temples. Avoid eyes. This preparation can also be placed inside a warm wet cloth and placed at back of neck and forehead simultaneously. Leave on until cloth cools.

Reflexology spritzer

Mix 4 ozs. of witch hazel and 2 drops lemon, lime, or orange oil. Place in mister or spray bottle with light mist setting and spray on feet before beginning the session. Wrap feet with towels dipped in warm Perrier or other mineral water. Let rest until towels cool, then proceed with session. On hot days or for a person who stands on his feet all day, a spritz of peppermint (1 drop to 4 ozs. of witch hazel) can be used at the finish of the session. Always check for allergies before using. Never spray open wounds or fungal irritations.

Nasal congestion

Place 1 drop of eucalyptus oil onto center of tissue. Fold over and hold under nose (not touching) for a few seconds. Tissue can be placed in plastic bag, sealed, and reused.

Motion sickness

Place 1 drop peppermint oil, and 1 drop clove oil onto hankerchief or tissue and fold over. Hold under nose (not touching for several seconds). Tissue can be placed in plastic bag, sealed, and reused.

PMS soother

olive oil (light, cold pressed)

3 drops rose

3 drops jasmine

2 drops clary sage

Can be placed, about 6 drops of mixture to warm bath water. Or can be used with warm wet towels, dipped in mixture and placed on abdomen. Can also be warmed and massaged onto abdomen.

Invigorating Oil Blends

For bath or inhalation from steam

sweet almond (base oil)

4 drops mandarin

2 drops orange

4 drops neroli

2 drops lemon

Calming rub

sweet almond (base oil)

5 drops rose

5 drops sandalwood

4 drops jasmine

4 drops ylang-ylang

Deep relaxation enhancement

sweet almond (base oil)

3 drops geranium (for women; for men, use sandlewood)

3 drops rose

2 drops lavender

Use for massage or in warm bath water for a soothing soak before bed.

Chakras and Their Corresponding Herbal Component

Each herb associated with a chakra can be used for the physiological and psychological function.

Chakra	Herb/Essential oil
Root	Sage, sandalwood, cinnamon
Sacral	Jasmine, neroli, orange blossom
Solar Plexus	Lemon, grapefruit, juniper, calendula
Heart	Foxglove, rose, carnation, lily of the valley
Throat	Gardenia, ylang-ylang, chamomile
Brow	Sweet almond, orange blossom, camphor
Crown	Lotus, lavender, elemi

Herbal Body Wraps Formulas

Most spas use a commercial product line that has premixed herbal products for use in an herbal wrap session; however, you can make herbal body wraps. Here are the categories and possible mixtures for a homemade wrap. Usually a combination of four herbs is used.

To detoxify the body

Black pepper, clove, eucalyptus, ginger, grapefruit, juniper, rosemary, sage

To relax the body

Chamomile, clary sage, jasmine, lavender, marjoram, peppermint

To reduce cellulite and water retention, and to tighten the skin

Ginger, grapefruit, juniper, lavender, orange, peppermint; parafango (paraffin and mineral muds) is used to reduce inches.

To invigorate and stimulate

Chamomile, clary sage, geranium, lemon grass, orange, peppermint, rosemary, ylang-ylang

Thalassotherapy

Seaweed (powdered), mineral muds

Quick Guide G *Commonly Prescribed Medications*

Before a session with a client who has listed medication use on his intake form, check a drug or medication reference book or a website to get a better understanding of the medication. A call to the client's physician is necessary if the client is on multiple medications for several different conditions. Medications in combination can greatly change the outcome of the massage.

Common Herbs and Supplements

Herb	Uses
Aloe vera	Topical use for minor burns, irritation
Black cohosh	PMS, menopause symptoms
Capsaicin	Topical use for pain, neuralgia, arthritis
Chamomile	Used as a tea for insomnia, anxiety, nausea
Echinacea	Helps strengthen immune system; cold and flu symptoms
Ephedra	Relieves nasal congestion
Evening primrose oil	Hormone balance, irritable bowel syndrome
Flaxseed oil	Constipation, colon cleansing
Feverfew	Migraines, fever reducer
Garlic	Lowers blood pressure, reduces cholesterol, boosts immunity
Ginger	Nausea, migraines, stomach inflammation, flu
Gingko	Alzheimer's, improves memory, tinnitus
Ginseng	Stress and anxiety, improves stamina
Glucosamine	Anti-inflammatory for arthritis
Kava kava	Anxiety and insomnia
Licorice	Menopause, colds and cough, peptic ulcers
Melatonin	Insomnia, jet lag, boosts immune system
Saw palmetto	Benign prostatic disease
Slippery elm	Colds, cough, chest congestion
Soy	Menopause symptoms, cancer prevention
St. John's wort	Depression
Valerian	Anxiety, insomnia

Category	Medication	Action	Contraindications/Remarks
Analgesic	Tylenol, Aspirin MS-Contin, Percocet	Pain reliever	Avoid all heat therapies; avoid stretching techniques; closely monitor duration and intensity; postural hypotension can occur
Analgesic (topical)	Lydoderm, Oraquix, Duranest, Marcaine, Raropin, Procaine	Topical pain reliever	Avoid applying heat to treated area including stone massage, heat pads, etc.
Antacid	Tums, Nexium, Previcid, Carafate	Relieves indigestion Coats ulcerative tissue	Client goals may be compromised by side effects; caution—client lying flat or face down may have reflux
Antiarrhythmic	Norpace, Inderal	Normalizes heartbeat	Postural hypotension; limit exposure to heat; medications may contribute to muscle weakness
Antibiotic	Amoxicillin, Zythromax Ceclor, Cipro, Biaxin	Kills microorganisms	Side effects may cause joint pain and numbness in hands or feet; avoid all heat or cold therapies; avoid circulatory massage; bruising likely
Anticholinergic	Bentyl, Atropine	Blocks PNS impulse	Side effects may cause flushing, dry skin, and decreased sweating; avoid heat, pressure
Anticoagulant	Lovenox, Hep-Loc, Coumadin (Warfarin)	Prevents blood from clotting	Avoid client lying prone; avoid deep tissue, abdominal massage, heat; postural hypotension likely
Anticonvulsant	Klonopin, Depakote, Dilantin	Controls seizures	Schedule appointment when medications are at a peak; side effects of medications include edema; avoid heat and deep pressure
Antidepressant	Elavil, Prozac, Paxil, Zoloft	Relieves depression	Medications may dry skin, making it fragile; avoid stretching techniques; sensory feedback compromised
Antifungal	Diflucan, Mycostatin, Lamisil	Kills fungi	Do not massage treated areas as skin will be easily broken; oral antifungals can cause joint pain and postural hypotension
Antihistamine	Zyrtec, Benadryl, Allegra, Claritin	Relieves allergies	Avoid heat therapies including sauna or steam; side effects include fatigue; postural hypotension possible
Antihypertensive	Apresoline, Lopressor, Inderal, Tenormin, Toprol XL, Cardizem	Reduces blood pressure	Avoid all heat therapies; avoid client lying prone, abdominal massage, deep tissue; limit duration; postural hypotension possible
Anti-inflammatory			

Classification	Examples	Action	Massage Considerations
Steroid	Decadron, Medrol, Prednisone	Reduces inflammation	Avoid heat or cold; use light and energy techniques; avoid injection sites, stretching
Nonsteroidal	Clinoril, Vioxx, Relafen, Motrin		Avoid heat therapies; monitor duration and intensity; postural hypotension possible
Antipsychotic	Haldol, Resperdal, Thorazine	Controls psychotic symptoms	Avoid heat therapies; postural hypotension possible; achieving client goals limited
Antipyretic	Tylenol, aspirin	Reduces fever	Avoid heat, deep tissue, and stretching techniques
Antitussive	Codeine, Tussar, Robitussin	Inhibits cough	Avoid heat and cold therapies; postural hypotension possible
Bronchodilator	Albuterol, Epinephrine	Dilates bronchi	Avoid heat or cold, lying client prone or flat
Decongestant	Afrin, Sudafed	Relieves congestion	Avoid heat or cold, lying client flat; edema may be present
Diuretic	Bumex, Lasix, Mannitol, Diazide, Maxide	Increases urine output	Avoid heat or cold, lying client flat; deep tissue, and abdominal massage; postural hypotension and bruising possible
Expectorant	Mucinex, Humabid LA, Robitussin	Liquefies mucus	Avoid heat or cold therapies, client lying flat
Hemostatic	Amacar, vitamin K, Thrombin	Stops bleeding	Avoid heat or cold, limit duration and pressure; bruising possible
Hormone replacement	Insulin (Humulin), Synthroid, Premarin, Evista	Counters hormonal deficiency	Massage may change the amount of insulin or synthroid needed by client; avoid heat and cold with diabetics; edema may be present with this class of medications
Muscle relaxant	Soma, Flexeril, Valium	Relaxes muscles	Avoid all heat therapies, deep tissue and neuromuscular techniques; bruising likely; muscle tone and elasticity compromised
Vasoconstrictor	Levophed, Aramine	Constricts blood vessels; increases blood pressure	Avoid heat and cold, deep tissue and vigorous techniques, circulatory massage
Vasodilator	Vasotec, Prinivil, Nitrostat	Dilates blood vessels; decreases blood pressure	Avoid heat and cold, deep tissue and vigorous techniques, circulatory massage

Glossary

A

ABCs of CPR Airway, breathing, and circulation

abduction movement of a body part away from the body or away from the midsagittal line

actin protein that make up the lighter bands on a skeletal muscle

acupressure points along the meridians that are stimulated with pressure

adaptation the process the body goes through in accepting the stresses placed on its systems

adduction movement of a body part toward the body or toward the midline

Adson's test/Allen's test requires the client to look up and over the affected shoulder while the tester feels for changes in the radial pulse; test for thoracic outlet syndrome

agonist prime mover; occurs when a muscle causes movement by concentric action

AIDS acquired immune deficiency syndrome

American Association of Masseurs and Masseuses the earliest professional association of massage practitioners in the United States established in 1943 by graduates of the College of Swedish Massage in Chicago

American Massage Therapy Association (AMTA) the largest professional organization for massage therapists and the modern version of its forerunner, the American Association of Masseurs and Masseuses

amino acids naturally occurring organic compounds found in plant and animal foods used to build and maintain tissue

Amma or *Anma* a bodywork method thought to have originated in the Chinese practice of rubbing and pressing cold hands and feet to warm them. *Amma* is built on a knowledge of pressure points and organized around the concept of Qi; an Asian bodywork technique based upon the *Nei Jing* and literally means "push-pull."

amphiarthrotic or cartilaginous joints joints that allow only slight movement; joints connected by cartilage; can be synchondroses or symphyses

anatomical position standing erect with the feet slightly separated, the arms hanging relaxed at the sides, and the palms of the hands facing forward

anatomy structure of the body of any living thing and the study of that structure

animal helpers animal spirits that help a shaman in receiving information on how to aid the patient/client

antagonist opposing muscle; occurs when the muscle opposes movement at a joint by eccentric action

anthropometry science that deals with body measurements, including size, shape, and weight

appendicular bones bones that comprise the extremities, including the shoulders, hips, arms, legs, hands, feet, fingers, and toes

areas of endangerment areas of the body where no pressure or no deep application of pressure is recommended because of underlying structures such as nerves, arteries, veins, and vital organs

aromatherapy using essential oils in treatments such as massage, facials, body wraps, and baths

arrector pili smooth muscle associated with each hair follicle; stimulates the skin to pucker around the hair in cold temperatures

artery blood vessel that carries blood away from the heart

articulation union site between two or more bones

asanas gentle stretching postures

assignment of benefits claim form a form signed by the client that requests the insurer to send payment to the therapist; this form also includes a release for records

asthma a chronic disease of the lungs in which the airways narrow

atrium (**atria,** plural) the upper, right and left, chambers of the heart

atrophy decrease in muscle size due to a decrease in the size of the muscle fibers

attention deficit hyperactivity disorder (ADHD) a disorder that manifests as hyperactivity, distractibility, inattention, and impulsivity

autism physical disorder of the brain in which a young child develops atypically; such atypical development may involve failure to develop normal social relationships, disturbances in communication, abnormal responses to sensory stimulation, and general developmental delays

autonomic nervous system (ANS) part of the peripheral nervous system that is involved in regulating cardiovascular, respiratory, endocrine, and other automatic body functions

Avicenna a Persian physician (980-1037 CE) who is largely responsible for popularizing modern pharmaceutical techniques (such as chemical preparation and distillation) and the use of medicines, such as camphor and iodine, bringing these practices to a wider audience. His 16-volume medical encyclopedia was a synthesis of Hippocratic and Arabic medical traditions, and its influence was considerable.

axes of motion imaginary reference points around which body segments move

axial bones bones that lie along the central, vertical axis of the body and support the head and trunk

Ayurveda "Arts of Life"; an ancient guide to healthy living that includes prescriptions for herbal treatments and massage techniques. Written around 1850 BCE, the *Ayurveda* is one of a set of sacred Sanskrit texts called the *Vedas*.

Ayurvedic medicine a system based on the idea of chakras (energy centers in the body) and *doshas* (general tendencies)

B

bacteria microorganisms that have both plant and animal characteristics

baroreceptors receptors that detect pressure changes

bathhouses public baths in ancient Greece. Massage was provided to patrons before or after a bath, and later, when the baths grew more elaborate, in conjunction with steam or hot water baths

Battle Creek Sanitarium established in 1866 in Battle Creek, Michigan, this was among the most well-known and respected facilities of its day. It was among the first to implement professional standards for massage and develop a rigorous training program for practitioners at the facility.

benefits specific services for which the insurance will pay on the client's behalf

bilaterally occurs on both sides

bile fluid secreted by the liver, stored in the gallbladder, and discharged into the duodenum, where it aids in the digestion of fats

blood-borne pathogens pathogens that are found in the blood and use blood loss or injury for transmission

blood brain barrier protective barrier that occurs naturally and functions by allowing tight cell-to-cell contact within the capillaries to prevent harmful substances from leaving the blood and entering the brain tissue

blood pressure the force of blood that is exerted against the walls of blood vessels

body's center of gravity point at which the frontal, horizontal, and sagittal planes intersect

bonding a unique relationship between two people that is specific and endures through time

bruxism teeth grinding; as in grinding one's teeth during sleep

bursa small sacs that are lined with synovial fluid and located at sites where friction occurs

business plan the map you need for setting up your massage business

C

capillaries microscopic blood valves

carbohydrates substances found in plant foods such as fruits, vegetables, and grains that the body breaks down into sugars, starches, cellulose, and gum

cardiac muscle a specialized type of muscle tissue found only in the heart; contracts to move blood through the body

carrier a host who has no symptoms of infection and is not aware that he is carrying and passing on a disease or infection-producing pathogen

C Corporation a separate entity from its owners or stockholders formed in accordance with state regulations

cell the basic unit of structure and function within the body; the basic unit of structure that groups to form tissues

cellular edema caused when water flows from the extracellular fluid into the cells

central nervous system (CNS) responsible for issuing nerve impulses and analyzing sensory data; includes the brain and spinal cord

cerebral palsy (CP) developmental disability that originates when the parts of the brain that control movement are damaged during gestational development, birth, and early infancy

Cerebrospinal Fluid Technique Massage (CSFTM) frees up the flow of cerebrospinal fluid around the cerebrospinal axis comprised of the brain and spinal cord

chakras energy wheels or centers

chemical name precisely describes the drug's atomic and molecular structure

circumduction circular movement around an axis of an extremity that combines flexion, extension, abduction, and adduction at a joint

client authority idea that the client is empowered by the caregiver's recognition that the client has authority over the caregiver

codes of ethics sets of standards that serve as guidelines for professional conduct

coenzymes work together with enzymes to activate chemical reactions that occur in order for the body to function appropriately

coinsurance with a coinsurance plan, the client will pay a percentage—usually 20% of the charges—and the insurance company will pay the remaining 80%, but only of the charges that the insurance company approves

colic a condition that may be due to a baby's underdeveloped gastrointestinal or nervous system

collagen therapy injection of collagen to fill out wrinkles and lines, usually done on the face

colon located in the lower part of the digestive system and used for elimination

complete proteins proteins that contain all nine essential amino acids

compression performed with the fist most often but can be applied with thumb, flat hand, elbows, or feet.

Compression is performed by pushing directly down into the tissue and may be accompanied by a slight twist.

concentric an isotonic contraction that results in shortening of a muscle

concentric action action that occurs when muscle shortening causes a change in joint angle

conductivity the quality of living matter responsible for the transmission of and progressive reaction to stimuli

considerations elements that dictate the specifics of each stroke, such as amount of pressure, the speed with which it is applied, and the length of time the stroke lasts

contact dermatitis allergic response that comes when skin is exposed to a harmful substance and the lymphatic vessels and cells try to stop the invasion

contagious disease a disease that can easily be transmitted to others

contaminated soiled or stained, particularly through contact with potentially infectious substances

contraction a shortening or increase in muscle tension

contusion also known as a muscle bruise

co-pay a small fee that clients with a coinsurance plan should pay at the beginning of each visit

corporation a legal organization whose assets and liabilities are separate from those of its owners

cortisol keeps the blood sugar at a higher than normal level so that extra energy for flight is available. It also slows metabolism to conserve energy

countertransference transference to the caregiver of the client's negative feelings; occurs when the therapist is unable to keep the therapist-client relationship separate and professional

coxa (**coxae,** plural) the hip joints

CPR (cardiopulmonary resuscitation) performing CPR provides ventilation and blood circulation to a person who has stopped breathing

cramp tonic muscle contraction that comes on rather suddenly; involuntary muscle twitches where the muscle spasm is related to mild myositis or fibromyositis

CranioSacral Therapy (CST) a very gentle, hands-on method for evaluating and enhancing the function of the craniosacral system

cross-stretch a myofascial release stretch that begins tissue release

cross-striations alternating dark and light bands on a skeletal muscle

cryokinetic ice therapy combined with movement

cryotherapy using ice or cooling agents to lower the body tissue temperature; the use of ice for an injury

cun a measurement that equals the width of the client's thumb at the middle joint

Current Procedural Terminology (CPT) a book with the most commonly used system of procedure codes. The federal Health Insurance Portability and Accountability Act (HIPAA) requires physicians and other health care providers to use these codes in coding procedures

cycle of infection made up of the five elements (a reservoir host, a means of exit, a means of transmission, a means of entrance, and a susceptible host) that must be present for infection to occur

D

DBA (doing business as) using a business name that is different from your own name

Dead Sea mud treatment mud from the Dead Sea is used to coat the body for detoxification and treatment of certain skin disorders

deductible a fixed dollar amount that the insured must pay or meet once a year before the insurance company will cover the charges

deglutition swallowing

dehydration an abnormal depletion of body fluids; occurs if we fail to ingest enough water or when water is lost through diarrhea, vomiting, hemorrhage, or other health conditions

dementia an irreversible neurological disorder involving a loss of reasoning power

depression moving the shoulder inferiorly; considered a condition of shortage of the neurotransmitters

depth or depth of pressure the amount of force a stroke applies to the tissue

dermabrasion an exfoliation procedure that uses microfine crystals of aluminum oxide to remove the top layer of skin and reduce the effects of minor skin irregularities

diaphysis central shaft of long bones

diarthrotic joints or synovial joints joints that are allowed to move freely; freely movable joints that are covered with hyaline cartilage; they are more complex than synarthrotic and amphiarthrotic

digestion the process of breaking down food

direction the path or track the stroke takes in its application

disconnection act of becoming withdrawn or detached from others

disinfection level of decontamination that is nearly as effective as sterilization; will destroy most viruses, fungi, and bacteria but will not usually kill the bacterial spores

divarication includes enhancing metabolic function with techniques that have a systemic effect

dorsiflexion toes pointed up

dosha or *tridoshas* the three fundamental energies of the body (*vata, pitta, kapha*)

Down's syndrome chromosomal disorder that results in mental retardation and physical abnormalities

drugs chemical substances taken into the body that affect body function

dry brush exfoliation used before mud and seaweed wraps to exfoliate the skin and improve surface circulation

dulse scrub in this treatment, the body is scrubbed with seaweed and oil to remove the top layer of skin and nourish the skin with vitamins and minerals

duration either the length of time each stroke lasts during its application or the length of time the stroke remains on any given body part

dynamics acceleration phase

E

eccentric action occurs when a muscle lengthens as it develops tension

ecchymosis bruising

edema swelling or accumulation of interstitial fluid in or around an area or joint

effleurage from the French word *effleurer*, meaning "to glide." Effleurage is considered a warming and gliding stroke and is used in many different ways.

EIN employer identification number obtained from the Internal Revenue Service

elasticity the ability of soft tissue to return to a resting length after a passive stretch

electroencephalogram (EEG) recording of the electrical currents in the brain

electrolytes sodium, chloride, and potassium

elevation movement of the shoulder in the superior direction

endocardium a thin serous membrane that lines the cavities of the heart

endochondral ossification process that turns soft, flexible cartilage into harder bone

endomysium connective tissue that surrounds the sarcolemma

entrainment synchronization to a rhythm as the massage therapist's movements coordinate with the client's breathing

entrepreneur usually refers to one who is ideologically a capitalist or industrialist, has a high tolerance for risk, and enjoys being his/her own boss

environmentally transmitted pathogen a pathogen that lives in the environment—in our food, water, and soil—and is picked up from direct contact with these surfaces

enzymes help digest food by breaking down proteins into essential amino acids

epicardium the outer membrane of the heart

epimysium connective tissue that surrounds skeletal muscle

epiphyseal plate (or epiphysis) where the growth of the bone occurs; sometimes called the "growth plate"

epithelial tissue the main tissue of the skin. Epithelial cells line the inner part of internal organs and cover the outside of the body

ergonomics the study of the anatomical, physiological, and psychological aspects of humans in the working environment

erythrocytes (red blood cells, RBCs) carry oxygen to the tissues and remove carbon dioxide waste

escherichia coli, (E. coli) bacteria a pathogen that is transmitted by ingestion and can cause severe food poisoning

essential nutrients the nutrients that can only be made available by the food we ingest

estrogen stimulates uterine growth and blood supply

eversion occurs when the sole of the foot is rotated outward

excitability an altered condition resulting from a neural or electrical stimulus

excretion elimination of by-products of drug metabolism from the body, essentially through the kidneys, intestines, and lungs but also through the skin in perspiration

exfoliate to remove the top layer of skin. This is done by a variety of techniques.

extension returning the body segment back to the anatomical position from flexion

extensors muscles that help to extend a bodily part

F

fascia areolar tissue that surrounds the bundles by covering the epimysium; a tough connective tissue that spreads throughout the body in a three-dimensional web from head to foot without interruption

fasciculi bundles of skeletal muscle cells

fatigue when muscle contractions grow weak from repeated stimulation; often causes a build up of lactic acid resulting from an oxygen debt

fats substances found in food we eat. Fats are not water-soluble and can be stored indefinitely within the body.

Federation of State Massage Therapy Boards organization established in 2005 that allows various massage therapy state boards to communicate with one another. It focuses on allowing state boards to give input into the national exam, creating a standard curriculum, and ensuring interstate portability of licenses.

Feldenkrais an approach to the body also called functional integration

femoral vein challenges the integrity of the valves of the femoral and saphenous veins already compromised by progesterone's relaxation of the smooth muscle walls

fiber the stringy and tough part of vegetables, fruits, and grains; helps in the treatment of constipation, hemorrhoids, diverticular disease, and especially irritable bowel syndrome

fibrinolysis the body's blood-clotting capacity

fibromyositis connective tissue inflammation

Field, Tiffany founder of the Touch Research Institute and leading authority on touch therapy

fight-or-flight response a complex system our bodies use to respond to changes that may be dangerous or life-threatening

fine tremulous classified by some texts as a shaking stroke, while others list it with vibration. Fingertips are gently placed on the skin with a light, quick, and steady movement stroking downward or outward.

five element theory entities in nature water, fire, metal, wood, and earth

flexion decreases the angle between the bones, forming a joint

flexors muscles that help to bend a bodily part

fontanels flexible cartilage membranes that connect skull (cranial) bones in infants

fossae indentions and depressions on the outer surface of a bone

frequency the number of times each stroke is performed

friction from the Latin word *frictio,* meaning "to rub"; friction often follows petrissage

frontal plane (also known as the coronal plane) splits the body vertically into front and back halves of equal weight

frost bite freezing of tissue due to exposure to cold temperatures for long periods of time

G

gallbladder organ that secretes bile

general partnership a business form in which partners share ownership and liability

generic (nonproprietary) **name** usually derived from chemical name but shorter and easier to remember; usually written in lower-case letters

glideability ease of movement over skin without drag

Gogli tendon organs proprioceptors in the musculotendinous junction that "register" the muscle contraction and gauge the degree of muscle tension

Golgi tendon reflex helps to prevent a tear within the muscle or in the muscle from the bone

Graham, Douglas a physician and historian trained in massage who played a key role in increasing public awareness of massage in the United States and popularizing the term *massage*. He wrote *Manual Therapeutics, A Treatise on Massage: Its History, Mode of Application, and Effects* (1902).

guided imagery method of taking the patient's brain and body through a preplanned outcome or a release of negativity. It is a state of autogenic meditation

gymnasiums in ancient Greece, athletes practiced, exercised daily, and perfomed in competitions at the gymnasium. Athletes employed personal assistants to provide their massage before and after training sessions and during competitions.

H

health insurance claim the documentation and forms submitted to an insurer requesting money to be paid for the services that the massage therapist has provided. Specific claim forms used are the CMS-15 for private practice and the UB-92 form for hospital charges such as massage in a cardiac rehabilitation setting.

Health Insurance Portability and Accountability Act (HIPAA) protects the privacy of patients and clients and confidentiality of health records from insurance companies, doctors, hospitals, and other health care individuals

Hellerwork consists of 11 one and one-half hour sessions that use deep tissue bodywork techniques to restore proper posture

hematoma an accumulation of blood and fluid as the body's first response to injury

herbal massage a unique practice of massage and anointing, and an ancestor of the contemporary custom

herbal wrap a warm herbal solution is spread over the body and then the body is wrapped to encourage perspiration or relaxation

Hippocrates Greek physician who lived from 460–377 BCE. Known as the "father of medicine," Hippocrates is considered the first physician in the modern tradition. He set diagnosis and treatment on a scientific—rather than mystical or spiritual—basis.

Hippocratic oath a pledge made by medical students and doctors that they will follow a professional code of ethics based on Hippocratic doctrine

Hippocratic tradition refers to philosophical tenets and ideals originating or popularized by Hippocrates and his followers. Many of these ideas have become an integral part of Western medical practice.

hold harmless clause a provision whereby a client does not have to pay a service provider if the provider does not file the insurance claim appropriately

horizontal or transverse plane divides the body into equal weight top and bottom halves

hospice helps view death as just a passageway during a human's journey depending on the philosophical conviction of the dying person and his or her family

hsueh the flow of Qi and the flow of blood and lymph fluids

human chorionic gonadotropin (HCG) prevents the mother's body from rejecting the embryo

Hydrocollator® a stainless steel tank that holds hot water

hydrotherapy the use of water whether it is via thermal, mechanical, or chemical application; the use of water for therapeutic purposes such as mineral baths, showers, herbal baths, and steam treatments

hyperemia condition in which an excess of red blood cells congests vascular tissues

hyperextension occurs when a body segment is moved in extension beyond the anatomical position

hypertension (HTN) elevated blood pressure

hyperthermia a body temperature higher than normal

hypertrophy an increase or broadening of the muscle due to vigorous muscle activity or exercise

hypoglycemia an excess in insulin that causes a sudden drop in blood sugar; can cause a person to become weak, irritable, fatigued, and experience muscle cramping and vision problems

hypothalamus the regulator of thirst and hunger; stimulates the pituitary gland to excrete antidiuretic hormone

hypothermia a core body temperature lower than normal

I

immersion bath a bath wherein the body part is submerged in water. The bath may be used with cold, tepid, or very warm water, depending on the objective of treatment.

incubation period amount of time between exposure and infection of a pathogen and the first occurrence of symptoms of disease

indications and contraindications general guidelines that specify conditions under which massage is and is not performed

indirect transmission can occur when a susceptible host comes in contact with insects or inanimate objects such as towels, unclean massage table surfaces, and floors

inferior vena cava area that runs along the right side between the spine and the uterus

insulin hormone produced by the pancreas necessary for glucose metabolism

insurance carrier the insurance company that carries the coverage plan

International Classification of Diseases, Ninth Revision, Clinical Modification (ICD9-CM) code set that is based on a system maintained by the World Health Organization of the United Nations. The use of the ICD-9 codes in the health care industry is used for reporting diseases, conditions, and signs and symptoms.

intervention introducing psychological or medical help to a patient

intramembranous ossification process in which connective tissue membranes are replaced by calcium deposits to form bone

inversion occurs when the sole of the foot is rotated inward

ischemia lack of oxygenated blood

isokinetic contraction occurs when the movement of a joint is kept at a constant velocity

isometric action occurs when tension does not change the muscle's length

isometric contraction occurs when a muscle does not shorten and no movement is produced, such as when pushing against a wall

isotonic contraction occurs when muscle shortens and produces movement

J

Jensen, Kathryn a nurse who wrote *Fundamentals in Massage for Students of Nursing*. This text was based on the European model of massage instruction, which emphasized anatomical and physiological understanding, as well as theoretical and practical applications of massage.

K

Kegel exercises prevent or correct incontinence by strengthening the pelvic floor muscles

Kellogg, John Harvey (1852–1943) a young doctor at the Battle Creek Sanitarium in the 1870s and an energetic advocate of massage. Kellogg wrote a curriculum titled *The Art of Massage* in 1895.

kinematics describe the appearance of motion relative to space and time

kinesiology the study of the anatomical and mechanical bases of human movement

kinetics study of the forces causing motion

Kneipp baths European therapeutic treatment utilizing herbs and minerals created by Father Sebastian Kneipp

kyphosis an exaggerated curvature of the thoracic spine commonly seen in elderly persons. Also known as "hunchback."

L

lactic acid waste products that build up in muscles after exercise

lateral bending or lateral flexion sideways movement of the neck or the trunk in frontal plane

lateral rotation occurs when arms or legs are moved as a unit in the transverse plane away from the midline

laxity loose joint

leukocytes (white blood cells, WBCs) provide a defense against infectious agents

limited liability corporation (LLC) business form permitted in most states and generally must have at least two owners who are taxed as a partnership while their liability is limited as in a corporation

limited partnership business form that has partners who are invested in the business but do not play an active role

Ling, Per Henrik (1776–1837) introduced a system of movements called medical gymnastics to Europe in the early 1800s

liver chemical warehouse of the body. If the liver is not functioning properly—health and well-being, including mental health—cannot be possible.

Lomi lomi a Hawaiian massage modality

loofah the dried fibrous part of the luffa tree fruit, used as a washing sponge

loofah scrub a full-body scrub with a loofah sponge to exfoliate and increase circulation

lordosis an exaggerated curvature of the lumbar spine, known as "swayback"

lymphatic drainage a hands-on technique designed to attain and sustain proper functioning of the human fluid system

lymphocytes receive antigens to aid the body in fighting infections

M

macrophages located in the lymph nodes and tissues; aid the body in fighting infections

malocclusion poor alignment of the jaw

manual lymph drainage a therapeutic massage specifically designed to promote lymph drainage

manual medicine use of the hands to treat illness or physical damage

Maori massage traditional massage techniques practiced in New Zealand

massage flow the fluid movements of the massage therapist used to transition from one massage stroke to another or from one body part to another

massage sequence how the massage therapist decides to organize the massage in terms of order of strokes and areas of the client's body on which to work

massage therapist's intent a given therapist's personality, philosophy, and spirituality with respect to his work as a massage therapist

mastication the chewing process

maternity massage offers an opportunity for the massage therapist to provide adjunct physical and emotional support for clients during pregnancy and childbirth

McMillan, Mary a World War I nurse, she wrote *Massage and Therapeutic Exercise* (1921), a primer in basic anatomical and physiological information, to inform nonmedical personnel assisting in army hospitals throughout the United States

mechanoreceptors movement receptors

medial rotation occurs when arms or legs are moved as a unit in the transverse plane toward the midline

meditation any act of mind-body focus that causes an altering of the psychophysiological state of an individual that brings about the opposite of the usual reactions to stress

medullary cavity interior shaft of the bone filled with the yellow bone marrow that consists primarily of fat cells

meiosis the form of cell division that produces ovum and sperm; each cell contains 23 chromosomes

Meissner's corpuscles corpuscles located at the papillae of the dermis right underneath the epidermis or outer covering of the skin

meninges Saran Wrap-like membranes covering the brain and spinal cord

meridians energetic pathways

metacarpals bones that form the broad structure of the hand

metu the Egyptians considered the heart the center of all bodily function and compared the cardiovascular system to channels of the Nile River, called *metu*. They believed good health was dependent on free flow through these channels in the body, and sickness was the result of blocked *metu*.

micronutrients vitamins, minerals, and supplements

microorganisms simple life forms, usually made up of a single cell and so small that they may only be seen using a microscope

mitosis a form of division that involves asexual reproduction; a process that takes place in the nucleus of a dividing cell that results in the formation of two new nuclei that each have the same number of chromosomes as the parent

motor unit one motor neuron that innervates muscle cells

moxibustion the burning of a special herb called artemisia

multidimensional or dual relationships relationships in which the therapist plays more than one role in regard to the client

muscle atrophy a wasting away of the tissue due to necrosis (or cell reabsorption) where the size of the muscle fibers (cells) decreases

muscle tissue makes up muscle fibers that control movement by contraction

musculotendinous junction the point at which the muscle and tendon meet

myocardium the heart muscle that generates contractions

myofascial release an approach that evaluates the fascial system through visual analysis of the human frame three dimensionally in space, by palpating the tissue texture and various fascial layers, and by observing the symmetry, rate, quality, and intensity of strength of the craniosacral rhythm

myositis muscle tissue inflammation

N

negative behavioral patterns symptoms such as possessing a pervasive underlying anxiety, a severely damaged self-concept, and fear of intimacy sometimes resulting from abuse

Nei Jing *The Yellow Emperor's Classic of Internal Medicine*, a Chinese book containing the earliest known mention of massage

nerve stroke a light brushing and finishing stroke using the fingertips. It is sometimes considered an energy technique

nerve tissue neurons that react to stimuli and conduct an impulse, transmitting messages throughout the body; they make up the brain, nerves, and the spinal cord

networking communicating with other professionals or joining professional associations to enhance your image and directly increase the revenue of your business

neuromuscular massage specific work that corrects the shortening of the tendon, muscle, and tendon (T-M-T) unit

neuropeptides (nerve proteins) biochemicals that regulate almost all life processes on a cellular level, and thereby link all body systems; chemical messengers that allow the mind to release cortisol

nociceptors pain receptors

noncomedogenic does not clog pores of the skin

noncontrolled drugs nonprescription or over-the-counter drugs

nutrients chemical substances that are necessary to maintain life

O

opportunistic infection infection by microorganisms that can cause disease only when a host's resistance is low

opportunistically transmitted pathogen a pathogen that naturally occurs on the skin and in mucous membranes; changes in the body's "environment" render these pathogens disease-producing

oral tradition memorized and passed down by word of mouth from one designated individual in a generation to the next over many centuries

organs two or more types of tissue that have joined together to perform a certain bodily function

ossification formation of bones

osteoblasts cells that form bones; formed beneath the periosteum

osteoclasts cells that help reconstruct or remodel a broken bone

osteocytes mature bone cells

overload principle when an exercise program is begun at just above the maximum strength, flexibility, and mobility of the client, a gradual increase in the number of repetitions at a carefully controlled level of higher endurance is then applied

over-the-counter (OTC) self-prescribed drugs

oxygen facial a facial done with liquid oxygen sprays and oxygen-rich oils. This facial is usually done for clients with burned skin or skin showing advanced aging.

P

"pain-spasm-pain" cycle as the muscle goes into spasm and the body attempts to "splint" the injured area, more spasm and pain result

palliative care care directed toward easing pain and making the patient comfortable

palpation examination by touch; the art of observing with our eyes, touching with our hands, and identifying with our eyes and hands

pancreas organ that makes and secretes enzymes

papyrus a durable plant fiber preserved by the dry Egyptian climate that was used as paper

parafango specialty sea mud mixed with paraffin and spread on the body

parafin a white or colorless solid hydrocarbon mixture used to make candles, wax, lubricants, and sealing materials

parallel muscles contains fibers that are parallel to the muscle's longitudinal axis

parasympathetic part of the autonomic nervous system that regulates rest and digestion

Pare, Ambrose (1510–1590) a French physician who was famous for his innovative surgical techniques and known as one of the founders of modern surgery; Pare was also a strong advocate for massage training in medical schools

paresthesia tingling

pennate muscle fibers fibers that lie at an angle to the longitudinal axis of the muscle

pericardium a sac of serous membrane that secretes a lubricating fluid to prevent friction from the movement of the heart

perimysium layer of connective tissue that surrounds fasciculi

periosteum the external surface of the bone

peripheral nervous system (PNS) part of the nervous system that contains cranial (12) nerves and spinal nerves (3); responsible for carrying nerve impulses to and from the body's many structures and includes the many craniospinal nerves that branch off the brain and spinal cord

person-to-person contact when pathogens are transmitted by handling an item of an infected person. An example would be shaking hands or using an infected person's pen. This is a common method of transmitting viruses such as colds and flu.

personal and professional boundaries are defined as areas or the parameters within which you work, live, and play

petrissage from the French word *patrir,* meaning to "knead"; petrissage is also referred to as "milking" or "wringing"

Phalen's test wrists are held in forced flexion for 60 seconds, eliciting pain; test for carpal tunnel syndrome

pharmacodynamics the study of the biochemical and physiological effects of drugs and the mechanisms of their actions

pharmacognosy deals with natural drugs and their constituents derived from plants, animals, and minerals

pharmacokinetics deals with the activity or fate of drugs in the body; includes absorption, distribution, metabolism, and excretion

pharmacology the study of drugs, their origins, nature, properties, and effects on living organisms

pharmacotherapeutics the study of the uses of drugs in the treatment of disease

physician or doctor referral a referral for therapeutic massage made by a chiropractor, physical therapist, or medical doctor

physiology science that deals with the function of the body

phytoceuticals plant-derived medications, vitamins, and supplements

pituitary gland stimulates the other glands to secrete hormones to maintain homeostasis

placebo a substitute for an actual medication that is prescribed for the mental affect rather than a physical one

placebo effect the improvement of a patient that occurs in response to treatment but cannot be considered due to the specific treatment used

plane two-dimensional flat surface that divides the body in half by mass or weight

plantar flexion toes pointed downward

plasticity the tendency of soft tissue to assume a greater length after the stretch force has been stopped

polarity therapy a method of energy-based bodywork that includes diet, exercise, and self-awareness

positional release or strain-counterstrain an effective way to relieve cramping and pain associated with it by moving the closest joint

post traumatic stress disorder (PTSD) development of symptoms following an extreme traumatic stressor that involves actual, perceived, or threatened death, serious injury, or other threat to the integrity of a person

posture reflects the ability of a person to maintain balance and muscular coordination with the least amount of energy expenditure

prana see *Qi*

preauthorization getting approval from the insurance company for payment before services are rendered

prefix a word element added to the beginning of a word to change that word's meaning

PRICE Prevention/Protection, Rest, Ice, Compression, Elevation

professional corporation a C corporation that is taxed at a higher rate than other corporations and has limited liability for its owners

progesterone the "pregnancy" hormone; increases energy storage by promoting fat disposition in pelvic area, quadriceps, hamstrings, and gluteal muscles and around internal organs

pronation inward rotation of the forearm, or palm facing down

prone face down

proprioceptive neuromuscular facilitation (PNF) a neuromuscular reeducation technique

proteins amino acids that are the main structural building blocks of the body. They constitute a major part of bone and muscle tissue and are an important component to blood, body cells, and enzymes.

protraction movement of a body part forward (anteriorly) in the horizontal plane

psychoneuroimmunology a valid field of science and a method of treatment that understands the depth of the mind-body interaction

psychotropic drugs medications that act on the mind by causing therapeutic effects in emotions or behavior

Q

Qi or *prana* "life force" or "universal life force energy"; an energy or life force traveling through pathways, or meridians, in the body

qi gong Chinese exercise combining energy and movement

R

radicular compressed nerve causing pain along the nerve pathway

Rawlins, Maude a nurse who wrote *A Textbook of Massage for Nurses and Beginners* in the early 1930s; this text was used in teaching the required 16 credit hours of practical massage needed for matriculation in New York

reciprocal inhibition PNF method that is the most effective way to alleviate muscle cramping using an isometric contraction of the antagonist or opposing muscle

reciprocal interaction each partner, as in the process of bonding, has a role in facilitating each stage

red blood cells erythrocytes; they contain hemoglobin and carry oxygen to the tissues of the body

referred or radiating pain pain that is experienced or occurs at a distance from the trigger point; painlike sensation that originates in a region of the body that is not the source of the pain stimulus

reflexive response stimulation or inhibition of cutaneous receptors, muscle spindle receptors, proprioceptors, or superficial skeletal muscle due to massage

reflexology a system of stimulating the body to heal by applying pressure to points on the body that affect organs or their functions

Reiki a Japanese healing energy work that involves energy flow through the chakras of the physical body. Mikao Usui trained the first modern-day Reiki masters and passed the traditions to the West through his students.

relaxation response the state reached by having a calm mind. During this state, the blood pressure drops, your muscles lose their tension, and the neuropeptides stop transmitting messages, which cause the heart and breath rate to slow down.

relaxin hormone that softens the ligament of the pelvic joints in order to increase the capacity of the pelvis, making it more pliable to open for delivery

Renaissance a cultural transformation that began in Europe around the late 1400s. Also known as the Enlightenment, the Renaissance was characterized by a revival in intellectual curiosity

respiration overall exchange of gases between the air, blood, and cells

retinaculum fibrous band across the wrist

retraction movement of body part backward (posteriorly) in the horizontal plane

retraumatization occurs when the victim experiences a situation similar to an abuse or traumatic situation they had earlier in life

rhythm the regularity or constancy with which a stroke is applied. As with speed, rhythm can be executed slowly or quickly, depending on the desired result.

RICE Rest, Ice, Compression, Elevation

right of refusal a client's right to refuse treatment

right to privacy a client's right not to have personal information shared with other clients, a client's friends and relatives, or even with other medical professionals

rocking a stroke often used at the completion of the massage to gently soothe the client by affecting the nervous system

Rolfing an approach that takes the body from a structurally imbalanced and stressed position or "randomness" to a place of alignment and balance based on the inherent design of the body

Roth, Mathias a renowned English physician who was a student of Henrik Ling

rugae layered folds that line the stomach

S

sagittal plane (also known as the median plane) divides the body vertically into right and left halves. Midsagittal divides the body into equal right and left halves

salt rub (glow) a body rub using coarse salt to exfoliate the skin and improve circulation

sanitariums a third alternative in health care, sanitariums shared qualities of both health spas and hospitals. Like health resorts today, they varied widely in philosophical approach, the quality of their health-related services, recommended diet and exercise programs, accommodations, and other amenities, including massage.

sanitation the method of decontamination used in all massage clinics and public facilities. Sanitation involves pathogens on a surface and is performed by using soap and general detergents to clean an area.

sarcolemma cell membrane that surrounds a muscle cell or fiber

sauna a hot, dry room used to detoxify the body by encouraging perspiration

Schedule C filed by sole proprietors to report business losses or profits

Schedule K-1 (form 1065) filed by a partner in a business to report his or her share of income, deductions, credits, etc.

Schedule SE form filed by sole proprietors to report self-employment tax if there are net earnings

scoliosis an exaggerated S curve in the spine

scope of practice the parameters within which a therapist may work; the professional therapeutic relationship

S Corporation (or Subchapter S Corporation) a corporation that meets specific Internal Revenue Service size and stock ownership requirements

Scotch hose a treatment in which a massage therapist uses alternating warm and cold water at high pressure to sooth aching and sore muscles

seaweed wrap a body wrap using seaweed applied to the skin, for detoxification

sen energy pathways in Thai massage similar to Chinese meridians

seven aural planes the seven levels of energy that surround the body in layers; from the top down, divine, monadic, spiritual, mental, emotional, etheric, and physical

sexual abuse includes but is not limited to incest, rape, sexual assault, child molestation, and sexual abuse by an authority figure

shaking a similar stroke to rocking. It is considered a gentler stroke than vibration. Shaking can encourage "letting go" when a client is holding onto tension; holding onto such tension can make it difficult to work on a body part.

shamans walkers between both the spiritual and physical worlds; early medicine men and women; these individuals were religious leaders, mystics, and physicians

shea or cocoa butter a natural lubricant helpful in lessening stretch marks

shiatsu a massage technique developed in Japan and based upon the *Nei Jing;* a bodywork modality that is also known as Japanese acupressure, shiatsu is a synthesis of Chinese and Japanese practice that evolved into its own independent discipline. Shiatsu stimulates the same pressure points used in acupuncture, but finger pressure is used in place of needles.

skeletal muscles a type of muscle tissue found in muscles attached to bones

skeletal striated muscles skeletal muscle that is characterized by alternating light and dark bands, or striations

skin rolling a stroke that addresses the skin and connective tissue. Skin rolling is performed by picking up the skin and connective tissue between the fingers and thumbs and rolling the tissue over the thumbs.

slow twitch fibers support activities requiring endurance

sole proprietorship a business form in which one person has ownership and liability of the business

soma all the cells and tissues in the body considered collectively, with the exception of germ cells, such as skin, fascia, and muscles

somatoemotional release ventilation of feelings or pent-up emotions from the body, characterized by spontaneous tears, laughter, and expressions of feelings, thoughts, or recall of traumatic events

somatotyping used to determine body type

spasms involuntary (convulsive) muscle contractions that develop slowly; the most commonly palpated muscle dysfunction, spasm involves a reflex reaction and occurs due to trauma in the musculoskeletal system

speed of the stroke how fast or slow a stroke is performed. Depending on the desired response—relaxation or invigoration—any stroke may be applied slowly or quickly.

sphygmomanometer commonly called a blood pressure cuff; used along with a stethoscope to measure blood pressure

splinting the body guarding against further injury

sprains injury to ligaments that occur as a result of being overstretched

stabilizer or fixator muscle that stabilizes a body part against a particular force

standardized a guarantee that the herbal content of a product is the same in every tablet, tea bag, or capsule

standard precautions rules and guidelines generally used by hospitals and medical clinical settings. These precautions apply to blood, all bodily fluids, secretions, and excretions (except sweat), nonintact skin, and mucous membranes

static not moving phase

statin a group of drugs that inhibit the production of cholesterol and promote the reduction of LDL in blood plasma

STDs sexually transmitted diseases

steam vapor state of water

sterilization the most thorough process for removing pathogens. This process destroys all living organisms on surfaces and equipment, including the spores of bacteria.

stone massage therapy a massage using smooth stones that are heated or chilled to relieve body conditions, restore energy, and promote relaxation in stressed individuals

strain a microscopic tear usually in the musculotendinous junction; tear in muscle or tendon that occurs as a result of overuse or being overstretched

streptococci bacteria common bacteria, with many species occurring naturally in the body

striations dark and light bands on muscles

suffix a word element added to the ending of a word to change the word's meaning

supination the outward rotation of the forearm, or palm facing up

supine face up

supine hypotensive syndrome a rapid decrease in blood pressure causing fainting and dizziness due to the weight of the uterus on the inferior vena cava

susceptibility a person's degree of immunity to infection by a particular organism

Swedish movement cure, Swedish treatment cure, or Swedish massage Ling's system of medical gymnastics. It had three main parts and used French terminology (learned from Dutch physician Johann Mezger [1839–1909]) to refer to many of the movements.

Swiss shower a shower stall with usually four showerheads that can be aimed where water is needed on the client

sympathetic promotes fight-or-flight responses such as those experienced in stressful situations leading to increased heart rate and increased rate of respiration

synarthrotic or fibrous joints unite two bones by fibrous tissue with no joint cavity in between and with almost no movement

system a group of organs that work together to perform a vital bodily function

T

tai chi a system that uses meditation and internal concentration to channel the Qi and manifest it physically

talking stones a process in which the person holds a stone while in a meditative state and listens to what the stone says concerning the cause of an illness

tapotement derived from the Old French term *tapir*, meaning "light blow." Tapotement is a percussion stroke with the blow being immediately pulled off the muscle as soon as the hand strikes the tissue.

Taylor, Charles Fayette a New York physician who was among the first individuals to introduce modern massage techniques in the United States. Dr. Taylor opened an orthopedic practice specializing in the Swedish movement cure, based on the teachings of Mathias Roth.

tendinoskeletal junction the point at which the tendon attaches to bone

tendonitis inflammatory condition

tendons tough fibrous structures that attach muscles to bones

tense-relax method PNF method that is the most effective way to increase range of motion by utilizing the body's own stretch reflex

tetanic contractions sustained contractions that result from repeated stimuli without any rest

tetonic contracture occurs in muscle tissue and results in continuous muscular contractions due to tonic or sustained spasm or fibrosis

Thai massage the ancient massage of Thailand that "manipulates" the body's muscular and connective tissue structures using acupressure-style massage combined with passive yoga stretches

thixotropic ground substance that moves from a gel-like state to a more liquefied state when worked or massaged and then returns to the gel-like state afterward

three phases of effects stages that most sexual abuse survivors experience

thumb presses Originate from the Eastern modalities such as Thai massage and shiatsu and are used to hold pressure points. Thumb presses are performed with the pad of the thumb close to the nail (but not the nail).

Tinel's test finger-tapping over the nerve elicits symptoms; test for carpel tunnel syndrome

tissues groups of cells

tonic contraction continuous partial contraction that does not create movement

topical administration applied to the skin

touch can be perceived in different ways, depending on childhood experience, context, cultural factors, and therapy experience

touch relaxation involves the parent/caregiver stopping at a point of tension, taking the child's body part in their hands, and molding to it, gently bouncing or just holding still, and using a calm voice to encourage the baby to "relax and let go"

Touch Research Institute conducted the most recent and specific study of massage for laboring women

toxicology the study of poisons and their actions, detection, and treatment of the conditions produced by them

trade (brand) name selected by the manufacturing company after it is ready for commercial distribution; always spelled beginning with a capital letter and usually followed by a superscript®

Trager uses gentle, nonintrusive movements such as rocking to release deeply held patterns

transference occurs when the client personalizes the professional therapeutic relationship

trigger point a hyperirritable spot in the muscle or the fascia that is painful when compressed

U

unilaterally occurs on one side

universal precautions rules and guidelines set forth by the US Department of Health and Human Services Centers for Disease Control and mandated by the Occupational Safety and Health Act. These rules are for the protection of health workers and designed to save lives and prevent injury.

V

veins blood vessels that carry blood toward the heart

ventricle the lower, right and left, chambers of the heart

vibration from the Latin term for shaker; vibration is a stroke that ranges from quick shaking to rhythmic rocking

Vichy shower a shower that sprays while the client lies on a cushioned mat placed on a special table

virus a class of submicroscopic organisms that are pathogenic agents capable of causing disease

viscera the internal organs of the body such as those contained within the dorsal and ventral cavities

visceral or smooth muscle moves fluids, waste, and other products through the organs of the body

vitalism doctrine that life cannot be explained fully in terms of chemical and physical forces alone

W

Wright's test a diminished radial pulse is felt when the arm is abducted; test for thoracic outlet syndrome

wringing a form of petrissage, wringing is actually considered a sports massage stroke

Y

yang indicates the "sunny side of a hill" and represents male

yin means the "shady side of a hill" and represents feminine

yoga the union of mind, body, and spirit

Contributors' Biographies

Dr. Medhat Alattar, MB.BCh, DC, MS

Dr. Medhat Alattar, a contributor for chapter 6, earned his medical degree in 1980 from Ain Shams University College of Medicine in Cairo, Egypt. He earned his doctor of chiropractic degree from Life Chiropractic College in 1987 and a master's degree in sport health in 1995. Dr. Alattar traveled to and lectured about chiropractic in several countries. Currently, he teaches at Palmer College of Chiropractic in Port Orange, Florida.

Don Ash PT CST-D

Don Ash, contributor for the CranioSacral Therapy section for chapter 16, has been a seminar instructor and lecturer in CranioSacral Therapy for the Upledger Institute for eight years. A physical therapist with over 25 years' experience in acute care, rehabilitation, hospice care, and private practice, he developed "breath venting," a gentle technique empowering people to use their breath to reduce tension and stress. He lectures internationally, with recent venues including the New Hampshire chapter of APTA, National Medical Association Conference, Beyond the Dura Conference, and the International Symposium on the Science of Touch. He has a private practice specializing in CranioSacral Therapy located at 243 Rochester Hill Rd., Rochester, NH 03867; (603) 332-1881; ASHPT@aol.com.

John F. Barnes, PT

John F. Barnes, PT, a contributor for chapter 16, graduated from the University of Pennsylvania as a physical therapist in 1960. He holds physical therapy licenses in Pennsylvania, Arizona, New Jersey, Delaware, Colorado, and Hawaii.

He is on the Counsel of Advisors of the American Back Society, an Editorial Advisor of the *Journal of Bodywork and Movement Therapies,* and a member of the American Physical Therapy Association.

John lectures internationally, presenting the "John F. Barnes Myofascial Release Approach" seminar series and "Advances in Spinal Diagnosis and Treatment for the 21st Century" for the American Back Society.

He wrote *Myofascial Release: The Search for Excellence* in 1990. He has also been the "Therapeutic Insight" columnist for *Physical Therapy Forum,* contributes the "Mind & Body" column to *Physical Therapy Today,* and has written several articles for the *Advance for Physical Therapists,* the most recent titled, "Alternative No More!" John also wrote *Healing Ancient Wounds: The Renegades Wisdom,* published in 2000.

John was named one of the most influential persons in the therapeutic professions in the last century in the national *Massage Magazine's* featured article "Stars of the Century."

He was also the featured speaker, presenting his Myofascial Release Approach, at the American Back Society's 2006 meeting, the theme of which was the most important advances in health care of this century.

Donna Cerio

Since 1979, Donna C. Cerio's years as an alternative health care professional have included personal and organizational development, health care, and stress management. Donna wrote her section in chapter 12 based on her years of research and practice. She offers health care and education in private practice, academic, and medical settings, as well as the public arena. Donna has developed and refined Intentional Touch™, a body of work that addresses the needs of people recovering from sexual abuse and other traumatic experiences, suffering from serious illness, or dealing with chronic emotional, physical, and/or mental pain.

Donna is a member of the Zero Balancing Association, American Massage Therapy Association, Soul Lightening, Inc., and International Association of Health Care Practitioners. She has a degree in social work and certifications in therapeutic massage, process acupressure, zero balancing, anatomy/physiology, holistic health education, and transpersonal integration. At present, she is a PhD candidate in health sciences and a zero balancing faculty member.

Currently, Donna is the director and principal provider at the Cerio Institute in Santa Cruz County, CA. The Cerio Institute is an organization dedicated to providing a therapeutic and educational resource for the local and global community. She is the author of several articles and manuals on the subject of delivering health care to survivors of sexual abuse. Donna delivers educational seminars and on-site services locally and across the nation.

Donna can be reached at dccerio@thecerioinstitute.com or (831) 475-5472. Visit her websites at www.thecerioinstitute.com and www.intentionaltouch.com.

Bruno Chikly, MD, DO (Hon.)

Bruno Chikly is a graduate of the medical school at Saint Antoine Hospital in France, where his internship in general medicine included training in endocrinology, surgery, neurology, and psychiatry. Dr. Chikly developed the modality of Lymphatic Drainage Therapy in chapter 16. Over the years, he trained extensively in a number of manual and osteopathic disciplines, including lymphatic techniques, CranioSacral Therapy, cranial osteopathy, visceral manipulation, mechanical link, muscle energy, strain/counterstrain, myofascial release, zero balancing, process acupressure, neuromuscular therapy, and orthobionomy.

Of these studies, it was Dr. Chikly's work in traditional medicine, osteopathy, and lymphology that primarily impacted his creation of lymph drainage therapy. In 1994, he earned the prestigious Medal of the Medical Faculty of Paris VI for his exhaustive research on the lymphatic system and lymph drainage therapy.

Dr. Chikly has conducted workshops and lectured in France, Belgium, Germany, Switzerland, Tunisia, Israel, Brazil, China, Canada, and the United States. He is a member of the International Society of Lymphology. He is an associate member of the American Academy of Osteopathy and the Cranial Academy. And he is listed in the Millennium Edition of *Marquis' Who's Who in the World*. Dr. Chikly resides in Arizona with his wife and teaching partner, Alaya Chikly, CMT.

Dr. Chikly created the first lymphatic dissection video in North America, providing an unprecedented view of major lymph nodes, vessels, and viscera. He is also the author of the first comprehensive book in North America on the lymphatic system and lymphedema: *Silent Waves: Theory and Practice of Lymph Drainage Therapy—With Applications for Lymphedema, Chronic Pain and Inflammation* (I.H.H. Publishing, 2001).

Don Curry, LMT, Certified Advanced Rolfer

Donald Curry passed his Florida state massage boards in 1976 and received certification as a Rolfer in 1978 and advanced Rolf training in 1985. He contributed his knowledge for the Rolfing section in chapter 16 of this text. He completed a two-year training at the Gestalt Therapy Institute of Florida and practiced developmental play therapy, a Gestalt technique developed by Dr. Vi Brody, working with language-disabled emotionally disturbed children for the Palm Beach County School System.

Donald served as the chairman of the Southeast Region Rolf Association and as vice president of the Palm Beach County Massage Association. He taught massage for "Foundations of Bodywork," the pre-Rolf training class for the Rolf Institute in Boulder, Colorado. He also developed and taught a series of workshops on "Understanding Structure" for continuing education credits for the Florida State Massage Board.

Don Curry now divides his time between a practice in South Florida and San Jose del Cabo, Baja California Sur, Mexico.

Carla DiMauro, LMT

Carla DiMauro, LMT and certified infant massage instructor, researched and wrote material for chapters 10 and 11. She maintains a private massage practice, Touching Tradition, Inc., serving families from Dade to Palm Beach County, Florida, throughout all of the cycles of life. She received her formal training at the American Institute of Massage Therapy in 1993 and is currently an instructor and continuing education provider of classes in her specialities of prenatal, infant, and geriatric massage.

Carla began her career providing massage therapy to abused, neglected, and special needs children. The transformations she witnessed in the lives of these children fueled her interest and love for this work. She continues to research and gather data to support the obvious benefits of loving touch to individuals, families, and communities as a whole.

Her work has taken her as far as Uzbekistan, where she presented the Western approach of nurturing touch to orphanage administrators and provided massage therapy to hundreds of special needs children. Carla continues to speak out on the importance of infant massage for enhanced growth and development as well as the critical role pregnancy massage plays in utero, where the bonding process begins.

She lives in Fort Lauderdale, Florida, close to her mother, sisters, brother, nephews, and nieces.

Dr. Donald J. Glassey, MSW, DC, LMT, NCTMB

Dr. Donald J. Glassey was born in 1946 in Brooklyn, NY, and educated at Michigan State University (BA with honor), the University of Pennsylvania (MSW), and Pennsylvania College of Straight Chiropractic (DC), where he subsequently taught chiropractic technique, history, and philosophy. He is a former national staff instructor for Network Chiropractic seminars, a Reiki Master, and has taught Toggle Recoil chiropractic technique nationally.

Dr. Glassey's many writing contributions to this text include philosophical foundations of massage (chapter 1), muscle palpation (chapter 4), *Ayurveda* (chapter 15), and Cerebrospinal Fluid Technique Massage (chapter 16).

After studying and researching many forms of body and energy work for over 10 years, he developed Cerebrospinal Fluid Technique Massage (CSFTM) in 1996. Dr. Glassey has been teaching CSFTM seminars throughout the United States, Canada, and Mexico for over nine years. He recently retired from 15 years of active chiropractic practice to devote his time to teaching and advancing CSFTM, including development of a CSF massage procedure with his teaching staff.

Dr. Glassey is also a graduate of the Florida Academy of Massage. He recently developed the curriculum for a new massage program at the International Academy in South Daytona, Florida. He is a member of the Florida Chiropractic Society. Dr. Glassey is also past president of the SW chapter of the FSMTA and current vice president of the Flagler/Volusia chapter, as well as a member of the National Certification Board for Therapeutic Massage and Bodywork. His seminars are approved for continuing education units with the National Certification Board for Therapeutic Massage and Bodywork for Category "A" and "B," the Florida and Louisiana Boards of Massage Therapy, and the South Carolina Massage Therapy Panel.

Daniel A. Heidel, BS, LMT

Dan Heidel, contributor for chapter 19, Western principles of movement section, is currently an adjunct professor and clinical instructor for massage at Delgado Community College in New Orleans, Louisiana. Dan received his bachelor of science degree in exercise science/physical education from the University of South Alabama. He received his diploma in massage therapy in 2000 from Blue Cliff College of Mobile. He has also been working as a clinical specialist in operating rooms throughout Louisiana and Mississippi.

As a faculty member of Delgado Community College, Dan lectures in anatomy and physiology, kinesiology, and pathology, and has designed and prepared course manuals on anatomy/physiology, kinesiology, and Swedish massage. He has also taught foundations and methods for Swedish, deep tissue, sports, and special populations massage.

Dan has worked in massage therapy as an independent contractor, owning his own business, Fitness Solutions. While working with his clients, he works primarily with integrative therapies, especially deep tissue, orthopedic, neuromuscular, sports, and proprioceptor neuromuscular facilitation techniques. Dan began his work in health and wellness care as a physical therapy technician for the Tenet Healthcare Systems Corporation in 1997.

Peter Joachim, LMT, NCTMB

Peter Joachim is a native of the Republic of Trinidad and Tobago. Peter contributed the chair massage routine in chapter 4 and T'ia Chi/Martial Arts to chapter 19. He is a martial arts instructor with 25 years' martial arts experience in the Chinese systems of Tiger and Crane Gung Fu, *xingyiquan*, tai chi, and *chin na* (the art of seize and control). Peter graduated valedictorian from Keiser College, West Palm Beach Campus (Florida) with an AS degree in massage therapy.

Deane Juhan, MA

Deane Juhan majored in English Literature from 1963 to 1973, attending Colorado University (B.A.), Michigan University (M.A.), and the University of California at Berkeley. Deane contributed the section on Trager in chapter 16. During the summer of 1973, one year before completing his PhD candidacy at Berkeley, he went for a retreat to Esalen Institute in Big Sur, California. This excursion proved to be the initiation of a major career change. He discovered a natural gift and a deep love for bodywork, and within a month was working full time on the Esalen Massage Crew, where he continued his practice over the next 17½ years.

At Esalen he had the opportunity to study with many of the innovative bodyworkers who were proliferating during that time. Most significantly, he met Dr. Milton Trager in 1974 and studied his work until the time of Dr. Trager's death in 1999. He is a senior Trager practitioner, an instructor for its certification program, developer and chair of the Anatomy Training Track for that program, and teaches a broad variety of continuing education courses ("Somatic Explorations") for the Trager Institute and for many other bodywork training programs in the US, Canada, Europe, and Japan.

During his time at Esalen he became deeply interested in the biological and psychological roots of the power of touch and movement, seeking to develop a scientific basis for the remarkable changes he was witnessing regularly. His survey of the clinical literature over a nine year period led to his writing *Job's Body: A Handbook for Bodywork,* which is now in its third edition and has become a standard textbook for many schools and training programs.

His most recent publication is *Touched by the Goddess: The Physical, Psychological and Spiritual Powers of Bodywork,* a collection of essays focusing on the potential social and cultural impact of touch and movement as bodywork continues to be the fastest growing alternative or complimentary approach to health care and personal development.

He currently resides in Mill Valley, California, where he has a private practice.

Marc Kalmanson, BSN, MSN, ARNP, LMT, RYT

Marc Kalmanson contributed his knowledge of Eastern practices in chapter 15. He is an advanced nurse practitioner with over 40 years of combined experience in the emergency department, labor and delivery, health care, and massage; he also has been chief flight nurse for a major aeromedical transport company.

Marc is a member of the faculty at Dragon Rises College of Oriental Medicine, a continuing education provider for the Florida Board of Massage Therapy, and has been on the faculty at Florida International University, Broward Community College. He has lectured both here and abroad on emergency nursing, massage, aeromedical transport, and altitude physiology.

Marc is a member of Sigma Theta Tau, the honorary scholastic nursing society.

Dan Rowlands, LMT, NCTMB

Dan Rowlands, contributor for chapter 21, has a BA in business administration and economics from Westminster College, New Wilmington, Pennsylvania. He is a graduate of Atlantic Vocational Technical Center, Coconut Creek, Florida, and sits on the Advisory Board of the Atlantic & Sheridan Technical Centers for Massage Therapy. As a massage therapist, he is proficient in deep tissue, Swedish, Swe-Thai®, NMT, Reiki, aromatherapy, and chair massage. As a Reiki Master, Dan leads Reiki Healing Circles every Tuesday evening and conducts Reiki I, II, and III classes at the Center for Optimal Health, Fort Lauderdale, Florida; he is also a continuing educational unit provider for the state of Florida.

Linda Rowlands, LMT, NCTMB

Linda Rowlands is co-owner/massage therapist at the Center for Optimal Health in Fort Lauderdale, Florida. She wrote a short piece based on her work with seniors in her practice for chapter 11. All Linda's treatments are client-based and include a mix of the following modalities: Reiki, reflexology, lymphatic drainage, acutonics, Swedish, Lomi lomi, deep tissue, and aromatherapy. Her purchase of the business in 1998 included a part-time office in a seniors' community. The practice has grown over the years so that the majority of Linda's clients are healthy, active geriatric individuals who value quality of life. Linda keeps fit with massage, acupuncture, exercise, biking, and yoga; creates through baking, painting, and writing; and explores through books, classes, shamanic studies, and astrology, to name a few. Being a participant in life enhances Linda's massage to help create balance and health for her clients.

Lewis Rudolph, BS, AAS, LMT

Lewis Rudolph was licensed in the state of Florida in 1992. Since 1993, he and his wife have been in private practice, working primarily on patients with injuries related to sports or accidents. He developed and contributed his work for neuromuscular therapy in chapter 16. Lewis has taught throughout Florida, most recently at Palm Beach Community College in Boca Raton. For additional information, call Lewis at Southern Rehab and Therapy, Inc., West Palm Beach, Florida, (561) 684-2624.

Valerie Wohl

Valerie Wohl, a writer and researcher for chapter 1, is president of Wohl Research and Consulting, Inc. Educated at the University of Michigan in Ann Arbor (undergraduate), and the School of Education and Social Policy at Northwestern University in Evanston, Illinois (graduate), she focuses on educational writing; sociocultural, behavioral, and economic research; and issues of social and public policy.

Christian M. Wright, DC, BsHB

Dr. Christian M. Wright, contributor for chapters 5 and 22, is a graduate of the National University of Health Sciences with a doctorate in chiropractic. Dr. Wright also has a bachelor of science degree in human biology and completed a family practice residency. He is currently a member of the faculty at Blue Cliff College of Gulfport, Mississippi, and continues to teach anatomy and physiology to both massage and medical assisting students.

As a chiropractor, Dr. Wright evaluates and treats his clients with a focus on anatomic and physiological function and its role in healing and wellness. He has always worked to promote the integration of Eastern and Western medicines while communicating the need for empowering patients in their own health.

Credits

Chapter 1

Figure 1.3: ©Bettmann/Corbis; 1.4: © Bettmann/Corbis; 1.5: © Corbis; 1.6: © Brown Brothers; 1.7: Courtesy Willard Library; 1.8: © Corbis.

Chapter 2

Figure 2.1–2.14: © The McGraw-Hill Companies, Inc./Shaana Pritchard, photographer; 2.15, 2.16: © The McGraw-Hill Companies, Inc./Chris Kerrigan, photographer; 2.17a-e, 2.20a-c, 2.21a-c: © The McGraw-Hill Companies, Inc./Jan L. Saeger, photographer.

Chapter 3

Figure 3.1, 3.3a, b, 3.7, 3.8: © The McGraw-Hill Companies, Inc./Shaana Pritchard, photographer.

Chapter 4

Figure 4.1a, b: © The McGraw-Hill Companies, Inc./Jan L. Saeger, photographer; 4.2–4.9: © The McGraw-Hill Companies, Inc./Shaana Pritchard, photographer; 4.10: © The McGraw-Hill Companies, Inc./Joe DeGrandis, photographer; 4.11–4.22: © The McGraw-Hill Companies, Inc./Shaana Pritchard, photographer.

Chapter 6

Figure 6.1, 6.2: © The McGraw-Hill Companies, Inc./Shaana Pritchard, photographer; 6.3: © The McGraw-Hill Companies, Inc./Joe DeGrandis, photographer; 6.5–6.7: © The McGraw-Hill Companies, Inc./Shaana Pritchard, photographer; 6.8a, b: © The McGraw-Hill Companies, Inc./Timothy L. Vacula, photographer; 6.9, 6.10: © The McGraw-Hill Companies, Inc./Shaana Pritchard, photographer, 6.11: © The McGraw-Hill Companies, Inc./Timothy L. Vacula, photographer; 6.12: © The McGraw-Hill Companies, Inc./Shaana Pritchard, photographer; 6.13: © The McGraw-Hill Companies, Inc./Timothy Vacula, photographer; 6.14a,b: © The McGraw-Hill Companies, Inc./Shaana Pritchard, photographer; 6.15a,b: © The McGraw-Hill Companies, Inc./Timothy Vacula, photographer; 6.16a,b: © The McGraw-Hill Companies, Inc./Shaana Pritchard, photographer; 6.17: © The McGraw-Hill Companies, Inc./Timothy Vacula, photographer; 6.18: © The McGraw-Hill Companies, Inc./Jan L. Saeger, photographer; 6.20, 6.21: © The McGraw-Hill Companies, Inc./Shaana Pritchard, photographer.

Chapter 7

Figure 7.1: © SPL/Photo Researchers, Inc.; 7.2, 7.3: © The McGraw-Hill Companies, Inc./Joe DeGrandis, photographer; 7.32a,b: © Richard Anderson.

Chapter 8

Figure 8.2, 8.3: © Ed Reschke; 8.4: © The McGraw-Hill Companies, Inc./Dennis Strete, photographer; 8.8a-d: © The McGraw-Hill Companies, Inc./Joe DeGrandis, photographer; p. 220, p. 221: © The McGraw-Hill Companies, Inc./Joe DeGrandis, photographer.

Chapter 10

Figure 10.1–10.3: Courtesy Jay D. Robare; 10.4–10.10: Courtesy Peter Joachim.

Chapter 11

Figure 11.1: © Vol. 113 PhotoDisc/Getty Images;11.2: Courtesy Edward Lloyd; 11.3: Courtesy Jay D. Robare; 11.4: Courtesy Nancy Harris; 11.5: © Pixtal RF/age fotostock; 11.6: © The McGraw-Hill Companies, Inc./Jan L. Saeger, photographer; 11.7: Courtesy Jay D. Robare; 11.8: Courtesy of Wayne Spangler.

Chapter 12

Figure 12.1: © Stockbyte/PunchStock; 12.2, 12.3: © Corbis Royalty-Free; 12.4: © Vol. 83 PhotoDisc/Getty; 12.5: © The McGraw-Hill Companies, Inc./Lars A. Niki, photographer; 12.6: © Dynamic Graphics/JupiterImages.

Chapter 13

Figure 13.1–13.15: © The McGraw-Hill Companies, Inc./Shaana Pritchard, photographer; 13.16, 13.17: © The McGraw-Hill Companies, Inc./Jan L. Saeger, photographer.

Chapter 14

Figure 14.6: Photo courtesy of Cosmopro, Inc.; 14.7 - 11: Courtesy Peter Joachim; 14.12 -16: © The McGraw-Hill Companies, Inc./Jan L. Saeger, photographer.

Chapter 15

Figure 15.17, 15.18, 15.20: © The McGraw-Hill Companies, Inc./Shaana Pritchard, photographer.

Chapter 16

Figure 16.1–16.4: © The McGraw-Hill Companies, Inc./Jan L. Saeger, photographer; 16.8: Courtesy of Deane Juhan; 16.9: Photograph courtesy of Upledger Institute/Heather Stanish, photographer; 16.10: Courtesy of Christian Orano; 16.11: Courtesy of Don Ash.

Chapter 17

Figure 17.2: © The McGraw-Hill Companies, Inc./Jan L. Saeger, photographer; 17.3a-b, 17.4: © Corbis RF; 17.6: © Pavel Filatov/Alamy RF.

Chapter 18

Figure 18.1a: (bread): © Vol. 83/Corbis; 18.1b: (potatoes): © Vol. 83/Corbis; 18.1c: (apples): © Vol. 83/Corbis; 18.1d: (oil): © PhotoDisc/EO006/Getty Images; 18.1e: (steak): © Vol. 83/Corbis; 18.1f: (eggs): © Vol. 83/Corbis; 18.1g: (beans): © Vol. 83/Corbis; 18.1h: (water): © Vol. 30/Corbis; 18.1i: (broccoli): © Vol. 83/Corbis; 18.1j: (strawberries): © Vol. 83/Corbis; 18.1k: (lettuce): © Corbis RF website; 18.1l: (milk): © Vol. 83/Corbis; 18.1m: (cereal): © Corbis RF website; 18.1n: (bananas): © Vol. 83/Corbis; 18.1o: (tofu): © OS49 PhotoDisc/Getty; 18.1p: (salmon): © Vol. 83/Corbis; 18.1q: (nuts): © OS49 PhotoDisc/Getty; 18.1r: (wheats/flour): © Corbis RF website;18.3: © Corbis RF; 18.4: © The McGraw-Hill Companies, Inc./Elite Images; 18.5a: © Vol. 12 PhotoDisc/Getty; 18.5b: © DV 23/Getty; 18.7: © PhotoDisc website/Getty.

Chapter 19

Figure 19.1a-c: © The McGraw-Hill Companies, Inc./Shaana Pritchard, photographer; 19.3: © ImageSource RF/Jupiter Images; 19.4–19.28: © The McGraw-Hill Companies, Inc./Shaana Pritchard, photographer.

Chapter 20

Figure 20.1: © The McGraw-Hill Companies, Inc./Jan L. Saeger, photographer; 20.2, 20.3: © Royalty-Free/Corbis; 20.5: © The McGraw-Hill Companies, Inc./Jan L. Saeger, photographer.

Chapter 21

Figure 21.5: © The McGraw-Hill Companies, Inc./Jan L. Saeger, photographer.

Chapter 22

Figure 22.1: © PhotoDisc/Getty website; 22.3, 22.4a-c, 22.5: © Corbis RF; 22.6: © PhotoAlto RF/PictureQuest/; 22.7: © The McGraw-Hill Companies, Inc./Ken Karp, photographer; 22.8: © Vol. 12 PhotoDisc/Getty; 22.9: © SS04 PhotoDisc/Getty.

Chapter 23

Figure 23.1–23.9, 23.11: © The McGraw-Hill Companies, Inc./Jan L. Saeger, photographer.

Illustration Credits

Chapter 16:

Figure 16.5-Reprinted with permission-Rehabilitation Services, Inc. Paoli PA/John F. Barnes, PT

Figure 16.6-Reprinted with permission-Rehabilitation Services, Inc. Paoli PA/John F. Barnes, PT

Figure 16.7-Reprinted with permission-Rehabilitation Services, Inc. Paoli PA/John F. Barnes, PT

Chapter 18:

Figure 18.2-Illustration by William Ober

Index

Page numbers followed by *b* indicate boxed text; *f*, figures; and *t*, tables.

A

Abbreviations, 66–67
ABCs (airway, breathing, circulation) of CPR, 41
Abdomen, muscles of, 201, 206*t*
Abdominal cavity, 156, 156*f*, 157, 157*t*, 158*f*
Abdominal massage, 101, 101*f*, 270
Abdominopelvic cavity, 156, 156*f*, 157*t*
Abduction, 137, 139*f*
ABMP. *See* Associated Bodyworkers and Massage Professionals
Absorption, 488
Abuse, survivors of sexual, 307–318
   categories of clients, 313–316
      one, 313–314, 313*f*, 314*b*
      three, 315–316, 316*b*
      two, 314–315, 314*f*, 315*b*
   client authority, 312
   consequences of, 316–317
   disconnection, 312
   effects of, 309–311, 310*f*
   indicators (signs) of, 317–318, 318*f*
   intervention, 311
   licensed professionals, team of, 313–314
   post-traumatic stress disorder, 311
   prevalence, 308–309
   retraumatization, 316
   special needs, 311
   therapeutic relationship and recovery, 312–313
Accident report form, 43, 43*f*
Achilles tendon
   rupture, 355
   stretching, 332*f*, 333*f*
   tendinitis, 355
Acidosis, 480
Acne facials, 377
Acquired immunodeficiency syndrome (AIDS), 50, 244, 296
Acrimal gland, 255*f*
Acromioclavicular sprain (separation), 350
Acronyms, 66
Actin, 196–197
Action, 198
Active inhibition, 522*b*, 524*b*
Active range of motion (AROM), 336, 336*t*
Acupressure
   criteria for applying, 405, 408–409
   physiological effects of, 126
   points
      on foot, 93, 94*f*
      on hand, 102*f*, 103

      on head and neck, 105*f*–106*f*
      for headaches, 409
      for low back and hip pain, 409–410
      for nausea, 409
      on upper back, 105*f*
Acute phase, 342
Acutonics, for senior clients, 298*b*
Adaptation, 514
Adduction, 138, 139*f*
Adductor brevis, action of, 212*t*
Adductor longus, action of, 212*t*
Adenosine triphosphate (ATP), 122*b*, 123*f*, 200
ADH (antidiuretic hormone), 480
ADHD (attention deficit hyperactivity disorder), 294
Adhesions, friction stroke for breaking up, 84
Adhesive capsulitis, 350
Adrenal glands, 239*t*, 240, 274
Adson's Test, 590, 591*f*
Advertising. *See also* Marketing
   in local media, 557
   professionalism, 540
Agonist, 143, 198
AIDS (acquired immunodeficiency syndrome), 50, 244, 296
Air circulation, massage room, 38
Ajna, 471
Alcohol
   for disinfection, 48
   as recreational drug, 577
Alexander Technique, 276, 449
Allen's Test, 590
Allergic rhinitis, 244
Allergies
   to lubricants, 36
   as lymphatic system disorder, 244
   treating clients with, 384
Alveoli, 250, 250*f*
Alzheimer's disease, 297
Ambience, 38
American Association of Masseurs and Masseuses, 19
American Massage Therapy Association (AMTA), 19–20, 358–359, 363, 532, 533*b*
American Medical Association, 19
American Physical Therapy Association, 19
Americans with Disabilities Act, 51
Amino acids, 486, 486*f*
Amma, 10, 21, 411
Amnesia, reversible, 443
Amphetamines, 577–578
Amphiarthrotic joints, 173–174
AMTA. *See* American Massage Therapy Association
Amylase, 245
Anahata, 471

Analgesic, topical, 575
Anatomical planes, 155, 155*f*
Anatomical position, 135, 135*f*
Anatomical positioning, 154–155, 155*f*
Anatomy
   cells
      description, 158, 159
      division, 161–162
      structure, 160*f*, 161
   definition, 154
   organs, 163
   terms and concepts
      abdominal regions, 157, 158*f*, 159*f*
      anatomical planes, 155–156, 155*f*
      anatomical position, 154–155, 155*f*
      body cavities, 156, 156*f*, 157*t*
      directional terms, 155–156
      tissues, 162–163, 162*t*
Anatripsis, 12
Ankle
   anatomy, 184, 185
   range of motion, 336*f*
   sprains, 340
Ankle circumduction, 522
Ankle rotation, 423*f*
Ankylosing spondylitis, 189
Anorexia nervosa, 490
Antacid, 487
Antagonist, 143, 198
Anterior (directional term), 156
Anthropometry, 134, 145
Antidiuretic hormone (ADH), 480
Antimicrobial disinfecting solution, 34
Anus, 248, 248*f*
Aorta, 227*f*, 229, 230*f*, 231*f*
Aortic valve, 227, 229, 231*f*
Appendicular skeleton, 166
Appendix, 247, 248*f*
Arabic tradition, 14–15
Areas of endangerment, 74, 76, 77*f*, 78*b*
Aristotle, 21
Arm
   bones, 179–181, 180*f*, 181*f*
   injuries
      elbow, 352–353, 353*f*
      shoulder, 350, 351*f*, 352*f*
   muscles, 206, 210*f*–211*f*
   supine massage sequence, 101, 102*f*, 103
Arndt-Schultz law, 442
AROM (active range of motion), 336, 336*t*
Aromatherapy
   description, 383
   history of, 382–383
   for senior clients, 298*b*
   use with steam, 373
Arrector pili, 254, 254*f*
The Art of Massage, 18

Arteries
   connecting to the heart, 227*f*
   definition, 224
   of the human body, 226*f*
   of importance to massage therapy, 229–230
Arthritis, 188
Articulation, 173
Asanas, 501–512
Ashtanga, 497, 498
Asia, history of massage in
   ancient world, 10–11
   Middle Ages, 15
Asperger's syndrome, 293
Assessment, 61–66
   client file
      client intake form, 56–57, 57*f*, 62
      corrections, 65
      documentation, 68–69
      history form, 56, 62, 65*f*
      insurance, 68–69, 69–72, 71*f*
      narrative report, 66, 66*b*
      posttreatment assessment, 66
      postural analysis, 62–63, 62*f*, 63*f*, 64*b*
   posttreatment, 66
Assignment of benefits claim form, 71, 71*f*
Associated Bodyworkers and Massage
      Professionals (ABMP), 20,
      532, 533*b*–534*b*
Assyrians, 7
Asthma, 244, 295–296, 296*f*
ATP (adenosine triphosphate), 122*b*, 123*f*, 200
Atrioventricular valves, 227, 231*f*
Atrium, 227
Atrophy, muscle, 79, 198, 200
Attention deficit hyperactivity disorder
      (ADHD), 294
Auckett, Amelia, 281
Aura, 420
Aural planes, 470, 471*f*
Autism, 293–294, 293*f*
Autonomic (involuntary) nerves, 237
Autonomic nervous system (ANS)
   anatomy, 232
   blood vessel diameter, 115, 116*f*
   parasympathetic branch, 119, 119*b*,
      121*f*, 235*f*, 267
   in pregnancy, 267
   sympathetic branch, 119, 119*b*, 120*f*, 234*f*
Autonomic pathway, 124*f*
Aversion, to touch, 316
Avicenna, 14–15, 14*f*
Axes of motion, 136
Axial skeleton, 166
Axillary artery, 229
Axons, 233
Ayur Veda, 11, 21
Ayurveda
   charting human constitution, 413*t*
   description, 10, 411–412
   doshas, 411*t*, 412, 413, 415*b*, 415*f*
   massage, 412–414

B

Babylonians, 7
Back
   anatomy, 357*f*
   effleurage, 325*f*
   injuries, 356–357
   massage routine, 357–358

   muscles, 208*t*–209*t*
   quacking, 327*f*
   table massage sequence, 96, 97*f*–98*f*, 99
Bacteria, 44
Balance, 255
Balancing the spirit, 470
Ball-and-socket joint, 176*f*
Baroreceptors, 116, 232
Bathhouses
   Greek, 12
   prostitution in, 13, 16
   Roman, 13, 13*f*, 14
Battle Creek Company, 21
Battle Creek Sanitarium, 18, 18*f*
Benefits, health insurance, 70
Bernard, Claude, 22
Biceps, action of, 206
Biceps brachii
   anatomy, 351*f*
   muscle test, 337
Bicuspid (mitral) valve, 227, 229, 231*f*
Bik Ram, 498
Bilateral presentation, 588
Bile, 246–247, 488, 489
Bindegewebmassage, 444
Binge eating disorders, 490*f*
Biomechanics of movement, 133–150
   anthropometry, 145
   body movements and ranges of motion,
      137–142, 137*f*–142*f*
   connective tissue, 143
   ergonomics, 145
   gait, 146–148, 147*f*
   injury prevention, 148, 149*f*
   joints, 144–145
   kinesiology, 145–146
   massage and, 149–150
   muscle, 143–144
   posture, 146
   terminology, 134–147
      anatomical reference axes, 136
      anatomical reference planes,
         135–136, 135*f*
      anatomical reference position,
         135, 135*f*
      directional terms, 136–137, 136*f*
      functional position, 135, 135*f*
Biotin, 482*t*
Black Death, 14
Bladder, 251
Bleach, 34, 48
Blood, elements, 225, 229*f*
Blood-borne pathogens, 46–47
Blood-brain barrier, 490
Blood flow, 115–116
Blood pressure
   description, 115–116
   hypertension, 116
   normal values, 230
   in pregnancy, 268, 269
   regulation, 230, 232
   supine hypotensive syndrome, 272, 272*f*
Blood vessel diameter, 115–116, 116*f*
Blumenbach, Johann Fredrich, 21
BNI (Business Network International), 558
Boat pose (Navasana), 508, 510*f*
Body mass index (BMI), 493*b*
Body mechanics, 89–92
Body-mind connection, 465–475
   balancing the spirit, 470
   energy levels (aural planes), 470, 471*f*
   fight-or-flight response, 466–467, 466*f*

   indigenous massage practices, 472–474
   methods of connection
      chakra balancing, 470–472
      energy work, 472
      guided imagery, 472, 473*b*
      meditation, 468–470, 469*f*
      yoga, 468*f*
   placebo effect, 467–468
Body temperature
   heat exhaustion, 345
   heat stroke, 345
   hyperthermia, 345
   hypothermia, 346
Bolstering
   during massage, 58, 60
   for postural deviations, 59*f*
Bolsters, 31–32, 32*f*
Bonding, 280
Bone, Dr. Roger C., 299
Bongers, 33
Bony landmarks, 172–173, 174*f*
Boundaries
   personal, 543–544
   professional, 543
Bow (Dhanurasana), 509, 511*f*
Brachial artery, 229–230
Brachial plexus, 237, 590
Brachioradialis muscle, 206
Brain, 237
Brain nutrition, 490
Brain waves, 470
Breast cushions, 32, 32*f*, 60
Breathing
   chakra balancing, 470–472
   deep, rhythmic during massage, 95
   in yoga, 498–501
British Medical Association, 19
Brochure, 553, 555*f*
Bronchi, 249*f*, 250
Bronchioles, 250, 250*f*
Bruxism, 593
Bubonic plague, 14
Bulimia, 490
Bunions, 187
Bursa, 341
Bursitis
   definition, 189
   elbow, 341, 353
   knee, 341
   shoulder, 341, 350
Business card, 553, 555*f*
Business development. *See also*
      Professionalism
   business name, selecting, 560
   business plan, 550–551
   entrepreneurs, 548–549
   external communication model, 549–550
   facilities and services agreement, 552*f*
   flyer, 557*b*
   goal-setting, 550–551
   insurance, 551, 553
   keys to success, 548
   marketing, 553–558
      brochures, 553, 555*f*
      business cards, 553, 555*f*
      coupons, 557, 557*f*
      networking, 558
      résumé, 553, 554*f*
      through chair massage, 553,
         555–556, 557*b*
      via local media, 557–558

questions to ask yourself, 549
start-up costs, 551
types of business, 558–560
    choosing, 558
    corporation, 559–560
    partnership, 559
    sole proprietorship, 558, 559
Business license, 559
Business Network International (BNI), 558
Business plan, 550–551
Butterfly technique, 302

C

C corporation, 559
Caesar, Julius, 12
Calcaneus, 186, 187f
Calf
    massaging, 93, 94f–95f, 96
    petrissage, 325f
    stretch, 519–520, 521f
Cannon, Walter B., 22
Capillaries, 224
Carbohydrates, 484–485, 484f
Carbon dioxide, effect on CSF circulation,
        456–457
Cardiac muscle, 194, 195f
Cardiovascular system
    anatomy and physiology, 224–232, 225f
        arteries of importance to massage
                therapy, 229–230
        baroreceptors, 232
        blood components, 225, 229f
        blood pressure, 230, 232
        heart, 226–229, 227f, 229f, 230f, 231f
        heart rate, 232
        vessels, 224–225, 226f, 228f,
                229–230
    changes in pregnancy, 275
    effects of massage on, 115–117, 116f
Caregiver, massage for, 303
Carpal tunnel syndrome (CTS), 189, 588,
        589f, 590b
Carpals, 181, 182f
Carrier
    disease, 45
    insurance company as, 71
Cart, rolling table, 28–29, 29f
Cartilage, classification and properties, 176
Cartilaginous joints, 144
Caudal (directional term), 155
Cell membrane, 161
Cells
    description, 158, 159
    division, 161–162
    of lymphatic system, 244
    structure, 160f, 161
Cellular edema, 480
Celsus, Aulus Cornelius, 12–13, 15
Center of gravity, 89–90, 136, 146, 274
Central nervous system (CNS), 118, 232
Centrosome, 161
Cerebral palsy, 282b, 292–293, 292f
Cerebrospinal Fluid Technique Massage
        (CSFTM)
    neuropeptides, 456–457
    philosophy and science, 452–454
    procedure, 454–456
Cervical plexus, 237
Cesarean section, 279
CEUs (continuing education units), 553

Chair massage
    benefits of, 556
    corporate stress management,
            555, 555f
    marketing through, 553, 555–556, 557b
    personal care for the massage
            therapist, 556b
    sequence, 107, 108f–109f
    at sporting event, 346f
    tutorial, 556
Chairs, massage
    description, 30–31, 31f
    dolphin, 31f
Chakras, 10, 38, 470–472
Chartered Society of Massage and Medical
        Gymnastics, 17
Chartered Society of Physiotherapy, 17
Chemical name, 569
Chemoreceptors, 114b
Cherokee massage, 472–474
Chest, massage sequence, 103–104, 103f
Chewing, muscles for, 366
Chi. See Qi
Children
    in hospice, 303–304
    infant and pediatric massage, 279–287
    orphans, 282b
    special needs, 290–296
        AIDS, 296
        asthma, 295–296, 296f
        attention deficit hyperactivity
                disorder (ADHD), 294
        autism and autism spectrum
                disorders, 293–294, 293f
        benefits of massage, 290
        cerebral palsy, 292–293, 292f
        colic, 290–291, 291f
        Down's syndrome, 294–295, 294f
        hearing impairments, 295
        preterm infants, 291–292
        visual impairments, 295
China
    Longshan culture, 20
    massage in ancient, 10–11
Chinese medicine
    diagnostics, 391–392
    five element theory, 401, 404–405,
            408f, 408t
    meridian system, 394–397, 395f–407f,
            400–401
    philosophical concepts in, 390–391
    Qi (Chi), 390, 392
    yin and yang, 390, 391, 392–394, 393f,
            393t, 394t
Chiropractors, 535, 536f
Cholesterol, 485, 489
Choline, 482t
Chordae tendineae, 227
Choroid, 255
Choroid plexus, 453
Chromatin, 161
Chronic phase, 342
Circular friction, for temporomandibular
        joint dysfunction, 594f
Circular strokes, 417
Circulatory system. See Cardiovascular
        system
Circumduction, 139, 141, 142f
Clavicle, 179, 180f
Clay, 377
Cleanliness. See Hygiene
Client authority, 312

Client file
    client intake form, 56–57, 57f, 62
    corrections, 65
    documentation, 68–69
    history form, 56, 62, 65f
    insurance, 69–72, 71f
    narrative report, 66
    posttreatment assessment, 66
    postural analysis, 62–63, 62f, 63f, 64b
    SOAP notes, 63–64, 65f
Client Information/Intake form, 568f
Clients
    greeting, 56–57, 56f
    intake form, 56, 57f, 62
Clinical pathology, of the skeletal system,
        187–189, 188f–189f
Clotting, 225, 275
CNS (central nervous system), 118, 232
Co-pay, 72
Cobra (Bhujangasana), 508, 511f
Cocaine, 577
Coccyx, 182
Cochlea, 255, 256f
Cocoa butter, 274
Codes of ethics, 532–535
    American Massage Therapy Association
            (AMTA), 533b
    Associated Bodywork & Massage
            Professionals (ABMP),
            533b–534b
    International Massage Association
            (IMA), 534b
    National Certification Board for
            Therapeutic Massage and
            Bodywork (NCBTMB),
            534b–535b
    overview, 532, 535
Coenzymes, 481
Coinsurance, 72
Cold
    benefits, 376
    effects of, 343
    friction bath, 376, 376b
    hydrotherapies, 126, 127, 127f
    overview, 375–376, 376b
    stone therapy, 378, 380, 381
Cold laser, 34
Colic, 290–291, 291f
College of Swedish Massage, 19
Colon, 247–248, 248f, 489
Color, 38
Common carotid artery, 230
Communication, during massage, 60
Complete proteins, 486
Compression
    with back of fist, 86f
    description, 86
    reflexology, 421–423, 422f, 423f
    sports massage, 327, 328f
    for temporomandibular joint
            dysfunction, 594b, 594f
Compression-broadening
    for carpal tunnel syndrome, 590b
    for feet and legs, 93, 94f–95f, 96, 99, 101
    sports massage, 328, 329f
Compression-torque with thumbs, sports
            massage, 330
Compressive active movement, sports
            massage, 330
Concentric action, of muscle, 143
Conception vessel, 394, 401
Condyloid joint, 176f

Confidentiality, 51
Cong-Fou of the Tao-Tse, The, 21
Connective tissue
    biomechanics of, 143
    defined, 162–163, 162*t*
    rolling stroke for, 329*f*
Connective Tissue Massage, 444
Consent, informed, 540
Considerations, definition, 74
Constantine (Roman Emperor), 14
Constipation, 276–277
Contact dermatitis, 244
Contagious disease, 45
Contamination, 47
Contemporary Pulse Diagnosis, 391
Continuing education units (CEUs), 553
Contractions, 198–200
    all or none response, 197
    causes, 197
    effects of, 198, 200
    fast-twitch, 200
    slow-twitch, 200
    types, 198
        isokinetic, 198
        isometric, 198
        isotonic, 198
        tetanic, 198
        tonic, 198
Contracture
    in cerebral palsy, 292, 292*f*
    description, 216, 522*b*
Contraindications, 74, 75–76
Controlled drugs, 573, 576*t*
Contusion, 79, 353
Cornea, 255, 255*f*
Cornstarch, 286
Coronal plane (directional term), 156
Corporate stress management, 555, 555*f*
Corporation, 559–560
Corpse post (Savasana), 502, 502*f*, 510
Corrections, to files, 65
Cortisol, 466
Costs, start-up, 551
Countertransference, 470, 544
Coupon, 557, 557*b*
CPR (cardiopulmonary resuscitation), 41, 42*f*
Cramp, muscle
    description, 79, 216, 341
    reciprocal inhibition for alleviating,
        335, 335*f*
Crane's Neck (Qi Gong exercise), 512
Cranial (directional term), 155
Cranial cavity, 156, 156*f*, 157*t*
Cranial nerves, 236, 236*f*, 236*t*
CranioSacral Therapy (CST)
    for ADHD child, 294
    benefits of, 458–459
    overview, 457–458
    working with, 459
Creep, 442
Crèmes, 36
Cross-fiber friction, sports massage, 326, 326*f*
Cross-stretch, 86, 87*f*
Cross-striations, 196
Crown chakra (Sahasrara), 499*t*
Cryokinetic therapy, 342, 345
Cryotherapy
    cryokinetic therapy, 342, 345
    description, 342, 343–344, 375
    ice application, 344–345
    sources, 33, 33*f*
    use with Trigger Point Therapy, 429*b*

CSFTM. *See* Cerebrospinal Fluid Technique
    Massage
CST. *See* CranioSacral Therapy
CTS. *See* Carpal tunnel syndrome
Cubital tunnel syndrome, 189
Cun, 409
Cupping, 411
Cure Autism Now foundation, 293
Current Procedural Terminology, 72
Cushions, 31–32, 32*f*, 273
Cycle of infection, 45
Cyriax, Dr. James, 326
Cytoplasm, 161

D

Da Vinci, Leonardo, 154
Dance, 496*f*
Daybreak Geriatric Massage, 302
DBA (doing business as), 560
De Humani Corporus Fabrica, 154, 154*f*
De Medicina, 12–13, 15
De Sanitate Tuenda, 13
DEA (Drug Enforcement
    Administration), 573
Dead Sea mud treatment, 383
Decoction, 583*t*
Decontamination, methods of, 48
Deductible, 72
Deep femoral arteries, 230
Deep tissue massage
    physiological effects of, 125–126
    use in pregnancy, 271
Deglutition, 245
Dehydration, 480
Deltoid, anatomy, 351*f*
Dementia, 297
Dendrites, 233
Depression, 140, 140*f*, 577
Depth, stroke, 80–81
Depth of pressure, 80–81
Dermatophytes, 44
Dermis, 253–254, 254*f*
Diabetes, 241*b*
Diaphragm, action of, 205*t*
Diaphysis, 169, 169*f*
Diarthrotic joints
    description, 144
    overview, 174–175
    structure, 175
    types, 176*f*
Diets
    alternative, 491
    American, 491–492, 492*f*
Diffusion, 224
Digestion, 486–489, 487*f*
Digestive system
    anatomy and physiology, 245–248,
        245*f*–248*f*
    changes in pregnancy, 276–277
    diseases and disorders, 245
DiMauro, Carla, 282*b*
Direct or sustained pressure, sports
    massage, 327, 328*f*
Direct transmission, 46
Direction, stroke, 81
Directional terms, 76, 155
Disconnection, 312
Disempowerment, 312
Disinfection, 48
Distal (directional term), 156
Dopamine, 115

Dorsal (directional term), 156
Dorsal body cavity, 156, 156*f*, 157*t*
Dorsiflexion, 140, 141*f*
Doshas, 10–11, 38, 412, 413, 414*t*,
    415*b*, 415*f*
Down's syndrome, 294–295, 294*f*
Dragon's Head (Qi Gong exercise), 512
Draping, during massage, 58, 59*f*, 60
Draping materials, 34–35, 34*f*
Dress, 542, 542*f*
Drug Enforcement Administration
    (DEA), 573
Drugs. *See also* Medications
    classifications, 573–579
        controlled drugs, 573, 576*t*
        drug categories, table of, 574*t*–575*t*
        noncontrolled drugs, 573
        psychotropic medications, 577
        recreational drugs, 577–578, 578*f*
        topical medications, 573, 577
    definition, 573
    excretion, 573
    names, 569
    routes of administration, 570, 570*t*,
        571*f*, 572, 572*t*
    schedules, 576*t*
    sources of, 570
Dry brush exfoliation, 375
Dual relationships, 544
Dubos, Rene, 22
Dulse scrub, 375
Duodenum, 247, 247*f*
Dura mater, 440
Duration, stroke, 81
Dynamic flexibility, 522*b*
Dynamic phase, 134

E

Ear
    anatomy, 255, 256*f*
    muscles, 366
Ear pull, 106*f*
Eastern practices, 389–418
    acupressure, 405, 408–410
    amma, 411
    Ayurveda, 411–414, 413*t*, 414*t*, 415*b*, 415*f*
    Chinese medicine
        diagnostics, 391–392
        five element theory, 401, 404–405,
            408*f*, 408*t*
        meridian system, 394–397,
            395*f*–407*f*, 400–401
        philosophical concepts in, 390–391
        Qi (Chi), 390, 392
        yin and yang, 390, 391, 392–394,
            393*f*, 393*t*, 394*t*
    Cupping, 411
    Jin Shin Do, 410–411
    lomi lomi, 418
    moxibustion, 391, 411
    overview, 390
    shiatsu, 410
    Thai massage, 414, 416–418
        methodology, 417
        overview, 414, 416
        practicing and receiving, 416–417
        techniques, 417–418, 419*f*
Easy pose (Sukhasana), 502–503, 503*f*
Eating habits, 490, 490*f*
Ebers Papyri, 10
Eccentric action, of muscle, 143

Eccymosis, 339
Ectomorphy, 145
Edema
    cellular, 480
    lymphedema, 450, 452
    relief through massage, 275
EEG (electroencephalogram), 470
Effleurage
    application, 82, 82f
    for asthma in children, 295
    for back, 96, 97f, 99
    for carpal tunnel syndrome, 590b
    in Cerebrospinal Fluid Technique
        Massage (CFTM), 454
    for chest, 103, 103f
    for colic relief, 291
    considerations, 83
    definition, 81
    for feet and legs, 93, 94f–95f, 96, 99,
        100f, 101
    for fibromyalgia, 595
    for hands and arms, 101, 102f, 103
    in infant massage, 284, 285f
    for neck and head, 104–105, 105f, 106f
    physiological effects, 83
    in sports massage, 324, 325f
    for thoracic outlet syndrome, 591b
    for torticollis, 593b
Egypt, ancient, 7, 10
Elastic cartilage, 176
Elasticity, 524b
Elastocollagenous fibers, 442
Elbow
    bursae, 341
    flexion and extension, 137f
    injuries, 352
    joint anatomy, 180–181, 181f
    massage routine, 352–353
    muscles of forearm, 353f
Elbow press, 418
Elderly clients, working with, 296–298,
        297f, 298b
Electrical stimulation devices, 34
Electroencephalogram (EEG), 470
Electrolytes, 480
Elevation, 140, 140f
Elimination, 489
Elliptical training, 517f
Emotional release, 544–545
Endocardium, 227, 231f
Endochondral ossification, 168
Endocrine system
    changes in pregnancy, 274
    hormones, 238–239, 240t
    main glands, 239–241, 239f
    overview, 237–238, 238f
    pancreas, 239–241
Endomorphy, 145
Endomysium, 196, 196f
Endoplasmic reticulum, 161
Endorphins, 115
Energy levels, 470, 471f
Energy work
    description, 472
    polarity therapy, 423–424
    reflexology, 421–423, 422f, 423f
    Reiki, 418, 420–421, 421f, 421t
    for senior clients, 298b
Enkephalins, 115
Entamoeba histolytica, 45
Entrainment, 60
Entrepreneur, 548

Enveloping the body, 300f
Environment
    air circulation, 38
    color and ambience, 38
    creating warm and friendly, 36, 36f
    lighting, 37
    music, 37
    for outcalls, 38–39
    safety, 37, 39–41
    size of room, 37
    Vastu or Feng Shui, 37, 37b
Environmentally transmitted pathogen, 45
Enzymes, 481
Epicardium, 227, 231f
Epidermis, 254, 254f
Epimysium, 196
Epinephrine, 466
Epiphyseal plate (epiphysis), 169, 169f
Epithelial tissue, defined, 162t, 163
Equilibrium, 146
Equipment, 25–52
    care, 34
    chairs, 30–31, 31f
    cryotherapy sources, 33, 33f
    cushions and bolsters, 31–32, 32f
    draping materials, 34–35, 34f
    history of, 20–21
    lubricants, 35–36
    mat, massage, 30, 30f
    moist heat hydrotherapy sources,
        32–33, 33f
    oils, crèmes, lotions, and gels, 36
    sanitation of, 384
    supplemental, 34
    table, massage, 26–30, 27f–29f
    tools, massage, 33
Erector spinae, muscle test, 339
Ergonomics, 145
Erythrocytes (red blood cells), 225, 229f
Erythropoietin, 251
Escherichia coli, 47
Esophagus, 245
Essential nutrients, 479
Essential oils, 383. See also Aromatherapy
Esthetician, 362, 363
Estrogen, 274
Ether, 17
Ethics. See Codes of ethics
Europe, history of massage in
    Middle Ages, 14
    nineteenth century, 15
Eversion, 140, 142f
Excretion, drug, 573
Exercise consultation form, 523b
Exfoliation, 375
Exocrine glands, 238
Extension, 137, 137f, 138f
Extensor carpi radialis
    anatomy, 353f
    muscle test, 338
Extensor carpi ulnaris
    anatomy, 353f
    muscle test, 338
External abdominal oblique
    action of, 206t
    anatomy, 207t
External communication model, 549–550
External intercostals, action of, 205t
Exteroceptors, 114b
Extracts, 581
Eye muscles, 366
Eyes, 255, 255f, 366

F
Face
    aging, changes from, 364, 364b
    muscles of, 201, 204f, 205f, 365–367, 365f
Face cradle, 27, 35, 58
Facial massage
    overview, 367
    procedure, 367b
        cleanser removal, 369f
        cleansing, 368f
        items use, 367
        technique, 370f–371f
Fanning, sports massage, 330
Fascia
    anatomy and physiology of, 196,
        439–441, 441f
    myofascial release, 438–444, 439f, 441f
    responsiveness to energy, 435
Fasciculation, 218
Fasciculi, 196
Fast twitch muscles, 143, 200
Fatigue, muscle, 200
Fats, 485
Federation of State Massage Therapy
        Boards (FSMTB), 20, 535
Feldenkrais, 449
Female reproductive system, anatomy and
        physiology, 251–252, 252f
Femoral vein, 275
Femur
    anatomy, 184, 185f
    muscles of, 206, 209, 212f–214f, 212t
Feng Shui, 37
Fiber, 484–485, 489
Fibrillation, 218
Fibrinogen, 225
Fibrinolysis, 275
Fibrocartilage, 176, 182
Fibromyalgia, 217, 595, 595f, 596b, 596f
Fibrous joints, 144
Fibula, 184, 186f
Field, Tiffany, 20, 280
Fight-or-flight response, 119, 240, 267, 466
Fine tremulous, 86
Finger and wrist stretch, 519, 520f, 521f
Fingers
    abduction and adduction of, 139f
    bones, 181, 182f
Finish, 105
Five element theory, 401, 404–405, 408f, 408t
Fixator, 143, 198
Flat bones, structure of, 169f, 170f, 171
Flexibility, 522b
Flexion, 137, 137f, 138f
Flexor carpi radialis
    anatomy, 353f
    muscle test, 338
Flexor carpi ulnaris
    anatomy, 353f
    muscle test, 338
Flow, massage, 89
Fluffing technique, 302
Flyer, 557b
FMS (fibromyalgia syndrome), 595, 595f,
        596b, 596f
Folate (folic acid), 482t
Folic acid, 491
Fomenteks®, 32–33
Fontanels, 166
Food. See Nutrition

Food pyramid, 491–492, 492f
Foot
    bones, 186–187, 187f
    muscles of, 209, 217f
    prone massage sequence, 93–96,
        94f–95f
    reflexology, 421–423, 422f, 423f
    stretching, 333f
    supine massage sequence, 99, 100f, 101
    tripod of, 90, 92f
Foramen magnum, 178
Foramina, 178–179
Forearm
    muscles, 206, 210f, 353f
    supination and pronation of, 142f
Forearm roll, 96, 418
Forearm work, for back, 96, 97f–98f, 99
Forward Bending pose (Uttanasana),
        504, 505f
Fossae, 172, 174f
Fracture, 187, 188f
Fragrance, of essential oils, 383
Francisco, Patricia Weaver, 308
Frequency, stroke, 81
Friction
    application, 84f, 85
    for asthma in children, 295
    for carpal tunnel syndrome, 590b
    in Cerebrospinal Fluid Technique
        Massage (CFTM), 454
    considerations, 85
    definition, 84
    for feet and legs, 93, 94f, 96
    in forearm massage, 103
    physiological effects, 85
    in sports massage, 325–326, 326f
    for temporomandibular joint
        dysfunction, 594b
    for thoracic outlet syndrome, 591b
    for torticollis, 593b
Friction bath, 376, 376b
Frontal plane
    definition, 136, 156
    movements in, 138–139
Frostbite, 376
FSMTB (Federation of State Massage
        Therapy Boards), 20, 535
Functional position, 135, 135f
Fundamentals in Massage for Students of
        Nursing, 19
Fungi, 44–45

G

Gait
    abnormal, 147–148
    normal, 146–147
    phases of, 147f
Galenus, Claudius, 13, 21
Gallbladder, 246, 247f, 487f, 488
Gallbladder meridian, 396, 401, 406f
Gallstones, 489
Gastric juice, 488
Gastrocnemius muscle
    action of, 209
    anatomy, 355f
    friction stroke, 326f
    injury to, 355–356
    muscle test, 338
    reciprocal inhibition, 335f
    stretching, 332f
Gastroesophageal sphincter, 245

Gastrointestinal system, changes in
        pregnancy, 276–277
Gate theory, 114–115
Gels, 36
Gemellus inferior, action of, 212t
Gemellus superior, action of, 212t
General partnership, 559
Generic (nonproprietary) name, 569
Geriatric massage
    methodology, 297–298
    toolbox of modalities, 298b
Gestational diabetes, 241b
Giardia lamblia, 45
Glideability, 36
Gliding, along Achilles tendon, 93, 94f
Gliding joint, 176f
Gloves, 49, 49f
Glucagon, 246
Gluteals
    anatomy, 206, 212t, 213f–214f
    beating, 327f
    massaging, 95f, 96
    muscle test, 339
Glycogen, 200, 247
Goal-setting, 550–551
A God Within, 22
Golfer's elbow, 352
Golgi apparatus, 161
Golgi tendon organs, 331, 334
Golgi tendon reflex, 331, 334
Gomphosis, 173
Goniometer, 145, 146f
Gout, 187
Governing Vessel, 394, 401
Graham, Douglas, 17
Grapeseed oil, 286
Greece, massage in ancient, 11–12
Ground substance, 143
Guided imagery, 472, 473b
Gutenberg printing press, 15
Gymnasiums
    Greek, 12
    Roman, 13, 14

H

Hacking/quacking
    of leg, 96
    sports massage, 326–327, 327f
Half squats, 521, 521f
Hamstring muscles
    action of, 209
    anatomy, 356f
    compression, 328f
    injuries, 356
    massaging, 95f, 96, 356
    muscle test, 338
    stretching, 333f, 348f
    supine big toe/hamstring stretch, 502, 503f
Hand
    bones, 181, 182f
    cryotherapy, 344f
    supine massage sequence, 101, 102f, 103
Hand washing, 39, 40b
Hatha yoga, 497, 498
Hawaiian cultural medicine, 418
Hay fever, 244
HCG (human chorionic gonadotropin), 274
Head
    muscles of, 201, 204f, 205f
    supine massage sequence, 104–105,
        104f–107f

Healing Touch, 299f
Health department, 41, 43
Health insurance claim, 70
Health Insurance Portability and
        Accountability Act (HIPAA),
        532, 538–539, 539b
Hearing, 255
Hearing impaired children, massage for, 295
Heart, anatomy, 226–229, 227f, 229f–231f
Heart chakra (Anahata), 499t
Heart meridian, 396, 397, 400f
Heart rate, 232
Heartburn, 276
Heat
    effects of, 343
    heating pads, 373
    hydrotherapies, 126, 127–128, 127f
    immersion bath, 375
    infrared radiation, 373
    moist heat therapy, 345, 373
    overview, 372–373
    sauna, 374
    sources, 32–33, 33f
    steam bath, 373
    stone therapy, 378, 380, 381
    Swiss shower, 374
    transfer, 343
    types, sources, and applications, 373b
    Vichy shower, 374, 374f
    water temperatures for treatments, 375t
Heat exhaustion, 345
Heat stroke, 345
Hedge clipper action, 330, 358
Heels-to-buttocks stretch, 332f
Hellerwork, 438
Hemoglobin, 225
Hepatitis, 50–51
Herbal massage, Assyrian use of, 7
Herbal wraps, 383–384, 384b
Herbs, 580–582, 581f, 582f, 583t, 584t
Hernia, 217–218
Hinge joint, 176f
Hip
    bones, 184
    dislocation, 189
    muscles of, 206, 209, 212f–214f, 212t
    sprain, 218
Hip flexor stretch, 332f, 348f
HIPAA. See Health Insurance Portability and
        Accountability Act
Hippocrates, 11, 11f, 12
Hippocratic oath, 11
Hippocratic tradition, 11, 12, 21
History, 5–23
    ancient world, 6–13, 10f
        Asia, 10–11
        Egypt, 7, 10
        Greece, 11–12
        Mesopotamia, 7
        Rome, 12–13
    Middle Ages, 14–15
    nineteenth century, 15–18
    philosophical foundation of massage,
        21–22
    regulation of massage, 16–17
    Renaissance, 15
    timeline, 8f–9f
    twentieth century, 19–21
The History of Massage, 12
HIV (human immunodeficiency virus),
        50, 244
Hoku point, 596b

Hold harmless clause, of insurance contract, 70
Homeostasis, 22, 237
Horizontal plane, 136. *See also* Transverse plane
Hormones, 238–239, 240*t*
Hospice and palliative care, 299–304
    caregiver, massage for, 303
    children, 303–304
    indications, 300–301
    massage technique, 302–303
    overview, 299–300
    precautions, 301
    training, 301–302
Housemaid's knee, 189, 341
Hsueh, 397
Human chorionic gonadotropin (HCG), 274
Human immunodeficiency virus (HIV), 50, 244
Humerus
    anatomy, 179, 180*f*
    medial and lateral rotation of, 141*f*
Hyaline cartilage, 176
Hydrocollator, 33, 33*f*, 373
Hydrotherapy
    cold applications, 126, 127, 127*f*
    cold effects, 343
    cryotherapy, 343–345
    definition, 342
    heat applications, 126, 127–128, 127*f*
    heat effects, 343
    heat transfer, 343
    moist heat therapy, 345
    physiological effects of, 342
    in pregnancy, 269
    Swiss shower, 374
    temperature ranges for, 342, 343*t*
    Vichy shower, 374, 374*f*
    water temperatures, 375*t*
Hygiene
    decontamination methods, 48
    disease transmission, 45–48
    hand washing, 39, 40*b*
    massage room, 37, 39–41
    pathogens, 43–45
    personal, 39
Hyoid bone, 173
Hyperemia, 117
Hyperextension, 137, 138*f*
Hypertension, 116
Hyperthermia, 345
Hypertrophy, muscle, 79, 198
Hypodermis, 253, 254*f*
Hypoglycemia, 488
Hypothalamus, 480, 481*f*
Hypothermia, 346
Hysteresis, 442

I

IASI (International Association of Structural Integrators), 438
Ice
    application, 344
    cryokinetic therapy, 345
    sensations of application, 344–345
Ice packs, 33, 33*f*
Ida channel, 498
Ileocecal valve, 247, 248*f*
Ileum, 247
Iliacus, action of, 212*t*
Iliocostalis cervicis, action of, 208*t*

Iliocostalis lumborum, action of, 208*t*
Iliocostalis thoracis, action of, 208*t*
Iliopsoas stretch, 334*f*
Iliotibial tract band, muscle test, 339
Illium, 184
IMA (International Massage Association), 20, 532, 534*b*
Immersion bath, 375
Impingement syndrome, 350
Incubation period, 48
India, massage in ancient, 11
Indian milking, 283
Indications, 74–75
Indigenous massage practices, 472–474
Indigestion, 276
Indirect transmission, 46
Infant and pediatric massage, 279–287
    benefits of tactile stimulation, 279
    bonding, parent-child, 280
    as global practice, 281
    massage routine
        child, 286–287, 286*f*–287*f*
        infant, 282–286, 283*f*–285*f*
    orphan children, 282*b*
    procedure and technique, 281–282
    reciprocal interaction, 282–286
    as resource for family ties, 281
    touch deprivation, harmful effects of, 280–281
Infections
    cycle of infection, 45–46, 46*f*
    decontamination methods, 48
    entrance into host, 47
    health crises, 50–51
    incubation, 47–48
    pathogens, 43–45
    precautions, universal and standard, 48–49, 49*f*
    transmission
        airborne, 46
        blood-borne, 46–47
        direct and indirect, 46
        environmental, 45
        by ingestion, 47
        opportunistic, 45
        person-to-person contact, 45
        primary, 45
        sexual, 47
        by touch, 47
Inferior (directional term), 155
Inferior vena cava, 275
Inflammation response, 117
Informed consent, 540
Infrared radiation, 373
Infraspinatus
    anatomy, 351*f*
    massaging, 96, 98*f*
    muscle test, 337
Infusion, 583*t*
Injury
    pathology
        acute *versus* chronic phase, 341–342
        bursitis, 341
        cramps, 341
        four-step healing process, 340–341
        pain-spasm-pain cycle, 339, 341
        spasms, 341
        splinting, 339
        sprains, 339–341
        strains, 340–341
        tendonitis, 341

rehabilitative/maintenance massage, 331*b*, 347, 350–358
    anterior lower leg injuries, 354–355, 354*f*
    hamstring injuries, 356, 356*f*
    knee injuries, 358
    low back problems, 356–358, 357*f*
    posterior lower leg injuries, 355–356, 355*f*
    quadriceps injuries, 353–354, 354*f*
    shoulder injuries, 350, 351*f*, 352
    tennis and golfer's elbow, 352–353, 353*f*
    therapy
        cryotherapy, 343–345, 344*f*
        heat therapy, 345
        hydrotherapy, 342–343, 343*t*
INM. *See* Intuitive Neuromuscular Massage
Innate intelligence, 22
Insertion, 198
Insomnia, in pregnancy, 268
Insulin, 246, 484
Insurance
    business, 551, 553
    claims, filing, 69–70, 71, 71*f*
    coding, 71–72
    deductibles, co-pays, and coinsurance, 72
    terms, 70–71
Intake form, client, 56–57, 57*f*, 62
Integrity, 311
Integumentary system
    anatomy, 252–253, 253*f*, 254*f*
        dermis, 253–254, 254*f*
        epidermis, 254, 254*f*
        hypodermis, 253, 254*f*
    changes in pregnancy, 274
    functions, 253
Intent, massage therapist's, 89
Intentional Touch™, 311
Intercostals
    action of, 205*t*
    massaging, 96, 101, 101*f*
Internal abdominal oblique
    action of, 206*t*
    anatomy, 207*t*
International Association of Infant Massage, 281, 291
International Association of Structural Integrators (IASI), 438
International Classification of Diseases, Ninth Revision, Clinical Modification (ICD9-CM), 72
International Massage Association (IMA), 20, 532, 534*b*
International Spa Association, 20
Intervention, 311
Intervertebral disc, 182
Intramembranous ossification, 168
Intuitive Neuromuscular Massage (INM)
    approach, 431–433, 431*f*, 432*f*, 433*b*
    history, 430–431
    overview, 430, 430*f*, 434
Inversion, 140, 142*f*
Irregular bones, structure of, 170*f*, 171
Ischemia, 341
Ischium, 184
Isokinetic contraction, 198
Isometric contraction, 143, 198
Isotonic contraction, 198

IT band
    massage of, 358
    syndrome, 354

J

Jack hammer's shoulder, 341
Jejunum, 247, 247f
Jensen, Kathryn, 19
Jin Shin Do, 410–411
John F. Barnes Myofascial Release
        Approach, 438–439, 439f
Joint movements, use in pregnancy, 271
Joints. *See also specific joints*
    biomechanical properties of, 144–145
    classification
        amphiarthrotic, 173–174
        diarthrotic (synovial), 174–175, 176f
        synarthrotic, 173, 175f
Jones, Dr. Lawrence, D.C., 336
Jumper's knee, 354

K

Kahun Medical Papyrus, 10
Kellogg, John Harvey, 18, 19f
Keratin, 254
Ki, 22
Kidney meridian, 396, 400, 403f
Kidneys, 250–251, 251f
Kinematics, 134, 145
Kinetics, 134, 145–146
Kneading, 324. *See also* Petrissage
Knee
    anatomy, 186, 186f
    bursae, 341
    injuries, 358
    massage routine, 358
    sprains, 340
Knee flexion/calf stretch, 519–520, 521f
Knee/Head pose (Janu Sirsasana), 508, 509f
Knee press, 418, 419f
Knee-to-chest stretch, 332f
Knobbles, 33
Knuckling, sports massage, 330, 330f
Kundalini energy, 500
Kupffer's cells, 246
Kyphosis, 59b, 59f, 187, 189f

L

Labor, 278–279
Lacteals, 244
Lactic acid, 200, 323
Lantry, Heather, 302
Large intestine, 247–248, 248f, 487f, 489
Large Intestine meridian, 395, 397, 397f
Larynx, 249, 249f
Laser, cold, 34
Lateral (directional term), 156
Lateral bend (Parvatasana in Tadasana), 504
Lateral bending, 140
Lateral flexion, 140, 591b
Lateral glide, for temporomandibular joint
        dysfunction, 594b
Lateral rotation, 140, 141f
Lateral rotators, muscle test, 339
Laws governing massage, 532, 535
Laxity, 340
LDL (low-density cholesterol), 485

LDT. *See* Lymphatic Drainage Therapy
Leasing office space, 551
Leg
    bones, 184–187, 185f–187f
    clots in vessels, 275
    cryotherapy, 344f
    injuries
        anterior lower leg, 354–355, 354f
        hamstring, 356, 356f
        knee, 358
        posterior lower leg, 355–356, 355f
        quadriceps, 353–354, 354f
    muscles of, 209, 213f–216f
    prone massage sequence, 93–96, 94f–95f
    supine massage sequence, 99, 100f, 101
Leukocytes (white blood cells), 225, 229f
Levator scapulae, massaging, 98f, 99, 104f
Lever, 246–247, 247f
License, business, 559
License massage practitioners (LMP), 532
License massage therapists (LMT), 532
Lifting techniques, proper, 148, 149f
Ligaments
    healing, 340
    in pregnancy, 278
    sprains, 339–340
Lighting, massage room, 37
Limbs, abduction and adduction of, 139f
Limited liability corporation (LLC), 559
Limited partnership, 559
Linea alba, separation of, 274
Linens, 35
Ling, Per Henrik, 15–16, 16f, 80
Liniment, 583t
Lipids, 485, 485f
Liver, 487f, 488, 489
Liver meridian, 396, 401, 407f
LLC (limited liability corporation), 559
LMP (license massage practitioners), 532
LMT (license massage therapists), 532
Lomi-balls, 21
Lomi lomi, 6, 418
Lomi-lomi sticks, 21
Long bones, structure of, 169, 169f, 170f, 171
Longissimus cervicis, action of, 208t
Longissimus thoracis, action of, 208t
Longitudinal axis, 140
Lordosis, 59b, 59f, 187, 189f
Lotions, 36
Low-density cholesterol (LDL), 485
Lubricants
    storage, 36
    types, 35–36
Lumbar plexus, 237
Lumbosacral stretch, 270, 270f, 349f
Lung meridian, 395, 396f, 397
Lungs, 249f–250f
Lying spinal twist (Bharadjasana), 509, 511f
Lying spinal twist stretch, 333f, 348f
Lymph, 242
Lymph nodes, 242–243, 245
Lymphadenitis, 245
Lymphangioscintigraphy, 452
Lymphatic drainage, for senior clients, 298b
Lymphatic Drainage Therapy (LDT),
        449–452
    areas of application, 451–452
    benefits of, 450–451
    how it is performed, 450
    importance of lymph drainage, 449
    Manual Lymphatic Mapping (MLM), 452
    overview, 449–450, 450f

Lymphatic system, 241–245
    cells, 244
    digestive system and, 244
    diseases of, 244–245
    effect of massage on, 118
    function, 117–118, 118f
    lymph, 242
    lymph nodes, 242–243
    lymphatic vessels, 242, 243f
    in pregnancy, 267
    overview, 24f, 241–242
    sking and, 244
    spleen, 243–244
    thymus gland, 244
    tonsils, 243
Lymphedema, 450, 452
Lymphocytes, 244
Lymphofascia Release, 451
Lymphoma, 245
Lysol®, 48
Lysosomes, 161
Lysozyme, 245

M

Male reproductive system, anatomy and
        physiology, 251–252, 252f
Malocclusion, 593
Manipura, 470, 471
Mantra, 470–471
Manual lymph drainage massage,
        physiological effects of, 126
Manual Lymphatic Mapping (MLM), 452
Manual medicine, 6
*Manual Therapeutics, A Treatise on Massage:
        Its History, Mode of
        Application, and Effects,* 17
Maori massage, 6
Marijuana, 578
Marketing, 553–558
    brochures, 553, 555f
    business cards, 553, 555f
    coupons, 557, 557f
    networking, 558
    professionalism, 540
    résumé, 553, 554f
    through chair massage, 553,
            555–556, 557b
    via local media, 557–558
Martial arts movements, 496f, 516f–517f
Masks, 377
Massage and Therapeutic Exercise, 19
Massage table. *See* Table, massage
Massage therapy, biomechanics of, 149–150
Mastication
    description, 245
    muscles of, 366
Mat
    massage, 30, 30f
    yoga, 501
Maternity massage, 266–279
    benefits of, 268–269
    contraindications and precautions,
            270–271
        abdominal massage, 270
        deep tissue techniques, 271
        joint movements, 271
        reflex massage, 270–271
        Swedish massage, 271
    high-risk pregnancies, 271
    hydrotherapy, 269

labor, 278–279
overview, 266
pain reduction, techniques for, 269–270
physiological changes, 267–269
postpartum, 279
system changes massage
circulatory, 275
endocrine, 274
gastrointestinal, 276–277
integumentary, 274
musculoskeletal, 277–278
respiratory, 275–276
urinary, 276–277
trimester positioning and
recommendations
first trimester, 271–272
second trimester, 272–273,
272f, 273f
third trimester, 273
McClure, Vimala Schneider, 281, 282, 285, 291
McMillan, Mary, 19
Mechanoreceptors, 115
Medial (directional term), 156
Medial rotation, 140, 141f
Median nerve, 590
Median plane (directional term), 156
Medical massage, 537–538
Medical terminology
abbreviations and acronyms, 66–67
prefixes, suffixes, and root words, 67–68
Medical wellness spas, 362
Medications, 565–586
body's response to, 568f, 569
classifications, 573–579
controlled drugs, 573, 576t
drug categories, table of, 574t–575t
noncontrolled drugs, 573
psychotropic medications, 577
recreational drugs, 577–578, 578f
topical medications, 573, 577
contraindication, 578–579
guide, 583b
herbs, 580–582, 581f, 582f, 583t, 584t
listing on Client Information/Intake
form, 568f
over-the-counter (OTC), 567, 576f
overview, 566
pharmacokinetics, 567, 572
pharmacology
basics, 567
branches, 567
terminology, 569
routes of administration, 570, 570t,
571f, 572, 572t
sources of, 570
vitamins and minerals, 579–580, 579f
Meditation
description, 468–470, 469f
yoga, 498, 500–501, 501f
Medullary cavity, 169f, 171
Meiosis, 162
Meissner's corpuscles, 80, 257
Melissa supreme, 294
Membranes, 157t
Memory dissociation, 443
Meninges, 454
Meniscus, 186, 186f, 358
MENTASTICS®, 445–446
Meridians
anatomical position, 395f
Conception Vessel (Ren), 394, 401
energy flow, timing of, 395–397

Gallbladder, 396, 401, 406f
Governing Vessel (Du), 394, 401
Heart, 396, 397, 400f
in Jin Shin Do, 411
Kidney, 396, 400, 403f
Large Intestine, 395, 397, 397f
Liver, 396, 401, 407f
Lung, 395, 396f, 397
overview, 394
Pericardium, 396, 400, 404f
Small Intestine, 396, 400, 401f
Spleen, 395, 397, 399f
Stomach, 395, 397, 398f
Triple heater (San jiao), 396, 400, 405f
Urinary Bladder, 396, 400, 402f
Mesomorphy, 145
Mesopotamia, 7
Metabolism, 114
Metacarpals, 181, 182f
Metaphysics, 21
Meth, 577
Metu, 7
Mezger, Johann, 80
Micronutrients, 481, 578, 578f, 579
Microorganisms, 46
Microvilli, 488
Middle deltoid, muscle test, 337
Midsagittal plane, 155f, 156
Midwives, 14
Miesler, Dietrich W., 302
Might Stance (Utkatasana), 504–505, 505f
Milking. See Petrissage
Mind-body connection, 119
Minerals, 484, 580
Miscarriage, risk of, 269, 271
Mitochondria, 161
Mitosis, 161–162
Mitral (bicuspid) valve, 227, 229, 231f
MLM (Manual Lymphatic Mapping), 452
Modalities
Alexander Technique, 449
Bindegewebmassage, 444
Cerebrospinal Fluid Technique Massage
(CFTM), 452–457, 454f
CranioSacral Therapy (CST), 457–459
Feldenkrais, 449
Hellerwork, 438
Intuitive Neuromuscular Massage
(INM), 430–434, 430f, 431f,
432f, 433b
Lymphatic Drainage Therapy (LDT),
449–452
Myofascial Release, 438–444, 439f, 441f
neuromuscular massage therapy, 429
rolfing, 434–438, 436f
Trager, 444–448, 445f
Trigger Point Therapy, 428–429, 429b
Moist heat
hydrotherapy sources, 32–33, 33f
packs, 373
therapy, 345
Molds, 44
Money sign, 329, 592b, 593b, 594b
Montague, Ashley, 20, 22
Morning sickness, 268, 271, 276
Moshou, 21
Motor/efferent nerves, 237
Motor unit, 197
Mountain pose (Tadasana), 503–504, 504f
Mouth
digestion in, 486, 487f
muscles, 365–366

Movement, eastern and western principles
of, 495–526
Moxibustion, 391, 411
Mucin, 245
Mud, 377–378, 383
Muladhara, 470
Multidimensional relationships, 544
Multifidus, action of, 209t
Multiple sclerosis, 216
Murrell, William, 16
Muscle(s). See also Muscular system;
specific muscles
biomechanics of, 143–144
for chewing (mastication), 366
ear, 366
eye, 366
facial, 365–367, 365f
mouth, 365–366
neck, 365
nose, 366
scalp, 367
spasm, 78–79, 84, 341, 432f, 433
strength, 514, 517, 518f
tears, 217
tissue, defined, 162t, 163
Muscle testing
biceps brachii, 337
description, 337
erector spinae, 339
extensor carpi radialis, 338
extensor carpi ulnaris, 338
flexor carpi radialis, 338
flexor carpi ulnaris, 338
gastrocnemius, 338
gluteals, 339
hamstrings, 338
hip rotators, 339
iliotibial tract band, 339
infraspinatus, 337
middle deltoid, 337
pronator, 338
quadratus lumborum, 339
quadriceps, 338
soleus, 338
subscapularis, 337
supinator, 338
supraspinatus, 337
tensor fasciae latae, 339
teres minor, 337
tibialis anterior and posterior, 338
Muscular dystrophy, 214
Muscular rheumatism, 216
Muscular system, 193–218
anatomy, 194, 195f, 196–197, 196f
anterior aspect, 202f
arm muscles, 206, 210f, 211f
face and head muscles, 201, 203f, 205f
foot muscles, 209, 217f
hip and femur muscles, 206, 209,
212f, 212t, 213f, 214f
leg muscles, 209, 213f, 214f, 215f, 216f
posterior aspect, 203f
torso muscles, 201, 205t, 206, 206t,
207f, 208f, 208t, 209t
attachments, 200–201
contractions, 198–200
effects of, 198, 200
fast-twitch, 200
slow-twitch, 200
types, 198
functions, 197–198
massage effects on, 123

Muscular system (continued)
movement terminology, 198
naming muscles, 198, 199t
palpation, 217b
pathologies, 214–218
properties of muscle cells, 197
role of, 122–123
Musculoskeletal system
changes in pregnancy, 277
injuries, prevention of, 148, 149f
Music, massage room, 37
Myalgia, 216
Myasthenia gravis, 215
Mycobacterium tuberculosis, 51
Myocardium, 227, 231f
Myofascial Release
development of approach, 438–439, 439f
fascia
anatomy and physiology,
439–441, 441f
function, 441–442
technique for facilitation of a release,
443–444
unwinding, 443
Myofascial unwinding, 443
Myosin, 196–197
Myositis, 216
Myositis ossificans, 189, 353
Myostatic contracture, 522b

N

Nadi Sodhna, 499
Nadis, 498
Narrative report, 66, 66b
National Certification Board for
Therapeutic Massage and
Bodywork (NCBTMB), 532,
534b–535b
Native American practices, 472–474
Neck
massaging, 99
muscles, 365
rotation of, 141f
supine massage sequence, 104–105,
104f–107f
Neck stretch, lateral, 107f
Neck traction, 106f, 591b, 591f
Negative behavioral patterns, 308
Nei Jing, 10
Nephrons, 251
Nerve proteins, 456–457
Nerve stroke, 86
Nerve tissue, defined, 162t, 163
Nervous system
anatomy and physiology, 232–237, 232f
autonomic nervous system (ANS), 232
brain, 237
central nervous system (CNS), 232
cranial nerves, 236, 236f, 236t
overview, 232–233
parasympathetic pathways, 235f
peripheral nervous system (PNS), 232
spinal nerves, 233f, 237
sympathetic pathways, 234f
autonomic nervous system (ANS)
parasympathetic branch, 119, 119b,
121f, 235f, 267
sympathetic branch, 119, 119b,
120f, 234f
massage effects on, 122

reflex mechanisms, 123–124, 123f
role of, 118
Networking, 558
Neuromuscular massage. *See also*
Intuitive Neuromuscular
Massage (INM)
description, 429
physiological effects of, 125
Neuromuscular Therapist (NMT), 536
Neurons, 233
Neuropeptides, 456–457, 466
Niacin, 481t
Nicolas V, Pope, 15
Nicotine, 578, 578f
NMT (Neuromuscular Therapist), 536
Nociceptors, 114b, 115
Noncomedogenic lubricants, 35–36
Noncontrolled drugs, 573
Nose
anatomy, 256–257
muscles, 366
Nuad Bo-Rarn. *See* Thai massage
Nucleolus, 161
Nucleus, 161
Nutrients
definition, 479
essential, 479
micronutrients, 481
Nutrition, 477–494
body mass index (BMI), 493b
carbohydrates, 484–485, 484f
classes of nutrients, 478t–479t
diets
alternative, 491
American, 491–492, 492f
digestion, absorption, and metabolism,
486–489, 487f
elimination, 489
essential nutrients, 479
fats and lipids, 485, 485f
micronutrients, 481, 579
minerals, 484, 580
mind, food and, 490–491
pathology, 489–490, 490f
proteins, 486, 486f
satiety, 481f
vitamins, 481, 481t–483t, 579–580, 579f
water, 479–481

O

Obturator externus, action of, 212t
Obturator internus, action of, 212t
Occupational Safety and Health
Administration (OSHA),
43, 48
Ohashiatsu, in pregnancy, 277
Oils
herbal, 581, 583t
massage, 36
plant, 485f
use in infant massage, 286
Olecranon bursitis, 189
Olfactory sense, 256–257, 257f
"Open a book" move, 283
Opportunistic infection, 50
Opportunistically transmitted pathogen, 45
Oral tradition, 6
Organ systems
cardiovascular, 224–232
digestive, 245–248

endocrine, 237–241
integumentary, 252–254
lymphatic, 241–245
muscular, 193–218
nervous, 232–237
reproductive, 251–252
respiratory, 248–250
senses, 254–258
skeletal, 163–189
urinary, 250–251
Organelles, 161
Organs, 158, 163
Origin, 198
OSHA (Occupational Safety and Health
Administration), 43, 48
Ossicles, auditory, 255, 256f
Ossification, 166, 168
Osteoarthritis, 187
Osteoblasts, 168, 170f
Osteoclasts, 168–169, 170f
Osteocytes, 168–169, 170f
Osteomalacia, 216
Osteoporosis, 187
Out-calls, 540–541, 541b
Ovaries, 239f, 241
Over-the-counter (OTC) medications,
567, 576f
Overload principle, 514
Overstretching, 522b

P

Pacinian corpuscles, 257
Pain
perception, 114–115
reduction in pregnancy, 269–270
referred (or radiating), 428
Pain-spasm-pain cycle, 339, 341
Palliative care, 299. *See also* Hospice and
palliative care
Palm pressing, 417
PALPATE acronym, 79
Palpation, 76–80
bony landmarks, 171–172, 172b
chair massage, 217b
contusion, 79
cramps, 79
methodology, 79–80
muscle atrophy, 79
muscle hypertrophy, 79
overview, 76, 78
spasm, 78–79
strains, 79
table massage, 217b
Pancreas, 239f, 240–241, 246, 247f, 487f, 488
Panthothenic acid, 482t
Papyrus, 7
Parafango, 377–378, 379b, 380f
Paraffin, 377, 378b
Parallel muscles, 143
Paranasal sinuses, 249
Paraspinals
direct pressure on, 328f
massaging, 96, 97f
palm press, 349f
Parasympathetic system, 119, 119b, 121f,
235f, 267
Parathyroid gland, 239t, 240
Pare, Ambrose, 15
Paresthesia, 588
Parkinson's disease, 216

Partnership, 559
Passive flexibility, 522b
Passive range of motion (PROM), 336, 336t
Patella, 184, 185f, 186
Patella tendinitis, 354
Patella tendon rupture, 353
Pathogens, 43–45
Pathologies
    massage routines for, 587–597
        carpal tunnel syndrome (CTS), 588,
            589f, 590b
        fibromyalgia, 595, 595f, 596b, 596f
        overview, 588
        temporomandibular joint
            dysfunction, 593, 594b, 594f
        thoracic outlet syndrome (TOS), 590,
            591b–592b, 591f, 592, 592f
        torticollis, 592, 593b
    of muscular system, 214–218
Payment, 61
Pectoral girdle, 179, 179f, 180f
Pectoralis
    massage, 103–104, 103f
    stretch, 332f
Pediatric massage. See Infant and pediatric
        massage
Pelvic cavity, 156, 156f, 157t
Pelvic tilts, 276
Pelvis
    bones, 184
    comparison of the male and female,
        166, 166f
Pennate muscles, 143
Peppermint oil, 58
Pepsin, 246, 487
Percolation, 583t
Pericardial cavity, 156f, 157t
Pericardium, 227, 231f
Pericardium meridian, 396, 400, 404f
Perimysium, 196
Periosteum, 169f, 171
Peripheral nervous system (PNS), 118, 232
Peristalsis, 101, 245, 276
Person-to-person contact, 45
Personalization, 544
Pervasive developmental delay:not otherwise
        specified (PDD:NOS), 293
Pes planus, 187
Petrissage
    application, 83f, 84
    back, 96
    in Cerebrospinal Fluid Technique
        Massage (CFTM), 454
    considerations, 84
    definition, 83
    for feet and legs, 93, 94f, 96, 99, 100f
    for hands and arms, 101, 103
    physiological effects, 84
    in sports massage, 324–325, 325f
    for thoracic outlet syndrome, 591b
Peyer's patches, 244
Phagocytosis, 243, 246
Phalanges, 181, 182f, 187
Phalen's Test, 588, 589f
Pharmacodynamics, 567
Pharmacognosy, 567
Pharmacokinetics, 567, 572
Pharmacology. See also Medications
    basics, 567
    branches of, 567
    definition, 567
    terminology, 569

Pharmacotherapeutics, 567
Pharynx, 245, 249, 249f
Philosophical foundation of massage, 21–22
Photoreceptors, 114b
Physiological effects, 113–128
    on body systems, 115–123
        cardiovascular system, 115–117, 116f
        lymphatic system, 117–118, 118f
        nervous system, 118–122, 119b,
            120f–121f
    chemical, 114
    hydrotherapy, 126–128, 127f
        cold applications, 126, 127, 127f
        heat applications, 126, 127–128, 127f
    of massage techniques, 125–126
        eastern techniques, 126
        western techniques, 125–126
            deep tissue massage, 125–126
            manual lymph drainage
                massage, 126
            neuromuscular massage, 125
            Swedish massage, 125
    mechanical, 114–115
    pain perception, 114–115
    reflex mechanisms, 123–124, 124f
    reflexive response, 115
Physiology, definition, 154
Phytoceuticals, 580
Picket fence movement, 593b
Pillow, 35
Pincher palpation
    sports massage, 329
    for temporomandibular joint
        dysfunction, 594b
    for thoracic outlet syndrome, 592b, 592f
    for torticollis, 593b, 593f
Pineal gland, 239f, 241
Pingala channel, 498
Pinocytic vesicles, 161
Piriformis, action of, 212t
Pituitary gland, 237, 239, 239t
Pivot joint, 176f
Placebo, 467–468
Placebo effect, 468
Planes, anatomical reference, 135–136, 135f
Plantar flexion, 140, 141f
Plasma, 225
Plasticity, 524b
Platelets, 225, 229f
Pleural cavity, 156f, 157t
Plexus, 237
PNF (proprioceptive neuromuscular
        facilitation), sports massage,
        331, 334f
PNS (peripheral nervous system), 118, 232
Points of attachment, muscle, 200–201
Polarity therapy, 423–424
Polynesia, 6
Positional release, sports massage, 336
Positioning, during the massage, 58, 60
Post-traumatic stress disorder (PTSD), 311
Postdelivery massage, 279
Posterior (directional term), 156
Postevent massage, 324, 331b, 347
Postural analysis, 62–63, 62f, 63f, 64b
Postural deviations, bolstering for, 59b,
        59f, 60
Postural retraining, in pregnancy, 276
Posture
    during chair massage, 556b
    definition, 146
    maintaining good, 148

Poultice, 583t
Power Yoga, 497, 498
Prakruti, 412, 413t
Prana, 22, 390, 498
Pranayama, 498
Prayer on forehead, 105, 107f
Prayer stroke, sports massage, 330
Preauthorization, 70
Precautions, universal and standard,
        48–49, 49f
Preevent massage, 324, 331b, 346–347
Prefixes, 67–68
Pregnancy. See also Maternity massage
    high-risk, 271
    labor, 278–279
    miscarriage risk, 269, 271
    physiological changes of, 267–268
    postdelivery massage, 279
    system changes during, 274–278
Pregnancy cushions, 31, 32f
Pregnant women, bolsters for, 60
Preterm infants, 291–292
Prevention/Protection, Rest, Ice,
        Compression, and Elevation
        (PRICE), 341
Primary respiratory mechanism, 455
Prime mover, 198
Privacy, right to, 538–540, 538f, 539b
Professional corporation, 560
Professionalism
    appearance, 542–543, 542f
    codes of ethics, 532, 533b–535b, 535
    demeanor, 543
    emotional release, 544–545
    for female therapists, 542
    informed consent, 540
    for male therapists, 541–542
    marketing and advertising, 540
    multidimensional relationships, 544
    office location, 540
    out-calls, 540–541, 541b
    personal boundaries, 543–544
    professional boundaries, 543
    right of refusal, 540
    right to privacy, 538–540, 538f, 539b
    scope of practice, 535–540, 537f,
        538f, 539b
Progesterone, 274, 275
Prolapsed disc, 189
PROM (passive range of motion), 336, 336t
Pronation, 140, 142f
Pronator
    muscle test, 338
    in tennis elbow, 352
Prone, table massage sequence, 93–99,
        93f–95f, 97f–98f
Prone position, 88
Proprioceptive neuromuscular facilitation
        (PNF), sports massage,
        331, 334f
Proprioceptors, 114b
Prostitution, 13, 16
Proteins, 486, 486f
Protoplasm, 158
Protozoa, 45
Protraction, 139
Proximal (directional term), 156
Psoas major, action of, 212t
Psychoneuroimmunology, 466
Psychotropic drugs, 577
PTSD (post-traumatic stress disorder), 311
Ptyalin, 487

Pubis, 184
Pulmonary trunk, 228–229
Pulmonary valve, 227, 228, 231f

Q

Qi (Chi), 10, 22, 390, 392, 513–514
Qi Gong, 512
Quacking, 96, 326–327, 327f, 417
Quadratus femoris, action of, 212t
Quadratus lumborum
    action of, 209t
    massaging, 96, 97f
    muscle test, 339
Quadriceps
    action of, 209
    anatomy, 354f
    injuries, 353–354
    massage routine, 354
    massaging, 99, 100f
    muscle test, 338

R

Radiating pain, 428
Radicular nerve, 590
Radius, 179–180, 181f
Range of motion (ROM), 271, 335–336,
    336f, 336t
Rawlins, Maude, 19
Receptors, sensory, 114b
Reciprocal inhibition, 335, 335f
Reciprocal interaction, in infant massage,
    282–286
Recreational drugs, 577–578, 578f
Rectum, 248, 248f
Rectus abdominis
    action of, 206t
    anatomy, 207t
Rectus femoris
    anatomy, 354f
    strain, 353
Red blood cells (RBCs), 225, 229f
Referrals, from medical professionals, 68
Referred pain, 258, 258f, 428
Reflex arcs, 237
Reflex massage, in pregnancy, 270–271
Reflex mechanisms of massage, 123–124, 123f
Reflexive response, 115
Reflexology, 283, 421–423, 422f, 423f
Regulated massage therapist (RMT), 532
Regulation, in nineteenth century, 16–17
Reiki
    levels, 420
    overview, 418, 420, 421f, 472
    symbols and meanings, 421t
Relaxation
    body-mind connection, 468–472
    parasympathetic system and, 267
    visualization/guided imagery technique
        for, 473b
Relaxation response, 468
Relaxin, 274, 277, 278
Release
    emotional, 544–545
    myofascial, 438–444, 439f, 441f
    somatoemotional, 457
Renaissance, 15
Renin, 251

Renting office space, 551
Respiration
    definition, 249
    muscles of, 201, 205t
    processes, 250
Respiratory system
    anatomy and physiology, 248–250,
        249f–250f
    changes in pregnancy, 275–276
Rest, Ice, Compression, and Elevation
    (RICE), 341
Résumé, 553, 554f
Retina, 255
Retinaculum, 590b
Retraction, 139
Retraumatization, 316
Rett's disorder, 293
Rhabdomyosarcoma, 215
Rheumatoid arthritis, 187, 188f
Rhomboids, massaging, 96, 97f
Rhythm, stroke, 81
Rib cage, 181–182
Riboflavin, 481t
RICE (Rest, Ice, Compression, and
    Elevation), 341
Rickets, 187
Right of refusal, 540
Right to privacy, 538–540, 538f, 539b
Rigor mortis, 218b
RMT (regulated massage therapist), 532
Rocking, 86, 328
Rolfing
    goal of structural integration, 435–436
    history, 434–435
    sessions, 436–437
    training, 437–438
Rollers, wooden, 33
ROM. See Range of motion
Rome, massage in ancient, 12–13
Roofer's knee, 189
Root/Base chakra (Muladhara), 499, 499t
Root words, 67–68
Rotational movements, 139–140
Rotator cuff injury, 218
Rotator cuff tendinitis, 350
Roth, Mathias, 20
Routes of administration, 570, 570t, 571f,
    572, 572t
Ruffini's corpuscles, 257
Rugae, 246, 246f
Runner's knee, 354

S

S corporation (Subchapter S
    corporation), 560
Sacral plexus, 237
Sacral/Splenic chakra (Svadisthana), 499t
Sacroiliac joint, 278
Sacrum, 182
Saddle joint, 176f
Safety
    accidental injury reports, 43
    CPR, 41, 42f
    decontamination methods, 48
    disease transmission, 45–48
    first aid, basic, 41
    hand washing, 39, 40
    health crises, 50–51
    health department criteria, 41, 43

    massage room, 37, 39–41
    pathogens, 43–45
    personal hygiene, 39
    precautions, universal and standard,
        48–49, 49f
Sagittal plane
    definition, 136, 156
    movements in, 137
Sahasrard, 471
Saliva, 245, 256, 487
Salivary glands, 245
Salt glow, 375
Salt rub, 375
Sanitariums, 17–18
Sanitation, 48, 384
Sarcolemma, 196, 196f
Sarcomere, 197
SARS (severe acute respiratory syndrome), 51
Sartorius, action of, 209
Satiety, 480f
Sauna, 374
Sawing technique, 276
Scalenes
    massaging, 104f
    stretching, 334f
Scalp
    massage, 106f, 371, 372f
    muscles, 367
Scapula
    anatomy, 179, 179f
    elevation and depression of, 140f
    massaging, 96, 97f
Scar Release Therapy, 451
Schedule C tax form, 559
Schedule K-1 (form 1065), 559
Schedule SE tax form, 559
Sciatic nerve, pressure on during
    pregnancy, 268
Sciatica, 357
Sclera, 255
Scoliosis, 59b, 59f, 187, 189f
Scope of practice
    medical massage, 537–538
    outside of, 537, 537f
    overview, 535–536
    right to privacy, 538–540, 538f, 539b
    working within, 536–537
Scotch hose, 375
Sea mud, 377–378
Seated spinal twist (Bharadjasana),
    507–508, 508f
Semicircular canals, 255, 256f
Semilunar valves, 227, 231f
Semireclining position, in maternity
    massage, 272f, 273, 275
Sen, 416
Senses, 254–258
    balance, 255
    hearing, 255
    referred pain, 258, 258f
    smell, 256–257, 257f
    taste, 255–256
    touch, 257
    vision, 255
Sensory/afferent nerves, 237
Sensory receptors, 114b
Sequence, massage. See also specific techniques
    overview, 88–89
    table
        overview, 92–93
        prone, 93–99, 93f

back, 96, 97f–98f, 99
feet and legs, 93, 94f–95f, 96
supine
abdominals and intercostals, 101, 101f
chest, 103–104, 103f
feet and legs, 99, 100f, 101
hands and arms, 101, 102f, 103
neck and head, 104–105, 104f–107f
turning the client, 99
Serotonin, 115
Serratus posterior inferior, action of, 208t
Serratus posterior superior, action of, 208t
Sesamoid bones, structure of, 171
Session, massage therapy, 55–72
bolstering for postural deviations, 59, 59f, 60
communicating during massage, 60
completion of massage, 60–61, 61f
draping and positioning, 58, 59f, 60
greeting the client, 56–57, 56f
history form, 56, 62, 65f
intake form, 56–57, 57f, 62
Seven aural planes, 470, 471f
Severe acute respiratory syndrome (SARS), 51
Sexual abuse. See Abuse, survivors of sexual
Sexually transmitted diseases (STDs), 47
Shaking, 86, 328
Shamans, 7, 473f
Share personal information, 538f, 540
Shea butter, 274
Sheets, 35
Shiatsu, 15, 126, 410
Shin splints, 189, 354–355
Short bones, structure of, 170f, 171
Shoulder
anatomy, 179, 180f
bursae, 341
hyperextension and flexion, 138f
injuries, 350
massage routines, 350, 352
muscles, 351f
Shoulder shrugs, 519, 520f
Shoulder stretch, 519, 520f
Siberian ritual for healing, 473f
Side-lying position, in maternity massage, 272, 273, 273f, 275
Simispinalis cervicis, action of, 209t
Simispinalis thoracis, action of, 209t
Sinuses, 178–179
SITS (supraspinatus, infraspinatus, teres minor, and subscapularis) muscles, 350
Skeletal muscle, 76–80, 194, 195f, 196–197, 196f
Skeletal system
adult skeleton, 167f
arm and hand bones, 179–181, 180f, 181f, 182f
articulation, 173
bone formation and growth, 168–169, 170f
bony markings and landmarks, 172–173, 174f
cartilage classification and properties, 176
classification
flat bones, 169f, 170f, 171
irregular bones, 170f, 171
long bones, 169, 169f, 170f, 171

sesamoid bones, 171
short bones, 170f, 171
clinical pathology, 187–189, 188f, 189f
function, 166–168
gender and age differences, 166, 166f
joints
amphiarthrotic, 173–174
diarthrotic (synovial), 174–175, 176f
synarthrotic, 173, 175f
legs, 184–187, 185f, 186f, 187f
overview, 163–165, 163f, 167f
palpation, 171–172, 172b
pectoral girdle, 179, 179f, 180f
pelvis, 184
rib cage, 181–182
skull, 165f, 176–179, 177f, 178f
spine, 182–183, 183f, 184f
table of bones, 164t
Skin, immune response and, 244
Skin rolling
description, 86, 87f
sports massage, 328, 329f
for temporomandibular joint dysfunction, 594b
Skull
divisions, 177–178
overview, 176–177, 177f
sinuses, 178–179
sutures, 178, 178f
Sleeping habits, 148
Sliding filament theory, 197
Slow twitch muscles, 143, 200
Small Business Administration, 548
Small intestine, 247, 247f, 487–488
Small Intestine meridian, 396, 400, 401f
Smell, 256–257, 257f
Smoking, 578, 578f
Smooth (visceral) muscle, 194, 195f
SOAP notes, 63–64, 65f
Society of Trained Masseuses, 17
Solar Plexus chakra (Manipura), 499, 499t
Sole proprietorship, 558–559
Soleus
action of, 209
injury to, 355–356
muscle test, 338
Soma, 123
Somasomatic reflex, 124
Somatic (voluntary) nerves, 237
Somatic pathway, 124f
Somatoemotional release, 457
Somatotyping, 145
Somatovisceral reflex, 124
Spa therapy, 361–384
allergies, treating clients with, 384
aromatherapy, 382–383
cold applications, 375–376, 375t, 376b
face massage, 364–367, 364b, 367b, 368f–371f
heat applications, 372–375, 373b, 374f, 375t
herbal wraps, 383–384, 384b
masks, 377
parafango, 377–378, 379b, 380f
paraffin treatments, 377, 378b
rules for success, 363, 363b
sanitation of equipment, 384
scalp massage, 371, 372f
stone therapy, 363, 378, 380–382, 380f, 381f, 382f
Swedish massage, 363

types of spas, 362–363
cruise ship/resort, 363
day, 363
fitness and beauty, 363
medical, 362
weight-loss, 363
Spasm, muscle, 78–79, 84, 341, 432f, 433
Special needs children. See Children, special needs
Speed, stroke, 81
Spheno-basilar junction, 455
Sphygmomanometer, 230
Spinal cord, 233
Spinal nerves, 233f, 237
Spinalis cervicis, action of, 208t
Spinalis thoracis, action of, 208t
Spine
extension and flexion, 138f
regions, 157t
rotation of, 141f
vertebrae, 182–183, 183f, 184f
Spleen, 243–244
Spleen meridian, 395, 397, 399f
Splinting, 339
Spores, mold, 44
Sports massage, 321–359
applications, 323
contraindications, 324
defined, 322–323
at events, 346–347, 348f–349f
postevent massage, 324, 331b, 347
preevent massage, 324, 331b, 346–347
indications, 323–324
injury pathology
acute versus chronic phase, 341–342
bursitis, 341
cramps, 341
four-step healing process, 340–341
pain-spasm-pain cycle, 339, 341
spasms, 341
splinting, 339
sprains, 339–341
strains, 340–341
tendonitis, 341
injury therapy
cryotherapy, 343–345, 344f
heat therapy, 345
hydrotherapy, 342–343, 343t
muscle testing
biceps brachii, 337
description, 337
erector spinae, 339
extensor carpi radialis, 338
extensor carpi ulnaris, 338
flexor carpi radialis, 338
flexor carpi ulnaris, 338
gastrocnemius, 338
gluteals, 339
hamstrings, 338
hip rotators, 339
iliotibial tract band, 339
infraspinatus, 337
middle deltoid, 337
pronator, 338
quadratus lumborum, 339
quadriceps, 338
soleus, 338
subscapularis, 337
supinator, 338
supraspinatus, 337

Sports massage *(continued)*
  muscle testing *(continued)*
    tensor fasciae latae, 339
    teres minor, 337
    tibialis anterior and posterior, 338
  physiological effects, 323–324
  rehabilitative/maintenance massage,
    331*b*, 347, 350–358
    anterior lower leg injuries,
      354–355, 354*f*
    hamstring injuries, 356, 356*f*
    knee injuries, 358
    low back problems, 356–358, 357*f*
    posterior lower leg injuries,
      355–356, 355*f*
    quadriceps injuries, 353–354, 354*f*
    shoulder injuries, 350, 351*f*, 352
    tennis and golfer's elbow,
      352–353, 353*f*
  stretching, 331–336, 332*f*–336*f*
    positional release, 336
    range of motion (ROM), 335–336,
      336*f*, 336*t*
    reciprocal inhibition, 335, 335*f*
    tense-relax method, 331, 334–335
  strokes, 324–330
    compression, 327, 328*f*
    compression-broadening, 328, 329*f*
    compression-torque with thumbs, 330
    compressive active movement, 330
    effleurage, 324, 325*f*
    fanning, 330
    friction, 325–326, 326*f*
    knuckling, 330, 330*f*
    petrissage, 324–325, 325*f*
    pincher palpation, 329
    prayer, 330
    preevent and postevent, 324
    pressure, direct or sustained, 327, 328*f*
    rocking and shaking, 328
    skin rolling, 328, 329*f*
    tapotement, 326–327, 327*f*
    thumb-stripping, 329
    uncoiling, 330
    vibration, 327
  timing parameters, 330, 331*b*
Sports massage cream, 324
Sprain
  common, 340
  definition, 188, 339
  elbow, 353
  grades, 339–340
  healing process, 340–341
Stabilizer, 143, 198
Standardized, 581
Start-up costs, 551
Static phase, 134
STDs (sexually transmitted diseases), 47
Steam baths, 373
Sterilization, 48
Sternocleidomastoid muscle, 201, 592,
  593*b*, 594*b*
Sternum, 181
Stomach, 246, 246*f*, 487–488, 487*f*
Stomach meridian, 395, 397, 398*f*
Stone massage therapy, 363, 378, 380–382,
  380*f*, 381*f*, 382*f*
Stool, 29–30, 29*f*
Strain
  description, 79, 340
  healing process, 340–341

quadriceps, 353
rotator cuff, 350
Strain-counterstrain, 336. *See also*
      Positional release, sports
      massage
Strap, yoga, 501
Streptococci bacteria, 47
Stress
  management, corporate, 555, 555*f*
  reduction in pregnancy, 267–268
Stretch weakness, 522*b*
Stretching
  adapting stretches for a client, 523*b*–525*b*
  benefits of, 519
  exercises, 519–522
    ankle circumduction, 522
    finger and wrist stretch, 519,
      520*f*, 521*f*
    half squats, 521, 521*f*
    knee flexion/calf stretch, 519–520, 521*f*
    shoulder shrugs, 519, 520*f*
    shoulder stretch, 519, 520*f*
  muscle maintenance program, 519
  overstretching, 522*b*
  passive, 522*b*, 524*b*
  precautions and contraindications, 525*b*
  selective, 522*b*
  sports massage, 331–336, 332*f*–336*f*
    positional release, 336
    range of motion (ROM), 335–336,
      336*f*, 336*t*
    reciprocal inhibition, 335, 335*f*
    tense-relax method, 331, 334–335
  terminology, 522*b*
  therapeutic methods, 518–519
  traditional western, 514–525
Striations, 194, 196
Strigil, 20
Stripping, for thoracic outlet syndrome, 591*b*
Strokes. *See also specific applications*
  applying, considerations in, 80–81
    depth of pressure, 80–81
    direction, 81
    duration, 81
    frequency, 81
    rhythm, 81
    speed, 81
  compression, 86, 86*f*
  cross-stretch, 86, 87*f*
  effleurage, 81, 82*f*, 83
  fine tremulous, 86
  friction, 84–85, 84*f*
  nerve stroke, 86
  petrissage, 83–84, 83*f*
  rocking, 86
  shaking, 86
  skin rolling, 86, 87*f*
  sports massage, 324–330
    compression, 327, 328*f*
    compression-broadening, 328, 329*f*
    compression-torque with thumbs, 330
    compressive active movement, 330
    effleurage, 324, 325*f*
    fanning, 330
    friction, 325–326, 326*f*
    knuckling, 330, 330*f*
    petrissage, 324–325, 325*f*
    pincher palpation, 329
    prayer, 330
    preevent and postevent, 324
    pressure, direct or sustained, 327, 328*f*

rocking and shaking, 328
skin rolling, 328, 329*f*
tapotement, 326–327, 327*f*
thumb-stripping, 329
uncoiling, 330
vibration, 327
  tapotement, 85
  thumb presses, 88
  vibration, 85–86
  wringing, 86, 87*f*
Structural Integration, 434–438
Student's elbow, 341
Subacute phase, 342
Subclavian artery, 229
Subscapularis, muscle test, 337
Suffixes, 67–68
Sumerians, 7
Superior (directional term), 155
Supination, 140, 142*f*
Supinator
  muscle test, 338
  in tennis elbow, 352
Supine, table massage sequence, 99–105,
  100*f*–107*f*
Supine big toe/hamstring stretch (Supta
  Padangusthasana), 502, 503*f*
Supine hypotensive syndrome, 272, 272*f*
Supine position, 88
Supplements, 584*t*
Supraspinatus
  anatomy, 351*f*
  massaging, 96, 98*f*
  muscle test, 337
Supraspinatus tendon, 350
Susceptibility, to infection, 47
Sushumna channel, 498, 499, 501
Suture, 173, 178, 178*f*
Svadisthana, 470
Swallowing, 245
Swedish massage
  for elderly clients, 301
  for hearing impaired children, 295
  infant massage, 283
  origin of, 15–16, 80
  physiological effects of, 125
  postpartum, 279
  in pregnancy, 271, 275, 277
  for senior clients, 298*b*
  spa therapy, 363
  strokes
    applying, considerations in, 80–81
      depth of pressure, 80–81
      direction, 81
      duration, 81
      frequency, 81
      rhythm, 81
      speed, 81
    effleurage, 81, 82*f*, 83
    friction, 84–85, 84*f*
    petrissage, 83–84, 83*f*
    tapotement, 85
    vibration, 85–86
  for visually impaired children, 295
Swedish Treatment Cure. *See* Swedish
      massage
Swiss shower, 374
Sympathetic system, 119, 119*b*, 120*f*,
  234*f*, 267
Symphysis, 144, 174, 175*f*
Synarthrotic joints, 144, 173, 175*f*
Synchondrosis, 144, 174

Syndesmosis, 173
Synergist, 198
Synovial joints
    overview, 144, 174–175
    structure, 175
    types, 176f
Synovitis, 188

T

T Band, PNF technique for, 334f
T-bar, 33, 326f, 429b
T lymphocytes, 244
Table, massage
    cart, rolling, 28–29, 29f
    cost, 28, 29
    coverings, 26–27, 34–35
    description, 26–28, 27f
    face cradle, 27
    height, 92, 271
    history of use, 21
    hydraulic, 27–28, 28f
    mat as substitute for, 30, 30f
    portable, 27f, 28
    selection criteria, 28–30
    stools for, 29–30, 29f
Table massage, at sporting event, 346f
Tactile stimulation, benefits of, 279, 281
T'ai Chi, 513–514, 515f
Tapotement
    application, 85
    in Cerebrospinal Fluid Technique
            Massage (CFTM), 454
    considerations, 85
    definition, 85
    of gluteals, 96
    physiological effects, 85
    sports massage, 326–327, 327f
Tarsal bones, 186, 187f
Taste, 255–256
Taylor, Dr. Charles Fayette, 20
Teas, 581
Techniques, 73–110. See also specific
            techniques
    areas of endangerment, 76, 77f, 78b
    body mechanics, 89–92, 91f
    contraindications, 74, 75–76
    flow, 89
    indications, 74–75
    palpation, 76–80
        contusion, 79
        cramps, 79
        methodology, 79–80
        muscle atrophy, 79
        muscle hypertrophy, 79
        overview, 76, 78
        spasm, 78–79
        strains, 79
    physiological effects of, 125–126
    sequence
        chair, 107, 108f–109f
        overview, 88–89
        prone, 93–99, 93f
            back, 96, 97f–98f, 99
            feet and legs, 93, 94f–95f, 96
        supine
            abdominals and intercostals,
                101, 101f
            chest, 103–104, 103f
            feet and legs, 99, 100f, 101

        hands and arms, 101, 102f, 103
        neck and head, 104–105,
            104f–107f
    turning the client, 99
    strokes
        applying, considerations in, 80–81
            depth of pressure, 80–81
            direction, 81
            duration, 81
            frequency, 81
            rhythm, 81
            speed, 81
        effleurage, 81, 82f, 83
        friction, 84–85, 84f
        petrissage, 83–84, 83f
        tapotement, 85
        vibration, 85–86
Teeth, 177, 179
Temporomandibular joint dysfunction
            syndrome, 189, 593, 594b, 594f
Tendinitis
    Achilles, 355
    description, 216, 341
    patella, 354
Tendon, muscle, and tendon (T-M-T)
            unit, 429
Tendons, 201
Tennis elbow, 352
Tense-relax method, 331, 334–335
Tensor fasciae latae
    action of, 212t
    muscle test, 339
Teres minor
    anatomy, 351f
    muscle test, 337
Terminology
    abbreviations and acronyms, 66–67
    pharmacology, 569
    prefixes, suffixes, and root words, 67–68
Testes, 239f, 241
Tetanic contraction, 198
Tetanus, 216–217
Tetrahydrocannabinol (THC), 578
A Textbook of Massage for Nurses and
            Beginners, 19
Thai massage
    methodology, 417
    overview, 414, 416
    practicing and receiving, 416–417
    techniques, 417–418, 419f
Therapeutic relationship, recovery from
            abuse and, 312–313
Therapy session. See session, massage therapy
Thermophores®, 32–33, 33f
Thermoreceptors, 114b
Thiamin, 481t
Third Eye chakra (Ajna), 499t
Thixotropic, 143
Thompson test, 355
Thoracic cavity, 156, 156f, 157t
Thoracic outlet syndrome (TOS), 277, 353,
            590, 591b–592b, 591f, 592, 592f
Three phases of effects, sexual abuse,
            309–311
Throat chakra (Vishuddha), 499t
Thrombi, 275
Thumb circles, for neck and head, 104–105,
            104f, 105f
Thumb glides
    for back, 96, 97f–98f, 99
    for chest, 103

    for feet and legs, 93, 94f–95f, 99, 100f, 101
    for hands and arms, 101, 102f, 103
    for neck and head, 104–105, 104f
    for temporomandibular joint
            dysfunction, 594b
Thumb presses, 88
Thumb stripping
    sports massage, 329
    for temporomandibular joint
            dysfunction, 594b
    for thoracic outlet syndrome, 591b
    for torticollis, 593b
Thumb walk, 417
Thymus gland, 239f, 241, 244, 274
Thyroid gland, 239–240, 239t, 274
Tibia, 184, 186f
Tibialis anterior
    anatomy, 354f
    injury to, 354–355
    massaging, 99
    muscle test, 338
Tibialis paeriostitis, 354
Tibialis posterior
    injury to, 354–355
    muscle test, 338
Tinctures, 581, 583t
Tinea capitis (scalp fungus), 44
Tinea corporis (ringworm), 44
Tinea cruris (jock itch), 44
Tinea pedis (athlete's foot), 44
Tinel's Test, 588, 589f
Tissue memory, 443
Toe boogie, 423f
Tomb of the Physician, 10
Tongue, 255–256, 256f
Tonic contraction, 198
Tonsils, 243
Tools, massage, 33. See also Equipment
Topical administration, 572
Topical medications, 573, 577
Torso, muscles of, 201, 205t, 206, 206t,
            207f–208f, 208t, 209t
Torticollis, 592, 593b, 593f
TOS. See Thoracic outlet syndrome
Touch
    benefits, of tactile stimulation, 279
    deprivation, harmful effects of,
            280–281
    perception by abuse survivor, 311, 312f
    receptors, 257
Touch relaxation, 285, 291
Touch Research Institute, 268, 280,
            291, 295
Touching, 22
Toxicology, 567
Trace minerals, 484, 580
Trachea, 249–250, 249f
Trade (brand) name, 569
Traditional Chinese Medicine, 10, 390. See
            also Chinese medicine
Trager®
    application of approach, 447–448
    elements of session, 445–447
    overview, 444–445, 445f
    for senior clients, 298b
Transference, 470, 544
Transverse friction, sports massage, 326
Transverse plane
    definition, 136
    directional terms, 155
    movements in, 139–140

Transversus abdominus
  action of, 206*t*
  anatomy, 207*t*
Trapezius, massaging, 96, 98*f*, 99, 104, 104*f*
Tree pose (Vriksasana), 507, 507*f*
Triceps
  action of, 206
  stretch, 333*f*
Trichomonas vaginalis, 45
Tricuspid valve, 227, 231*f*
Trigger Point Therapy
  description, 428–429
  methodology, 429, 429*b*
Triple heater or San jiao meridian, 396,
    400, 405*f*
Trochanteric bursitis, 189
Tsubo point, 410
Tuberculosis, 51
Tui Na, 390. *See also* Chinese medicine
Turning the client, 94
Tympanic membrane, 255, 256*f*
Type 1 diabetes, 241*b*
Type 2 diabetes, 241*b*

U

Ulna, 179–180, 181*f*
Ulnar nerve, 590
Ulnar neuritis, 353
Ultrasound equipment, 34
Unani medicine, 15
Uncoiling, sports massage, 330
Undergarment, tucking drape under, 58
Unilateral presentation, 588
Universal precautions, 48
Urea, 251
Ureter, 251, 251*f*
Urethra, 251
Urinary Bladder meridian, 396, 400, 402*f*
Urinary system
  anatomy and physiology, 250–251, 251*f*
  changes in pregnancy, 276–277
U.S. Department of Agriculture (USDA)
      food guide pyramid,
      491–492, 492*f*
Uterine prolapse, 218

V

Valves, heart, 227–229, 231*f*
Varicose veins, 272, 275
Vasoconstriction, 127, 127*f*, 343, 376
Vasodilation, 116, 127*f*, 128, 343, 373
Vastu, 37, 37*b*
Vastus intermedius muscle, strain, 353
Vastus lateralis, anatomy, 354*f*
Vastus medialis, anatomy, 354*f*
Vedas, 11
Vegetarian diet, 491
Vein, 224, 228*f*
Vena cavae, 228, 230*f*, 231*f*
Ventral (directional term), 156
Ventral body cavity, 156, 156*f*, 157*t*

Ventricle, 227
Vertebral column
  bones, 182–183, 183*f*, 184*f*
  curvature
    abnormal, 189*f*
    normal, 183*f*
  muscles of, 208*f*, 208*t*–209*t*
  regions, 157*t*
Vertebral nerve, 590
Vesalius, Andrea, 154
Vestibule, 255, 256*f*
Vibration
  application, 85
  considerations, 86
  definition, 85
  physiological effects, 86
  sports massage, 327
Vichy shower, 374, 374*f*
Villi, 488
Viruses, 44
Viscera, 123
Visceral (smooth) muscle, 194, 195*f*
Visceroceptors, 114*b*
Viscerosomatic reflex, 124
Viscerovisceral reflex, 124
Viscous flow phenomenon, 442
Vishuddha, 471
Vision, 255
Visualization, 472, 473*b*
Visually impaired children, massage for, 295
Vitalism, 21–22
Vitamins
  fat-soluble, 483*t*, 580
  overview, 481, 579–580
  supplements, 579*f*
  water-soluble, 481*t*–482*t*, 580
Vodder, Emil, 449, 451

W

Warrior pose (Virabhadrasana II), 505, 506*f*
Waste products, removal by urinary system,
    250–251
Water, 479–481
Water temperatures for spa treatments, 375*t*
Wedge bolsters, 31, 32*f*
Weight-loss spas, 363
Weight lifting, 514, 518*f*
Whiplash, 189
White blood cells (WBCs), 225, 229*f*
The Wisdom of the Body, 22
Witch hazel, 36
Wrap, herbal, 383–384, 384*b*
Wright's test, 590
Wringing. *See also* Petrissage
  description, 86, 87*f*
  sports massage, 324–325, 325*f*
  thigh muscles, 96, 101
Wrist
  cryotherapy, 344*f*
  hyperextension, extension, and
      flexion, 138*f*
  sprains, 340
Wrist stretch, 519, 520*f*, 521*f*

Wryneck, 592, 593*b*, 593*f*
Wu Shu, 513

Y

Yang
  contrasting aspects of yin and yang, 393*t*
  description, 390, 391, 392–394
  expressed as signs and symptoms, 394*t*
  organs, 394*t*
  symbol, 393*f*, 513
Yin
  contrasting aspects of yin and yang, 393*t*
  description, 390, 391, 392–394
  expressed as signs and symptoms, 394*t*
  organs, 394*t*
  symbol, 393*f*, 513
Yoga
  asanas, 501–512
    Boat pose (Navasana), 508, 510*f*
    Bow (Dhanurasana), 509, 511*f*
    Cobra (Bhujangasana), 508, 511*f*
    Corpse post (Savasana), 502,
        502*f*, 510
    Easy pose (Sukhasana),
        502–503, 503*f*
    Forward Bending pose (Uttanasana),
        504, 505*f*
    Knee/Head pose (Janu Sirsasana),
        508, 509*f*
    Lateral bend (Parvatasana in
        Tadasana), 504
    Lying spinal twist (Bharadjasana),
        509, 511*f*
    Might Stance (Utkatasana),
        504–505, 505*f*
    Mountain pose (Tadasana),
        503–504, 504*f*
    overview, 501, 512
    Seated spinal twist (Bharadjasana),
        507–508, 508*f*
    Supine big toe/hamstring stretch
        (Supta Padangusthasana),
        502, 503*f*
    Tree pose (Vriksasana), 507, 507*f*
    Warrior pose (Virabhadrasana II),
        505, 506*f*
  Ashtanga, 497, 498
  Bik Ram, 498
  for body-mind connection, 468*f*
  chakras, 498–500, 499*t*, 500*f*
  Hatha, 497, 498
  meditation, 498, 500–501, 501*f*
  overview, 497–498
  prana, 498
Yoga Alliance, 498
Yoga mat, 501
Yoga strap, 501